DICTIONARY OF
MEDICAL
BIOGRAPHY

EDITORIAL BOARD

DICTIONARY OF MEDICAL BIOGRAPHY

Volume 5, S–Z

Edited by

W. F. Bynum *and* Helen Bynum

GREENWOOD PRESS

Westport, Connecticut • London

Library of Congress Cataloging-in-Publication Data

Dictonary of medical biography / edited by W. F. Bynum and Helen Bynum.
     p.   cm.
    Includes bibliographical references and index.
    ISBN 0–313–32877–3 (set : alk. paper) — ISBN 0–313–32878–1 (v. 1 : alk. paper) —
    ISBN 0–313–32879–X (v. 2 : alk. paper) — ISBN 0–313–32880–3 (v. 3 : alk. paper) —
    ISBN 0–313–32881–1 (v. 4 : alk. paper) — ISBN 0–313–32882–X (v. 5 : alk. paper)
  1. Medicine—Biography. 2. Healers—Biography. I. Bynum, W. F. (William F.), 1943– . II. Bynum, Helen.
R134.D57   2007
610—dc22   2006022953

British Library Cataloguing in Publication Data is available.

Library of Congress Catalog Card Number: 2006022953
ISBN: 0–313–32877–3 (set)
        0–313–32878–1 (vol. 1)
        0–313–32879–X (vol. 2)
        0–313–32880–3 (vol. 3)
        0–313–32881–1 (vol. 4)
        0–313–32882–X (vol. 5)

First published in 2007

Greenwood Press, 88 Post Road West, Westport, CT 06881
An imprint of Greenwood Publishing Group, Inc.
www.greenwood.com

Printed in the United States of America

The paper used in this book complies with the
Permanent Paper Standard issued by the National
Information Standards Organization (Z39.48–1984).

10   9   8   7   6   5   4   3   2   1

CONTENTS

CONTRIBUTORS

Göran Åkerström
Academic Hospital, Uppsala, Sweden
Sandström

Seema Alavi
Jamia Millia University, New Delhi, India
Aziz

Angelo Albrizio
Institut d'Histoire de la Médecine et de la Santé,
Geneva, Switzerland
De Giovanni

W. R. Albury
University of New South Wales, Sydney,
Australia
Bichat, Broussais, Corvisart des Marets, Magendie

Marta de Almeida
Museu de Astronomia e Ciências Afins,
Rio de Janeiro, Brazil
Ribas

Cristina Álvarez Millán
UNED, Madrid, Spain
*Ibn Buṭlān, Al-Majūsī, Ibn al-Nafīs, Al-Rāzī, Ibn Rushd,
Ibn Zuhr*

Stuart Anderson
LSHTM, London, England
Beecham, Holloway, Squibb

Warwick Anderson
University of Wisconsin–Madison, Madison, WI,
USA
Burnet, Cleland

Jon Arrizabalaga
CSIC, Barcelona, Spain
Laguna, Sanches, Torrella

S. N. Arseculeratne
University of Peradeniya, Peradeniya,
Sri Lanka
M. Paul, Wickramarachchi

Mikel Astrain
Universidad de Granada, Granada, Spain
Lardizábal Dubois

Guy Attewell
Wellcome Trust Centre for the History of Medicine
at UCL, London, England
*Medical Traditions in South Asia, Abd ul-Hamīd,
M. Ajmal Khān, M. A'zam Khān, Saīd*

Nara Azevedo
Casa de Oswaldo Cruz, Fundação Oswaldo Cruz,
Rio de Janeiro, Brazil
Cruz

Søren Bak-Jensen
Medical Museion, Copenhagen, Denmark
*Fibiger, Friderichsen, Gram, Hagedorn,
Pindborg, Salomonsen*

Martha Baldwin
Stonehill College, Easton, MA, USA
Dionis

Marta Aleksandra Balinska
Institut national du cancer, Paris, France
Hirszfeld, Rajchman, Śniadecki

Rosa Ballester
Universidad Miguel Hernández, Alicante-Valencia, Spain
Martínez Vargas

Scott Bamber
UNICEF, Bangkok, Thailand
Jivaka

Richard Barnett
Wellcome Trust Centre for the History of Medicine
at UCL, London, England
Godlee, Knox, Long, W. Morton, Read, Simpson, Wakley

Josep Lluís Barona
Universidad de Valencia Blasco, Valencia, Spain
Ramón y Cajal, Trueta i Raspall

Penelope Barrett
Wellcome Trust Centre for the History of Medicine
at UCL, London, England
Li Shizhen

Alexander R. Bay
Chapman University, Orange Campus, CA, USA
Takaki

Elaine Beale
Cherhill, Wiltshire, England
Ingen Housz

Norman Beale
Cherhill, Wiltshire, England
Ingen Housz

Denise Best
California State University, Fresno, CA, USA
Pokrovskaia

Anne-Emanuelle Birn
University of Toronto, Toronto, ON, Canada
Morquio

Carla Bittel
Loyola Marymount University, Los Angeles, CA, USA
Baker, A. Jacobi, M. P. Jacobi, Van Hoosen

Johanna Bleker
ZHGB, Institut für Geschichte der Medizin,
Berlin, Germany
Henle, Schoenlein

Michael Bliss
University of Toronto, Toronto, ON, Canada
Cushing, Dandy

Hans Blom
Erasmus Universiteit, Rotterdam, the Netherlands
Mandeville

Michel Bonduelle
University of Paris, Paris, France
Duchenne de Boulogne, Guillain

Christopher Booth
Wellcome Trust Centre for the History of Medicine
at UCL, London, England
Haygarth, Hurst, Lettsom, Sherlock

Cornelius Borck
McGill University, Montreal, QC, Canada
Berger

Mineke Bosch
Universiteit Maastricht, Maastricht,
the Netherlands
Jacobs

David Bradley
LSHTM, London, England
Macdonald

Gunnar Broberg
University of Lund, Lund, Sweden
Linnaeus

Alejandra Bronfman
University of British Columbia, Vancouver,
BC, Canada
Finlay y Barres, Guiteras Gener

Linda Bryder
University of Auckland, Auckland, New Zealand
Gordon, King, Liley

Chris Burton
University of Lethbridge, Lethbridge, AB,
Canada
Burdenko, Fedorov, Semashko, Solev'ev

Helen Bynum
Shadingfield, Suffolk, England
Halsted, Harinasuta, Rogers, Snow, Steptoe

Ricardo Campos
CSIC, Madrid, Spain
Rubio Gali

Franco Carnevale
Azienda Sanitaria di Firenze, Florence, Italy
Devoto, Ramazzini

Ana María Carrillo
UNAM, Mexico City, Mexico
Montoya Lafragua

Ian Carter
University of Auckland, Auckland, New Zealand
M. Bell

Ramón Castejón-Bolea
Universidad Miguel Hernández, Alicante, Spain
Azúa y Suárez

Rafael Chabrán
Whittier College, Whittier, CA, USA
Hernández

Iain Chalmers
The James Lind Initiative, Oxford, England
Cochrane

Joël Chandelier
Ecole française de Rome, Rome, Italy
Gentile da Foligno

Rethy Chhem
University of Western Ontario, London, ON,
Canada
Yajnavaraha

Indira Chowdhury
Tata Institute of Fundamental Research,
Mumbai, India
*Chopra, Dharmendra, Mukerji, Pandit,
Ramalingaswami, P. Sen, Vakil*

Charlotte Christensen-Nugues
University of Lund, Lund, Sweden
Harpestreng

Amy Eisen Cislo
Washington University, St Louis, MO, USA
Gilbert the Englishman

Catherine S. Coleborne
Waikato University, Hamilton, New Zealand
Manning

Andrea Contini
University of Paris XII, Paris, France
Basaglia

Roger Cooter
Wellcome Trust Centre for the History of Medicine
at UCL, London, England
Braid, Charnley, Gall, R. Jones, Treves, Wells

Anne Cottebrune
Ruprecht-Karls-Universität Heidelberg,
Heidelberg, Germany
Fischer, Wagner

Christopher Crenner
KUMC, Kansas City, KS, USA
*Bowditch, Codman, Edsall, J. Jackson, Jarvis,
Minot*

Anna Crozier
University of Edinburgh, Edinburgh, Scotland
Atiman, Cook, Kasili, Spoerry, C. Williams

Ivan Crozier
University of Edinburgh, Edinburgh, Scotland
*Dickinson, Ellis, Haire, Hirschfeld, C. Mosher,
E. Mosher, Reich, Sanger, Stopes*

Marcos Cueto
Universidad Peruana Cayetano Heredia,
Lima, Peru
*Balmis, Candau, Horwitz Barak, Houssay,
Monge Medrano, Núñez Butrón, Paz Soldán,
Soper*

Michael Z. David
University of Chicago, Chicago, IL, USA
Pavlovskii, Sklifosovskii

Rosalie David
University of Manchester, Manchester,
England
Imhotep

Annemarie de Knecht-van Eekelen
CITO International, Arnhem, the Netherlands
De Lange

Ana Cecilia Rodríguez de Romo
Universidad Nacional Autónoma de México,
Mexico City, Mexico
*Arias de Benavides, Bernard, Bustamante
Vasconcelos, Chávez Sánchez, Izquierdo
Raudón, Liceaga, Martínez Báez, Montaña
Carranco*

Michelle DenBeste
California State University, Fresno, CA, USA
Pokrovskaia

Michael Denham
Wellcome Trust Centre for the History of Medicine
at UCL, London, England
M. Warren

Sven Dierig
Max-Planck-Institut, Berlin, Germany
Brücke, Ludwig

Derek A. Dow
University of Auckland, Auckland, New
Zealand
Buck, Gillies, Hercus, G. Robb, Scott

Alex Dracobly
University of Oregon, Eugene, OR, USA
Fournier, Ricord

Jean-Jacques Dreifuss
Centre Médical Universitaire, Geneva,
Switzerland
Coindet, Prevost

Ariane Dröscher
University of Bologna, Bologna, Italy
*Bassini, Bizzozero, Cotugno, Lombroso, Perroncito,
Rasori, Rizzoli*

Jacalyn Duffin
Queen's University, Kingston, ON, Canada
Laennec

Marguerite Dupree
University of Glasgow, Glasgow, Scotland
Anderson, Blackwell, Jex-Blake

Achintya Kumar Dutta
University of Burdwan, West Bengal, India
Brahmachari

William Eamon
New Mexico State University, Las Cruces, NM, USA
Nicholas of Poland

Myron Echenberg
McGill University, Montreal, QC, Canada
Brazil, Girard, A. Gregory, Jamot, Simond, Yersin

Wolfgang U. Eckart
Ruprecht-Karls-Universität Heidelberg,
Heidelberg, Germany
*Büchner, Dietl, Domagk, Sachs, Sauerbruch, Schwalbe,
Sennert, Skoda, Wundt, Zeiss*

Flávio Coelho Edler
Casa de Oswaldo Cruz, Fundação Oswaldo Cruz,
Rio de Janeiro, Brazil
Wucherer

Martin Edwards
Wellcome Trust Centre for the History of Medicine
at UCL, London, England
Balint

Kristen Ann Ehrenberger
University of Illinois, Urbana-Champaign, IL, USA
Drake

Antoinette Emch-Dériaz
University of Florida, Gainsville, FL, USA
Tissot

Eric J. Engstrom
ZHGB, Berlin, Germany
Kraepelin

Gunnar Eriksson
Uppsala Universitet, Uppsala, Sweden
Rudbeck

Bernardino Fantini
Institut d'Histoire de la Médecine et de la Santé,
Geneva, Switzerland
*Baglivi, Bovet, Celli, Dubini, Fabrizi da Acquapendente,
Golgi, Grassi, Lancisi, Pacini, Puccinotti, Redi, Sanarelli*

F. N. Fastier
University of Otago, Dunedin, New Zealand
Smirk

Morten Fink-Jensen
University of Copenhagen, Copenhagen, Denmark
Bartholin

Michael A. Flannery
University of Alabama at Birmingham,
Maylene, AL, USA
*J. Jones, Lloyd, McDowell, Newton, Nott, E. Warren,
D. Williams*

Yajaira Freites
IVIC, Caracas, Venezuela
Balmis, Beauperthuy, Gabaldón, Razetti

Charlotte Furth
University of Southern California, Los Angeles,
CA, USA
Zhu Zhenheng

Namrata R. Ganneri
Independent scholar, Mumbai, India
Joshi, Rakhmabai, Scudder

Michelle Garceau
Princeton University, Princeton, NJ, USA
Chauliac, William of Saliceto

Amy Gardiner
LSHTM, London, England
Burkitt

Nina Rattner Gelbart
Occidental College, Los Angeles, CA, USA
Du Coudray

Toby Gelfand
University of Ottawa, Ottawa, ON, Canada
*Bayle, Bernheim, Bourneville, Charcot, Desault, Hayem,
Lapeyronie, Lasègeu, Péan, Petit, Sée*

Jacques Gélis
University of Paris, Paris, France
Baudelocque

Dario Generali
Edizione Nazionale delle Opere di Antonio Vallisneri,
Milan, Italy
Vallisneri

Norman Gevitz
Ohio University, Athens, OH, USA
A. Still

James Gillespie
University of Sydney, Sydney, Australia
Argyle, Cilento

Florence Eliza Glaze
Coastal Carolina University, Conway, SC, USA
Constantine the African, Gariopontus

Christopher Goetz
Rush University Medical Center, Chicago, IL,
USA
Déjerine, Marie

Asaf Goldschmidt
Tel Aviv University, Tel Aviv, Israel
*Li Gao, Liu Wansu, Qian Yi, Wang Weiyi,
Xu Shuwei*

Christoph Gradmann
University of Oslo, Oslo, Norway
Klebs, Koch, Pettenkofer, Rabinowitsch-Kempner

John L. Graner
Mayo Clinic, Rochester, MN, USA
C. Mayo, W. Mayo

Joanna Grant
London, England
Wang Ji

Monica H. Green
Arizona State University, Tempe, AZ, USA
Trota

Samuel H. Greenblatt
Brown University, Pawtucket, RI, USA
Broca

David Greenwood
University of Nottingham, Nottingham,
England
Florey

Alberto Alonso Guardo
Universidad de Vallodolid, Vallodolid, Spain
Bernard of Gordon

Patrizia Guarnieri
Università degli Studi de Firenze, Florence, Italy
*Bufalini, Cerletti, Chiarugi, Concetti, De Sanctis,
Morselli, Mya*

Annick Guénel
LASEMA, Villejuif, France
Tùng Tôn Thất

Anita Guerrini
University of California, Santa Barbara, CA,
USA
G. Cheyne

Anne Y. Guillou
L'Université de Haute-Bretagne, Rennes, France
Pen

Bert Hall
University of Toronto, Toronto, ON, Canada
Guido da Vigevano

June Hannam
University of the West of England, Bristol, England
R. Paget

Caroline Hannaway
NIH History, Bethesda, MD, USA
Alibert, Cruveilhier, Dunglison, Dupuytren, Louis, Parran

Signe Lindskov Hansen
Copenhagen, Denmark
Finsen

Marta E. Hanson
Johns Hopkins University, Baltimore, MD, USA
Wu Youxing, Ye Gui, Zhang Jiebin

Susan Hardy
University of New South Wales, Sydney, Australia
Gillbee

Mark Harrison
Wellcome Unit for the History of Medicine, University of Oxford, Oxford, England
Carter, Christophers, Fayrer, Martin, Parkes, Ross

Joy Harvey
Independent scholar, Somerville, MA, USA
Bert, Bertillon, Brès, Edwards-Pilliet, Littré, Rayer, Tardieu, Trousseau, Vulpian

Mike Hawkins
Wellcome Trust Centre for the History of Medicine at UCL/Imperial College, London, England
Willis

E. A. Heaman
McGill University, Montreal, QC, Canada
Fleming, Sanderson, Wright

R. van Hee
Universiteit Antwerpen, Antwerp, Belgium
Depage, Vesalius

Jürgen Helm
Martin Luther Universität, Halle-Wittenberg, Halle, Germany
Brunfels, Erxleben, Frank, Gersdorff, Hoffmann, Stahl

John Henry
University of Edinburgh, Edinburgh, Scotland
Caius, Dubois, Fernel, Harvey, Linacre, Lower, Turquet, Winsløw

Volker Hess
ZHGB, Berlin, Germany
Behring, Frerichs, Kraus, Leyden, Traube, Wunderlich

Martha Hildreth
University of Nevada, Reno, NV, USA
Brouardel, Grancher

Caroline Hillard
Washington University, St Louis, MO, USA
Del Garbo, Mondino de' Liuzzi

Gilberto Hochman
Casa de Oswaldo Cruz, Fundação Oswaldo Cruz, Rio de Janeiro, Brazil
Barros Barreto, Chagas, Cruz, Fraga, Penna, Pinotti, Ribas, Wucherer

Hans-Georg Hofer
University of Manchester, Manchester, England
Krafft-Ebing, Wagner-Jauregg

Eddy Houwaart
Vrije Universiteit Medisch Centrum, Amsterdam, the Netherlands
Ali Cohen

Joel D. Howell
University of Michigan, Ann Arbor, MI, USA
Elliotson, Flick, Gerhard, Heberden, Herrick, Lewis

Elisabeth Hsu
University of Oxford, Oxford, England
Chunyu Yi

Christian Huber
Sigmund Freud-Privatstiftung, Vienna, Austria
Breuer, Jung

Rafael Huertas
CSIC, Madrid, Spain
Orfila i Rotger, Rodríguez Lafora

Teresa Huguet-Termes
Universitat Autònoma de Barcelona, Barcelona, Spain
Cardenal Fernández

Frank Huisman
University Medical Center, Utrecht/Universiteit Maastricht, Maastricht, the Netherlands
Einthoven, Hijmans van den Bergh, Loghem, Sylvius

Marion Hulverscheidt
Ruprecht-Karls-Universität Heidelberg,
Heidelberg, Germany
Basedow, Hegar

J. Willis Hurst
Emory University, Atlanta, GA, USA
White

Erik Ingebrigsten
Norwegian University of Science and Technology,
Trondheim, Norway
Holst

Lorentz M. Irgens
University of Bergen, Bergen, Norway
Hansen

Mark Jackson
University of Exeter, Exeter, England
Blackley, Down, Floyer, Freeman, Seguin, Tredgold

Bengt Jangfeldt
Center for the History of Science, Royal Academy of
Science, Stockholm, Sweden
Munthe

Mark Jenner
University of York, York, England
*Chamberlen, Clowes, Glisson, D. Turner, Wiseman,
Woodall*

William Johnston
Wesleyan University, Middletown, CT, USA
*Gotō Konzan, Hanaoka, Manse, Sugita, Yamawaki,
Yoshimasu*

Peter Jones
King's College Library, Cambridge, England
Arderne, Yperman

Eric Jorink
Constantijn Huygens Instituut, the Hague,
the Netherlands
*J. Heurnius, O. Heurnius, Lemnius, Piso,
Swammerdam*

Robert Jütte
Robert Bosch Stiftung, Stuttgart, Germany
*Auenbrugger, Hahnemann, Hirsch, Hufeland, Kaposi,
Rolfink, Rubner*

Oliver Kahl
University of Manchester, Manchester, England
Ibn at-Tilmīdh

Harmke Kamminga
University of Cambridge, Cambridge, England
Eijkman

Amalie M. Kass
Harvard Medical School, Boston, MA, USA
Cabot, Channing, Churchill, Dameshek, Kelly, Sims

Matthew Howard Kaufman
University of Edinburgh, Edinburgh, Scotland
Ballingall, C. Bell, Brodie, Guthrie, Liston, McGrigor

Amy Kemp
Indiana University, Bloomington, IN, USA
Souza

Helen King
University of Reading, Reading, England
*Agnodice, Archagathus, Hippocrates, Machaon,
Podalirius*

Stephanie Kirby
University of the West of England, Bristol, England
Nightingale

Rina Knoeff
Universiteit Maastricht, Maastricht,
the Netherlands
G. Bidloo, Boerhaave

Carl Henrik Koch
University of Copenhagen, Copenhagen,
Denmark
Stensen

Peter Koehler
Wever Hospital, Heerlen, the Netherlands
Babinski, Brown-Séquard, Winkler

Luuc Kooijmans
Universiteit van Amsterdam, Amsterdam,
the Netherlands
Ruysch

Maria Korasidou
Panteion University of Athens, Athens, Greece
Geroulanos, Goudas, Papanicolaou, Vouros, Zinnis

Jan K. van der Korst
Loosdrecht, the Netherlands
Camper, Swieten

Samuel Kottek
Hebrew University, Jerusalem, Israel
Astruc

Simone Petraglia Kropf
Casa de Oswaldo Cruz, Fundação Oswaldo
Cruz, Rio de Janeiro, Brazil
Chagas

Howard I. Kushner
Emory University, Atlanta, GA, USA
Gilles de la Tourette

Ann F. La Berge
Virginia Tech, Blacksburg, VA, USA
Parent-Duchâtelet, Villermé

Paul A. L. Lancaster
University of Sydney, New South Wales, Australia
Gregg

Øivind Larsen
University of Oslo, Oslo, Norway
Schiøtz

Christopher Lawrence
Wellcome Trust Centre for the History of
Medicine at UCL, London, England
*Cheselden, Culpeper, Lind, Mead, Pott, Pringle,
Salk, Sydenham, Trotter*

Sean Hsiang-lin Lei
National Tsing-hua University, Hsinchu, Taiwan
Yu Yan

Efraim Lev
University of Haifa, Haifa, Israel
Asaph

Milton James Lewis
University of Sydney, Sydney,
Australia
Cumpston

Shang-Jen Li
Institute of History and Philology, Academia
Sinica, Taipei, Taiwan
*Bruce, Hobson, Leishman, Lockhart, Manson,
Parker*

Kai Khiun Liew
Wellcome Trust Centre for the History of Medicine
at UCL, London, England
Chen Su Lan

Vivienne Lo
Wellcome Trust Centre for the History of Medicine
at UCL, London, England
Medicine in China

Stephen Lock
Aldeburgh, Suffolk, England
*The Western Medical Tradition, Beecher, Cooper,
Crile, Dale, Doll, Ferrier, Fishbein, Gull, Hart,
Hastings, G. Holmes, Keynes, Mitchell,
Pappworth, Pickles, Ryle, Saunders, Trudeau*

Winifred Logan
Glasgow, Scotland
Stephenson

Brigitte Lohff
Medizinische Hochschule Hannover,
Hannover, Germany
Autenrieth, Baer, Blumenbach, Müller, Oken, Reil

Jorge Lossio
University of Manchester, Manchester, England
Carrión, Espejo, Unanue

Ilana Löwy
CERMES, Villejuif, France
Aleksandrowicz, Bieganski, Biernacki, Korczak

Kenneth M. Ludmerer
Washington University, St Louis, MO, USA
Flexner

Joan E. Lynaugh
University of Pennsylvania Nursing School,
Philadelphia, PA, USA
L. Dock, L. Richards, I. Robb

Kan-Wen Ma
Wellcome Trust Centre for the History of Medicine
at UCL, London, England
Bian Que

Helen MacDonald
University of Melbourne, Carlton, Victoria,
Australia
W. MacKenzie

Andreas-Holger Maehle
University of Durham, Durham/Wolfson Research
Institute, Stockton, England
Moll

Susanne Malchau
Aarhus Universitet, Aarhus, Denmark
Mannerheim, Reimann

John Manton
University of Oxford, Oxford, England
Johnson, Lambo, Schweitzer

Predrag J. Markovic
Institute for Contemporary History, Belgrade, Serbia
*Batut, Djordjević, Lazarević, Kostić, Nešić, Štampar,
Subbotić*

Shula Marks
SOAS, London, England
Gale, Gear, Gillman, Gluckman, Kark, Waterston

José Martínez-Pérez
Universidad de Castilla-La Mancha, Albacete, Spain
Calandre Ibáñez, Jiménez Díaz, Marañón Posadillo

Àlvar Martínez-Vidal
Universidad Autónoma de Barcelona, Barcelona,
Spain
Gimbernat i Arbós, Giovannini

Romana Martorelli Vico
Università di Pisa, Pisa, Italy
Lanfranc, Ugo Benzi

J. Rosser Matthews
Williamsburg, VA, USA
Biggs, Bouchard, Bouchardat, Chapin, Greenwood, Hill

Janet McCalman
University of Melbourne, Melbourne, Australia
*Balls-Headley, Bryce, Campbell, Macnamara,
Scantlebury Brown*

Louella McCarthy
University of Sydney, Sydney, New South Wales,
Australia
D'Arcy

Laurence B. McCullough
Baylor College of Medicine, Houston, TX, USA
Hooker, Rush

Susan McGann
RCN Archives, Edinburgh, Scotland
Fenwick

James McGeachie
University of Ulster, Newtownabbey, Northern Ireland
Corrigan, Graves, W. Jenner, M. Mackenzie, Stokes, Wilde

Alessandro Medico
Washington University, St Louis, MO, USA
Peter of Abano

Rosa María Medina-Doménech
Universidad de Granada, Granada, Spain
Goyanes Capdevila, Guilera Molas

Alfredo Menéndez
Universidad de Granada, Granada, Spain
Casal Julián

Sharon Messenger
Wellcome Trust Centre for the History of Medicine
at UCL, London, England
Livingstone

Alexandre Métraux
Dossenheim, Germany
S. Freud, Goldstein

Dmitry Mikhel
Saratov State University, Saratov, Russia
Botkin, Erisman, Manassein, Molleson, Ostroumov, Zakhar'in

Bridie Andrews Minehan
Bentley College, Waltham, MA, USA
Ding Fubao, Yen

Consuelo Miqueo
Universidad de Zaragoza, Zaragoza, Spain
Piquer Arrufat

Néstor Miranda Canal
Universidad El Bosque y de la Universidad de Los Andes,
Bogotá, Colombia
Vargas Reyes

Jorge Molero-Mesa
Universidad Autònoma de Barcelona, Barcelona, Spain
Sayé i Sempere

Laurence Monnais
Université de Montréal, Montreal, QC, Canada
*Medical Traditions in Southeast Asia: From Syncretism to
Pluralism*

Maria Teresa Monti
CSPF-CNR, Milan, Italy
Spallanzani

Francisco Moreno de Carvalho
Independent scholar, São Paulo, Brazil
Amatus Lusitanus, Orta

Edward T. Morman
Baltimore, MD, USA
*Bartlett, H. Bigelow, J. Bigelow, Billings, Da Costa, Pepper,
Thayer, Welch*

Barbara Mortimer
Edinburgh, Scotland
Sharp

Anne Marie Moulin
CNRS-CEDEJ, Cairo, Egypt
Bordet, Davaine, Laveran, Netter, Roux, Widal

Wolf-Dieter Müller-Jahncke
Hermann-Schelenz-Institut für Pharmazie und
Kulturgeschichte, Heidelberg, Germany
Paracelsus

Jock Murray
Dalhousie University, Halifax, Nova Scotia, Canada
*Abbott, Banting, Bethune, Gowers, Grenfell, Huggins,
J. H. Jackson, Macphail, Osler, Parkinson, Penfield, Selye*

Takeshi Nagashima
Keio University, Tokyo, Japan
Gotō Shinpei, Kitasato, Miyairi, Nagayo, Noguchi, Shiga

Michael J. Neuss
Columbia University, New York, NY, USA
Al-Anṭākī

Michael Neve
Wellcome Trust Centre for the History of Medicine
at UCL, London, England
Beddoes, Gully, Head, Prichard, Rivers, Winslow

Malcolm Nicolson
University of Glasgow, Glasgow, Scotland
Alison, Baillie, Donald, J. Hunter, W. Hunter, Lister, Smellie

Ingemar Nilsson
University of Gothenburg, Gothenburg, Sweden
Acrel

Sherwin Nuland
Yale University, New Haven, CT, USA
Beaumont, Bloodgood, Kubler-Ross, McBurney, Mott, Murphy

Eva Nyström
University of Uppsala, Uppsala, Sweden
Rosén von Rosenstein

Ynez Violé O'Neill
UCLA, Los Angeles, CA, USA
Paré

Diana Obregón
Universidad Nacional de Colombia Edificio Manuel
Ancizar, Bogotá, Colombia
Carrasquilla, García-Medina

Ambeth R. Ocampo
National Historical Institute, Manila, Philippines
Rizal

Guillermo Olagüe de Ros
Universidad de Granada, Granada, Spain
García Solá, Nóvoa Santos, Urrutia Guerezta

Jan Eric Olsén
University of Lund, Lund, Sweden
Gullstrand, Holmgren

Todd M. Olszewski
Yale University, New Haven, CT, USA
Cannon, D. Dock

Willie T. Ong
Makati Medical Center, Makati, Philippines
Acosta-Sison

Giuseppe Ongaro
Ospedale di Padova, Padova, Italy
*Aranzio, Aselli, Bellini, Benivieni, Berengario da Carpi,
Borelli, Cardano, Cesalpino, Colombo, Cornaro,
Da Monte, Eustachi, Falloppia, Malpighi, Mattioli,
Mercuriale, Morgagni, Santorio, Scarpa, Severino,
Tagliacozzi, Valsalva, Zacchia*

Ooi Keat Gin
Universiti Sains Malaysia, Penang, Malaysia
Danaraj, Lim Boon Keng, Wu Lien-Teh

Teresa Ortiz-Gómez
Universidad de Granada, Granada, Spain
Arroyo Villaverde, Soriano Fischer

Abena Dove Osseo-Asare
University of California, Berkeley, CA, USA
Ampofo, Barnor, De Graft-Johnson, C. Easmon

Nelly Oudshoorn
Universiteit Twente, Enschede,
the Netherlands
Laqueur

Caroline Overy
Wellcome Trust Centre for the History of
Medicine at UCL, London, England
Livingstone

Steven Palmer
University of Windsor, Windsor, Ontario,
Canada
*Calderón Guardia, Durán Cartín,
Fernández y Hernández*

José Pardo-Tomás
CSIC, Barcelona, Spain
Monardes

Lawrence Charles Parish
Jefferson Medical College, Philadelphia, PA, USA
Bateman, Duhring, Gross, Hutchinson, Shippen, Willan

Eldryd Parry
Tropical Health and Education Trust, London, England
Burkitt

Adell Patton Jr.
University of Missouri, St Louis, MO, USA
Boyle, J. Easmon, Odeku, Togba

Harry W. Paul
University of Florida, Gainesville, FL, USA
Pasteur, Rothschild

John Pearn
University of Queensland, Brisbane, Australia
Bancroft, Beaney, Coppleson, Fairley, Halford, MacGregor

Steven J. Peitzman
Drexel University College of Medicine, Philadelphia, PA, USA
Addis, Bright, A. Richards, Scribner

Kim Pelis
National Institutes of Health, Bethesda, MD, USA
Barker, Councilman, Gorgas, Hammond, Nicolle, Reed, T. Smith

Concetta Pennuto
Université de Genève, Geneva, Switzerland
Ficino, Fracastoro

José Morgado Pereira
Universidade de Coimbra, Coimbra, Portugal
Egas Moniz

Jacques Philippon
Salpêtrière-Pitié Hospital, Paris, France
Mondor

Howard Phillips
University of Cape Town, Rondebosch, South Africa
Abdurahman, Barnard, Barry, Naidoo, Orenstein, Xuma

Jean-François Picard
CNRS, Paris, France
Debré, Delay, Hamburger, Leriche, Roussy, Vincent

Mikhail Poddubnyi
Voenno-meditsinskii Zhurnal, Moscow, Russia
N. Bidloo, Buial'skii, Dobroslavin, Gaaz, Inozemtsev, Pirogov, Pletnev

Hans Pols
University of Sydney, Sydney, Australia
Beard, Beers, Bowlby, Burton-Bradley, Grinker, Klein, Laing, Stillé

María-Isabel Porras-Gallo
University of Castilla-La Mancha, Madrid, Spain
Obrador Alcalde

Patricia E. Prestwich
University of Alberta, Edmonton, AB, Canada
Magnan, Moreau de Tours, Morel

Lawrence M. Principe
Johns Hopkins University, Baltimore, MD, USA
Helmont

Armin Prinz
Medizinische Universität Wien, Vienna, Austria
Wenckebach

Cay-Ruediger Pruell
Albert-Ludwigs-Universität, Freiburg, Germany
Aschoff, Cohnheim, Conti, Ehrlich, Rokitansky, Virchow

Constance Putnam
Independent scholar, Concord, MA, USA
Balassa, Bene, Duka, O. W. Holmes, Korányi, Markusovszky, Meigs, Morgan, Semmelweis, G. Shattuck, N. Smith, J. Warren

Emilio Quevedo
Universidad Nacional de Colombia, Bogotá, Colombia
Franco

Sean Quinlan
University of Idaho, Moscow, ID, USA
A. Louis, Quesnay

Camilo Quintero
University of Wisconsin–Madison, Madison, WI, USA
Mutis y Bosio

Roger Qvarsell
University of Linköping, Linköping, Sweden
Huss

Karina Ramacciotti
Universidad de Buenos Aires, Buenos Aires, Argentina
Carrillo, Mazza, Rawson

Mridula Ramanna
SIES College, University of Mumbai, Mumbai, India
Bentley, Choksy, Jhirad, Khanolkar, Lad, Morehead, J. Turner

Matthew Ramsey
Vanderbilt University, Nashville, TN, USA
Civiale, Desgenettes, Fourcroy, Portal, Richerand, Velpeau,
Vicq d'Azyr

Ismail Rashid
Vassar College, Poughkeepsie, NY, USA
Fanon, Horton

Carole Reeves
Wellcome Trust Centre for the History of Medicine
at UCL, London, England
Abt, Battey, Buchan, Budd, Cole, Darwin, Holt, Keen,
Lane, S. Morton, Prout, Rock, Sabin, Scharlieb, Seacole,
Spock, Tait

C. Joan Richardson
University of Texas Medical Branch, Galveston, TX,
USA
Barton

Philip Rieder
Université de Genève, Geneva, Switzerland
Bonet, De La Rive, Le Clerc, Odier, Reverdin, Tronchin

Ortrun Riha
Universität Leipzig, Leipzig, Germany
Isaac Israeli

Julius Rocca
University of Birmingham, Birmingham, England
Aëtius, Aretaeus, Aristotle, Asclepiades, Caelius Aurelianus,
Celsus, Dioscorides, Empedocles, Erasistratus, Herophilos,
Pliny, Scribonius Largus, Soranus, Whytt

Julia Rodriguez
University of New Hampshire, Durham, NH, USA
Aráoz Alfaro, Coni, Grierson, Ingenieros

Esteban Rodríguez-Ocaña
Universidad de Granada, Granada, Spain
Ferrán y Clúa, Pittaluga Fattorini

Volker Roelcke
Justus-Liebig Universität, Giessen, Germany
Alzheimer, Bleuler, Kretschmer, Mitscherlich, Rüdin

Hugo Röling
Universiteit van Amsterdam, Amsterdam,
the Netherlands
Rutgers

Naomi Rogers
Yale University, New Haven, CT, USA
Kenny

Anastasio Rojo
University of Valladolid, Valladolid, Spain
Bravo de Sobremonte, Mercado, Valles

Nils Rosdahl
Medical Museion, Copenhagen Denmark
Madsen

Barbara Gutmann Rosenkrantz
Harvard University, Cambridge, MA, USA
Hardy, L. Shattuck

Leonard D. Rosenman
UCSF, San Francisco, CA, USA
Frugard

Fred Rosner
Mount Sinai School of Medicine, New York,
NY, USA
Maimonides

Lisa Rosner
Richard Stockton College, Pomona, NJ, USA
Bennett, Brown, Christison, Cullen, Ferriar, J. Gregory,
Laycock, Monro, Percival, Withering

Frederic Roy
Université de Montréal, Montreal, QC,
Canada
Suvannavong

Marion Maria Ruisinger
Friedrich-Alexander-Universität,
Erlangen-Nuremberg, Germany
Heister

Han van Ruler
Erasmus Universiteit, Rotterdam,
the Netherlands
Blankaart, Bontekoe, Graaf

Andrea Rusnock
University of Rhode Island, Kingston,
RI, USA
Arbuthnot, Bond, Boylston, E. Jenner, Jurin, Sutton,
Waterhouse

Fernando Salmón
Universidad de Cantabria, Santander, Spain
Arnald, López Albo

Lutz D. H. Sauerteig
University of Durham, Durham/Wolfson
Research Institute, Stockton, England
Blaschko

Walton O. Schalick III
Washington University, St Louis, MO, USA
*Gilles de Corbeil, Henry of Mondeville, John of
Gaddesden, John of Saint-Amand, Peter of Abano, Peter
of Spain, Richard the Englishman, Taddeo, William of
Brescia*

Volker Scheid
University of Westminster, London, England
Ding Ganren, Fei Boxiong, Yun Tieqiao

Aina Schiøtz
Universitetet i Bergen, Bergen, Norway
Evang

William Schneider
Indiana University, Indianapolis, IN, USA
Hirszfeld, Pinard, Richet, Tzanck

Heinz Schott
Rheinische Friedrich-Wilhelms-Universität,
Bonn, Germany
Mesmer

Andrew Scull
University of California San Diego, San Diego, CA,
USA
*Brigham, Cotton, Dix, Earle, Haslam, Meyer, Ray,
Tuke*

Nikolaj Serikoff
The Wellcome Library, London, England
*The Islamic Medical Tradition, Aḥmad, Ibn al-Bayṭār,
Al-Bīrūnī, Clot Bey, Foley, Ḥaddād, Ibn al-Haytham,
Mahfouz, Ibn al-Māsawayh, Meyerhof, Ibn Sīnā, Sournia,
Van Dyck, Waldmeier, Al-Zahrāwī*

Jole Shackelford
University of Minnesota, Minneapolis, MN, USA
Severinus

Sonu Shamdasani
Wellcome Trust Centre for the History of Medicine
at UCL, London, England
*Adler, Forel, A. Freud, Gesell, Janet, Menninger, Putnam,
Sullivan*

Patrick Henry Shea
Rockefeller Archive Center, Sleepy Hollow, NY, USA
Carrel

Sally Sheard
University of Liverpool, Liverpool, England
*Bevan, Beveridge, Chadwick, Farr, Newman, Newsholme,
Shuttleworth, T. S. Smith*

Dongwon Shin
Korean Advanced Institute of Science and
Technology, Taejon, Korea
Choe Han'gi, Heo, Sejong, Yi Jema

Barry David Silverman
Northside Hospital, Atlanta, GA, USA
Taussig

Mark E. Silverman
Emory University, Atlanta, GA, USA
Flint, Hope, J. Mackenzie

Jelena Jovanovic Simic
Zemun, Serbia
*Batut, Djordjević, Lazarević, Kostić, Nešić, Štampar,
Subbotić*

P. N. Singer
London, England
Galen

Kavita Sivaramakrishnan
Public Health Foundation of India, New Delhi,
India
G. Sen, P. Sharma, T. Sharma, Shukla, Vaid, Varier

Morten A. Skydsgaard
University of Aarhus, Aarhus, Denmark
Panum

Jean Louis De Sloover
Erpent (Namur), Belgium
Dodonaeus

David F. Smith
University of Aberdeen, Aberdeen, Scotland
Orr

F. B. Smith
Australian National University, Canberra, Australia
W. Thomson

Thomas Söderqvist
Medical Museion, Copenhagen, Denmark
Jerne

Marina Sorokina
Russian Academy of Sciences, Moscow, Russia
*Al'tshuller, Briukhonenko, Haffkine, Ilizarov, Iudin,
Negovskii, Semenovskii*

David Sowell
Juniata College, Huntingdon, PA, USA
Perdomo Neira

Eduard A. van Staeyen
Leiden, the Netherlands
Guislain

Frank W. Stahnisch
Johannes Gutenberg-Universität, Mainz, Germany
Graefe, Griesinger, His, C. Vogt, O. Vogt, Warburg,
Wassermann

Ida H. Stamhuis
Vrije Universiteit Amsterdam, Amsterdam,
the Netherlands
Quetelet

Darwin H. Stapleton
Rockefeller Archive Center, Sleepy Hollow, NY, USA
Hackett

Jane Starfield
University of Johannesburg, Bertsham, South Africa
Molema, Moroka

Martin S. Staum
University of Calgary, Calgary, AB, Canada
Cabanis

Hubert Steinke
University of Bern, Bern, Switzerland
Haller

Oddvar Stokke
National Hospital, Oslo, Norway
Følling, Refsum

Michael Stolberg
Universität Würzburg, Würzburg, Germany
Bartisch, Fabricius, Fuchs, Platter, Rösslin, Scultetus

Marvin J. Stone
Baylor University Medical Center, Dallas, TX, USA
Coley, Ewing, Farber, E. Graham, Hodgkin, Wintrobe

Hindrik Strandberg
Helsinki, Finland
Willebrand, Ylppö

Karin Stukenbrock
Martin-Luther-Universität Halle-Wittenberg,
Halle, Germany
Brunfels, Erxleben, Frank, Gersdorff, Hoffmann,
Stahl

Charles Suradji
Jakarta, Indonesia
Soedarmo

Akihito Suzuki
Keio University, Yokohama, Japan
Medicine, State, and Society in Japan, 500–2000,
Asada, Baelz, Conolly, Hata, Mori, Ogata, Pompe van
Meerdervoort, Siebold, Yamagiwa

Mika Suzuki
Shizuoka University, Shizuoka, Japan
Ogino, Yoshioka

Victoria Sweet
UCSF, San Francisco, CA, USA
Hildegard of Bingen

Simon Szreter
University of Cambridge, Cambridge,
England
McKeown

Cecilia Taiana
Carleton University, Ottawa, ON, Canada
Lacan

Ian Tait
Aldeburgh, Suffolk, England
Browne

Jennifer Tappan
Columbia University, New York, NY, USA
Trowell

Robert Tattersall
University of Nottingham, Nottingham,
England
Abel, Addison, Albright, Doniach, Hench, Horsley,
Joslin, Minkowski, Starling

Kim Taylor
Kaimu Productions, Shanghai, China
Hatem, Zhu Lian

Manuela Tecusan
University of Cambridge, Cambridge, England
Alcmaeon, Anaximander, Andreas, Democedes,
Democritus, Diocles, Diogenes, Oribasius, Paul
of Aegina, Philistion, Plato, Praxagoras, Rufus

Bert Theunissen
Universiteit Utrecht, Utrecht, the Netherlands
Donders

Michel Thiery
Stichting Jan Palfyn en Museum voor
Geschiedenis van de Geneeskunde, Ghent, Belgium
Palfyn

C. Michele Thompson
Southern Connecticut State University,
New Haven, CT, USA
Lán Ông, Tuệ Tĩnh

Carsten Timmermann
University of Manchester, Manchester, England
*Bauer, Grotjahn, McMichael, Pickering, D. Richards,
Rosenbach*

Tom Treasure
St George's Hospital Medical School, London,
England
*Beck, Blalock, C. E. Drew, C. R. Drew, Favaloro, Gibbon,
Hufnagel*

Ulrich Tröhler
University of Bern, Bern, Switzerland
*Bergmann, Billroth, Kocher, Langenbeck,
Mikulicz-Radecki, Nissen, Quervain*

Arleen Marcia Tuchman
Vanderbilt University, Nashville, TN, USA
Zakrzewska

Marius Turda
Oxford Brookes University, Oxford, England
Babeş, Cantacuzino, Ciucă, Marinescu

Trevor Turner
Homerton University Hospital, London, England
Maudsley

Peter J. Tyler
Edgecliffe, New South Wales, Australia
*W. Armstrong, Bland, Fiaschi, Mackellar, Skirving,
Stuart, Thompson*

Michael Tyquin
Making History, Darlington, New South Wales,
Australia
Dunlop

Tatiana Ul'iankina
Institute of the History of Science and Technology,
Moscow, Russia
Mechnikov, Sechenov

G. van der Waa
Rotterdam, the Netherlands
Gaubius

Lia van Gemert
Universiteit Utrecht, Utrecht, the Netherlands
Beverwijck

Maria Vassiliou
University of Oxford, Oxford, England
Belios, Livadas

Jan Peter Verhave
UMCN, Nijmegen, the Netherlands
Swellengrebel

Joost Vijselaar
Trimbos-Instituut, Utrecht, the Netherlands
Schroeder van der Kolk

Jurjen Vis
Amsterdam, the Netherlands
Foreest

An Vleugels
National University of Singapore, Singapore
Kerr

Hans de Waardt
Vrije Universiteit Amsterdam, Amsterdam,
the Netherlands
Wier

Keir Waddington
Cardiff University, Cardiff, Wales
*Abernethy, Brunton, Garrod, Gee, Lawrence,
J. Paget*

Lisa K. Walker
University of California, Berkeley, CA, USA
Khlopin, Teziakov

John Walker-Smith
Wellcome Trust Centre for the History of
Medicine at UCL, London, England
G. Armstrong, G. Still, Underwood, West

Paul Weindling
Oxford Brookes University, Oxford, England
Verschuer

Dora B. Weiner
UCLA, Los Angeles, CA, USA
Esquirol, Larrey, Percy, Pinel, Tenon

Kathleen Wellman
Southern Methodist University, Dallas, TX, USA
La Mettrie, Patin, Renaudot

Ann Westmore
The University of Melbourne, Parkville, Victoria,
Australia
Cade

James Whorton
University of Washington, Tacoma, WA, USA
Eddy, S. Graham, Kellogg, Lust, B. Palmer, D. Palmer,
S. Thomson, Trall

Ann Wickham
Dublin City University, Dublin, Ireland
A. Jones

Elizabeth A. Williams
Oklahoma State University, Stillwater, OK, USA
Boissier de la Croix de Sauvages, Bordeu

Sabine Wilms
Paradigm Publications, Taos, NM, USA
Ge Hong, Sun Simiao, Tao Hongjing

Warren Winkelstein, Jr.
University of California, Berkeley, CA, USA
Emerson, Frost, Goldberger, Hamilton, Kinyoun,
Lane-Claypon, Park, Paul, Wynder

Michael Worboys
University of Manchester, Manchester, England
Allbutt, Bristowe, W. W. Cheyne, Moynihan, Simon, Syme

Jill Wrapson
University of Auckland, Auckland,
New Zealand
Barnett

Marcia Wright
Columbia University, New York, NY, USA
Park Ross

Rex Wright-St Clair (deceased)
Huntingdon, Hamilton, New Zealand
A. Thomson

Henrik R. Wulff
Medical Museion, Copenhagen, Denmark
Hirschsprung

Ronit Yoeli-Tlalim
Warburg Institute, London, England
Sangye Gyatso, Yuthog Yontan

William H. York
Portland State University, Portland, OR,
USA
Despars, Valesco of Tarenta

Benjamin Zajicek
University of Chicago, Chicago, IL, USA
Bekhterev, Korsakov, Pavlov

Soledad Zárate
Universidad de Chile, Santiago, Chile
Cruz-Coke Lassabe

Alfons Zarzoso
Museu d'Història de la Medicina de Catalunya,
Barcelona, Spain
Pedro-Pons, Puigvert Gorro

Franz Zehentmayr
Salzburg, Austria
Zhang Yuansu

Barbara Zipser
Wellcome Trust Centre for the History of Medicine
at UCL, London, England
Al-Mawṣilī

Patrick Zylberman
CERMES, Villejuif, France
Sand

ABBREVIATIONS

AMA	American Medical Association
ANB	*American National Biography*
BA	Bachelor of Arts
BCE	Before Common Era
BCG	Bacillus Calmette-Guérin (tuberculosis vaccination)
BM	Bachelor of Medicine
BMA	British Medical Association
BMJ	*British Medical Journal*
CBE	Commander, The Most Excellent Order of the British Empire
CE	Common Era
ChB	Bachelor of Surgery
ChD	Doctor of Surgery
ChM	Master of Surgery
CIE	Companion, The Most Eminent Order of the Indian Empire
KCIE	Knight Commander, The Most Eminent Order of the Indian Empire
CM	Master of Surgery
CMB	Combat Medical Badge (U.S. Army)
CMG	Companion, The Most Distinguished Order of St Michael and St George
CMO	Chief Medical Officer
CMS	Church Missionary Society
CSI	Companion, The Most Exalted Order of the Star of India
CSIRO	Commonwealth Scientific and Industrial Research Organization (Australia)
DAMB	*Dictionary of American Medical Biography*
DAuB	*Dictionary of Australian Biography* (available online)
DBE	Dame of the British Empire
DBI	*Dizionario Biografico degli Italiani*
DGMS	Director General Medical Service (military)

DMed	Doctor of Medicine
DNZB	*Dictionary of New Zealand Biography* (available online)
DPM	Diploma of Psychological Medicine
DSB	*Dictionary of Scientific Biography*
DSO	Distinguished Service Order (military British)
ECT	Electo-convulsive Therapy
EEG	Electroencephalogram
FAO	Food and Agriculture Organization (United Nations)
FRCP	Fellow Royal College of Physicians
FRCPEdin/FRCPEd	Fellow Royal College of Physicians Edinburgh
FRCS	Fellow of the Royal College of Surgeons
FRCSEdin/FRCSEd	Fellow Royal College of Surgeons Edinburgh
FRS	Fellow of the Royal Society
FRSEdin/FRSEd	Fellow of the Royal Society of Edinburgh
GBH	General Board of Health (England and Wales)
GMC	General Medical Council (UK)
GP	General Practitioner
ICN	International Council of Nursing
ICS	Indian Civil Service
IHB	International Health Board (Rockefeller Foundation)
IMS	Indian Medical Service
IOC	Institute Oswaldo Cruz
JAMA	*Journal of the American Medical Association*
KCSI	Knight Commander, The Most Exalted Order of the Star of India
LLD	Doctor of Laws
LMS	Licentiate in Medicine and Surgery
LRCP	Licentiate of the Royal College of Physicians
LRCPEdin/LRCPEd	Licentiate of the Royal College of Physicians Edinburgh
LRCSEdin/LRCSEd	Licentiate of the Royal College of Surgeons Edinburgh
LRFPS	Licentiate of the Royal Faculty of Physicians and Surgeons of Glasgow
LSA	Licentiate of the Society of Apothecaries
LSHTM	London School of Hygiene and Tropical Medicine
LSMW	London School of Medicine for Women
MA	Master of Arts
MB	Bachelor of Medicine
MBCM	Bachelor of Medicine Master of Surgery
MC	Military Cross
MD	Doctor of Medicine
mg	milligram
MMed	Master of Medicine
MO	Medical Officer
MoH	Medical Officer of Health
MRC	Medical Research Council
MRCNZ	Medical Research Council of New Zealand
MRCOG	Member of the Royal College of Gynaecologists
MRCP	Member of the Royal College of Physicians
MRCS	Member of the Royal College of Surgeons
MS	Multiple Sclerosis
NHMRC	National Health and Medical Research Council (Australia)
NSDAP	National Socialist Party (Nazi Germany)
NSW	New South Wales (Australia)
OAS	Organization of American States
OBE	Officer, The Most Excellent Order of the British Empire
Oxford DNB	*Oxford Dictionary of National Biography* (UK)
PASB	Pan American Sanitary Bureau

PhD	Doctor of Philosophy
QVJIN	Queen Victoria Jubilee Institute of Nursing
RACP	Royal Australasian College of Physicians
RACS	Royal Australasian College of Surgeons
RAMC	Royal Army Medical Corps (UK)
RBNA	Royal British Nurses Association
RCP	Royal College of Physicians
RCPEdin	Royal College of Physicians of Edinburgh
RCS	Royal College of Surgeons
RCSEdin	Royal College of Surgeons of Edinburgh
RMO	Resident Medical Officer
RSTMH	Royal Society of Tropical Medicine and Hygiene
SA	Sturm Abteilung [Storm Section] (Nazi Germany)
SLSAA	Surf Lifesaving Association of Australia
SS	Schutzstaffel [Protective Squadron] (Nazi Germany)
STD	Sexually Transmitted Diseases
UCH	University College Hospital (London, England)
UCL	University College London (England)
UNICEF	United Nations Children's Fund
UNRRA	United Nations Relief and Rehabilitation Administration
WHO	World Health Organization
YMCA	Young Men's Christian Association

LIST OF ENTRIES

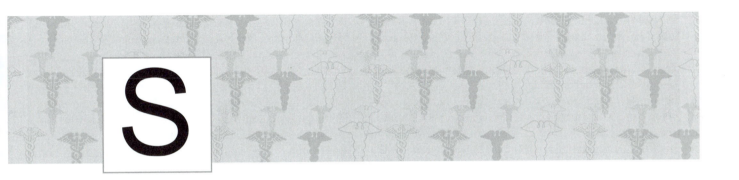

S

SABIN, ALBERT BRUCE (b. Bialystok, Russia, 26 August 1906; d. Washington, D.C., USA, 3 March 1993), *medicine, virology, immunology, epidemiology.*

Sabin, one of four children, emigrated to the United States (1921) from Russia with his parents, Jacob and Tillie, settling in Paterson, New Jersey, where Jacob worked in the silk and textile business. Graduating from Paterson High School (1923), he enrolled at New York University dental school but soon switched to medicine. At New York University College of Medicine, he devised a fast, accurate system for typing *Pneumococci.* Later, he pioneered a sensitive diagnostic dye test for toxoplasma antibody. Awarded an MD (1931), he interned at New York's Bellevue Hospital (1931–34). Here he isolated and characterized the herpes B virus from a colleague who had died after a monkey bite (1932). A research post at the Lister Institute, London (1934–35), was followed by a Fellowship at the Rockefeller Institute for Medical Research (1935–39) to study virology, notably the neuro-invasiveness of viruses, with Peter K. Olitsky. They grew poliovirus in human embryonic nervous tissue (1936). Appointed to the University of Cincinnati College of Medicine and Children's Hospital Research Foundation (1939), Sabin was associate professor (1943–45) and then distinguished service professor of pediatrics (1945–69). He married Sylvia Tregillus (1935), and they had two daughters.

During World War II, Sabin served in the Pacific as a lieutenant colonel in the U.S. Army Medical Corps. Achievements included isolation of the sandfly fever virus as well as vaccines for dengue fever and Japanese B encephalitis, against which he immunized 65,000 military personnel at Okinawa. His postwar research included autopsies on everyone dying of poliomyelitis within a 400-mile radius of Cincinnati. He showed that poliovirus invaded the digestive tract before attacking nerve tissue. When John Franklin Enders and colleagues succeeded in growing poliovirus in non-nervous tissue (1949), vaccine production became a possibility. Sabin worked on a live attenuated oral vaccine that would multiply in the intestinal tract while Jonas Salk, University of Pittsburgh, experimented with an injectable killed-virus vaccine. Salk's vaccine was backed by the National Foundation for Infantile Paralysis (March of Dimes), although early success was marred by contamination with virulent live virus, causing polio in vaccinated children (1955). By spring 1957 Sabin had obtained a trivalent vaccine (containing attenuated strains of all three types of poliovirus) and had given it to over 100 volunteers, including his wife and children. He also sent a batch to the Soviet Union at the request of Anatoli A. Smoridentsev of the Virus Research Laboratories, All Union Institute of Experimental Medicine, Leningrad. Collaboration with Soviet virologists resulted in their immunization of 87 million Russian people (1959–60), which more than compensated for the difficulty in obtaining large-scale clinical trials in the United States (by then committed to the Salk vaccine). The massive uptake of Sabin's vaccine in Communist countries established it internationally, resulting in approval for manufacture by the U.S. Public Health Service. On 'Sabin Sundays' about 100 million Americans received the vaccine (1962–64) free of charge, many physicians providing their service gratis. People who were fed oral vaccine shed weakened virus in their feces, boosting local immunity and reducing numbers susceptible to polio. Sabin donated his poliovirus strains to the World Health Organization for use in developing countries (1972). He remained committed to global eradication of polio and measles, for which he developed an aerosol vaccine.

Sabin was a meticulous researcher and was eloquent and decisive in debate, hard to defeat in scientific argument, competitive, and occasionally dogmatic but with great warmth, courage, and wisdom. After Sylvia's death (1966) and a brief marriage to Jane Warner (1967–71), he wed Heloisa Dunshee de Abranches (1972), who survived him. A recipient of numerous awards and honorary degrees, Sabin served as president of the Weizmann Institute of Science, Israel (1970–72), consultant to the U.S. National Cancer Institute (1974), distinguished research professor of biomedicine, Medical University of South Carolina (1974–82), and senior expert consultant for the Fogarty International Center for Advanced Studies in the Health Sciences, National Institutes of Health (1984–86). He was interested in the viral etiology of cancer, in controlling influenza epidemics, and later, in the HIV virus.

Bibliography

Primary: 1945. (with Schlesinger, Robert Walter) 'Production of Immunity to Dengue with Virus Modified by Propagation in Mice.' *Science* 101 (2634): 640–642; 1960. (with Ramos-Alvarez, Manuel, José Alvarez-Amezquita, et al.) 'Live, Orally Given Poliovirus Vaccine.' *JAMA* 173: 1521–1526; 1987–88. 'Role of My Co-operation with Soviet Scientists in the Elimination of Polio.' *Perspectives in Biology and Medicine* 31: 57–64; 1993. 'Reflections on the Qualitative and Quantitative Aspects of Neurovirulence of Different Polioviruses.' *Developments in Biological Standardization* 78: 3–7.

Secondary: Chanock, Robert M., 1996. 'Reminiscences of Albert Sabin and His Successful Strategy for the Development of the Live Oral Poliovirus Vaccine.' *Proceedings of the Association of American Physicians* 108: 117–126; Beale, John, 1993. 'Obituary, Albert Sabin.' *Lancet* 341 (8846): 685; Grouse, Lawrence D., 1993. 'Obituary, Albert Bruce Sabin, MD.' *JAMA* 269: 2140; Koprowski, Hilary, 1993. 'Obituary, Albert B. Sabin (1906–1993).' *Nature* 362 (6420): 499; Benison, Saul, 1982. 'International Medical Cooperation: Dr Albert Sabin, Live Poliovirus Vaccine and the Soviets.' *Bulletin of the History of Medicine* 56: 460–483; The Legacy of Albert B. Sabin. Sabin Vaccine Institute, www.sabin.org

Carole Reeves

SACHS, HANS (b. Kattowitz, Upper Silesia [now Katovice, Poland], 6 June 1877; d. Dublin, Ireland, 25 March 1945), *immunology.*

Sachs was the son of Jewish parents, Flora Haussdorf and Elias Sachs. He went to school in Kattowitz. From 1895 until 1900 he studied medicine at Freiburg, Breslau (Wroclaw), and Berlin, where he passed his final examinations and gained a doctorate one year afterward. In this very year he started his scientific career. He volunteered at the pathological institute Senckenberg in Frankfurt am Main until he was appointed as an assistant in 1901. In 1905 he became assistant to Paul Ehrlich at the Royal Institute for Experimental Therapy at Frankfurt am Main, too. In 1907 Sachs was appointed titularprofessor and held the post of vice director before he was awarded a full professorship and made director of the scientific department at the Institute for Experimental Cancer Research at Heidelberg.

Sachs mainly concentrated on immunity and serum research, a field that he significantly influenced in Germany during the 1920s and early 1930s. His treatise on immunobiological pathophysiology (1928) and his extensive work 'Antigene und Antikörper' (1930) were both of fundamental importance. Together with Ernst Witebsky, Sachs worked on tests about the importance of lipoids for cancer immunity. During this time he built up the reputation as a leading serologist in Germany and even in Europe. Being Jewish, however, he was 'relieved of his duties' soon after the Nazi takeover in 1933. By the intervention of Richard Siebeck, dean of the medical faculty of Heidelberg University at that time, and Ludolf Krehl, head of the clinic for internal medicine, this leave was canceled temporarily. Yet his definite removal from office took place on 15 January 1936. Sachs emigrated to England and finally to Ireland. He died on 25 March 1945 at Dublin.

Because of his excellent achievements in the field of serum research, he received significant awards. From 1928 he was a corresponding member of the Vienna Society for Microbiology. In 1930 he was awarded the Ludwig Darmstätter prize with the Paul Ehrlich medal for his studies on immunity and serology; moreover, he joined the Akademie der Naturforscher Leopoldina [academy of natural scientists] at Halle-on-Saale. In 1905 Sachs married Adelheid Sophie Charlotte Grelling, and with her, he had two children, Werner and Ilse.

Bibliography

Primary: 1902. *Die Hämolysine und ihre Bedeutung für die Immunitätslehre* (Wiesbaden); 1928. *Probleme der pathologischen Physiologie im Lichte neuerer immunbiologischer Betrachtung* (Vienna); 1930. 'Antigen und Antikörper' in Oppenheimer, Carl, ed., *Handbuch der Biochemie* 1 (2nd edn., 1933).

Secondary: Wagner, G., and A. Mauerberger, 1989. *Krebsforschung in Deutschland. Vorgeschichte und Geschichte des Deutschen Krebsforschungszentrums* (Berlin and Heidelberg); Drüll, D., 1988. *Heidelberger*

Gelehrtenlexikon 1803–1932 (Berlin, Heidelberg, New York, and Tokyo); Mussgnug, Dorothee, 1988. *Die vertriebenen Heidelberger Dozenten—zur Geschichte der Ruprecht-Karls-Universität nach 1933* (Heidelberg).

Wolfgang U. Eckart

SAĪD, MUHAMMAD (see under ABD UL-HAMĪD and SAĪD, MUHAMMAD)

SALK, JONAS

(b. New York, New York, USA, 28 October 1914; d. La Jolla, California, USA, 23 June 1995), *virology, poliomyelitis vaccination.*

Salk was the oldest of the three sons of Russian-Jewish immigrants, Daniel B. Salk, a lady's clothing designer, and his wife, Dora, neither of whom had received a formal education. Salk was the first member of his family to go to college. He attended Townsend Harris High School, Upper Manhattan, and the City College of New York. He first intended to study law but switched to medicine. While at college, Salk met his future wife, Donna Lindsay. They married in the year Jonas graduated, 1939. They had three children: Peter, Darrell, and Jonathan. Jonas and Donna divorced in 1968. In 1970 Salk married Françoise Gilot. In 1938, while still attending medical school, Salk spent a year researching influenza with Thomas Francis. Salk recalled that the basic ideas he used to create his polio vaccine were formed at this stage. After graduating, Salk worked as a staff physician at the Mount Sinai Medical School. In 1942 he became a research fellow, again with Francis, who was now a department head at the newly formed School of Public Health at the University of Michigan.

In 1947 Salk moved to Pittsburgh, where he directed a virus research laboratory. Although still working on influenza, he turned his attention at this time to poliomyelitis. At the beginning of the twentieth century, the killer epidemic bacterial diseases of industrial societies, such as diphtheria, typhoid, and cholera, began to decline. However, by the interwar years, seemingly new, viral disorders, often affecting the central nervous system, such as influenza, encephalitis lethargica, and poliomyelitis, were apparently taking their place. America suffered a severe epidemic of the latter disease in 1916, and in New York City alone, more than 9,000 cases were reported. The disease also took center stage in the United States because Franklin Roosevelt had contracted polio at age thirty-nine and developed irreversible paralysis. In 1938 Roosevelt founded March of Dimes, a national health charity, as the National Foundation for Infantile Paralysis. At Pittsburgh, Basil O'Connor, president of the foundation, supported Salk's research.

During his Pittsburgh years Salk developed, tested, and refined his polio vaccine. When he started his work, it was generally held that immunity was conferred only by infection with a live virus. Salk worked on the theory that it was possible to acquire immunity through contact with inactivated virus. Using formaldehyde, Salk rendered the poliovirus inert but kept it intact enough to trigger the necessary immune response. His vaccine was first tested in monkeys and then in humans, at the D. T. Watson Home for Crippled Children. After successful trials, in 1952, Salk tested his vaccine on volunteers, including himself, the laboratory staff, his wife, and his children. In 1954 testing in the United States was begun on one million children, ages six to nine, who were known as the Polio Pioneers (one group of children received a placebo). On 12 April 1955, it was announced that the results showed that the vaccine was safe and effective.

Statistics supported the vaccine's efficacy. In 1952 57,628 cases of polio were recorded in the United States. After the vaccine became available, recorded polio cases fell by 85–90 percent in only two years. In 1979 only ten cases were reported. Later, the oral, or Sabin, vaccine came into use. This had the advantage (besides its less aggressive mode of administration) of transmitting an attenuated live virus and protecting unvaccinated children. In 1962 Salk established the Salk Institute for Biological Studies in La Jolla, California.

Bibliography

Primary: 1963. *Biological Basis of Disease and Behavior* (New York); 1985. *The Virus of Poliomyelitis: From Discovery to Extinction* (Chicago); 1985. *Considerations in the Preparation and Use of Poliomyelitis Virus Vaccine* (Chicago).

Secondary: Oshinsky, David M., 2005. *Polio: An American Story* (Oxford); Kluger, Jeffrey, 2004. *Splendid Solution: Jonas Salk and the Conquest of Polio* (New York); Meldrum, Marcia, 1998. "'A Calculated Risk': The Salk Polio Vaccine Field Trials of 1954.' *British Medical Journal* 317: 1233–1236.

Christopher Lawrence

SALOMONSEN, CARL JULIUS

(b. Copenhagen, Denmark, 6 December 1847; d. Copenhagen, 14 November 1924), *bacteriology.*

Salomonsen grew up in a wealthy and cultured Jewish family, the only son of Martin Salomonsen, a general practitioner and medical officer of health, and Eva Henriques. He studied medicine at the University of Copenhagen (1865–71), and upon graduation he worked at the public maternity hospital, Fødselsstiftelsen, there observing the effects of Listerian antiseptics, and later as an assistant at the pathology department of Almindelig Hospital (1872). He then entered a position as house physician at a combined medical and surgical department at Kommunehospitalet (1873–75).

In late 1873 Salomonsen performed the first clinical bacteriological examinations and experiments in Denmark, quickly earning a reputation as a promising researcher in bacteriology. His thesis (1877) focused on pyemic processes and on the natural history of the bacteria involved, providing support for Ferdinand Cohn's view that bacteria were distinct species. More originally, Salomonsen demonstrated a method for growing bacteria in pure cultures using capillary tubes, an important innovation in cultivation methods before Robert Koch's introduction of transparent solidifiable media in 1881.

Salomonsen spent the summer of 1877 in Breslau (Wroclaw) working with Julius Cohnheim and meeting with leading German experimental pathologists. Together with Cohnheim, he demonstrated the specificity of tuberculosis (1878); he continued his work in this field upon his return to Denmark, while also publishing results from clinical experiments of bacteria in pus accumulations. He worked as prosector at Kommunehospitalet (1877–79) and started giving private lectures, thus founding a strong interest in teaching.

In March 1882 Salomonsen visited Robert Koch in Berlin and returned to Copenhagen with a strengthened belief in the future of bacteriology. He saw a need for teaching in this field, and in 1883 Salomonsen was offered a temporary position as lecturer in bacteriology at the University of Copenhagen, the first university in Europe to establish such a chair. He taught in the basement of the Botanical Museum and gained a strong following among young physicians and veterinaries. He published a textbook on experimental technique and bacteriological methodology (1889), which appeared in several editions and was translated into English and French. Salomonsen was appointed professor of pathology in 1893 and moved to new laboratory facilities. A new building was constructed for the institute of pathology in 1910 in connection with the new university hospital, Rigshospitalet.

In addition to his teaching, Salomonsen continued research and displayed an interest in a variety of subjects. He was instrumental in reforming the Danish smallpox vaccination service in 1886, replacing human lymph with vaccine from calves. Inspired by the results of serum therapy against diphtheria, he set up production of serum in connection with his university laboratory (1895). Salomonsen soon acknowledged the need for better production facilities and suggested the establishment of a separate institute for this purpose. This opened in 1902 as the State Serum Institute, which became one of the world's leading serum institutes. Salomonsen headed the institute until 1909, with Thorvald Madsen as his closest associate and successor. He served as Rector of the University of Copenhagen (1909–10) and retired in 1920.

Salomonsen outlived both his wife Ellen (née Henriques, a distant relative of his mother), whom he married in 1880, and their only child. During most of his academic career, Salomonsen maintained a large private practice primarily serving the Jewish community in Copenhagen. In his younger years, he was a part of progressive literary and political circles, and he decided upon a career in bacteriology at a time when the prospects of this field were hotly debated. He maintained a broad cultural and historical interest throughout his life, and he launched a series of attacks on the 'dysmorfia' of modern art in his later years. In 1907 he cofounded the Museum of Medical History (now the Medical Museion) in Copenhagen.

Bibliography

Primary: 1891. *Bacteriological Technology for Physicians* (Copenhagen).

Secondary: Lautrop, Hans, 1983. 'Carl Julius Salomonsen og bakteriologiens begyndelse i Danmark.' *Bibliotek for Læger* 175: 97–146; Thomsen, Oluf, 1925. 'Carl Julius Salomonsen.' *Festskrift udgivet af Københavns Universitet i anledning af Universitetets Aarsfest* November: 75–81; Bang, Bernhard, 1924. 'Carl Julius Salomonsen.' *Ugeskrift for Læger* 86: 913–15.

Søren Bak-Jensen

SANARELLI, GIUSEPPE (b. Monte San Savino, Arezzo, Italy, 24 September 1864; d. Rome, Italy, 6 April 1940), *medicine, parasitology, virology, hygiene.*

After obtaining his degree in medicine and surgery from the University of Siena (1889), Sanarelli worked with Camillo Golgi (1843–1926) in Pavia, studying the natural immunity against anthrax and introducing a new technique for ultrafiltration of microorganisms (viruses) using a colloidal membrane. In 1890 he visited Max von Pettenkofer in Munich and spent two years in Paris, where he studied with Louis Pasteur, Émile Duclaux, Elie Mechnikov, and Emile Roux. This period was fundamental for his scientific career, and he was always considered a 'Pasteurian'. During his Paris years, Sanarelli published his results on the pathogenesis of typhoid fever, proposing the theory of a general infection of hematogenic origin, with a secondary, localized infection in the intestine.

Back in Italy, he was appointed professor of hygiene at the University of Siena (1893), before accepting an invitation from the Uruguay government to join the University of Montevideo and organize a new Institute of experimental hygiene.

During this period he studied the etiology of yellow fever, working in Brazil and Uruguay, isolating in 58 percent of autopsies a bacterium (*Bacterium icteroides*), which he considered to be the cause of the disease. He believed that yellow fever was an intoxication resulting from a factor produced by *B. icteroides*. One major barrier for studying the disease was that it only affected humans. With no animal model to use, the researchers were obliged to do all their experiments on people. Sanarelli reported that he reproduced the disease by injecting formaldehyde-inactivated broth cultures into five humans (three of whom died). That was strongly criticized by William Osler (1849–1919), who considered it 'criminal . . . to deliberately inject a poison of known high degree of virulency into a human being, unless you obtain that man's sanction'.

This bacterial theory, at first confirmed by several medical authorities, was finally refuted when the ultrafilterable nature of the contagious agent and the role of *Stegomya* mosquitoes as its vector were demonstrated.

In 1896 Sanarelli observed a very peculiar disease in some laboratory rabbits imported from Brazil (*Oryctologus*) and used for the microbiological research. He described the disease's pathognomonic manifestations, including its specific lesions in the ears and eyes, which produced what he called a 'lion head'. Sanarelli searched without success for bacteria in diseased tissues and organs and attributed the cause of the disease to an ultrafilterable virus, which he named 'myxomatogenic virus' and considered analogous to the filterable virus of rabies studied by Pasteur. In 1897 Moses was able to reproduce the infection using the filtrate of a tumor produced by the virus. Sanarelli undertook an extensive survey of the disease, and he showed the causative agent's specificity for rabbits, given that he was unable to infect other animals, including dogs, rats, and monkeys. He demonstrated also that surviving animals were made resistant to the infectious agent (acquired immunity). He presented his results in 1898 at the 9th Congress of Hygiene and Demography in Madrid and published them in the *Centralblat für Bakteriologie*.

In 1898, after marrying Maria Carmen Pons, Sanarelli returned to Italy, becoming professor of hygiene at the University of Bologna and starting a long political career. He was elected to Parliament five times and was also for three years (1906–09) Under-secretary of State for Agriculture, Industry, and Commerce. This political activity stopped his scientific research, until 1912, when he delivered his classic lecture on the hereditary immunity to tuberculosis at the international congress on tuberculosis in Rome, published as a book the following year. Sanarelli refuted the classical idea of a 'hereditary predisposition' to tuberculosis, reversing the concept and suggesting the idea of a 'hereditary resistance', linking the diffusion of the disease to socioeconomic conditions. This idea was developed further, especially in two books published in 1930 (*Il fattore editario nella tuberculosi*) and 1931 (*L'hérédité et la contagion dans la tuberculose*).

After the sudden death of Angelo Celli (1857–1914), creator of the Institute of Hygiene in Rome and the leading Italian hygienist, Sanarelli offered to withdraw from political activity if nominated to the chair of hygiene at Rome University. He was nominated in 1914. In a series of papers published between 1916 and 1924, he discussed the pathogenesis of cholera, demonstrating the marked gastric enterotropism of the cholera bacillus. He observed also the hemorrhagic allergy (Sanarelli's phenomenon) implicated in choleric algidity.

In 1920 he was elected Senator of the Kingdom of Italy for his scientific achievements.

Bibliography

Primary: 1898. 'El virus mixomatògeno—Contribuciòn al estudio de los virus no organizados por el Prof. Dr. José Sanarelli.' *Anales de la Universidad de Montevideo* 13p; 1900. *Per la storia di una scoperta. Il bacillo della febbre gialla ed i suoi critici* (Città di Castello);

1926. *Les entéropathies microbiennes* (Paris); 1930. *Il fattore ereditario nella tubercolosi* (Rome) [French trans., 1931, *Hérédité de la contagion dans la tuberculose* (Paris)].

Secondary: Vitali, E. D., 1975. 'Sanarelli, Giuseppe' in *Scienziati e tecnologi dalle origini al 1875*, vol. 2 (Milan) p. 80; Puntoni, V., 1965. 'In memoria di Giuseppe Sanarelli nel 25° della sua morte.' *Nuovi Annali d'Igiene e di Microbiologia* 16: 81–87; Agrifoglio, L., 1953. *Ricordando Giuseppe Sanarelli (1864–1940)* (Rome); *DSB*.

Bernardino Fantini

SANCHES, ANTÓNIO NUNES RIBEIRO   (b. Penamacor, Beira-Baixa, Portugal, 7 March 1699; d. Paris, France, 14 October 1783), *medicine.*

Member of a family of 'new Christians' (baptized Jews) who often suffered the Inquisition's harassment, Sanches studied arts at the University of Coimbra (1716–19) and medicine at the University of Salamanca (1720–24), where he took the degree of bachelor in arts and medicine in April 1724.

Sanches began to practice medicine in the Portuguese cities of Guarda, Benavente, and Lisbon. Yet the difficulties he coped with as a result of his lineage, including a denunciation of crypto-Judaism to the Inquisition Court of Lisbon, led him to leave Portugal in 1726. Settling then in London under the protection of an uncle who was a physician and practicing Jew, he practiced medicine for two years among the Portuguese Marrano community in addition to following the anatomical lessons of James Douglas (1675–1742), visiting hospitals, and privately teaching Latin and history to a teenager of a well-off family of that community.

During the years 1728 and 1729 he traveled through France and Italy, having visited Paris, Montpellier, Marseille, Livorno, Pisa, Genoa, and Bordeaux. In early 1730, after a short stay in London, he accompanied his former private student to study medicine at the University of Leiden. There Sanches followed Herman Boerhaave's lectures and soon became his close student. Thanks to Boerhaave's references, a year and a half later Sanches was contracted by the Tsarina Anna Ivanovna to work in Russia.

In October 1731 Sanches began a professional stay of seventeen years in Russia, first in Moscow as a senate-physician and city-physician. From 1733, in St Petersburg, he was successively physician of the chancellery (1734), of the imperial army—having participated as such in military campaigns against Poland (1735) and Turkey (1736–1737)—of the Imperial Body of Cadets (*c.* 1737), and of the tsarist court (1740) in the service of Anna Ivanovna (d. 1740) and of her heir. In 1741, however, after a military revolt and the enthronement of the new Tsarina Elisabeth Petrovna (r. 1741–52), Sanches was accused of crypto-Judaism, and his career as imperial court physician cut short, although he did not leave Russia until 1747.

By late 1747 Sanches moved to Paris, where he devoted himself for the rest of his life to medical practice and to writing on a broad range of topics, including medicine, education, economy, politics, morals, and religion, with the help of a personal library that contained over 1,100 volumes by the time of his death. His wide intellectual concerns reflect not only his medical concerns, but also a vocation of *philosophe* who cultivated a close contact, from a distance, with the reformist elites of the Russian and Portuguese Enlightenment. Six of his writings were printed while he was alive, and two more soon after his death, but there are many others in about twenty manuscripts scattered over libraries of Paris, Madrid, Lisbon, Braga, Vienna, and Leiden.

In his medical writings Sanches paid particular attention to 'venereal disease' (three printed works in addition to his article 'Maladie vénérienne inflammatoire chronique' for the *Encyclopédie*, vol. XVII, 1765, pp. 83–84), to 'passions of the soul' (for the *Encyclopédie Méthodique*, 'Médecine', vol. I, 1787, pp. 245–277), to hygiene ('people's health', military health, steam baths, and thermal waters), to the reform of medical teaching, and to the control of health practices and practitioners.

A member of several scientific societies—the Imperial Academy of Sciences of St Petersburg (1747), the Societé Royale de Médecine (1778), and the Academia Real das Sciencias de Lisboa (1780), among others—Sanches from the 1760s was pensioned by the king of Portugal and by the Tsarina Catalina II.

Bibliography

Primary: 1959–1966, *Obras* 2 vols. (Coimbra); 1751. *A dissertation on the origin of the venereal disease* (London) [French edns.: Paris 1752, Leiden 1778, along with *Examen historique sur l'apparition de la maladie vénérienne en Europe, et sur la nature de cette épidémie* (Lisbon, 1774)]; 1756. *Tratado da conservação da saúde dos povos* (Paris) [Lisbon, 1757; Spanish edn.: Madrid, 1781]; 1763. *Metodo para aprender e estudar a medicina, illustrado com os apontamentos para estabelecerse huma universidade Real naqual deviam aprender-se as sciencias humanas de que necessita o Estado civil e politico* (Paris); 1779. *O Parnych Rossijskich Banjach* (St Petersburg) [Moscow, 1782] [French mss original version: *Memoire sur les bains de vapeur de Russie* (c. 1771)].

Secondary: Willemse, David, 1966. *António Nunes Ribeiro Sanches—élève de Boerhaave—et son importance pour la Russie* (Leiden); Lemos, Maximino, 1911. *Ribeiro Sanches. A sua vida e a sua obra* (Porto).

Jon Arrizabalaga

SAND, RENÉ (b. Ixelles, Belgium, 30 January 1877; d. Brussels, Belgium, 23 August 1953), *social medicine.*

Son of Hubert Sand, a tile layer from Luxembourg, and Julie Lévêque, a school teacher in Maubeuge, France, Sand was first tempted to study embryology and marine zoology. Interning in Brussels (1899), he obtained his MD degree in 1900. He traveled to Berlin (1902) and Vienna (1904), where he studied anatomical pathology and neurology.

In 1901 he married Marie-Thérèse Joris, with whom he had four children. He was assistant (1903) and then chief (1910–20) in the anatomical pathology laboratory of Professor Rommelaere at the Free University of Brussels (ULB), and he obtained the agrégation in 1906. A consulting physician for an insurance company (1905) and expert for the courts, he was invited in 1911 to teach industrial hygiene and occupational accidents. In 1912 he founded the Belgian Association of Social Medicine. In 1919 he created the Belgian Society of Eugenics, which he renamed ten years later the Belgian Society of Preventive Medicine and of Eugenics.

His teaching contributed strongly to the development of social medicine in Belgium. After the success of his book *Health and Human Progress* (1934–35), he was entrusted with a course in social medicine at the School of Criminological Sciences at the ULB (1936). He delivered lectures on the fundamentals of social medicine at the medical school (1938–40), where he created an Institute of Hygiene (1938). After the war, he sat on the supervisory committee of the Solvay Sociology Institute. Most importantly, and with help from the Rockefeller Foundation, the ULB created the chair of social medicine and history of medicine for him in 1945.

His important administrative responsibilities were evidence of his influence. Medical inspector in the Ministry of Labor from 1919, he was designated on 16 June 1936 as technical consultant to the new Ministry of Public Health. He was also a member of the cabinet of the socialist Emile Vandervelde, and on 1 January 1937, he was appointed secretary general to the ministry (honorary in 1945). The former president of the Belgian Medical Federation was thus able to negotiate the creation of an Order of physicians (25 July 1938) and lay the foundations for the future law on public health insurance adopted after World War II.

Following World War I he became deeply involved in international work. The League of the Red Cross Societies called upon him to be General Secretary (1921–27), and he organized the first International Conference of Social Services in 1928 in Paris. He participated in the foundation of many international medical associations. However, he concentrated his efforts on the international organization of public health. He sat from 1932 to 1936 on the Child Welfare Committee of the League of Nations and from 1934 to 1936 on the LN's Health Committee. In April 1946 his diplomatic talents led to his chairing the Technical Preparatory Committee that produced the preamble to the WHO constitution, which includes the celebrated definition of health (authored by Andrija Štampar) as 'a state of complete physical, mental and social well-being and not merely the absence of disease and infirmity'. In 1951 he was given the chairmanship of the WHO's Expert Committee on Medical Education. At the same time, the 4th World Health Assembly awarded him the Léon Bernard Foundation Prize. Sand was a member of numerous medical bodies (among them the British Medical Association).

It was less because of a penchant for reform than because of the spectacle of a medical profession closed to all social aspects of health and illness that Sand turned toward social medicine. Sand was initially influenced by Alfred Grotjahn and Rudolf Goldscheid, and for him, social medicine covered 'everything that interests the sociologist in medicine and hygiene, [and] everything that interests the physician in social sciences'. Products of a period when progress was embodied in medicine and public health, his work on the history of social medicine (1952) are nothing less than a mine of relevant information today.

Bibliography

Primary: 1934. *L'Economie humaine par la médecine sociale* (Paris) [English trans. 1935, *Health and Human Progress* (London)]; 1948. *Vers la médicine sociale* (Paris) [English trans. 1952, *The Advance to Social Medicine* (London)].

Secondary: Zylberman, P., 2004. 'Fewer Parallels than Antitheses: René Sand and Andrija Stampar on Social Medicine, 1919–1955.' *Social History of Medicine* 17: 77–92; Anciaux, A., 1988. *Le Docteur René Sand ou la culture des valeurs humaines* (Brussels).

Patrick Zylberman

SANDERSON, JOHN SCOTT BURDON   (b. Jesmond, near Newcastle upon Tyne, England, 21 December 1828; d. Oxford, England, 23 November 1905), *physiology.*

One of six children born to devout Evangelical parents, lawyer Richard Burdon and Elizabeth Sanderson, John's childhood was austere but happy. He chose medicine over the law as a profession and in 1847 obtained an MD and gold medal from the University of Edinburgh, an important center of laboratory physiology. His teachers sent him to Paris, where he studied physiology under Claude Bernard (1813–78), whom he described as 'the most inspiring teacher, the most profound scientific thinker, and the most remarkable experimental physiologist that he had ever known'.

Burdon Sanderson returned to England in 1852 with a calling—science—but with limited opportunities to pursue it. Pressure was compounded by marriage (childless) to Ghetal Herschell (August 1853). Already he was supplementing his private practice by serving as medical registrar at St Mary's Hospital, Paddington, London, and from 1854 he lectured there. He also obtained an appointment as physician to the Western General Dispensary and, in 1856, became the first medical officer of health for Paddington, with responsibilities that included collecting vital statistics; inspecting unhealthy trades and buildings, as well as food and drink for adulteration; and investigating epidemics. Meanwhile, Burdon Sanderson continued to pursue a hospital career, becoming assistant physician to the Brompton Hospital for Consumption (1859) and the Middlesex Hospital (1863).

The sanitary work rather than the hospital work inaugurated a truly scientific career for Burdon Sanderson. His reports on Paddington pleased John Simon (1816–1904), the chief medical officer of the Privy Council, who commissioned Burdon Sanderson to investigate diphtheria (1857), vaccination practices across the country during the early 1860s, meningitis in Poland (1865), and other outbreaks. In 1865 a royal commission on the cattle plague asked Burdon Sanderson to study transmission, which he discovered did occur from animal to animal. This investigation was a turning point for Burdon Sanderson and indeed for the country: henceforth, the state would find funds for important medical and veterinary research, and Burdon Sanderson would rely primarily on science rather than on medicine to advance his career. Burdon Sanderson continued to investigate the transmission of disease in tuberculosis, cholera, and smallpox. In 1864 he began to do physiology work and research at University College Hospital, in 1866 he was appointed lecturer in physiology at the Middlesex Hospital, and in 1867 he was elected FRS and gave the society's Croonian lecture, speaking on respiration and circulation, based on his vivisection experiments with dogs performed at UCL as well as on his experiments with the sphygmograph.

In 1867 Burdon Sanderson resigned as medical officer of health, and in 1870 he gave up medicine entirely, becoming professor of practical physiology and histology at University College London (1870). He became director of the Brown Institute for animal pathology in 1872 and the Jodrell professor of human physiology at UCL in 1874. Burdon Sanderson had finally become a professional scientist to stand alongside his old teacher, his name a watchword for science ('Burdon-Sanderson's physiology' was touted by Bram Stoker's *Dracula* as the height of professional knowledge) and a bugbear to the antivivisectionists. Burdon Sanderson spent these years continuing his researches into inflammation and transmission—with mixed conclusions both for and against the new germ theory emerging from Paris—and investigating plant physiology, after Charles Darwin (1809–82) queried him about the role of electricity in the Venus flytrap. In 1883 he transferred to Oxford, as Waynflete professor of physiology, but his plans to establish a school of physiology were thwarted by conservative graduates of the university. The final decade of his life was spent as regius professor of medicine.

Bibliography

Primary: 1873. (ed., with Klein, E., and M. Foster) *Handbook for the Physiology Laboratory* (London); 1911. (Burdon Sanderson, G., J. S. Haldane, and E. S. Haldane, eds.) *Sir John Burdon Sanderson: A Memoir, with Selections from His Papers and Addresses* (London).

Secondary: Romano, T. M., 2002. *Making Medicine Scientific: John Burdon Sanderson and the Culture of Victorian Science* (Baltimore); *DSB; Oxford DNB.*

E. A. Heaman

SANDSTRÖM, IVAR VIKTOR (b. Stockholm, Sweden, 22 March 1852; d. Uppsala, Sweden, 2 June 1889), *anatomy.*

Ivar Viktor Sandström was born in 1852 in Stockholm. In 1872 he began medical studies at the University of Uppsala, where he became medicine candidate in 1878. He supported his medical studies by working as assistant to Professor Clason in the anatomy department. He was made responsible for histology and was praised for his succinct lecturing and use of the microscope in medical training. During 1879–80 he was appointed Prosector in the Anatomy Department. In 1881 he became extra teacher in histology, and he remained in that position until 1886 while he continued his medical studies. In 1886 he became a medical licentiate, and in 1887 he finished his medical studies and obtained his diploma as a physician. In 1886–89 he was appointed as a doctor at Sala County Hospital north of Uppsala. He married Anna in 1885; they had two children. The family was poor, and Sandström had to split his time between teaching, research, his own medical studies, and earning a living for the family. His wife was distressed with his hard work, and the family's poor economic state, and she finally returned to her parents together with the two children. Sandström had a mental disability, possibly inherited from his mother's family, became mentally ill and depressed, and had to stay in hospital for a short time. Thereafter, when he continued to be alone, his depression increased, leading to his death by suicide in 1889 at the age of thirty-seven.

Sandström's great contribution to medical science, the discovery of the parathyroid glands, represents a milestone in the history of medicine. The discovery was made at the anatomy department in Uppsala in 1877, when he was still only a medical student and anatomy assistant. Sandström first detected the glands in dissections of a dog and understood after microscopical examination that it was an organ with a structure entirely different from that of the neighboring thyroid. He completed his investigations during the winter of 1879–80 and confirmed the existence of the gland in man and several animal species. He named the new structures 'glandulae parathyroideae' and made detailed anatomical and histological studies after dissection of the glands in fifty human autopsy cases.

Three years later he published his observations (in Swedish) in an article entitled 'On a new gland in man and several animals' in a local journal, *Uppsala Läkareförenings förhandlingar.* The manuscript was initially offered to a German journal but was refused because it was considered too long. The paper was appreciated in Sweden, and Sandström was awarded the Hwasser prize of the Medical Society of Uppsala and the Florman prize from Stockholm. In 1880 he reported his discovery at a Scandinavian meeting for natural sciences in Stockholm. However, few noted or were interested in the finding, and Sandström was very disappointed with the lack of recognition of his discovery. Anatomy Professor Clason tried in vain to arrange a professorship for Sandström. Before his death Sandström wrote in a letter to his sister, 'it would have been nice to become a professor and get a name'.

He never became a professor, but he certainly acquired a name to be remembered in the history of medicine. The recognition and comprehensive description of the parathyroid glands is often claimed as the last anatomical discovery, and Sandström's scientific work has been repeatedly praised for its accuracy. It was reported to the world in 1880 in a brief summary in German by the Swedish professor G. Retzius. This was recognized, and Sandström's work was deservedly acknowledged when the parathyroid glands were discovered for the second time, in England in 1892. Welsh in 1898 wrote, 'I cannot too strongly emphasize the admirable precision and accuracy, which characterize this earliest record of these glands in man.' Decades later, Sandström's findings turned out to be of considerable physiological and clinical importance, when the glands were realized to be crucially important for calcium regulation and calcium regulatory disorders.

Bibliography

Primary: 1879–80. 'Om en ny körtel hos menniskan och åtskilliga däggdjur.' *Uppsala Läkareförenings förhandlingar* 15: 441–471.

Secondary: Seipel, C. M., 1938. 'Ivar Sandström: An English Translation of Sandström's Glandulae Parathyreoideae.' *Bulletin of the History of Medicine,* 6 (3):192–222 (includes biography by Hammar, J. Aug.).

Göran Åkerström

SANGER, MARGARET LOUISE HIGGINS (b. Corning, New York, USA, 14 September 1879; d. Tucson, Arizona, USA, 6 September 1966), *birth control.*

Sanger was the sixth of eleven children of Michael and Anne Higgins. She attended Claverack College and Hudson River Institute before studying nursing at White Plains Hospital between 1900 and 1902. In 1902 she married draftsman and painter William Sanger, moving to Hastings and then, in 1910, to New York City. There the Sangers associated with intellectuals, including Emma Goldman and Upton Sinclair, and Margaret joined various political actions, including the Women's Committee of the New York Socialist Party. Her work as a visiting nurse, combined with her mother's premature death from exhaustion, focused her interest on sexual matters. Her sex-education column, 'What Every Girl Should Know', in *New York Call,* led to her first clashes with censors, who objected to her references to venereal diseases.

Sanger's interest in birth control was spurred by her work with poor women in the Lower East Side. Incited by the frequent sufferings of these women resulting from excessive childbirth, miscarriage, and abortion and encouraged in her social thinking by Goldman, Sanger argued for reproductive choices as a central tool through which working-class women could liberate themselves. Relief from the burden of unwanted pregnancy also fitted Sanger's feminist agenda. But, as with her other efforts to provide free information on sexual matters, Sanger clashed with the censors. She challenged the 1873 Comstock Law on obscene publications, arguing that information about family limitation was central to securing independence for women.

In March 1914 Sanger published her feminist journal *The Woman Rebel*, in which she framed the right to birth control as a feminist issue. Her publishing venture soon landed her in trouble. The first three issues of *The Woman Rebel* were banned because of the contraceptive information, and Sanger was indicted for violating the Comstock Law. Rather than risk imprisonment, Sanger sailed to London under the false name 'Bertha Watson'. As a parting gesture, she released 100,000 copies of a contraception information leaflet entitled *Family Limitation*. Soon after disembarking in England, Sanger contacted the leading British neo-Malthusians, who led her to emphasize the social and economic justifications of birth-control advice. She also met Havelock Ellis, whose arguments concerning the fundamental need for women's sexual enjoyment free from the fear of unwanted pregnancy appealed to Sanger.

In 1915 Sanger returned to New York to face charges for distributing *The Woman Rebel*, although charges were dropped. In the same year, she visited a Dutch birth-control clinic, which convinced her to advocate the use of a rubber diaphragm. In 1916 Sanger opened the first American family-planning clinic in Brooklyn, although this was raided after only nine days—leading to a thirty-day prison sentence for Sanger. Meanwhile, in keeping with her views on sexual liberation, Sanger divorced William and commenced a series of affairs with several men, including Havelock Ellis and H. G. Wells. In 1922 she married oil baron James Slee—although she maintained her sexual and financial freedom. Slee was the main financer of the birth-control movement in the United States until his death in 1943.

By 1917 Sanger's publishing included the monthly *Birth Control Review*, which was associated with the 1921 formation of the American Birth Control League. Through this body, Sanger gained the support of leading doctors, social workers, and eugenicists. Eugenics came to be an important part of Sanger's justification of contraception—and she supported sterilization of the mentally incapacitated. Ensuing organizations, such as the National Committee on Federal Legislation for Birth Control and the International Planned Parenthood Federation, took up much of Sanger's energy. Her aims to provide cheaper, effective birth-control methods led to her support of the American manufacture of Dutch-designed diaphragms, as well as developments of spermicidal jellies and eventually the Pill. Her efforts paid off in 1965, when the Supreme Court ruled in the case of *Griswold v. Connecticut* that contraception should be legal for married couples. Shortly after this ruling, Sanger died in Tucson, Arizona.

Bibliography

Primary: 2003. (Katz, Esther, ed.) *The Selected Papers of Margaret Sanger, Volume 1: The Woman Rebel* (Urbana, IL).

Secondary: Reed, Miriam, 2003. *Margaret Sanger: Her Life in Her Words* (Fort Lee, NJ); Cullen-DuPont, Kathryn, ed., 1999. *Margaret Sanger: An Autobiography* (New York) [orig. pub. 1938]; Kennedy, David M., 1970. *Birth Control in America: The Case of Margaret Sanger* (New Haven); *DAMB*.

Ivan Crozier

SANGYE GYATSO (aka SANGS RGYAS RGYA MTSHO) (b. ?, 1653; d. ?, 1705), *Tibetan medicine.*

Sangye Gyatso, regent of the fifth Dalai Lama (1617–82) and one of the most notable figures in Tibetan history, was a Buddhist scholar, a leading politician, and an eminent figure in the history of Tibetan medicine. A prolific writer, his works included treatises on Buddhism, history, medicine, astrology, and the history of medicine.

Sangye Gyatso became the regent of Tibet in the summer of 1679, a position that assigned to him the care of the Dalai Lama's temporal ruling rights. The Fifth Dalai Lama died in 1682, but Sangye Gyatso concealed his death until 1697, claiming that he was in a religious retreat.

Sangye Gyatso's epoch was a golden era of Tibetan culture in general and of Tibetan medicine in particular. Although not a physician himself, Sangye Gyatso either initiated or oversaw a number of monumental projects in the sphere of medicine that had a lasting effect on the history of Tibetan medicine. Like many other Buddhist scholars, Sangye Gyatso's medical training was an integral part of his Buddhist schooling: he studied medicine as one of the five Buddhist sciences, as theoretical knowledge.

Sangye Gyatso is generally credited with the foundation of the Tibetan medical colleges, as well as the Tibetan public health system. Based on the wish of his master, the Fifth Dalai Lama, Sangye Gyatso sought to codify the theory and practice of medicine. He thus founded, in 1696, the first Tibetan College of medicine, the Chagpori [lCags po ri or 'Iron Mountain'] College of Medicine, adjacent to the Potala Palace in Lhasa, as well as a number of others. Iron Mountain was the first medical college in Tibet that was open for both monks and laymen. The medical colleges he established later served as a model for similar establishments, such as in Labrang [bLa brang] and Kumbum [sKu 'bum], as well as medical colleges in Mongolia. Sangye Gyatso was personally involved in setting and supervising the curricula in these colleges, based on his medical writings. In setting the curricula, Sangye Gyatso emphasized the integrated study and practice of medicine and astrology.

Sangye Gyatsho is credited with composing some of the most frequently used Tibetan medical treatises. These include *Blue Beryl* [*Vaidurya sngon po*], a commentary on the medical *Four Tantras* [*rGyud bzhi*]; *White Beryl* [*Vaidurya dkar po*], an astrological work synthesizing various elements from Chinese astrology and serving as a main text for astro-medicine; *Practical Manual for Medical Treatment* [*lhan thabs*], focusing on the third of the *Four Tantras*; and *History of Tibetan Medicine* [*gso ba rig pa'i khog 'bugs legs bshad vaduu rya'i me long*]).

Sangye Gyatso also commissioned medical paintings to accompany the *Blue Beryl* (published by Parfionovitch, Meyer and Dorje in 1992). A parallel set was later commissioned for the *White Beryl* (published 2001).

Sangye Gyatso was killed in the autumn of 1705 because of his rivalry with the ruler of the Qosot Mongol tribe, Lhabzang Khan.

Bibliography

Primary: Sangs rgyas rgya mtsho. *Dpal ldan gso ba rig pa'i khog 'bugs legs bshad vaduu rya'i me long drang srong dgyes pa'i dga' ston*; Pasang Yonten, 1988. *Bod kyi gso ba rig pa'i lo rgyus kyi bang mdzod gyu thog bla ma dran pa'i pho nya* (Leh, Ladakh); Byams pa 'phrin las, 2000. *Gangs ljongs gso rig bstan pa'i nyin byed rim byon gyi rnam thar phyogs bsgrigs* (Beijing).

Secondary: Meyer, Fernand, 2003. 'The Golden Century of Tibetan Medicine' in Pommaret, Françoise, ed., Solverson, Howard, trans., *Lhasa in the Seventeenth Century: The Capital of the Dalai Lamas* (Leiden and Boston) pp. 99–117; Parfionovitch, Yuri, Fernand Meyer, and Gyurme Dorje, 1992. *Tibetan Medical Paintings: Illustrations to the Blue Beryl Treatise of Sangye Gyamtso (1653–1705)* (London); Lange, Kristina, 1976. *Die Werke des Regenten Sans rgyas rgya mc'o (1653–1705): Eine philologisch-historische Studie zum tibetischsprachigen Schrrifttum* (Berlin).

Ronit Yoeli-Tlalim

SANTORIO, SANTORIO (aka SANCTORIUS, SANCTORIUS)

(b. Capodistria, Italy (now Koper, Slovenia), 29 March 1561; d. Venice, Italy, 6 March 1636), *medicine, physiology.*

The son of Antonio Santorio, originally from Spilimbergo, and Elisabetta Cordonia, Santorio began his education in his native town and then went to Venice to further his learning as a guest of the Morosini family. In 1575 he began his studies of philosophy and medicine at the University of Padua. He remained in Padua after graduating (1582), working as a physician, and it was here that he began his systematic study of the variation of the weight of the human body considering various internal and external factors.

Between 1587 and 1599 Santorio worked as a physician for various noble families in Hungary, Croatia, and perhaps in Poland. After moving definitively to Venice, he formed friendships with Paolo Sarpi, Galileo Galilei (1564–1642) and Giovanfrancesco Sagredo. Santorio was the first to apply the quantitative method in biology and medicine, inventing for this purpose a series of measuring instruments. In fact, Galilei was one of the more than 10,000 subjects whom Santorio weighed on his chair scales.

In 1602 Santorio published his first book, dedicated to the method to be followed in order to avoid errors in the practice of medicine. Without breaking with the Galenic tradition, he took a critical approach to classical physiology, and expressed ideas anticipating the mechanistic explanations of the iatrophysical school. Santorio employed the analogy, later used by René Descartes (1596–1650), between the organism and a clock, the movements of which depend on the number, form, and disposition of its parts; thus, in his first work, he was already mentioning measuring instruments.

On 6 October 1611 Santorio was appointed professor of the first chair of theoretical medicine at the University of Padua, a position he held with great renown until 1624. In 1612 Santorio published *Commentaria in artem medicinalem Galeni*, containing the first printed reference to the air thermometer. In 1614 he published *De statica medicina*, the work that made him famous. 'Static medicine' meant medicine founded on weighing and therefore on the use of the scale. This work is based on a long series of experiments Santorio carried out over about thirty years using a special chair scale and other measuring instruments. The comparison between the weight of the body and the difference between the quantity of food ingested and the quantity of excrement eliminated allowed him to define the quantitative aspects of the *perspiratio insensibilis*, and the dependence of this on various internal and external factors—the basis of the modern study of metabolism. Compiled in the unusual form of aphorisms, the *De statica medicina* met with an extraordinary success, not only among the followers of the iatromechanical school, but also in practical medicine.

In 1624 Santorio abandoned teaching and settled in Venice. The following year he published the *Commentaria in primam fen primi libri Canonis Avicennae*, in which many of the instruments he had invented were described and represented. Some instruments were made to quantify and measure physical and biological phenomena, such as the chair scales, the *pulsilogium* (for measuring 'with mathematical certainty' the pulse rate), the thermometer, the hygrometer, the anemometer, and devices to measure the temperature of the moon, the strength of the wind, and the force of water currents. Other instruments were destined for clinical use, such as special trocars for abdominal and thoracic paracentesis and for tracheotomy, a tricuspid syringe for extracting bladder stones, a bathing bed, and a specially equipped bed.

Bibliography

Primary: 1660. *Opera omnia* 4 vols. (Venice); 1602. *Methodi vitandorum errorum omnium . . .* (Venice); 1612. *Commentaria in artem medicinalem Galeni* (Venice); 1614. *Ars . . . de statica medicina* [2nd edn., 1615] (Venice); 1625. *Commentaria in primam fen primi libri Canonis Avicennae* (Venice); 1629. *Commentaria in primam sectionem Aphorismorum Hippocratis* (Venice).

Secondary: Ongaro, Giuseppe, 2001. 'Introduction' in *Santorio's De statica medicina* (Florence) pp. 5–47; Ettari, Lieta Stella, and Mario Procopio, 1968. *Santorio Santorio. La vita e le opere* (Rome); Grmek, Mirko Drazen, 1952. *Santorio Santorio i njegovi aparati i instrumenti* (Zagreb); Castiglioni, Arturo, 1920. *La vita e l'opera di Santorio Santorio capodistriano, MDLXI–MDCXXXVI* (Bologna and Trieste) [reprinted 1987 (Trieste), English trans. 1931, 'The Life and Work of Sanctorius' *Medical Life* 38: 726–786]; *DSB*.

Giuseppe Ongaro

SAUERBRUCH, ERNST FERDINAND   (b. Barmen, Germany, 3 July 1875; d. Berlin, Germany, 2 July 1951), *surgery*.

As no other German doctor in the twentieth century, still in his lifetime, the surgeon Ernst Ferdinand Sauerbruch became the idol of his patients and of his audience in all sections of German society. He was at the center of what has been called the 'Sauerbruch myth', a myth of a 'demigod in white'. However, biographical transfiguration on the one hand and medical and political reality on the other have to be distinguished. Soon after the death of the famous Berlin surgeon on 2 July 1951, the memoirs of this much-adored doctor were published in the magazine *Revue*, followed by the film *Sauerbruch. Das war mein Leben*, one of the typical heroic medical dramas of the early 1950s. As with the autobiography, the film also was a tightrope walk between fiction and reality.

Born on 3 July 1875 at Barmen, Sauerbruch finished school at Elberfeld. The young Sauerbruch did his medical training at Marburg, Leipzig, and Jena and again at Leipzig, where he passed his final examinations on 25 February 1901. After his Habilitation under J. von Mikulicz-Radecki at Breslau (8 June 1905), he was briefly senior physician (12 October 1907) and associate professor of surgery (23 December 1908) at Marburg. He was director of the Chirurgische Universitätsklinik at Zurich from 15 December 1910 and held the same position at Munich (1918), and finally, on 3 December 1927, he was called to the chair for surgery at the Chirurgische Klinik of the Charité in Berlin, where he stayed until he was given emeritus status in 1949.

As a surgeon, Sauerbruch was brilliant in every field, but his special focus was thoracic surgery. Although he faced considerable difficulties and setbacks, his method of pressure difference inaugurated the development of modern thorax surgery and facilitated for the first time extensive operations of the lung and the open heart. Indisputable is his role as one of the pioneers of plastic surgery, remembered despite technical revolutions in prosthetics; he is known for his work on the hand prosthesis, named after him ('Sauerbrucharm'), and the cineplasty: a femur amputation, saving the lower leg. He was a distinguished surgeon and a popular lecturer. Moreover, Sauerbruch published and edited important surgical books. Soon after the Nazis seized political power in Germany, he approximated his nationalist ideas, which were of immense importance to his personal view of the world, to the ideological sphere of national socialism and frequently even agreed with it publicly, although reconstructing his private views on the new situation proves to be ambivalent. Altogether, the keynote was rather positive. In his 'Offener Brief an die Ärzteschaft der Welt' [open letter to the world's physicians], (3 September 1933), he praised Germany's exemplary national revival; 'all countries' would 'have to fight for fundamental ideological ideas prevalent in fascism and national socialism'. Nationalist declarations and confessions of loyalty toward Nazi ideology expressed by such a popular public person tended to be rewarded by Hitler. Together with August Bier (1861–1949), the surgeon with an inclination for homeopathy, Sauerbruch was awarded the first Deutscher Nationalpreis für Kunst und Wissenschaft [German National Award for Art and Science].

Sauerbruch never joined the NSDAP or any other Nazi organization; he did not agree with Nazi ideology and practice without reservation. He objected strongly to anti-Semitism. Still, he allowed the Nazis to use him for their purposes. Acting as a medical consultant for the Reichsforschungsrat [Reich Research Council] from 1933 until 1945, he approved research projects in concentration camps, such as the experiments of Otmar Freiherr von Verschuer (geneticist in Berlin) and his assistant Josef Mengele in Auschwitz in 1943. Furthermore, he had knowledge of the horrid sulfonamide experiments with women in the concentration camp of Ravensbrueck, carried out by Karl Gebhardt (physician of the SS), and he did not criticize them. From at least 1948, Sauerbruch suffered from cerebral arteriosclerosis, which led him to retire on 3 December 1949. He died on 2 July 1951.

Bibliography

Primary: 1937. *Thoracic Surgery* (London); 1953. *A Surgeon's Life, Ferdinand Sauerbruch* (London).

Secondary: Eckart, Wolfgang U., 2002. 'Ernst Ferdinand Sauerbruch (1875–1951)' in Fröhlich, Michael, ed., *Die Weimarer Republik—Portrait einer Epoche in Biographien* (Darmstadt) pp. 175–187.

Wolfgang U. Eckart

SAUNDERS, CICELY MARY STRODE   (b. Barnet, Hertfordshire, England, 22 June 1918; d. Sydenham, London, England, 14 July 2005), *terminal care*.

The eldest of three children, Saunders was born to a father who was a prosperous estate agent. Her father and mother were unhappy together (indeed, in 1945 her father made her tell her mother that the marriage was over), so for the first few years of her life, until her mother took her back home, she was boarded contentedly with an aunt. At the age of ten, she was sent to Roedean, an upper-class, single-sex boarding school, where she felt like an outsider: shy and taller than the other girls, she also had a slight curvature of her spine for which daily exercises were prescribed. In later life, Saunders said that this sense of alienation had probably made her always take the part of other outsiders.

Her wish had been to become a nurse, but her parents insisted on her going to Oxford, and after one failed attempt and attendance at a crammer, she went to the future St Anne's College to study the course in politics, philosophy, and economics. Nevertheless, in 1944 she enrolled as a student nurse at St Thomas's Hospital, London, only to be advised to abandon nursing because an operation had failed to cure her painful back, which was made much worse through lifting patients. Returning to Oxford, she took her degree and then went to Archway Hospital, London, after qualifying as a hospital social worker in 1947. Here and elsewhere, she became aware of the special needs of the dying, in terms of both pain control and spiritual comfort (on holiday around this time, she had abandoned her longstanding agnosticism and become a committed Christian). In particular, she formed a strong emotional bond with a friendless dying Polish waiter, David Tasma, a refugee from the Warsaw ghetto with no family. They discussed the possibility of setting up a special home for the terminally ill, with his cryptically asking to be 'a window' in this. He went on to leave her all his money, £500 (then a substantial sum), to help in this project.

While still a social worker and wanting to study firsthand the problems of the dying, Saunders enrolled as a part-time nurse, again at St Thomas's Hospital, choosing night duties because this would not entail heavy lifting work. She discussed the problems regarding the needs of the dying with Norman Barrett (1903–79), a distinguished thoracic surgeon, whose name is commemorated in the eponym 'Barrett's oesophagus'. He told her that little was likely to change unless the initiative came from somebody who was medically qualified and who would have the pharmacological knowledge to use drugs to achieve maximum pain relief. Hence, at the age of thirty-five, she entered the hospital's medical school, re-experiencing a sense of alienation given that she was ten years older than her fellow— and rather unfriendly—students, and qualifying in 1957. Thereafter, she did research into pain control at St Joseph's Hospital, Hackney, London, a hospice run by Roman Catholic nuns, also becoming a member of a research team studying the problem at St Mary's Hospital, London. But after seven years, she increasingly wanted to start her own unit, particularly after the death of another Polish patient with whom she had formed a strong relationship showed her that, as she stated, 'as the body becomes weaker, so the spirit becomes stronger'.

Her hospice was to be called St Christopher's, named after the patron saint of travelers, given that dying was itself a mode of travel. Her brother found a site for her in Sydenham, near the Crystal Palace location of the 1851 Great Exhibition, and a grant of £63,000 from the King's Fund enabled her to start building in 1965. She also lobbied other charities for funds and obtained the support of another grande dame Albertine Winner (1907–85), then Deputy Chief Medical Officer in the Government's health department (and subsequently to become chairman of St Christopher's). The charities insisted that the hospice should be nondenominational, though Saunders had originally wished it to have a Christian basis; her subsequent research showed that although atheists might die happily, the people who coped best were those with a shining faith. In any case, the time was right for a major initiative because think tanks such as the cancer charity Marie Curie Foundation and the Gulbenkian Foundation had produced reports emphasizing the unmet needs of patients who were hospitalized long-term or who had terminal cancer.

Opened in 1967, St Christopher's Hospice was different from a hospital. It encouraged patients to lead as full lives as possible, with activities such as creative writing courses and gardening, and it welcomed children as visitors and the presence of pets. Pain became controlled by continuous rather than intermittent medication, so that patients could remain conscious and retain their interests. Attention was also paid to other, often unmet, needs, such as the relief of constipation, bedsores, nausea, and breathlessness. Nor was the outcome necessarily fatal: several patients went home after a course of expert management. Such success increased support for those who, like Saunders, opposed voluntary euthanasia, arguing that the new methods in expert hands could always achieve relief of pain—a view that became accepted even though not all experts agreed.

A bright and cheerful building, with an ordinary window dedicated to Tasma, the Hospice contained fifty-four beds and soon added home care and research to its functions while acting as a resource for similar developments in Britain and elsewhere. Such were its obvious merits that by 1970 two-thirds of its running costs were being borne by the National Health Service, and Saunders was in great demand to lecture and advise all over the world as well as writing books on hospice practice. By 1993 almost 200 hospices had been created in Britain, which had recognized terminal care as a distinct medical specialty, and over 100 other countries had modeled their own units on St Christopher's.

Saunders herself retired from the directorate in 1985, but continued as president of St Christopher's until 2000. She received numerous awards and honors, being created a Dame (1980) and raised to the Order of Merit in 1989 (an award in the personal gift of the monarch and limited to twenty-four holders). Interested in the arts, she singled out for special places in her life Bach's *St Matthew Passion* (she had sung in the chorus at Oxford), the *Revelations of Divine Love* by Julius of Norwich, *The Lord of the Rings* by Tolkien, the poems of Gerard Manley Hopkins, and the *Blue Crucifixion*, an oil painting by the Polish artist Marian Bohusz-Szysko. After seeing this latter work in an art gallery window while driving through London, she went in and bought it; becoming friends with the rather older artist, she went on to marry him in 1975 at the death of his long-estranged Catholic wife, who had remained in Poland.

Together with Elisabeth Kubler-Ross (1926–2004), whose writings greatly influenced her, within a generation Saunders changed both public and professional attitudes about dying. When she qualified, even as a doctor, let alone as a nurse or a social worker, there was an embarrassed refusal to let patients know their true diagnosis. Medical staff tended to use weasel words, such as anemia for leukemia or ulcer for cancer. Moreover, the regimen to address both their mental distress and their need for pain relief was inadequate, often left to poorly trained junior doctors or nurses who were reluctant to provide powerful drugs in the right doses (fearing of all things that their patients might become addicted to them). With her expertise in all aspects of patients' needs, Saunders revolutionized attitudes and the efficacy of treatment. Her own mother died in St Christopher's in 1968, as did her husband in 1995. When asked how she herself would like to die, she replied that she would prefer a cancer that gave her enough notice to put her affairs in order. She was granted this wish, developing inoperable cancer of the breast and dying in the hospice she had created.

Bibliography

Primary: 1960. *Care of the Dying* (London); 1978. *The Management of Terminal Disease* (London); 1983. (with Baines, Mary) *Living with Dying* (Oxford); 2004. 'Palliative Care' in Lock, Stephen, et al., eds., *Oxford Illustrated Companion to Medicine* (Oxford) pp. 613–616.

Secondary: Richmond, C., 2005. 'Dame Cicely Saunders.' *Independent* (14 July); Du Boulay, S., 2002. *Cicely Saunders, Founder of the Hospice Movement: Selected Letters* (London); Zorza, V., 1980. *A Way to Die: Living to the End* (London).

Stephen Lock

SAYÉ I SEMPERE, LLUÍS   (b. Barcelona, Spain, 19 February 1888; d. Barcelona, 27 June 1975), *tuberculosis.*

Sayé oriented his professional career toward tuberculosis, motivated by the death of his three elder brothers from the disease. Upon graduating (1911), he opened an antituberculosis dispensary with Joan Darder i Rodés in the School of Medicine of Barcelona. That same year, in the University Hospital of Barcelona, with Cintó Reventós i Bordoy he used for the first time in Spain the artificial pneumothorax as a treatment for pulmonary tuberculosis.

After a stay in Hamburg with Ludolph Brauer in 1914, Sayé became interested in the collective prophylaxis of tuberculosis. In his view, a substantial decrease in tuberculosis mortality depended on the improvement of economic conditions, on the development of social legislation, and on measures of general hygiene, as well as on the proper use of epidemiological, diagnostic, prophylactic, and therapeutic resources in order to identify and eliminate the sources of contagion.

From a leading position in the Public Health organization of the Mancomunitat de Catalunya [federation of the four provincial councils of Catalonia], Sayé in 1921 put into practice those premises to create the Servei d'assistencia social dels tuberculosos de Catalunya. This scheme, located in Barcelona's most deprived district, started BCG vaccination in 1924 and was the first to employ visiting nurses. Thus Barcelona became the second big city in the world, following Paris, to implement large-scale BCG vaccination.

A self-educated man, Sayé combined his clinical private practice with research and teaching on tuberculosis, a field and subject he helped to consolidate in Spain. He founded the journal *Archivos Españoles de Tisiología* in 1919 and made a relevant scientific contribution, together with the Swiss René Burnand, by describing a new clinical form of chronic miliary tuberculosis in 1924, known as the 'Burnand-Sayé Syndrome'.

In 1931 Sayé was appointed as a member of the National Health Council, and during the entire Republican period (1931–36) he belonged to different institutions of the National Health Department aimed at organizing the antituberculosis campaigns throughout the country. In 1933 he founded the University Anti-tuberculosis Agency in the Autonomous University of Barcelona and made students undergo compulsory medical examination to prevent TB. As head of the Catalonian Anti-tuberculosis Service, he promoted a project to build an antituberculosis dispensary designed by the vanguard architects Sert, Subirana, and Torres Clavé. The dispensary, opened in 1937, became one of the most representative examples of modern architecture in Barcelona.

Sayé left Spain in 1936, heading into exile because of the Civil War, and accepted Albert Calmette's invitation to work at the Pasteur Institute in Paris. One year later he moved to Montevideo (Uruguay), and in 1942 he settled in Buenos Aires (Argentina) where he worked in the Central Hospital for Tuberculosis. In that period, he helped establish antituberculosis plans in Uruguay, Argentina, Peru and Chile. In 1950 he published his monograph on tracheo-broncho-pulmonary tuberculosis, a work that summarized the experience he had acquired during his stay in Latin America.

In 1951 Sayé returned to Spain where, as a former Republican, he was excluded from Franco's antituberculosis organization. He worked unpaid at the University Agency he had founded until he retired in 1958. In 1967 a stroke left him severely disabled. He died in 1975, ruined, and accompanied only by some close friends.

Bibliography

Primary: 1924. *Profilaxis de la tuberculosis* (Barcelona); 1938. *La Tuberculose pulmonaire chez les sujets apparemment sains et la vaccination anti-tuberculeuse* (Paris); 1950. *La tuberculosis traqueobroncopulmonar* 2 vols. (Buenos Aires).

Secondary: Cornudella, Raimond, 2000. *Història de la Pneumologia a Catalunya* (Barcelona); Molero Mesa, Jorge, 1989. *Historia social de la tuberculosis en España (1889–1936)* (Granada); Cornudella, Josep, 1979. *Estudio biográfico del Profesor Luis Sayé Sempere* (Barcelona).

Jorge Molero-Mesa

SCANTLEBURY BROWN, VERA (b. Linton, Victoria, Australia, 6 August 1889; d. Melbourne, Victoria, 14 July 1946), *infant welfare.*

Scantlebury Brown was the daughter of George James Scantlebury, a medical practitioner interested in psychiatry, and his wife Catherine Millington, née Baynes, both born in Victoria. Vera Scantlebury graduated (MB, BS, 1914) from the University of Melbourne and, soon after, the departure of medical men for World War I opened hospital residencies hitherto closed to women. In 1915 she joined the resident staff of the Children's Hospital, where she had two grueling years before sailing in 1917 to England. There she was attached to the Royal Army Medical Corps as assistant surgeon to Dr L. Garrett Anderson at Endell Street Military Hospital.

Returning to Australia in 1919, Scantlebury focused on the health and welfare of babies and children. She was given honorary appointments at the Queen Victoria Hospital for Women and Children, the Women's and Children's hospitals, the Victorian Baby Health Centres Association and, significantly, the Free Kindergarten Union of Victoria. She began regular medical inspections at girls' private schools, but it was her work with poor children that absorbed her. In 1921, while retaining her honorary responsibilities, she became part-time medical officer in charge of city baby health centers. Awarded the MD in 1924, Scantlebury visited New Zealand, Canada, and the United States to study child welfare work that year.

In 1925 the Victorian government asked her to make a survey, with Dr Henrietta Main, of the welfare of women and children, comparing Victoria with New Zealand. In 1926 the government created a section of infant welfare in the Health Department, and Scantlebury was appointed part-time director, a position she held until her death. In September 1926 she married Dr Edward Byam Brown, then lecturer, later associate professor of engineering, at the University of Melbourne. They had two children.

Scantlebury Brown's greatest achievement was the creation of an integrated system of infant and early childhood care and education in Victoria, and she was joined in this mission by a small group of progressive municipal health officers in Melbourne. As director of infant welfare for Victoria, she established liaison with obstetric hospitals so that expectant mothers could attend infant welfare centers for advice and support. Her administrative and political skills were matched by her attention to the detail of training infant welfare sisters, and while infant mortality had been falling steadily since the 1890s, that fall was uninterrupted by the economic afflictions of the 1930s. The integrated system of infant care from pregnancy to early school age that she developed endured until the economic rationalism of the 1990s.

In 1929 Scantlebury Brown published *A Guide to Infant Feeding,* in which, as in other publications, she was assisted by her husband, who made the measurements and calibrations for her. In 1937 she wrote a report for the National Health and Medical Research Council which prompted Commonwealth government funding of the Lady Gowrie Child Centres around Australia. In 1944 she added preschool children to the Victorian Health Department's responsibilities. Her 1929 publication was expanded to include the preschool child and was reissued in 1947 as *A Guide to the Care of the Young Child.*

Scantlebury Brown advocated a more relaxed regime of infant feeding and child care than did her New Zealand colleague, Sir Truby King. She was widely respected as a humane and visionary doctor, and was appointed OBE in 1938. Vera Scantlebury Brown died on 14 July 1946 of cancer, and was buried with Anglican rites in Cheltenham cemetery. Her papers are housed in the University of Melbourne Archives.

Bibliography

Secondary: Smith, Philippa Mein, 1997. *Mothers and King Baby: Infant Survival and Welfare in an Imperial World: Australia 1880–1950* (London); Reiger, K., 1985. 'Vera Scantlebury Brown' in Kelly, F., and M. Lake, eds., *Double Time: Women in Victoria* (Melbourne); Neve, M. H., 1980. *This Mad Folly* (Sydney); *AuDB.*

Janet McCalman

SCARPA, ANTONIO (b. Motta di Livenza, near Treviso, Italy, 19 May 1752; d. Pavia, Italy, 31 October 1832), *anatomy, pathological anatomy, neurology.*

The son of Giuseppe Scarpa and Francesca Corder, Antonio Scarpa received a sound general education under the guidance of his paternal uncle, the canon Paolo Scarpa. Toward the end of 1766 he enrolled at the University of Padua, where he became the favorite student of Giovanni Battista Morgagni (1682–1771), and from where he graduated on 31 May 1770. In October 1772 he was made professor of anatomy and institutes of surgery at the University of Modena. In 1781 he went on a research trip to Paris, where he met the anatomist Félix Vicq d'Azyr (1748–94), and from there he went to London, where he met the brothers William (1718–83) and John Hunter (1728–93). In 1783 he was called to Pavia to be professor of anatomy and surgical operations (later known as clinical surgery), where he built a spacious new anatomical amphitheater and increased the anatomical museum. In 1804 he gave up teaching anatomy and, in 1813, clinical surgery, remaining director of the Faculty of Medicine until his death.

Scarpa's most important contributions were those regarding descriptive anatomy. His research was mainly carried out by means of fine dissection, but he also carried out microscopic observations on nerve ganglia and bones (1799). A very accomplished draftsman, Scarpa produced his own anatomical drawings. His first research (1772), suggested by Morgagni and carried out while he was still at Padua, concerned the comparative anatomy of the ear. Subsequently (1789), he discovered the membranous labyrinth and the endolymph, describing with accuracy the semicircular membranous canals with their ampullae and the utricle. Scarpa was also the first to describe the vestibular nerve and its ganglion, which has been called Scarpa's ganglion. He accurately illustrated the course of the acoustic nerve from the cochlea to the rhombencephalon (hindbrain).

At the same time, Scarpa was involved in the study of the olfactory apparatus, publishing in 1785 the first illustrations of the human olfactory nerves, the olfactory bulbs, and olfactory tracts, as well as the pterygopalatine (or sphenopalatine) ganglion (or Meckel's ganglion), and the internal nasal nerves. Scarpa's research on the auditory and olfactory apparatus formed part of an extensive and systematic plan of research on the nervous system. He began publishing, in *De nervorum gangliis et plexubus* (1779), his anatomical and functional studies of the peripheral nervous system, distinguishing for the first time the spinal from the sympathetic ganglia. In 1787 he demonstrated that the accessory nerve also contains a part that has its origins in the medulla oblongata (accessory nerve of the vagus). Scarpa's masterpiece was the set of seven magnificent life-size plates (1794) that illustrated the glossopharyngeal, vagus, and hypoglossal nerves, and which provided the first proper delineation of cardiac nerves.

Scarpa was also an excellent surgeon. In his monumental atlas on hernia (1809), he masterfully described the exact structure of the inguinal canal and of the crural ring, as well as the disposition of the parts known today as the 'triangle of Scarpa'. His 1784 essay on freemartins (sterile female calves) was a pioneer study of hermaphroditism. His pathological works on diseases of the eye (1801) and on aneurysm (1804) were remarkable.

Bibliography

Primary: 1772. *De structura fenestrae rotundae auris, et de tympano secundario anatomicae observationes* (Modena); 1779. *Anatomicarum annotationum liber primus. De nervorum gangliis et plexubus* (Modena); 1785. *Anatomicarum annotationum liber secundus. De organo olfactus praecipuo . . .* (Pavia); 1789. *Anatomicae disquisitiones de auditu et olfactu* (Pavia) [2nd edn., 1794 (Milan)]; 1794. *Tabulae ad illustrandam historiam anatomicam cardiacorum nervorum . . .* (Pavia); 1809. *Memorie anatomico-chirurgiche sulle ernie* (Milan).

Secondary: Franceschini, Pietro, 1962. *L'opera nevrologica di Antonio Scarpa* (Florence); Ovio, Giuseppe, 1936. *L'oculistica di Antonio Scarpa e due secoli di storia* 2 vols. (Naples); Favaro, Giuseppe, 1933. 'Antonio Scarpa nella storia dell'anatomia.' *Monitore zoologico italiano* 43(suppl.): 29–43; Favaro, Giuseppe, 1932. *Antonio Scarpa e l'Università di Modena* (Modena); *DSB*.

Giuseppe Ongaro

SCHARLIEB, MARY ANN DACOMB
(b. London, England, 18 June 1845; d. London, 21 November 1930), *medicine, obstetrics, gynecology.*

Scharlieb was the only child of William Candler Bird, a merchant's clerk, and Mary Ann Dacomb, who died of puerperal fever within ten days of the birth of her daughter and namesake. Scharlieb's grandparents raised her until she reached the age of two, when she joined her father, who was living in Manchester. By the age of five, Scharlieb had acquired a stepmother and thereafter three sisters. A serious-minded child in a strict Evangelical household, which was nevertheless musical (a cousin was the organist Henry Bird), she was well-educated at schools in Manchester, Merseyside, and London. She married William Mason Scharlieb (19 December 1865) within months of their meeting and against the initial objections of her parents on account of her age and the fact that his home was in India. However, she claimed to know immediately that they were right for each other. Eighteen years her senior, William Scharlieb had recently qualified as a barrister and was due to return to practice in Madras, his family serving in the ICS. The couple arrived there in 1866, and their first son was born the same year, followed by another (1868) and a daughter (1870). Scharlieb settled into an expatriate life, running a household, adjusting to the climate, and helping her husband in his practice. He was a Roman Catholic, and she was soon received into the Faith. When her father's business failed, he and her stepmother joined them, along with one of her sisters (1875), and they all moved into a large airy house.

Midwifery and Medicine, Madras

Motherhood sharpened Scharlieb's awareness of sickness, childbirth, and postnatal care in the culture of seclusion (zenana) that prevailed among high-caste Hindu and Gosha (Muslim) women, who were allowed no contact with men other than their husbands. A particularly harrowing case affected her deeply. A very young girl was advanced in a difficult and unproductive labor when her husband, who could not bear to witness her suffering, sent for a European surgeon. The girl dragged herself to the door so that it could not be opened from without and lay there until she died, without intervention from her women companions. Using her connections and powers of persuasion and having exhausted her doctor's stock of obstetrical texts, Scharlieb began midwifery training (1872) at the

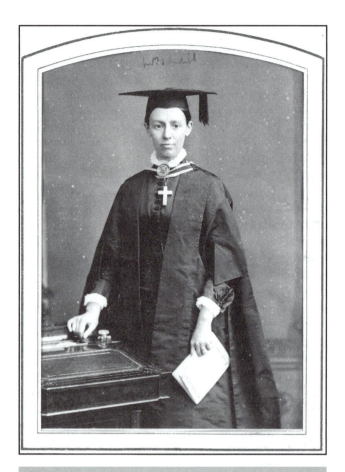

Mary Scharlieb, graduating from the London School of Medicine for Women, 1882. Photograph, Archives and Manuscripts, Wellcome Library, London.

Madras Lying-in Hospital, which admitted low-caste Indian and European mothers. After she had been working for a year with its superintendent, Surgeon-Major Cockerill, on duty from 6.00 A.M. to 6.00 P.M. (her husband having stipulated that she be home for dinner), her ambitions turned to medicine. It being impractical for her to return to England, she participated in a scheme whereby women intending to practice in India were admitted to Madras Medical College. Scharlieb enrolled (1874) along with three other European women, qualifying as a licentiate of medicine, surgery, and midwifery (1877). At this point, with her health weakened by the climate, which she always disliked, a return to London was essential. Her husband, meanwhile, remained in Madras.

Medical Training, London

She arrived in London in 1878, bringing her children to school and with introductions to Sir Henry Acland (1815–1900) and Florence Nightingale (1820–1910). Elizabeth Garrett Anderson (1836–1917) offered her a place at the London School of Medicine for Women (LSMW) when her

health had improved and she had passed the qualifying examination. At that time, the LSMW was affiliated to the Royal Free Hospital, the latter being the only London hospital to admit women to clinical practice on its wards. The BMA excluded women from membership. With her husband's consent, Scharlieb became a medical student, obtaining her MB (1882) and winning a gold medal for obstetrics along with a scholarship enabling her to study operative midwifery for six weeks at the Frauenklinik, Vienna. She also received support from missionary organizations. On her return to London (1883), she was joined by her husband for an audience at Windsor with Queen Victoria, who expressed interest in the intimate details of her subjects' sufferings in India and to whom Scharlieb outlined her mission to establish a hospital for caste and Gosha women. Despite the monarch's well-known opposition to women doctors, she appeared to accept the special needs of India and gave Scharlieb a photograph of herself that she might show to patients. Scharlieb noted in her autobiographical *Reminiscences* (1924) that although the British medical establishment was largely hostile to the idea of women becoming doctors, there was less antagonism if they expressed a wish to work abroad. Missionary medicine offered women opportunities for personal fulfillment and professional autonomy that they might not achieve at home, but nevertheless, such women needed to be well-trained and of very high caliber to deal with disease under tropical conditions without nearby assistance from colleagues and in ill-equipped buildings.

A New Hospital and Medical Practice, Madras

The Scharliebs returned to India in 1883, leaving their children at school in England and under the care of close friends, Edward Schäfer and his wife. With the help of Lady Grant Duff, wife of the governor of Madras, Surgeon-General Furness, and the leaders of the Indian community, a suitable house for a hospital was found that could be partitioned according to religion and caste. Queen Victoria agreed that it could be named the Royal Victoria Hospital for Caste and Gosha women (now the Kasturba Gandhi Hospital for Women and Children). For over a year, Scharlieb ran the hospital single-handedly with her sister acting as anesthetist and her maid, Mrs Franks, serving as surgical assistant to the best of her ability. During operations, the carbolic spray was kept going by the family's Muslim ayah. On one occasion she fainted, dropping the spray, and it was kicked by the patient's husband into the garden, where it safely exploded. From her experiences in this makeshift environment, Scharlieb later argued that no woman should be sent to work alone in the medical field because mistakes would inevitably jeopardize an entire project.

A second doctor, Mary Pailthorpe, who had recently graduated MB BS from Cambridge, joined the team (1885) en route to take charge of a mission hospital at Benares. Despite the extra pair of qualified hands, Scharlieb maintained a punishing schedule, rising at 5:30 A.M. for home visits; arriving at the hospital at 7:00 A.M. and seeing seventy patients before breakfast; lecturing at Madras Medical College between 12:00 P.M. and 1:00 P.M.; returning home to see patients; lunching, bathing, and changing at 4:00 P.M. before house visits to European patients; and arriving home at 8:00 P.M. for a walk on the beach with her husband, followed by supper. She also expected to be called out during the night. Although primarily an obstetrician and gynecologist, Scharlieb was obliged to widen her practice as necessary, treating children and a number of Indian men who called especially to see her, including one who walked miles leading a valuable cow as payment in kind. Her large private practice earned £2,000 a year. Although personally driven by a Christian vocation, Scharlieb argued against proselytizing, believing that conversion was more likely to be achieved by example.

Medical Practice, London

By 1887 Scharlieb was ready to turn her back on India, believing she could achieve nothing further and finding herself, once again, debilitated by the climate. The parting from her husband was amicable, and they were reunited during his visits to England. Her first appointment, through Garrett Anderson, was as lecturer in medical jurisprudence at the LSMW. She also was elected president of the University of London Women's Graduate Association (1888), lectured on physiology to the Queen's Jubilee Nurses, and joined the National Indian Association, through which she encouraged a number of Indian women to study medicine. She obtained her MD (1888) from London University, the first woman to do so, and became lecturer on women's diseases at the LSMW (1889). Encouraged by Sir James Paget (1814–99), she began contributing articles to the medical and lay press, notably *Lancet* and *The Queen* magazine, for which she wrote for thirty-five years. As one of the growing numbers of medical experts in the circle of information passing from woman to woman, her popular books, *A Woman's Words to Women* (1895), *The Seven Ages of Woman* (1915), *How to Enlighten our Children* (1926), etc., reflect her desire to influence opinion on women's health issues. She supported repeal (1886) of the Contagious Diseases Acts and argued for the role of doctors in social reform through the media. Involved in the rebuilding of the New Hospital for Women (1890, later the Elizabeth Garrett Anderson Hospital), she was appointed outpatients' physician and, when Garrett Anderson retired, surgeon. She became the hospital's senior surgeon and consultant (1892–1903), achieved her MS (1897), and became gynecologist to the Royal Free (1902) in competition with male applicants. A Harley Street practice (1887) provided additional security and a home for her parents and children, her son Herbert qualifying as a doctor (1892) and her husband dying of influenza while working on a legal case in London (1891).

Public Life

After retiring from hospital work (1905) but not private practice, Scharlieb took on various public duties. She helped establish medical inspection in schools and was a member of the Commission on the National Birth rate and also the Royal Commission on Venereal Disease (1913–16), following which she was a founder member of the National Council for Combating Venereal Disease (1916), established under the wide umbrella of the Eugenics Education Society. Although she supported public information on VD (especially for the young), free clinics, and anonymous treatment, she opposed the issue of prophylactic kits (largely disinfectants) to World War I servicemen (1917), arguing that it reinforced the double standard, condoned prostitution, and contravened Christian morality. Her views, publicly aired, made her in great demand as a public speaker. After declining (because of age) to take charge of a wartime women's hospital in Belgium, she offered instead to treat, free of charge, all officer's wives and Belgian women. She nevertheless became Chairman of the Midwifery Committee of the Council of War Relief, spending much time in its maternity hospital.

An interest in mental pathology stemmed from attendance at Charles Mercier's lectures to the LSMW, and she became a lunacy commissioner, under which institution she was appointed one of the first women magistrates (1920). She served in the Juvenile Court and as a visiting magistrate to the women's prison at Holloway, London. She was awarded a CBE (1917) and DBE (1926). Much of Scharlieb's public work centered on the issues of motherhood, imperialism, national efficiency, and race regeneration so prevalent in medical and political debate prior to World War I. Like many of her colleagues she promoted fertility among the educated middle classes, proclaiming that 'ours is a people . . . commissioned to carry the lamp of light and learning to the uttermost ends of the earth' (Scharlieb, 1911), but not among the worst elements of the wage-earning class. She supported the Mental Deficiency Bill (1911–12, also sponsored by the Eugenics Society) in its aim to control fertility of the feeble-minded by segregation in institutions, but was hostile to the birth-control movement. It was responsible, she believed, not only for lowering the middle-class birthrate, but also probably for subjecting women to increased sexual demands from their husbands. In a paper to the Anglo-Catholic Congress (1923), she contended that contraceptives were wrong morally, medically, and rationally. Although something of a 'new woman' herself and in favor of girls' education and exercise, both for their own well-being and that of the race, she voiced concern that the athletic 'neuter' type of girl would be unfitted and unwilling to embrace motherhood.

By the 1920s, a decade that disturbed her because of its relaxed social mores, some of her ideas began to seem old-fashioned to the new generation of medical women and to feminists in general. She viewed the increasing demand of women for sexual equality with distrust, believing that humanity would suffer if equality was gained at the cost of lowering women's moral standards. Her only novel, *Yet a More Excellent Way* (1929), written at the end of her life, can be read as Scharlieb's own spiritual journey through the ministry of healing.

Bibliography

Primary: 1895. *A Woman's Words to Women: On the Care of Their Health in England and India* (London) (2nd edn., 1905); 1898. *Women in the Medical Profession* (London); 1911. 'Recreational activities of girls during adolescence.' *Child Study* 4: 9–14; 1915. *The Seven Ages of Woman: A Consideration of the Successive Phases of Woman's Life* (London); 1916. *The Hidden Scourge* (London); 1917. (with Butts, Barbara) *England's Girls and England's Future* (London); 1919. *The Welfare of the Expectant Mother* (London); 1924. *Reminiscences* (London) (2nd edn., 1925); 1927. *The Psychology of Childhood: Normal and Abnormal* (London); 1929. *Yet a More Excellent Way* (London).

Secondary: Collinson, S. R., 1999. 'Mary Ann Dacomb Scharlieb: A Medical Life from Madras to Harley Street.' *Journal of Medical Biography* 7: 25–31; Jones, Greta, 1995. 'Women and Eugenics in Britain: The Case of Mary Scharlieb, Elizabeth Sloan Chesser, and Stella Browne.' *Annals of Science* 52: 481–502; Balfour, Margaret I., and Ruth Young, 1929. (with a foreword by Dame Mary Scharlieb) *The Work of Medical Women in India* (London and New York); *Oxford DNB*.

Carole Reeves

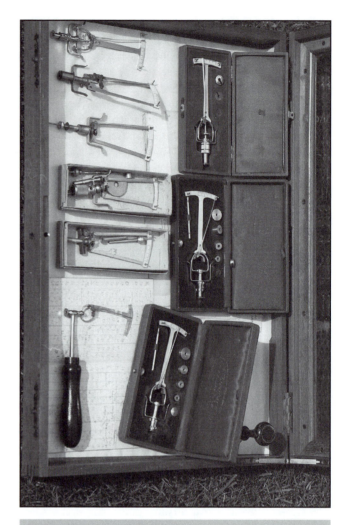

Schiøtz tonometers in a box with his own calibration notes. Photograph 1989, Ø. Larsen.

SCHIØTZ, HJALMAR (b. Stavanger, Norway, 9 February 1850; d. Oslo, Norway, 8 December 1927), *opthalmology.*

The Norwegian ophthalmologist Schiøtz attained a lasting international reputation for his important inventions, in particular the ophthalmometer (1881) for exact measurement of refraction disturbances in the eye, and the tonometer (1905) for the measurement of pressure within the eyeball. He was born in southwestern Norway and graduated as a medical doctor from the university of Oslo (then Kristiania) in 1877. After a few years of clinical practice in internal medicine and surgery at the National Hospital, and in general practice in the small village of Brevik, from 1879 on Schiøtz committed himself to ophthalmology.

He studied in Vienna and Paris, and became directeur adjoint at the ophthalmological laboratory at the Sorbonne under Louis Emile Javal (1839–1907), with whom he launched a substantially improved ophthalmometer. In 1881 he opened an ophthalmological practice in Kristiania, interrupted in 1886 by a study tour of eye clinics around Europe. He defended his doctoral thesis (1883) on optical properties of the cornea.

From 1881 onward, he was connected to the National Hospital and the university in Kristiania, working within ophthalmology, but also covering surgery and diseases of the ears and nose, in which fields he was very active. He is credited for having introduced aseptic surgery at the National Hospital in 1881. In 1888 he founded a private eye clinic in Kristiania together with a colleague. In 1901 he was appointed professor of ophthalmology, and could concentrate on this discipline and commit himself to building up a modern eye department.

Schiøtz's technical skills made him the father of diagnostic instruments of enduring value. Among his inventions were the Schiøtz-Javal ophthalmometer, of which a first version was presented to the international ophthalmological congress in Milan in 1880 and a final model in London the next year; this instrument became famous, allowing exact diagnostics of refraction failures in the cornea. He constructed an ophthalmoscope, an instrument to measure the color rings perceived by glaucoma patients, and a perimeter with a registration device to map the patient's field of vision.

Strabismus was a life long interest, and in the 1890s Schiøtz demonstrated a diagnostic prism instrument in various places, including Edinburgh (1894), Moscow (1897), and at home in Kristiania (1898). After a famous 1875 railway crash in Sweden, where color blindness was blamed for causing misinterpretation of signals, color perception became a core interest in ophthalmology. Colors should be perceived correctly by a pilot or a driver, including when light was just flashing and could not be observed and considered for some time. In 1916 Schiøtz introduced a diagnostic flashlight to properly test this important ability.

However, Schiotz's most memorable invention was his tonometer. It is still in use, a century after its introduction in 1905. This very simple, ingenious invention became a primary instrument in the handling of patients with glaucoma. The basic principle was that, when the pressure inside the eyeball is high, as in glaucoma, more counter pressure will be needed from the outside to make a measurable depression in the eyeball than if the internal pressure is normal. Schiøtz's small, elegant instrument is placed directly on the eyeball. A small piston, in original models loaded with tiny weights, records the pressure. The instruments were constructed based on complicated calculations, and had to be carefully calibrated to yield correct results.

Professor Hjalmar Schiøtz was a highly distinguished member of the national and international ophthalmological scientific community, publishing in Norwegian, German, English, and French between 1881and 1927.

Bibliography

Primary: 1882. *Om nogle optiske Egenskaber ved Cornea* (Stockholm); 1897. *Appareil prismatique* (Oslo); 1920. *Tonometry* (London).

Secondary: Johansen, Otto, 1999. *Hjalmar Schiøtz 1850–1927: vitenskapsmannen, øyelegen, mennesket* (Oslo).

Øivind Larsen

SCHOENLEIN, JOHANN LUKAS (b. Bamberg, Germany, 30 November 1793; d. Bamberg, 22 January 1864), *medicine.*

Schoenlein, who later adopted the second name Lukas, was the only child of Thomas Schoenlein, a well-to-do ropemaker, and Margarete Huemmel, the intelligent, warm-hearted, and strong-minded daughter of a miller, who decided that her son should be more than a craftsman. Schoenlein grew up in Bamberg, a prince-bishop's residence town, which fell to Bavaria in 1803. In the same year Bamberg's university was closed. It had harbored outstanding representatives of German 'romantic' medicine, who amalgamated enlightened plans for health care and medical education with idealistic theories on life and disease. They included Andreas Roeschlaub, who moved to the University of Landshut; Adalbert Friedrich Marcus, innovator and director of Bamberg's General Hospital; and the anatomist and embryologist Ignaz Doellinger, who after 1803 became Professor at Würzburg. These names mark the coordinates for Schoenlein's intellectual and medical education, while the Napoleonic wars, liberal hopes, and political repression mapped the general background.

From 1811 to 1816 Schoenlein studied medicine first at Landshut, then at Würzburg. His main interest lay in natural history (he was, and remained, a keen collector of rare or fossil plants), so he chose Doellinger as supervisor for his doctoral thesis. After his dissertation on the comparative anatomy of the brain was accepted in February 1816, he accomplished his practical training at the General Hospital at Bamberg. In autumn 1817, he obtained the right to lecture as a Privatdozent at Würzburg, and when in 1819 the professor for general and special pathology and therapy (and leading physician at the Würzburg Juliusspital) fell ill, Schoenlein was installed as his temporary replacement. In 1824 this temporary appointment turned into a full professorship, putting Schoenlein, barely thirty-one years old, in charge of one of Germany's largest and best organized general hospitals of the time.

In 1827 Schoenlein married Therese Haffner, daughter of a Würzburg magistrate, who would give birth to two daughters and a son. By this time the fame of the young clinical teacher had already spread throughout Germany, making (as a contemporary put it) Würzburg 'a place of pilgrimage' for medical students and doctors from all over the continent.

Hospital Experience as Source of Medical Science

In early nineteenth-century Germany, the university training of physicians was based on academic lectures. Academic hospitals were very small or even nonexistent. As a rule, the academic teacher lectured on the origin and nature of diseases, and on the significance of signs and symptoms as the basis of pathological theories, using bedside teaching only to demonstrate basic skills of examination and treatment. In turning this procedure upside down, Schoenlein originated what Rudolf Virchow would call 'the method of the German clinic'. He watched over the wards of the Juliusspital like a botanist considering a blossoming field. The medical cases were to be observed like growing plants that unfold their characteristic structures according to an underlying plan still hidden from the observer's eye. Similar cases should be compared, and their constant and essential characteristics should be used to abstract 'ideal effigies' of special diseases, in analogy to specimens in botany or zoology.

In further steps, the defined diseases should be grouped according to their essential features, thereby, step by step, forming species, families, and classes. In contrast to eighteenth-century nosology in the wake of Sydenham, Schoenlein's so-called natural history method embraced ideas from German early nineteenth-century natural philosophy. To him, diseases were not conditions but dynamic processes brought about by the efforts of the organism to overcome a morbific agent. Therefore, morbid phenomena had to be registered in the chronological order of their appearance, and could be read as results of functional and anatomical changes within the organism. These hidden causes could be subjected to physiological reasoning and checked by morbid anatomy. And since fever was now assessed as an unspecific reaction of the organism, the former class of fevers disappeared from nosology.

The advantage of Schoenlein's natural history approach was its principal openness to new findings in physiology, anatomy, and other basic sciences, as well as to all sorts of diagnostic tools. Schoenlein was one of the first German clinicians who made use of the stethoscope, the microscope, and chemical tests.

Würzburg (1819–32)

Thanks to Schoenlein's new method, the impact of walking the wards changed fundamentally from the mere acquisition of practical skills to embarking on medical research. At last the gap between medical practice and medical science seemed to be bridged. Moreover, young Schoenlein had the gift of inspiring his audience. He was a short man of ruddy complexion and unembarrassed manners, his speech animated and colorful. His audience felt they were participants in a great common endeavor. There was not a new dogma to be followed, but a method everybody could use, be it for practical purposes or with scientific intent. A considerable number of Schoenlein's students at Würzburg would achieve university careers, among them Conrad Heinrich Fuchs and Carl Canstatt.

However, Schoenlein had little inclination to put his ideas into print, so in 1832 students compiled their lecture manuscripts and had them published under the title *Allgemeine und spezielle Pathologie und Therapie. Nach J. L. Schoenlein's Vorlesungen von einem seiner Zuhörer.* In the second edition (also 1832), we find the first reference to Peliosis rheumatica, or Schoenlein-Henoch's disease (vol. 2, p. 68), and the first use of the term 'tuberculosis' (vol. 3, pp. 117–131). But great parts of the textbook are inconsistent and often barely understandable, misspelling personal names and technical terms, and obviously stemming from different sources. Nevertheless, the four-volume book became a bestseller, achieved (unaltered) six reprints by 1846, and was translated into Swedish (1837) and Italian (1850). Schoenlein wanted to inhibit its circulation, but the course of events prevented this.

In 1832 the German monarchies reacted with a wave of political persecution to a number of upheavals and demonstrations that followed the French revolution of 1830. Students and professors were especially suspected of subversive democratic activities. Many went to prison or were relegated. At Würzburg a large part of the academic staff was suspended, among them Schoenlein, who, although no political activist himself, frequently had met with members of the liberal movement at his favorite inn. Moreover, when rumor linked his name to a political assault, he reconsidered an offer made by the young university of Zurich and fled to Switzerland, where he arrived in spring 1833.

Zurich (1833–40)

Political persecution made Schoenlein a hero to the academic youth, and added to the appeal of his method. Soon young doctors trooped to Zurich to further their medical education. Schoenlein himself did not live up to his revolutionary image. He associated with other German scholars who, like him, had found exile in Switzerland, for only a short time. Yet soon he found out that he could turn his fame into money. The wealthy and the noble, among them the Belgian king, sought his advice. Although he refused to adopt the polished manners of the upper class, he lost the natural and amiable way of his Würzburg days. His style became self-assured and authoritative. On the other hand, the new university had few inpatient facilities. A larger general hospital that might have served for teaching and research was planned, but far from being finished. Accordingly, the material basis for Schoenlein's hospital-based approach was poor.

In this period the only two papers Schoenlein was ever to publish appeared, neither of them longer than a page, and both edited in Johannes Müller's renowned *Archiv für Anatomie, Physiologie und wissenschaftliche Medizin.* In both cases Schoenlein drew attention to microscopic phenomena that might be specific for certain diseases. The first paper described (1836) crystals that could be detected in the intestines in typhoid fever. Schoenlein, who according to the students' notes was the first in Germany to draw a firm line between epidemic typhus and typhoid fever, hoped the crystals would prove a pathognomonic sign for typhoid—which they did not. The second paper (1839) was on the 'fungus character' of favus (*Porrigo lupinosa,* ringworm), showing that the crusts in favus consist of the mycelium of a fungus. This was the first proof that a disease can be caused by a specific living organism. The fungus was later named *Achorion* (or *Trichophyton*) *schoenleinii.*

Despite his success, Schoenlein did not feel happy in Zurich. Apart from the inadequate hospital conditions, he felt offended by the anti-Catholic attitude of the Zurich magistrate who, in 1837, refused him the rights of citizenship. Therefore, when in 1838 the Berlin medical faculty inquired as to whether Schoenlein would be willing to come to Berlin, he agreed to do so.

Berlin (1840–58)

Negotiations to bring Schoenlein to Berlin took two years. On the one hand, the Prussian court and the ministry of culture and education favored other candidates; on the other, Schoenlein made conditions. Up to then, the Berlin Charité hospital was controlled by military medicine, reserving bedside facilities and internships for future military surgeons, while university medicine had only very limited access to the hospital wards. Moreover, university lectures still had to be read in Latin. Finally, Schoenlein was granted the use of sixty beds and free choice of patients for clinical teaching, the right to appoint at least one civilian assistant, and permission to use German in his lectures.

In spring 1840 Schoenlein arrived in Berlin and was greeted with enormous enthusiasm from the general public and the academic community. In 1841 Schoenlein was appointed counselor to the ministerial department of health, and in 1842 he became personal physician of Friedrich Wilhelm IV. No physician in Prussia could possibly rise higher. Yet, as Virchow would stress in his obituary, Schoenlein never misused his power.

Reaction to Schoenlein came promptly. Between 1840 and 1845 some 100 pamphlets were written for and against Schoenlein, who himself never contributed a single written word. The controversy was launched by ultraconservatives from Bavaria who denounced him for liberalism and shameless materialism, and was carried on by a group of younger physicians, led by Carl August Wunderlich and Wilhelm Griesinger, who stressed that Schoenlein's ideas were old-fashioned—full of nonsensical analogies describing imaginary disease entities as if they were parasites, instead of deducing them from secure scientific knowledge in terms of physical causation. The central question was whether bedside experience or laboratory knowledge should form the basis of medical science.

Although often hampered by his official duties, Schoenlein remained a fascinating medical teacher. But in contrast to his Würzburg days he did not form a school. Due to the strict military regime, students and young doctors were not permitted to enter the Charité outside of lecture hours. The few civilian assistant physicians Schoenlein managed to appoint joined the ranks of experimental medicine: Robert Remak developed galvanotherapy, and was in 1846 the first Jewish Privatdozent in Berlin. He was followed by Ludwig Traube, also a Jew, inventor of clinical thermometry and one of Berlin's famous clinicians of the 1860s.

Schoenlein kept himself aloof from Berlin society. If there was time, he met with old friends at Bamberg, where in the 1850s he started to build a house. Schoenlein's wife had died of typhoid fever in 1846; in 1856 his only son died on an expedition to West Africa at the age of twenty-two. In 1859 Schoenlein submitted his resignation and returned to Bamberg.

Bibliography

Primary: 1816. *Von der Hirnmetamorphose* (Würzburg); 1836. 'Ueber Crystalle im Darmkanal bei Typhus abdominalis.' *Archiv fuer Anatomie, Physiologie und wissenschaftliche Medicin* 258; 1839. 'Zur Pathogenie der Impetigines.' *Archiv fuer Anatomie, Physiologie und wissenschaftliche Medicin* 82.

Secondary: Bleker, Johanna, 1991. 'Johann Lukas Schoenlein (1793–1864)' in Engelhardt, Dietrich von, and Fritz Hartmann, eds., *Klassiker der Medizin* vol. 2 (Munich) pp. 81–94; Bleker, Johanna, 1983. 'Between Romantic and Scientific Medicine: Johann Lukas Schoenlein and the Natural History School 1825–1845.' *Clio medica* 18: 191–201; Bleker, Johanna, 1981. *Die naturhistorische Schule 1825–1845* (Stuttgart); Virchow, Rudolf, 1865. *Gedaechtnisrede auf Joh. Lucas Schoenlein* (Berlin).

Johanna Bleker

SCHROEDER VAN DER KOLK, JACOBUS LUDOVICUS CONRADUS (b. Wommels, the Netherlands, 14 March 1797; d. Utrecht, the Netherlands, 1 May 1862), *medicine, psychiatry, neurology.*

Jacobus van der Kolk belonged to a family of Frisian notables, his father being a medical doctor working as a town clerk. His mother descended from a family of German professors named Schroeder, who had recently migrated to Groningen in the Netherlands. To save the family name from extinction, his mother's name was joined to his father's, into Schroeder van der Kolk. At the age of fifteen, in 1812, Jacobus embarked on the study of medicine at Groningen University, with Gerbrand Bakker among his professors. At the time, Bakker was experimenting with animal magnetism and somnambulism, concluding that insanity was a curable disease. In 1820 Schroeder van der Kolk took his PhD with a thesis on the coagulation of the blood.

Local Reform

In November 1821 Schroeder van der Kolk was appointed resident physician of the Buitengasthuis of Amsterdam. This hospital, established in the seventeenth century as a pest house, catered for citizens suffering from contagious, venereal, and in general abhorrent diseases. The institution included a special ward for some 160 insane, living in conditions of filth, noise, unrest, idleness, and physical restraint. From the late eighteenth century onward, it had been the object of severe criticism. As the Belgium alienist Josef Guislain put it in 1842, 'The Buitengasthuis was a horrible place, an asylum of suffering and pain, a true hell.' Schroeder was one of the first to implement some reform, introducing occupation, rewards and punishments, some kind of 'psychological cure', and both medicines and therapeutic showers. At the same time, he reduced the use of straitjackets and corporeal punishment.

These initiatives of Schroeder should be seen against the background of the change of opinion regarding the care for the insane that manifested itself in these years in the Netherlands, as well as in the surrounding countries. In 1818 King William I made an appeal to the provincial authorities to close down inadequate madhouses and to build new therapeutic asylums. Led by these same motives, medical doctors in Amsterdam held a competition in 1821, asking for a treatise on the reform of psychiatry. The competition was won by Guislain. Hampered by the unwillingness of the board of trustees and a lack of money, Schroeder's attempts at reform in the Buitengasthuis failed, as did some large-scale designs conceived by the Home Office, which was responsible for the insane.

In 1826 Schroeder moved from Amsterdam to Utrecht, where he was appointed professor of anatomy and physiology, a chair that he held until his death in 1862. During this period, Schroeder—being a talented anatomist—conducted research on the eye, the lungs, the uterus, and the circulation and published on cancer and tuberculosis. His chief merits, however, lay in the fields of psychiatry, neurology, and neuroanatomy.

As early as May 1827, Schroeder became a member of the board of the local madhouse. Now holding responsibility, in contrast with his inferior position in the Amsterdam Buitengasthuis, he initiated reforms in this small institution, proceeding at a gradual pace because of a lack of financial means. Step by step, the building was renovated, creating separate wards for men and women, for the quiet and the disturbed, for paupers and the well-to-do. All kinds of labor as well as recreational activities were developed as part of the new systematic treatment. Cells were redesigned, and chains were replaced by straitjackets and restraining chairs. Schroeder introduced various forms of hydrotherapy (baths and several types of showers), as he had done in Amsterdam. The ongoing medical treatment was entrusted to a medical doctor, under close supervision of Schroeder.

Around 1834, the initial plans had been realized: with small means a very insufficient madhouse had effectively been changed into a therapeutic asylum, as Schroeder emphasized. He also pointed to the increasing number of patients leaving the asylum healed or improved. Although the changes in the Utrecht asylum were only small-scale and modest (as compared to systematic psychiatric reform in France or England), the initiative was unique in the Netherlands.

National Reform

In 1837 Schroeder criticized the inertia in the Dutch care system for the insane as vice-chancellor of the University of Utrecht in his *Oratio de debita cura infaustam maniacorum sortem emendandi mosques sanandi, in nostra patria nimis neglecta* [Address on the neglect of care required for the assuagement of the fate of the insane, and the cure of the same in our country]. In contrast to all other works of philanthropy the Netherlands could take pride in, psychiatry remained in a backward position, and the living conditions of the insane were a cause for embarrassment. He made an urgent appeal to all responsible administrators to stimulate reform of the Dutch asylums.

Schroeder's address—which was translated into Dutch in 1838—made psychiatry a national issue. Within a few months, cooperation was established between Schroeder and C. J. Feith, a high-ranking civil servant of the Home Department responsible for the care of the insane. Until Schroeder's death in 1862, they closely worked together toward reform, producing a blueprint in the years between 1837 and 1842. At the request of the department, Schroeder drew up a *Report on the best way to improve the asylums in the Netherlands* (1837), which was turned into a circular sent to all provincial authorities, save those of

Utrecht. In it, the provinces were admonished to fulfill their moral obligation toward the insane. This should be done by closing down the worst madhouses, reforming the others, and, ideally, establishing new provincial asylums. These asylums were to accommodate at least 100, but no more than 200 patients, and be located in or near a major city. In an appendix, Van der Kolk described the Utrecht asylum as the adequate model for reform.

The next step was to create a legal framework for reform and for admission procedures to the new asylums. In 1838 the Dutch parliament passed a new civil code, which only provided for the hospitalization of the incurable insane under legal restraint. This would be the chief obstacle to the projected reform of psychiatry, with the speedy admission of patients with acute cases to an asylum being regarded as a major precondition for recovery. In his *Thoughts on the legislation on the insane* (1838), Schroeder strongly advised the Home Department to follow the example of the French insanity law of the same year, which put responsibility for admission with medical doctors to the exclusion of the judiciary. According to Schroeder, magistrates were incapable of judgment in cases of mental illness. Feith and Schroeder actually prepared a concept for a law that mirrored the French statute almost to the letter. However, the Ministry of Justice objected, arguing that the judiciary should legitimize the restraint inherent in a forced admission to a mental institute.

In May 1841 the first insanity law was voted for by the parliament. The law indeed created an admission procedure in which the justice played the chief role in authorizing hospitalization. To stimulate reform, the statute provided the suppression of bad madhouses and the official recognition of therapeutic asylums for acute, curable cases and of 'nursing homes' reserved for the incurable. Provincial authorities were made responsible for the creation of sufficient places for pauper lunatics, although they were not obliged to establish asylums themselves, as required by the French law of 1838. Apart from the sections on the admission procedure, the new law bore the stamp of Schroeder van der Kolk's ideas.

To guarantee the implementation of the law, as well as the adequate provision of care, Schroeder van der Kolk and Feith were appointed inspectors for the asylums in 1842. That summer, they visited some twenty-eight madhouses, concluding that none of these met the legal standards. It 'was not without sad memories and a feeling of great pain that we have come to know many of these institutions as real holes of suffering', as they put it in their report. At the time, the inspectors were convinced that in due time, a considerable number of provinces would establish their own modern, therapeutic asylums. Until then, a number of old madhouses could be licensed temporarily.

However, during the next decade, Schroeder and Feith were disappointed in their expectations. Although by 1850 some sixteen madhouses were closed down, only one of the

Dutch provinces—Noord-Holland—had taken the initiative to build a new asylum: Meerenberg near Bloemendaal, soon recognized internationally as a model institution. In all of the other provinces, municipal authorities and the boards of asylums refused to close down old institutions. They preferred piecemeal and gradual renovation of existing facilities, with Schroeder's own 'Dolhuis' in Utrecht as the example to be emulated. Paradoxically, it was Schroeder's original small-scale initiative that in the end turned out to prevent thorough reform.

Lacking the legal means to compel authorities to create new facilities, the two inspectors had to acquiesce in this situation. Nonetheless, in the early 1850s, they prided themselves publicly upon the general improvement of Dutch psychiatry. This situation continued at least until the 1880s, although it met with severe criticism by a younger generation of psychiatrists.

Academic Psychiatry

In 1831 Schroeder started to teach psychiatry in private lectures at the request of some students, thus being the first in the Netherlands to lecture in mental science. He continued these lectures in intervals for the next thirty years.

Psychiatry as taught by Schroeder was founded on a strict dualism. His stance was close to the contemporary German *Somatiker*. According to Schroeder, the soul—the seat of reason, judgment, and (self) consciousness—was an immaterial entity that could not be ill. Adhering to vitalism, he thought the nerve force, the autonomous source of vitality in organisms, mediated between soul and body. In psychiatric illness, either the brain (idiopathic insanity) or other organs, foremost the intestines or the genitals (sympathetic insanity), were diseased, disturbing the transmission of sensations to the soul. Especially changes in the composition or the pressure of the blood could provoke psychopathology, high pressure leading to irritation of the nerve force, with dreams, delirium, and eventually delusions and madness as a result. Schroeder made the observation that only in rare cases did he not find in the corpses of the insane any material alterations corresponding to their mental illness.

Building on these premises, Schroeder's nosology distinguished between idiopathic insanity (such as mania, hallucinations, dementia, and idiocy) and sympathetic insanity (which included melancholia, intermittent mania, and melancholy). Although he did not discount psychological means such as moral treatment, he preferred a somatic approach using medication, bloodletting, or hydrotherapy. Schroeder's ideas on mental illness were published posthumously in 1863 by two of his pupils as the *Handboek van de pathologie en therapie der krankzinnigheid*, translated into English seven years later as *The Pathology and Therapy of Mental Diseases*.

In 1858 and 1859 Schroeder published neuroanatomical findings 'on the minute structure and functions of the spinal cord and the medulla oblongata'. These articles, in which he elucidated a source of epileptic attacks, brought him international renown in neurology.

Bibliography

Primary: 1858. *Over het fynere zamenstel en de werking van het verlengde ruggemerg en over de naaste oorzaak van epilepsie en hare rationele behandeling* (Amsterdam) [English trans., 1859. *On the Minute Structure and Functions of the Spinal Cord and the Medulla Oblongata and on the Proximate Cause and Rational Treatment of Epilepsy* (London)]; 1863. *Handboek van de pathologie en therapie der krankzinnigheid* (Utrecht) [English trans., 1870. *The Pathology and Therapy of Mental Diseases* (London)]; 1865. *Seele und Leib in Wechselbeziehung zu einander* (Braunschweig).

Secondary: Vijselaar, Joost, 1999. 'J. L. C. Schroeder van der Kolk (1797–1862), de eerste hervormer van de psychiatrie in Nederland.' *Jaarboek voor psychiatrie en psychotherapie* 6: 3–14; Vijselaar, Joost, 1985. 'Schroeder van der Kolk en de Krankzinnigenwetgeving van 1841.' *Maandblad geestelijke volksgezondheid* 40: 271–285; Binneveld, J. M. W., and M. J. van Lieburg, 1978. 'De eerste psychiatrische revolutie in Nederland, een revolutie die niemand wilde.' *Tijdschrift voor psychiatrie* 10: 517–534; Esch, Piet, van der, 1954. *Jacobus Ludovicus Conradus Schroeder van der Kolk 1797–1862. Leven en werken* (Amsterdam).

Joost Vijselaar

SCHWALBE, JULIUS   (b. Nakel, Posen, Germany, 13 June 1863; d. Berlin, Germany, 17 February 1930), *medical journalism.*

Schwalbe was descended from a Jewish family of bookbinders at Nakel, near Poznan. He studied medicine in Berlin (from 1881), as most of his Jewish college peers did. After his exams (1886) and a short period at the hospital Friedrichshain, he had his own surgery with a laboratory for clinical studies and diagnosis (1890–94). From 1882, researchers can trace back Schwalbe's interest in widely varying publications. He was head of the editorial staff of the journal *Fortschritte der Krankenpflege* (Enke) before he started his full-time publishing career at the publishing house Thieme in 1894.

Schwalbe obtained an excellent reputation among the German medical profession from his efforts for the medical press and as an editor at the *Deutsche medizinische Wochenschrift* (1894–1930). To strengthen the medical press and to improve their conditions of work—especially at congresses—Schwalbe in cooperation with Albert Eulenberg fought for a federation of the entire German medical press, including Austria and the German-speaking part of Switzerland. His objective being an international organization of the medical press, the example was France with its Association de la presse médicale, existing since 1889. On 25 September 1894, the Freie Vereinigung der deutschen medicinischen Fachpresse was founded at the 66th conference of the Versammlung deutscher Naturforscher und Ärzte in Vienna.

In addition to his extensive and nationwide journalistic commitment, Schwalbe was the publisher of important periodicals and anthologies such as the *Jahrbuch der practischen Medicin* (1894–1913); the *Reichs-Medizinal-Kalender* for Germany (1895–1930); the *Handbuch der practischen Medizin* (1898–1901); the first bibliography on Virchow, 1843–1901 (1901); and the *Gesammelte Werke von Robert Koch* (1912). He was the cofounder of the journals *La Medicina Germano-Ibero-Hispanio-America* (1923–24) and *Revista Médica Germano-Ibero-Americana* (1928). In many of his own articles, Schwalbe took up class problems of the medical profession. Considering himself the spokesman of a large part of the medical profession, in particular of internal medicine, he expressed his journalistic ambitions, loaded with his personal views, under the headline 'Kleine Mitteilungen', in the *Deutsche medizinische Wochenschrift*. Particularly his comments on World War I and on the November revolution (November revolution of 1918, which led to the first German republic), as well as on politics, social, and medical issues during the Weimar Republic, reflect the events of the day in relation to the interests of the medical profession. As to his political ideas, Schwalbe can be characterized as a national conservative. Besides, the distinguished medical journalist was working for different welfare organizations. Several foundations resulted from his initiative, such as the Robert-Koch-Stiftung zur Bekämpfung der Tuberkulose (1907), the Schwalbestiftung für notleidende Ärzte (1914), and the Aushilfsfonds der Notgemeinschaft deutscher Ärzte (1923). For the publishing house Thieme, Schwalbe was the dominant pillar for nearly forty years during difficult times of war and inflation, from the Empire to the agonizing Weimar Republic. For his special merits for German medical publishing, he was awarded the title 'Professor' as early as 1902. In 1911 he was appointed Geheimer Sanitätsrat at the age of forty-eight. Dying in 1930 at the age of sixty-seven, Schwalbe was spared a fate similar to that of his daughter Adelheid, who was forced by the Nazis to emigrate to Brazil six years later.

Bibliography

Secondary: Eckart, Wolfgang U., 1999. '"Ein Temperament griff hier zur Feder!"—Julius Schwalbe und die DMW, 1894–1930.' *Deutsche Medizinische Wochenschrift* 124: 1539–1540; Staehr, Christian, 1986. *Spurensuche: Ein Wissenschaftsverlag im Spiegel seiner Zeitschriften 1886–1986* (Stuttgart and New York).

Wolfgang U. Eckart

SCHWEITZER, ALBERT (b. Kaysersberg, Upper Alsace, Germany, 14 January 1875; d. Lambaréné, Gabon, 4 September 1965), *missionary medicine, humanitarianism.*

Schweitzer was the son of a Lutheran pastor from Alsace. He grew up in Gunsbach, and entered theological studies at the University of Strasbourg in 1893. Taking a doctorate in philosophy in 1899, he began to preach at St Nicholas Church in Strasbourg, while pursuing studies as an organist under Charles-Marie Widor. His accomplishments as a theologian and musician culminated in works on the eschatological views of Jesus and the music of Johann Sebastian Bach, and he was appointed principal of St Thomas theological college in 1903. The following year, attracted by an appeal in the Paris Missionary Society's magazine, Schweitzer decided to train as a physician and work as a missionary in Equatorial Africa.

He continued to teach theology while studying medicine at Strasbourg. In 1912 he married Helen Bresslau, a trained nurse, and concluded his studies with a course on tropical medicine in Paris and the submission of his medical dissertation. He sailed from Bordeaux in March 1913, arriving at the station of the Paris Mission at Lamberéné, Gabon, then a province of French Equatorial Africa, to begin constructing a hospital and surveying the medical needs of Africans and Europeans in the vicinity of the mission. His medical work was interrupted by the outbreak of war in 1914, and he practiced sporadically until he and his wife were interned in 1917 as German citizens and returned to Europe.

Following the Armistice, Schweitzer traveled, lectured, and gave concerts across Europe, publishing on the philosophy of civilization and on his experiences in Africa. In 1924 he returned to Lamberéné, and developed his hospital on a new site. He continued to direct and oversee the institution until his death. Numbering 400 beds, the hospital complex was extensive, laid out in a series of low-rise barracks arranged in compounds, leading up from the river Ogowe. Schweitzer deliberately kept the hospital simple and accessible, according to his interpretation of African vernacular village layout; workers, patients, and their families stayed on site.

Schweitzer was awarded the 1952 Nobel Peace Prize, cited for his 'reverence for that ineffable thing which is life' and his 'concept of brotherhood', and continued to periodically tour Europe as a missionary, theologian, scholar, and musician (Jahn, 1953). Greeted by a crowd of 20,000 well-wishers in Oslo, he raised double the Nobel prize money of $33,000, dedicating all monies to improving the care of leprosy patients housed at Lamberéné. As with the main hospital, leprosy work at Lamberéné proceeded on a residential basis, concentrating medical expertise in one location under Schweitzer's autocratic oversight, with little attempt to incorporate mid-twentieth-century developments in rural and primary health care.

Schweitzer used his writings and publicity to assiduously cultivate the notion of the missionary life as exemplary, and considered his work an expiation of, and restitution for, European colonial crimes. His longevity contributed in part to an increasing perception of Schweitzer as a paternalist devotee of benign colonialism, while his customary identification of Africa's best qualities with its sick and its poor was latterly often interpreted as racist in an era of rapid decolonization. He died in an independent Gabon in 1965; the humanitarian vision at the heart of his work continues to inspire medical, development, and missionary work.

Bibliography

Primary: 1910. *The Quest of the Historical Jesus* (London); 1911. *J.S. Bach* (London); 1923. *The Philosophy of Civilization* (London); 1933. *My Life and Thought: An Autobiography* (London); 1936. *Indian Thought and Its Development* (London).

Secondary: Brabazon, James, 2000. *Albert Schweitzer: A Biography* 2nd edn. (Syracuse, NY); Jilek-Aall, Louise, 1990. *Working with Dr. Schweitzer: Sharing His Reverence for Life* (Surrey, BC); Davenport, Manuel M., 1974. 'The Moral Paternalism of Albert Schweitzer.' *Ethics* 84(2): 116–127; Haberman, Frederick W., ed., 1972. *Nobel Lectures, Peace, 1951–1970* (Amsterdam); Jahn, Gunnar, 1953. 'The Nobel Peace Prize 1952. Presentation Speech.' English trans. at http://nobelprize.org/peace/laureates/1952/press.html

John Manton

SCOTT, JOHN HALLIDAY   (b. Edinburgh, Scotland, 28 December 1851; d. Dunedin, New Zealand, 25 February 1914), *anatomy, medical education.*

Scott, known as 'pussy' to generations of Otago Medical School students for his unobtrusive presence in the dissecting room, was the son of Andrew Scott, a lawyer, and his second wife, Marion Shaw Lidderdale. Scott began his medical training at Edinburgh University in 1870, shortly after Joseph Lister was appointed professor of surgery; he took first prize in junior surgery in 1872, and graduated MB CM in 1874.

After a time as demonstrator in anatomy, Scott was appointed professor of anatomy and physiology in Dunedin's recently established Otago Medical School, as successor to Millen Coughtrey (another of Lister's early students), who had failed to gain formal recognition for the school. Scott was permitted to delay his departure from Scotland until May 1877, to give him time to complete his MD. Shortly after his arrival in New Zealand, Edinburgh University announced that Scott had been awarded a gold medal for his thesis on the nervous system of the dog.

From 1877 until the appointment of John Malcolm to the chair of physiology in 1904, Scott was the only full-time staff member at Otago, assisted by a number of part-time lecturers. In its early days, the school taught only the first two years of the curriculum; it did not produce its first graduate until 1887. In 1891 Scott persuaded the authorities to establish a Medical Faculty, with himself in the combined role of dean/director and faculty secretary.

A talented artist who served as honorary secretary of the Otago Art Society (1881–1914), Scott had illustrated his own MD thesis and prepared many anatomical drawings which were still used by students long after his death. During a career spanning almost four decades he visited Britain only once, in 1883, where he married Helen Bealey, a New Zealander. His own teaching, although sound, became increasingly outdated. He himself may have realized this, for two of his sons traveled to Edinburgh for their medical education, graduating in 1907 and 1909, respectively.

Although Scott assumed a heavy administrative burden, his teaching duties were relatively light. In 1884 he had only twelve students; this number increased to thirty-one in 1887 and peaked at forty-three in 1898. By 1901 this figure had dropped back to twenty-two. Otago had produced only fifty-six graduates by this date, although an additional ninety had received a partial medical education before completing their studies in Britain.

In addition to teaching, Scott was credited in the 1960s as the founder of medical research in New Zealand for his 1893 study of Maori and Moriori bones, intended to demonstrate the mixed origins of the Maori people. This theory originated in Scott's 1885 presidential address to the Otago Institute, in which he commented upon the absence of any systematic study of Maori anthropometry—although Frederick Knox (brother of Robert, the infamous Edinburgh anatomist) had published his observations on a Moriori skeleton in 1872. While based on the earlier craniometry of Samuel Morton and others, Scott's work carried no pejorative overtones, and his research paved the way for further studies by German, Australian, and English anatomists. Scott himself produced nothing else of note after 1893, possibly as a result of his increased administrative commitments after 1891.

By 1911 Otago had established part-time chairs in bacteriology, medical jurisprudence and public health, ophthalmology, practice of medicine, pathology, and surgery. These additions testified to Scott's stewardship and persuasiveness, and laid the foundations for a home-grown medical profession.

Bibliography

Primary: Scott, J. H., 1893. 'Contribution to the Osteology of the Aborigines of New Zealand and of the Chatham Islands.' *Transactions & Proceedings of the New Zealand Institute*, 26: 1–64.

Secondary: Scott, J. H., 1996. *Without Parade or Fuss: A Biographical Memoir of John Halliday Scott, MD* (Christchurch); Hercus, C., and G. Bell, 1964. *Otago Medical School under the First Three Deans* (Edinburgh).

Derek A. Dow

SCRIBNER, BELDING H.   (b. Chicago, Illinois, USA, 18 January 1921; d. Seattle, Washington, USA, 19 June 2003), *nephrology.*

Scribner attended Williams College and the University of California and obtained his MD from Stanford University School of Medicine in 1945. There, he acquired an interest in diseases of the kidney through contact with Thomas Addis (1881–1949), a prominent authority from the 1920s. Scribner completed a 'rotating' internship at San Francisco Hospital (1944–45) and then from 1945 until 1950 did further postgraduate work in internal medicine there and at the Mayo Clinic in Rochester, Minnesota. He spent one year on the medical staff at Mayo. Choosing a career in academic medicine, he went to Seattle in 1951 as director of general medical research at the Veterans Administration Hospital in that city and as associate in medicine at the University of Washington School of Medicine. He became professor of medicine in 1962 and retired in 1992.

The medical subspecialty of nephrology in the United States in the 1950s (before the term was used) grew up around the accomplishments mainly of renal physiologists such as Homer W. Smith in New York and chemically oriented physicians such as John P. Peters of Yale. Scribner's early work and publications centered on problems of water and electrolyte balance, acid–base equilibrium, disturbances in potassium regulation, and bedside chemical determinations (an interest retained from his student days with Thomas Addis). Like all physicians who chose to make a specialty of nephrology, however, he confronted the inability to successfully treat patients with irreversible failure of overall kidney function. While at the Mayo Clinic, Scribner had heard a presentation by John P. Merrill of the Peter Bent Brigham Hospital in Boston, an early American figure in the utilization of the artificial kidney, or hemodialysis. Scribner initiated this technique in Seattle beginning in 1953; in that period, its main use was to temporarily replace renal function for persons with presumed acute, reversible injury to the kidneys. Occasionally, those few physicians and surgeons using the artificial kidney for this purpose would confront the awful dilemma of a very alert and otherwise reasonably well patient failing to regain native renal function, for at the time there was no way to repeatedly cannulate blood vessels in such a way as to repeat dialytic treatments indefinitely.

Working with engineer Wayne Quinton and surgeon David Dillard, Scribner, a sort of born 'tinkerer', utilized the newly available synthetic material Teflon to perfect an external arterial-venous 'shunt' that could be repeatedly connected to the dialysis machine, but left in place in the arm between treatments. In 1960 he and his coworkers initiated what came to be called 'maintenance dialysis' or 'chronic dialysis' for a limited number of persons with terminal renal failure. The first was a man named Clyde Shields; both he and his physician gained something like celebrity status as the joint adventurers in a wholly new form of medical treatment—the indefinite sustenance of life through dependence on an artificial organ. The very restricted availability of the new procedure led to the creation of a lay community-based selection committee to decide who, among medically suitable candidates, would be kept alive through its application; this controversial 'who will live' committee attracted as much, if not more, publicity than chronic dialysis itself.

Scribner next helped invent the chronic dialysis 'unit', a center to which patients needing long-term treatment could come from home, on a schedule, several days per week. The first opened in Seattle in 1962 (the Seattle Artificial Kidney Center, later Northwest Kidney Center). But in order to expand availability, he also developed and promoted dialysis at home, backed by a clinical team and training program. Scribner also endorsed an alternative modality, peritoneal dialysis, which could also be carried out by the patient. Eventually, however, free-standing dialysis units spread extensively in the United States, particularly following passage of legislation in 1972 that extended Medicare coverage to most persons in need of care for what came to be formally known as 'end-stage renal failure'. Chronic dialysis care in the United States entered the 'medical market place' with the advent of commercial dialysis units and 'chains'; Scribner, like some other pioneers of the artificial kidney, decried 'for-profit dialysis'.

Scribner served as president of the American Society for Artificial Internal Organs and the American Society of Nephrology. He received awards from the latter and also from the International Society of Nephrology. In 2002 he received the Albert Lasker Award for Clinical Medical Research. Scribner enjoyed fine wines and flying his radio-controlled model airplanes. For many years, he and his wife Ethel lived on a houseboat on Portage Bay, from which he canoed to work. He was the father of four children and three stepchildren. He was known for his sustained devotion to his family and to his patients.

Bibliography

Primary: 1960. (with Quinton, Wayne, and David Dillard), 'Cannulation of Blood Vessels for Prolonged Hemodialysis.' *Transactions of the American Society for Artificial Internal Organs* 6: 104–113; 1960. (et al.) 'The Treatment of Chronic Uremia by Means of Intermittent Hemodialysis: A Preliminary Report.' *Transactions of the American Society for Artificial Internal Organs* 6: 114–122; 1990. 'A Personalized History of Chronic Hemodialysis.' *American Journal of Kidney Disease* 16: 511–519.

Secondary: Fox, Renée C., and Judith P. Swazey, 2002. *The Courage to Fail: A Social View of Organ Transplants and Dialysis* (New Brunswick, NJ, and London: first published in 1974).

Steven J. Peitzman

SCRIBONIUS LARGUS (fl. *c.* 14–54), *medicine, ethics, pharmacology.*

A younger contemporary of Aulus Cornelius Celsus, the career of Scribonius Largus developed under Tiberius and flourished during Claudius's rule. Largus was Greek, possibly of Sicilian ancestry, as was certainly the case of one of his teachers, Apuleius Celsus from Centuripae. Celsus also taught Vettius Valens, himself an instructor of Largus (and who may have been the Valens executed for alleged adultery with Claudius's wife Messalina). Another of Largus's teachers was the surgeon Tryphon, who practiced in Rome and whom Cornelius Celsus praised for improving the practice and reputation of surgery. Largus traveled widely. In 43 he accompanied Claudius in the invasion of Britain, although it is not known in what capacity; he may have been attached to the imperial household as a supernumerary physician or assigned to medical duties in the expeditionary force.

Largus's *De Compositione Medicamentorum*, or *Compositiones* [Drug Recipes], was written in Latin (although some Greek terms and proper names are cited), and consisted of 271 compounds and remedies. Largus stated that, since he was abroad and without his library, the work was not comprehensive. It was dedicated to his patron, Caius Julius Callistus, an imperial freedman and secretary to Claudius. Largus was generous in his flattery both to his patron and to 'our divine Caesar' (*deus noster Caesar*). Largus's treatise included scattered allusions to the imperial family, ranging from the preparation of toothpaste for Messalina to medications used by Tiberius and Augustus. It was organized in three parts: diseases (listed *ad capite a calcem*) and their treatment (1–162); antidotes (163–78); and topical preparations, dressings and medicated plasters (179–271). The drugs were ranked from simple preparations to more complex derivatives. Largus gave six recipes for the treatment of trachoma, a common and debilitating eye disease, and provided an accurate and detailed description of its effects, especially its early stages. There were innovative treatments for headache and gout using the electric properties of the torpedo fish. Largus mentioned some doctors whose works are lost, and some who are otherwise unknown. These included Ambrosius of Puteolanus and his recipe for calculi; the medicated plasters of the surgeons Aristus, Glycon, Meges, and Tryphon; the antidotes of Apuleius Celsus (against hydrophobia); Cassius (snakebite); and the antidote of Marcianus, used by Augustus, which seems similar to Mithridation, the universal cure-all. Largus also refuted the charge leveled against Asclepiades of Bithynia that he failed to prescribe to those who were ill.

In his preface, echoing Herophilus, Largus stated that drugs were 'like divine hands' [*divum manus esse*]. To him, drug therapy was the oldest part of medicine, but there were those who sought to capitalize on the popularity of drug therapies by testing new agents on their patients. Some did not use drugs, either because they were ignorant (in which case they were greatly negligent) or, if they were adept in the use of drugs but kept such knowledge to themselves, because they were evil [*malus*]. A doctor was prohibited from prescribing dangerous medications, even to enemies of the state; but if occasion demanded, he could take up arms and defend the state like any good citizen.

Largus invoked Hippocrates, the 'founder of our profession' [*conditor nostrae professionis*]. The word *professio* did not refer to a medical profession in the modern sense, but was a declaration of allegiance to the duties of a doctor. These duties, for Largus, were focused in the Hippocratic oath, a model for the relief of suffering. The judicious use of drugs thus accorded with Hippocratic ethical precepts. Largus sought a moral basis for medical practice, and it is this aspect of his work in particular which remains relevant today.

Bibliography

Primary: Sconocchia, Sergio, 1983. *Scribonii Largi Compositiones* (Leipzig); Deichgräber, Karl, 1950. *Professio medici. Zum Vorwort des Scribonius Largus* (Mainz).

Secondary: Baldwin, Barry, 1992. 'The Career and Work of Scribonius Largus.' *Rheinisches Museum* 135: 74–82; Hamilton, J. S., 1986. 'Scribonius Largus on the Medical Profession.' *Bulletin of the History of Medicine* 60(2): 209–216.

Julius Rocca

SCUDDER, IDA SOPHIA   (b. Madras, India, 9 December 1870; d. Vellore, India, 24 May 1960), *medicine, surgery.*

Scudder, daughter of American missionary doctor John Scudder II and Sophia Weld Scudder, was born into a family of American missionaries who had devoted their lives to working in India. Scudder's grandfather John Scudder was one of the first missionaries sent by the Reformed Protestant Dutch Church, later known as the Reformed Church of America. The only sister of five brothers, Scudder had decided against becoming a doctor or pursuing missionary work. She completed her education at Northfield Seminary and attended Wellesley College at Massachusetts. A visit to India (1891) to tend to her ailing mother changed her plans. In a single night, three young women died in childbirth, their husbands having refused any help offered by the male doctors at John Scudder's clinic. The deaths of these women convinced her of the need for women doctors in India.

Scudder returned to the United States and enrolled in a medical college at Philadelphia (1895). She was one of the first women admitted to Cornell College of Medicine for her final year and obtained her MD in 1899. While in America she had raised money for a hospital in India. Her father died just months after she returned to India, leaving her alone to pursue her work. She began with a single-bedded clinic at Vellore, Madras Presidency, in January 1900. In 1902 she built the forty-bed Mary Taber Schell Memorial Hospital (named after the donor), which subsequently became the Christian Medical College.

Before the end of that year, she had performed twenty-one major operations, 428 minor ones, and treated more than 12,000 patients. Scudder's contribution was not only the provision of medical care to an increasing number of people, but also the creation of a medical infrastructure. Scudder began training compounders in 1903, and in 1909 she set up a school of nursing. In 1910 she started 'roadside' dispensaries, with the aim of reaching out to villagers who had difficulties accessing clinics. This concept, whereby the medical staff travel to surrounding rural communities in bullock carts carrying medical supplies to provide health care, has matured to a Community Health and Development Program commended by the World Health Organization.

In 1918 Scudder set up a medical school for women, called the Missionary Medical College, which trained licentiates. There were seventeen students in the first cohort. The College was financed and controlled by Missionary Societies in America and Britain. The representatives constituted the Board of Governors which sat in separate American and British sections. Scudder taught many courses in the early years and launched many successful medical careers.

Scudder visited the United States on fundraising tours, and there met her lifelong companion and friend, Gertrude Dodd. While on tour she performed surgery in India and Eastern Europe, and particularly acquired fame for performing operations to repair vesicovaginal fistulas. Her efforts were also directed toward the care and cure of leprosy patients, establishing the rural health center at Kavanur. Dr Paul Brand, the famous leprosy surgeon, chose to work at Vellore. In 1931 Scudder's niece and namesake, Dr Ida Belle Scudder, came from America as a missionary to work with her.

In 1938, to improve the qualifications offered by the school, the Board of Governors decided to appoint men as well as women to the faculty. The medical school became a medical college in 1942. The institution finally agreed to admit male students in 1947, a decision unpopular with some, and its name was changed to the Christian Medical College, Vellore. Scudder remained involved with the institution even after her official retirement in August 1946.

Bibliography

Secondary: Wilson, Dorothy Clarke, 1959. *Dr Ida: The Story of Dr Ida Scudder of Vellore* (London); Jeffery, Mary Pauline, 1938. *Dr Ida: The Life Story of Ida S Scudder* (New York).

Namrata R. Ganneri

SCULTETUS, JOHANNES (b. Ulm, Germany, 12 October 1595; d. Stuttgart, Germany, 1 December 1645), *surgery.*

Scultetus (Schultheiss, Schultes) was the oldest son of skipper Michael Schultheiss and his wife, Margarete. His parents died early, both within the space of a fortnight, and relatives and friends took care of Johannes and his seven siblings. He attended a local Latin school for six years, but because of financial constraints he was not able to proceed to an academic institution. Instead, for several years he was forced to make a living working in taverns, or as a bricklayer in various cities and towns along the Danube. During this period—perhaps in Vienna—he met the famous anatomist, Adriaan van den Spiegel, then professor of anatomy in Padua. The encounter changed his life.

From 1616 to 1623 Scultetus assisted Spiegel, and must have acquired extraordinary skills in performing operations and autopsies. Simultaneously, he studied medicine in Padua and received his doctoral degree in 1623. Appointed town physician by the magistrate in Ulm with an annual salary of 300 florins, Scultetus returned to Germany in 1625 and became a member of the local collegium medicum. In 1636 he married Maria Villinger; they had two children, both of whom died early. For the last twenty years of his life, Scultetus lived and worked in Ulm. He died from 'apoplexy' during a short absence in Stuttgart, where he had gone to visit and treat a high-ranking patient.

Scultetus counts among the few sixteenth-century and seventeenth-century physicians who combined learned medical knowledge and a doctoral degree with extensive theoretical and practical knowledge in surgery. His fame as a medical writer rests above all on his *Armamentarium chirurgicum*, published ten years after his death by his nephew, Johannes Scultetus. The implicit (and sometimes explicit) double message which runs through the book, and especially through the second part, is clear: addressing academic physicians, Scultetus proclaimed the outstanding importance of surgical expertise for medicine in general; and, turning to the simple barber surgeons, he praised the importance of extensive learned knowledge, from anatomy to pharmaceutics. The book's first and major part provided an extensive overview of the whole realm of surgery. It included numerous illustrations of surgical techniques and the instruments needed for the various interventions. The second part presented a hundred 'observations' and case reports from Scultetus's practice. These neatly complemented his surgical treatise. The treatment of complicated wounds and fractures was described in great detail, sometimes in day-by-day accounts.

Scultetus often combined external treatment with internal drug therapy. Purgatives, in particular, were almost routinely given to drive the harmful, corrupt humors out of the body, lest they accumulate in and around the diseased part. For analogous reasons, the body had to be carefully prepared before any surgical intervention, above all by means of purgatives. This careful preoperative cleansing of the body was outlined as one of the crucial differences between the diligent treatment of a skillful, learned surgeon and the simple barber surgeons who recklessly proceeded to their surgical interventions without preparation. Reports of unfavorable outcomes were virtually absent in Scultetus' observations. The few negative outcomes which Scultetus did mention had, as he claimed, either been correctly predicted by him, or were due to the misguided previous treatment of another healer, or to the fact that the patient had not followed Scultetus's regimen or therapeutic advice.

A striking feature of some of the case reports is also the great care with which Scultetus explained the nature and cause of the disease to patients and bystanders in scientific terms, and responded to their questions and doubts. When a patient died, Scultetus might even perform an autopsy in the presence of relatives and friends to provide them with direct evidence that his diagnosis had indeed been correct. On occasion he even made them feel with their own hands the large adherent bladder stone which was responsible for the fatal outcome, for which Scultetus was therefore in no way to blame.

Together with Ambroise Paré and Wilhelm Fabricius Hildanus, Scultetus helped to raise the social and scientific status of surgery, and to spread learned surgical knowledge among apprenticed surgeons and learned physicians alike. In Germany, a translation of the *Armamentarium* by Amadeus Megerlin, published in 1666 under the title *Wund-Arzneyliche Zeughaus*, became a standard textbook for more than a century. The work was also translated into English (*The chyrurgeon's store-house*, London 1674) and other European languages such as French and Dutch.

Bibliography

Primary: Bischoff, Ludwig, 1646. *ΕΥΘΑΝΑΣΙΑ, oder Selige Sterbkunst/ Christliche LeichPredigt/bey Volckreicher ansehenlicher LeichBestattung Deß Edlen/Ehrnvesten vnnd Hochgelehrten Herrn Johannes Sculteti, oder Schultes* (Ulm); 1655. *Χειροπλοτεκε, seu Joannis Sculteti Armamentarium chirurgicum* (Ulm); 1666. *Wund-Artzneyisches Zeug-Hauß* (Frankfurt).

Secondary: Seiz, Anneliese, 1974. *Johannes Scultetus und sein Werk. Biographie und Glossar* (Stuttgart).

Michael Stolberg

SEACOLE, MARY JANE   (b. Kingston, Jamaica, 1805; d. London, England, 14 May 1881), *nursing.*

Seacole (née Grant), daughter of a Scottish soldier and a Creole mother, was the eldest of three children. She learned traditional healing and nursing from her mother, a respected 'doctress' and owner of Blundell Hall, a hotel and convalescent home for garrisoned British officers and their families. Seacole visited London (*c.* 1821) for a year with Jamaican companions, returning on her own initiative (*c.* 1823) to trade West Indian preserves. Back in Kingston (*c.* 1825), she nursed soldiers stationed at Up-Park military camp and made trading visits to the Bahamas, Cuba, and Haiti. She married Edwin Horatio Hamilton Seacole (10 November 1836), an English-born doctor's son and godson of Lord Nelson, and they established a store at Black River. After Edwin's death (1844) and also her mother's, Seacole returned to Kingston, working alongside military surgeons during a cholera epidemic (1850). In 1851, joining her brother Edward in New Granada (Panama), she established a restaurant, store, and first-aid post, the British Hotel, catering for gold prospectors bound for California. On this lawless isthmus, she dealt mainly with cholera and gunshot wounds. Leaving Edward to manage the hotel, she returned to Kingston (1852), nursed patients through a severe outbreak of yellow fever (1853), and provided a nursing service for the hospital at Up-Park camp, earning her the nickname 'Mother Seacole'. She went back to New Granada (Spring 1854), and with Thomas Day, a relative of her husband, founded a trading company, Seacole and Day, in the mining community at Escribanos.

Following Britain's declaration of war with Russia (March 1854) and deployment to the Crimea, she (and later Day) booked passage for London, arriving about the same time as Florence Nightingale (1820–1910), and her nurses left to organize the hospital at Scutari (October 1854). Despite references from doctors in Jamaica, Seacole's application to join the next nursing contingent was refused. Undaunted, she and Day traveled to the Crimea (*c.* January 1855) with a shipment of stores and built a British Hotel at a spot she named 'Spring Hill' between Balaklava and Sevastopol, employing Jamaican cooks. Here, she rose before daybreak; prepared food, coffee, and medicines; tended to sick 'outpatients', many suffering from diarrhea and frostbite; took food and comforts to patients at the nearby Land Transport Corps Hospital; and fed officers in her restaurant. At Balaklava, she dispensed tea and medicines to casualties awaiting transport to Scutari. About three-quarters of Crimean deaths were from typhoid, cholera, and dysentery, diseases with which Seacole was readily familiar. On the battlefields at the Redan, Tchernaya, and Sevastopol, she was always present with food, wine, medicines, and bandages, but was equally adept at organizing lavish refreshments (including champagne) for off-duty games and entertainments. Florence Nightingale privately disapproved of Seacole's hotel while conceding that she was very kind to the men. Seacole styled herself as camp 'doctress, nurse, and "mother"' (Seacole, 1857, p. 110). Among her close friends throughout were the *Times* war correspondent William Howard Russell and Count Gleichen, a nephew of Queen Victoria, who sculpted her likeness (1871). She also met the chef Alexis Soyer, inventor of the field kitchen.

Seacole returned to London (summer 1856) a bankrupt heroine, having extended credit to many servicemen. A fund was established to pay off her debts and provide a comfortable annuity. Her autobiography, *Wonderful Adventures* (1857), sold well, and she apparently became a friend of Alexandra, Princess of Wales. Back in Kingston (*c.* 1860), she built a house and lived there for a time but had returned to London by 1870. At some point she became a Roman Catholic. Portraits of Seacole show her wearing medals, among which are the Crimea medal and the Légion d'Honneur, although it is uncertain whether these were 'official' awards. The Jamaican Order of Merit was bestowed on her in 1990. Seacole's importance lies in her contributions not only as a nurse and healer in the widest sense but also as a courageously independent, self-represented woman.

Bibliography

Primary: 1857. *Wonderful Adventures of Mrs. Seacole in Many Lands* (London) [reprint 2005, ed. and introd. Salih, Sara (London)]; Soyer, Alexis, 1857. *Soyer's Culinary Campaign: Being Historical Reminiscences of the Late War* (London and New York).

Secondary: Robinson, Jane, 2005. *Mary Seacole: The Charismatic Black Nurse Who Became a Heroine of the Crimea* (London); Hawthorne, Evelyn J., 2000. 'Self-Writing, Literary Traditions, and Post-Emancipation Identity: The Case of Mary Seacole.' *Biography* 23: 309–331; Goldie, Sue, 1997. *Letters from the Crimea, 1854–1856: Florence Nightingale* (Manchester and New York); Shepherd, John, 1991. *The Crimean Doctors: A History of the British Medical Services in the Crimean War* 2 vols. (Liverpool); Baylen, Joseph O., and Alan Conway, eds., 1968. *Soldier-Surgeon: The Crimean War Letters of Douglas A. Reid, 1855–1856* (Knoxville); *Oxford DNB*.

Carole Reeves

SECHENOV, IVAN MIKHAILOVICH (b. Teplyi Stan [now Sechenovo], Simbirsk *guberniia* [province—now Arzamas *oblast'*], Russia, 1 August 1829; d. Moscow, Russia, 2 November 1905), *physiology, physical chemistry, psychology.*

Sechenov was born into the nobility, receiving his early education from a German governess, then acquiring mathematics and the natural sciences during five years at the Military Engineering School in St Petersburg (1843–48). There, his honesty and directness often brought him into collision with the school administration.

After two years as a military engineer in Kiev, Sechenov became a graduate student at Moscow University in 1850, showing a special interest in comparative physiology and anatomy. Upon graduation in 1856, Sechenov went to Germany where, until 1860, he worked in various leading physiological laboratories. While abroad, Sechenov wrote his dissertation on the 'Future Physiology of Alcoholic Intoxication'. He defended it successfully in 1860 at St Petersburg Medico-Surgical Academy, where he was appointed professor (1860–64, adjunct professor; 1864–70, ordinary professor). He took the chair of physiology at St Petersburg University and founded the first Russian school of physiology. His students and followers included many outstanding Russian physiologists: Vvedenskii, Pavlov, Ukhtomskii, I. P. Tarkhanov, and Samoilov.

During the twelve years Sechenov worked at St Petersburg University, he carried out notable research, supplementing this with work in the Paris laboratory of Claude Bernard in 1862, where he discovered the phenomenon of inhibition in the central nervous system. This discovery led Sechenov to the theory of cerebral mechanisms, according to which all conscious and unconscious acts are reflexes, and provided the basis for the development in Russia of neurophysiology and psychology as a science. Sechenov established the principle of self-regulation and coordination between nerve centers.

Sechenov developed a new approach to the functions of the sensory organs in *Fiziologia organov chuvstv* [Physiology of the Sensory Organs] (1867). The signals of muscle sensation were the main source of information about the environment around the organism. The complete physiological mechanism consisted of a receptor and muscle activity. On the basis of this new 'reflexive' theory, Sechenov suggested a plan in 1873 for reorganizing psychology into a natural science studying the psychic regulation of behavior, instead of as an adjunct of physiology.

After resigning to protest the rejection of Elie Mechnikov (his candidate for chair of zoology), Sechenov took the chair at the Novorossisk University at Odessa from 1871 to 1876. While there, he edited and published Darwin's book, *The Descent of Man*. Sechenov applied Darwin's ideas and is considered to be the founder of evolutionary physiology and psychology.

In 1881 Sechenov established the existence of periodic spontaneous fluctuations of electricity in the brain. Having analyzed disorders of nerve and muscle activities (ataxia), he introduced the conception of muscle as a 'receptor' of sensory information. Signals reflecting the muscle effects are involved in the regulation of motor activity in animals and man. This was a precursor of the concept of feedback as an essential factor in the organization of behavior.

From 1888 to 1891 Sechenov was an assistant professor, then (1891–1901) an ordinary professor and the head of the chair of physiology at Moscow University and also, from 1896 to 1898, a distinguished professor and the director of the Physiological Institute of Moscow University. He investigated the chemistry of respiration; the physiology of respiration, particularly at reduced atmospheric pressure; and the physics and chemistry of solutions. His *A Survey of the Working Movements of Man* (1901) laid the foundation for later investigations into the physiology of work in Russia.

In 1901 Secjempv retired, but he continued his experimental work and teaching at Prechistenka Courses for workers (1903–04). He died of pneumonia on 2 (15) November 1905 at his summer cottage on the Oka river. Sechenov left the greater part of his fortune to the peasants of Teplyi Stan, the place where he was born.

Bibliography

Primary: 1860. *Materialy dlia budushchei fiziologii alkogol'nogo opianenia* [Data for the Future Physiology of Alcoholic Intoxication] (St Petersburg); 1862. *O zhivtnom electrichestve* [On Animal Electricity] (St Petersburg); 1863. 'Refleksy golovnogo mozga.' ['Reflexes of the Brain'] *Meditsinskii vestnik* 47–48; 1866. *Fiziologia nervnoi sistemy* [Physiology of the Nervous System] (St Petersburg); 1873. 'Komu i kak razrabatyvat psikhologiiu.' ['Who Must Investigate Psychology and How'] *Vestnik Evropy* 4; 1878. 'Elementi mysli.' ['The Elements of Thought'] *Vestnik Evropy* 3–4; 1879. *O pogloshchenii ugolnoi kisloty solianymi rastvorami i kroviu* [On Absorption of Carbon Acid by Salt Solutions and Blood] (St Petersburg); 1891. *Fiziologia nervnykh tsentrov* [Physiology of Nerve Centers] (St Petersburg); 1901. *Ocherk rabochihk dvizheny u cheloveka* [A Survey of the Working Movements of Man] (Moscow); Collections of Sechenov's writings are available in French as *Etudes psychologiques* (Paris, 1889) and in English as *Selected Works*, Subkov, A. A., ed. (Moscow and Leningrad, 1935).

Secondary: Iaroshevskii M. G. 1968. *I.M. Sechenov* (Leningrad); Vvedenskii, N. E., 1963. *I.M. Sechenov. Polnoe sobranie sochineni* [Complete Works], VII [contains a biography] (Leningrad); Koshtoyants, K. S., 1950. *I.M. Sechenov* (Moscow); *DSB.*

Tatiana Ul'iankina

SÉE, GERMAIN (b. Ribeauvillé, France, 6 March 1818; d. Paris, France, 12 May 1896), *medicine, therapeutics.*

Sée was the tenth of thirteen children born to Mayer Sée, a merchant and municipal official, and Rosine Lévy Schoningeim. The family traced its Jewish origins in Alsace back more than two centuries. After lycée schooling in Metz, Sée pursued medical studies in Paris. He won a hospital internship, and defended his MD thesis at age twenty-eight. In 1852 he placed first in the competition for a post of hospital physician, and in 1866 succeeded Armand Trousseau as professor of therapeutics, becoming the first Jew to hold that rank on the Paris medical faculty (there would not be another for thirteen years).

Sée's professorship occasioned protests by students and colleagues, ostensibly due to his being named by imperial patronage, in lieu of the usual route of passing the *aggregation*, or competition, for assistant professor. Within two years, derision turned to applause when Sée emerged as a champion of medical materialism. In 1868, he moved to a more prestigious professorship of clinical medicine, first at the Charité hospital and finally, in 1876, at the Hôtel Dieu where he spent the remaining twenty years of his career.

Sée's openness to laboratory medical science distinguished him from most French clinicians of his generation. He believed the physician should keep 'one foot in the hospital ward and the other in the laboratory' (1882, p. 911). An early advocate of Claude Bernard's experimental medicine, Sée believed the Paris school's reliance on observation and pathological anatomy had served its time. 'The clinic', he declared, 'that I should like to call physiological finds its indications in the physiological mechanisms underlying lesions and symptoms' (1869, pp. 14–15). Sée put forward physiological explanations for the action of various remedies whose use he pioneered in France. These included ergot for cardiovascular disease; salicylates for rheumatism, gout, and other inflammatory conditions; iodides for asthma; and bromides for epilepsy. Sée's therapeutic interventionism distinguished his practice from the reigning skepticism. Sée was one of the first Paris hospital physicians to appreciate the implications of the Pastorian revolution for medicine. His monograph, *De la phtisie bacillaire des poumons* (1884), appeared within two years of Robert Koch's demonstration of the tubercle bacillus. Knowledge of German, unusual for Paris physicians, gave Sée ready access to that rich medical scientific literature. His publications encompassed all fields of internal medicine; his multivolume textbook project resulted in monographs on diseases of the lungs, heart, and gastrointestinal system. He also published on chorea, anemia and blood diseases, infectious diseases in children, nutrition, and other subjects. He founded and edited the weekly periodical, *La médecine moderne.*

Sée had a vast private practice, one of the most extensive in the capital. His patients included Victor Hugo. In July 1870, he was called as a consultant to the bedside of Napoleon III. Had his correct diagnosis of bladder stone and bold recommendation of surgery been heeded, the Emperor might have been prevented from launching the disastrous war against Prussia. A controversial and contentious personality, Sée became a target for anti-Semites in the years leading up to the Dreyfus affair. Toward the end of his career, he vigorously denounced the notion of so-called Jewish diseases such as neurosis or diabetes. Despite advanced age and declining health, Sée never retired from his professorship or his hospital post.

In 1846 Sée married Adelaïde Lippmann, with whom he had two daughters. His wife and older daughter died of diphtheria in 1866. His other daughter married the prominent politician, Camille Sée, a distant relation.

Bibliography

Primary: 1898. *Oeuvres complètes* 7 vols. (Paris). [In English: 1885, *Bacillary phthisis of the lungs,* trans. Weddell, W. H. (London), and 1885, *Diseases of the lungs (of a specific not tuberculous nature),* trans. Hurd, E. P. (New York)]; 1869. *Leçon d'ouverture du cours de clinique médicale* (Paris); 1882. 'Ouverture du cours de clinique médicale.' *Le progrès médical* 10: 911.

Secondary: Gelfand, Toby, 1996–97. 'Dr. Germain Sée (1818–1896): "Israélite de cœur".' *Korot* 12: 9–33; Bianchon, Horace [Maurice de Fleury], 1891. 'Germain Sée' in *Nos grands médecins d'aujourd'hui* (Paris) pp. 409–420.

Toby Gelfand

SEGUIN, EDOUARD (b. Clamecy, France, 20 January 1812; d. New York, New York, USA, 28 October 1880), *mental deficiency, education, psychiatry.*

Seguin was educated at the collège d'Auxerre, close to his hometown of Clamecy, and at the lycée Saint-Louis in Paris. In 1837 he began studying medicine and surgery, initially under the tutorship of Jean Gaspard Itard, renowned for his attempts to educate the Wild Boy of Aveyron, and subsequently under the prominent alienist Jean-Etienne Esquirol. Inspired in particular by Itard, Seguin rapidly became committed to improving the education and training of 'les enfants arriérés et idiots'. He established his first school for 'idiot' children in 1839 and managed to convince the skeptical Esquirol that backward children could indeed learn with appropriate training.

After the deaths of Itard in 1838 and Esquirol in 1840, Seguin began to develop his own educational system for 'idiot' children, drawing on his experiences and observations both as head teacher at the Salpêtrière and as a private tutor.

During the early 1840s, having accepted a position at the Bicêtre, Seguin published several influential texts in which he set out his distinct system of educating idiot children. However, in 1843 tensions between Seguin and the medical authorities at the Bicêtre led to Seguin's dismissal. Between 1843 and 1850, Seguin continued to expand his private school and to publish the results of his observations. Two of his most influential books, *Traitement moral, hygiène, et éducation des idiots* and *Jacob-Rodrigues Pereire*, were published during his enforced exile from mainstream French education and medicine.

In 1850 Seguin emigrated to America, working first in Cleveland, Ohio, before moving in 1852 to Albany, New York, and then to New York City. In 1861 he graduated MD from the University Medical College of New York. After the death of his wife during that period, Seguin remained in New York for the remainder of his life, continuing to write extensively on the training and treatment of idiots, traveling occasionally to Europe and collaborating loosely with some of the large American educational institutions for children classified as 'idiots' and 'imbeciles'. In 1876 Seguin was elected the first president of the Association of Medical Officers of American Institutions for Idiotic and Feeble-Minded Persons.

Seguin's approach to the education and treatment of mentally defective children was based on a strong belief that so-called idiots and imbeciles were educable. Convinced that the development of motor and sensory skills would promote the development of mental and moral faculties, he devised a particular system of 'physiological education' that was aimed at strengthening muscles, improving coordination, educating the senses, and facilitating social integration. His work thus clearly drew upon and extended that of contemporary proponents of moral treatment of the insane in asylums. In addition, Seguin increasingly attempted to legitimize his pedagogic strategies by reference to the emergent language and approaches of neurology.

In addition to his pioneering work on the education of mental defectives, Seguin also studied 'animal heat' and invented a 'physiological thermometer' intended to facilitate more accurate clinical measurements of body temperature.

Although Seguin's particular brand of therapeutic optimism fell out of favor as fears of degeneration and national decline spread throughout Europe and North America during the closing decades of the nineteenth century, his approach to the education of mental defectives proved influential in many areas. In particular, his ideas provided the theoretical basis for the medico-pedagogic approaches to mental deficiency devised by British doctors and educationalists such as George Shuttleworth (1842–1928) and Fletcher Beach, as well as providing the inspiration for the 'scientific pedagogy' promoted by Maria Montessori (1870–1956) in Italy and the restorative educational programs for English working-class children developed by Margaret McMillan (1860–1931).

Bibliography

Primary: 1846. *Traitement moral, hygiène, et éducation des idiots et des autres enfants arriérés ou retardés dans leur développement* (Paris); 1856. 'Origin of the treatment and training of idiots.' *American Journal of Education* 2: 145–152; 1864. *Idiocy: Its Diagnosis and Treatment by the Physiological Method* (Albany, NY).

Secondary: Trent, James W., 1994. *Inventing the Feeble Mind: A History of Mental Retardation in the United States* (Berkeley); Pelicier, Yves, and Guy Thuillier, 1980. *Edouard Séguin (1812–1880), 'instituteur des idiots'* (Paris); *DAMB*.

Mark Jackson

SEJONG (KING OF KOREA) 世宗 (b. Korea, 1397; d. Korea, 1450), *Korean medicine.*

Among the Chosun (1392–1910) monarchs, the long reign of King Sejong 'the Great' (r. 1418–1450), styled as Korea's Golden Age, was a period of great cultural and intellectual accomplishment. A patron of research and development, Sejong sponsored young scholars, providing grants for research into the country's cultural, economic, and political heritage. Supporting initiatives in philosophy, music, linguistics, science, and medicine, Sejong's reign saw a range of technical achievements including the rain gauge, sundial, water clock, celestial globes, astronomical maps and clocks, and the orrery (mechanical model of the solar system).

King Sejong believed a synthesis of ancient Chinese and Korean medical knowledge would enhance imperial authority. In 1431 he ordered two scholars and one royal doctor to make a comprehensive and categorized record of locally produced drugs. The long-term dependence on Chinese medical knowledge and practice meant that scholarly Korean doctors had always relied on imported drugs, which were both expensive and difficult to obtain. In fact, each of the dynasties occupying Korean territory had also expressed interest in regional and local treatments. The first Korean medical book on local drugs, *Hyang'yakgugup'bang* 鄉藥救急方 [Emergency Remedies Using Locally Produced Drugs], was published in the years between 1192 and 1259. Thereafter, there was a gradual increase in remedy books that specialized in the use of locally produced drugs.

King Sejong also ordered a definitive collection of medical texts, and *Hyang'yakjipseong'bang* 鄉藥集成方 [Collected Remedies of Locally Produced Drugs] was published in 1433. This eighty-five-volume treatise included 959 entries on diagnosis, 10,706 prescriptions, 1,477 items on acupuncture therapy, and some original discussions on Korean drugs and their manufacturing processes.

Dispatching envoys and interpreters to China in 1437, King Sejong planned to add new Chinese medical titles to the hundreds archived in the Royal Library. During the previous dynasty, the rulers had been enthusiastic collectors of Chinese books from the Chinese Yuan Empire (1279–1368).

In 1443 King Sejong ordered seven scholars and two royal doctors to compile an encyclopedia summarizing the information from 151 Chinese medical books from the Han to Ming dynasties, and two Korean medical books. They finished the job in 1445 with the publication of the huge 365-volume *Ui'bang'yuchui* 醫方類聚 [Classified Collection of Medical Remedies]. The encyclopedia consisted of one part general discussion on medicine, and ninety-one parts devoted to physiology, pathology, diagnostics, internal medicine, treatments for external injures, otorhinolaryngology, obstetrics and gynecology, pediatrics, infectious diseases, acupuncture and moxibustion, and self-cultivation. Even proofreading the volumes required thirty-two years; the final 266-volume edition was eventually published in 1477, twenty-seven years after King Sejong's death. *Ui'bang'yuchui* was the largest medical encyclopedia in the world at that time. Today, it contains fifty-four entries from ancient Chinese medical books that are otherwise not extant.

In addition to *Hyang'yakjipseong'bang* and *Ui'bang'yuchui*, King Sejong contributed to the publishing, in 1438, of a two-volume treatise on forensic medicine entitled *Sin'jumu' wonrok* 新註無冤錄 [Washing Away Wrongs with a new commentary]. This book was a commentary on Wang Yu's 王與's *jumu'wonrok* 無冤錄 [Washing Away Wrongs], written in the Yuan period and designed as a manual for provincial and capital magistrates offices during the Choson dynasty to aid in determining criminality in cases of fatality.

Bibliography

Secondary: Dongwon, Shin, 2004. *Hoyelja, Choson'eul Seup'kyok'hada: Momkoa Ui'hak'ui Hankuksa* [Cholera Invaded Korea: A Korean History of Body and Medicine] (Seoul); Dujong, Kim, 1966. *Han'kuk'ui'hak'sa* [History of Korean Medicine] (Seoul); Sakae, Miki, 1962. *Chosen Iigakusi kyu Sitsubeisi* [History of Korean Medicine and of Disease in Korea] (Osaka).

Dongwon Shin

SELYE, HANS (b. Vienna, Austria, 26 January 1907; d. Montreal, Canada, 16 October 1982), *medicine, physiology.*

Born in Austria, Hans Selye was educated at the College of Benedictine Fathers in Kamarom, Czechoslovakia. He entered the University of Prague for medicine, taking some of his training in Paris and Rome, and graduated with his MD in 1929 and PhD in 1931. He received a Rockefeller Research Fellowship in 1931 and spent a year at Johns Hopkins University and a year at McGill University. Appointed a lecturer in biochemistry at McGill in 1933, he began his experimental research. He received a DSc from McGill in 1942. In 1945 he moved to the Université de Montreal as professor and director of the newly founded Institute of Experimental Medicine and Surgery.

As a medical student in Prague, he noticed that many people suffering from different disorders often manifested with the same general symptoms, a general pattern of 'being sick', no matter what the cause. His supervisor thought the idea was naïve, and Selye forgot it for a decade.

When searching for a new ovarian hormone in rats, he thought he was successful when he noted injections of extract were producing the same pattern of enlarged adrenal cortex, bleeding ulcers in the stomach and duodenum, and involution of the thymus and lymph nodes. His excitement faded when the same reaction occurred no matter what toxic substance was injected.

He considered abandoning the research but then hypothesized that the rats were developing the pattern of 'being sick' that he had noticed in patients with different disorders when he was a medical student. He published his initial observations in *Nature* in 1936. From this came his life work of studying the effects of 'noxious agents', later called stress, and the responses to maintain the homeostasis defined by Claude Bernard in the fight-or-flight situations described by Walter Cannon.

In his first publications he called the syndrome 'the alarm reaction' but then realized that the organism cannot be continuously in an alarm state. There was a second stage of 'adaptation or resistance' with lessening of the symptoms. If the stress continued, the adaptation and resistance failed, and a third stage, the stage of 'exhaustion', ensued because the capacity to adapt is finite. He called the phenomenon and its stages 'the general adaptation syndrome'.

Initially, his experimental concepts of the general adaptation syndrome were questioned, even by Walter Cannon, whose work he was expanding. Criticism continued when he argued that many physical disorders were the result of stress. He did years of experiments to describe the response of the nervous system to the initial alarm phase, the output of ACTH from the pituitary to stimulate secretion of large amounts of what he called 'corticoids' from the adrenal gland, and the effects of these on tissues. Because of the effects on glucose metabolism, he called the hormones ACTH, cortisone, and cortisol 'glucocorticoids'.

A prolific writer, and fluent in ten languages, he published more than 1,700 scientific papers and popular articles and thirty-three books, many of which were best sellers. He was a frequent speaker at scientific and public meetings, always denying that he had 'invented' stress. Some scientists thought him an unconventional popularizer, but he was a strong advocate for the importance of basic science.

After retirement in 1977, he founded the International Institute of Stress and the Hans Selye Foundation. Many honors came to him, including forty-three honorary degrees, fellowship in the Royal Society of Canada, honorary fellowships in sixty-eight scientific societies, and the highest decoration awarded by his adopted country, Companion of the Order of Canada.

Bibliography

Primary: 1950. *The Physiology and Pathology of Exposure to Stress: A Treatise Based on the Concepts of the General-Adaptation Syndrome and the Diseases of Adaptation* (Montreal); 1952. *The Story of the Adaptation Syndrome* (Montreal); 1956. *The Stress of My Life* (2nd edn., 1979) (New York); 1964. *From Dream to Discovery: On Being a Scientist* (New York).

Secondary: Viner, Russell, 1999. 'Putting Stress in Life: Hans Selye and the Making of Stress Theory.' *Social Studies of Science* 29: 391–410; Jasmin, Gaëtan, ed., 1968. *Endocrine Aspects of Disease Processes, Conference in Honor of Hans Selye* (London).

Jock Murray

SEMASHKO, NIKOLAI ALEKSANDROVICH (b. Livenskii, Orlov *guberniia* [province], Russia, 20 September [2 October] 1874; d. Moscow, Russia, 18 May 1949), *public health, social hygiene.*

Semashko, styled as the 'father' of Soviet public health, was born in 1874 to a family of *sluzhashchii* (white-collar worker) origin. He entered the medical faculty of Moscow University in 1891 but was arrested for his revolutionary involvement in 1895. Because of his political activities he was banned from residence in Moscow, so upon his release he studied at the medical faculty of Kazan University, from which he graduated in 1901.

Semashko spent the years until the 1905 Revolution working as a *zemstvo* (elective district council) physician, but was imprisoned in 1905. He then emigrated to Switzerland in 1906, living and working in several European countries in the years afterwards. He returned to Russia only in 1917 to head the Moscow department of public health. Semashko was truly an Old Bolshevik, being a personal friend of Lenin. His career peaked in 1918 when he became the first People's Commissar of Health for the Russian Republic, a position he retained until 1930. This appointment and that of Christopher Addison as Minister of Health in the UK in 1919 were the world's first ministerial-rank health care positions.

With the change of course of the first Five Year Plan, Semashko was dismissed as People's Commissar and considered himself to be in great danger during the Great Terror of 1937–38, going so far as to burn most of his personal papers; but he was not arrested. He maintained a position he had had since 1920, that of head of department for the organization of public health at the First Moscow Medical Institute. In the post–World War II years, he was given the directorship of the new All-Union Institute of Public Health in 1947, renamed for him upon his death in 1949.

Semashko's contributions to public health were considerable. Not only was he one of the world's first ministers of health, he was also instrumental in establishing the ministry itself. The administrative rationale he put forth helped sway the First All-Russian Congress of Medical-Sanitary Sections in 1918 to support organizational unity in Soviet medicine.

During his years as Commissar, Semashko guided and oversaw an array of public health innovations. His *Sotsial'naia gigiena v SSSR* [Social Hygiene in the USSR] helped define a distinctively Soviet variant of social hygiene. While originally envisaged in Germany as a blend of social and biological analysis—especially eugenics—to plan population growth, under the influence of Semashko and others, social hygiene in the Soviet Union became very heavily sociological. Identifying the social origins of disease and sickness became a major political objective in the early Soviet years, with the original emphasis of social hygiene on preventive medicine being carried much further. By the mid-1920s, under Semashko's tutelage, the social hygienists had advanced organizationally and theoretically. Semashko fostered the dispensary method as a solution to dealing with endemic 'everyday' diseases in the Soviet Union. Soviet dispensaries differed from normal clinics in that they were supposed to improve the everyday and working conditions of patients, as well as treat their symptoms.

Many of Semashko's writings were polemical attacks on nonsocialist medicine, but his polemics reflected the strong orientation toward preventive medicine, against which he distinguished bourgeois, reactionary medicine with its supposed reliance on clinical care only. Semashko was more politician than doctor, but his importance lies in clearly defining Soviet public health as highly centralized, statist, strongly oriented toward statistical analysis and social surveillance, and, in principle at least, toward preventive health care as well.

Bibliography

Primary: 1954. *Izbrannye proizvedeniia.* [Collected Works] (Moscow); RGASPI (Russian State Archive for Social and Political History) f. 17, op. 117, d. 822, l. 107.

Secondary: Mirskii, Mark Borisovich, 1995. 'N.A. Semashko (k 120-letiiu so dnia rozhdeniia).' *Gigiena i sanitaria* 4: 46–52; Potulov, Boris Mikhalovich, 1986. *N.A. Semashko—vrach i revoliutsioner.* [N. A. Semashko—doctor and revolutionary] (Moscow).

Chris Burton

SEMENOVSKII, PETR SERGEEVICH (b. Moscow, Russia, 9 December [21 December], 1883; d. Moscow, 1959), *forensic medicine.*

Born to the family of the sexton of the Nikolo-Golutvinskaia church in Moscow, Semenovskii studied at Donskaia church school from 1898 and in college from 1904. Like many young Russians of his time, he refused a religious career and entered the Medical Faculty of the Emperor Iur'ev (Derpt/Tartu) University (Estonia). As a student, Semenovskii proved his potential both as a medical researcher and forensic physician. Guided by Professor A. S. Ignatovskii, he prepared a paper, 'Sudebno-meditsinskoe issledovanie semennykh piaten' ['The Forensic Medical Study of Seminal Stains'], for which he won a gold medal from the university and, unusually for a student, the privilege to publish the paper in the *Transactions* of Iur'iev University in 1910. After graduating from the university with a gold medal, Semenovskii was retained there between 1910 and 1918 as an assistant prosecutor in the medical clinic and an assistant in the department for forensic medicine.

The Bolshevik Revolution and the ensuing Civil War (1917–21) utterly changed the life of the academic community in Russia. The young Soviet Republic welcomed the participation of specialists as experts in establishing the new state power. Semenovskii left Iuriev for Moscow and launched his 'Soviet' career in the agencies of the People's Commissariat (Ministry) of Internal Affairs (NKVD). In 1919 he was appointed the first head of the first Soviet department of criminology, the office of forensic examination of the Central Criminal Investigation Department. He later founded and headed the registration and fingerprint identification bureaus there.

At that time Semenovskii combined intensive organizational work and forensic examinations with scientific research in the field. As a forensic pathologist, he was permanently involved in different examinations. His scientific activities were mostly focused on the study of fingerprint identification. Based upon the idea of the inherited nature of dermatic patterns in the same family groups and between twins, he suggested a new method of kin identification (Semenovskii's method). He also devised a classification of fingerprints which is still in use in Russia. All these investigations were summed up by Semenovskii in his 1923 monograph on *Dactylography*.

By the middle of the 1920s, Semenovskii was the author of thirty scientific papers on forensic medicine, anthropology, and criminology. In 1927 he was elected an honorary member of the International Institute of Anthropology in Paris, and from 1930 to 1932, he chaired the Moscow Society of Forensic Medicine.

In 1931 the first State Research Institute for Forensic Medicine was established in the Soviet Union, and Semenovskii was appointed the senior researcher of the department of thanatology (the branch of medicine that studies changes in the organism just before and just after death, as well as the symptoms of death). Some results of the Institute's research works were used intensively against political opponents of Stalin's regime. Semenovskii was one of those physicians who were included on the special team of specialists working for the NKVD during the Great Purges of the 1930s. He contributed to the studies and practices of the secret NKVD research laboratory headed by G. Mairanovsky. It experimented directly on prisoners, and searched for different pharmacological, chemical, and medical methods of murdering without leaving any evidence. As a forensic physician Semenovskii signed many falsified death certificates for Soviet generals and diplomats, and foreign prisoners of war in the Lubianka and Lefortovo prisons. In 1943–44 he took part in the Commission of Soviet forensic examiners who prepared and signed the falsified documents for the medical examination of mass graves of the Polish officers in Katyn (near Smolensk). The title of 'Death Doctor' will forever be associated with the name of Semenovskii.

Bibliography

Primary: 1910. 'Sudebno-meditsinskoe issledovanie semennykh piaten.' ['The Forensic Medicine Study of Seminal Stains'] *Transactions of the Emperor Iur'iev University* Vols. 11–12 (Derpt); 1923, *Daktiloskopiia kak metod registratsii* [Dactylography as a Method of Criminal Registration] (Moscow).

Secondary: Birstein, V., 2001. *The Perversion of Knowledge: The True Story of Soviet Science* (Boulder, CO); Bobrenev, V., 1997. 'Doktor Smert", ili Varsonof'evskie prizraki ['Death Doctor', or Varsonofiev's Ghosts] (Moscow).

Marina Sorokina

SEMMELWEIS, IGNÁC FÜLÖP [IGNAZ PHILIPP]

SEMMELWEIS, IGNÁC FÜLÖP [IGNAZ PHILIPP] (b. Buda-Tabán, Hungary, 1 July 1818; d. Vienna, Austria, 13 August 1865), *obstetrics, gynecology, medical research.*

The fifth child of a large Catholic family in a section of Buda undergoing demographic change, Semmelweis was the son of a grocer; his mother was the daughter of one of Buda's richest merchants. They lived in comfortable quarters. Today Semmelweis's birthplace is Budapest's Museum of Medical History, named after him. Although Semmelweis considered himself Hungarian, many of his neighbors—as well as his parents—were descendants of Swabian German immigrants. As a result, he spoke a dialect of German that marked him as an outsider (especially when he studied and worked in Vienna). There is evidence that he spoke and wrote Hungarian with ease, however, and he definitely considered himself Hungarian. The family was not, as some writers have claimed or assumed, Jewish.

Semmelweis devoted his first year at the University of Vienna (1837–38) to the study of law (his parents' wish), but then enrolled in the medical faculty. The change may have been inspired by the large number of Hungarians studying medicine (a Vienna degree was valid throughout the Habsburg Empire, whereas a Pest degree permitted practice only in Hungary). Among them was Lajos Markusovszky, who became a close friend and shared rooms with Semmelweis. (Markusovszky would prove to be one of the earliest and most persistent supporters of Semmelweis's discovery of the etiology and prophylaxis of puerperal fever.) After two further years of study in Pest, Semmelweis returned for a final two in Vienna. There he came under the influence of the reform-minded stars of the medical faculty—Carl von Rokitansky, Joseph Skoda, and Ferdinand von Hebra—all supporters of Semmelweis. Awarded his MD in 1844 (with a dissertation entitled *De Vita Plantarum*), some months later Semmelweis also earned a Magister Obstetriciae following a short course on midwifery. He then spent fifteen months working with Skoda, developing his diagnostic skills and learning to employ statistical methods.

In July 1846 Semmelweis was appointed assistant in the First Obstetrical Clinic in Vienna's great teaching hospital, the famous Allgemeines Krankenhaus. He was charged with a large variety of medical tasks, serving in effect as house officer and being responsible for some lecturing. He worked under the direction of Johann Klein, who—although by no means one of the reformers and not enamored of statistics—was genuinely concerned about patient welfare. Semmelweis immediately noticed and was alarmed by the high mortality rate among women in the First Clinic. Others had observed, too, that the death rate from puerperal fever was much lower in the Second Clinic, where midwives rather than medical students were trained. No one had been able satisfactorily to explain the difference.

Semmelweis's career did not follow a smooth trajectory. After a few months in his new position, he was demoted to make room for his predecessor, Franz Breit (and then re-instated when Breit left for a position in Tübingen). The demotion came, apparently without warning, at a particularly bad time; shortly before, Semmelweis's father had died. According to Markusovszky, Semmelweis had in the meantime also become increasingly agitated over the staggering death figures in his clinic. Emotionally exhausted and temporarily jobless, Semmelweis went to Italy with Markusovszky in an effort to recoup his good spirits and energy.

Upon his return, Semmelweis learned to his distress that his friend, Jakob Kolletschka, professor of forensic medicine and another erstwhile Rokitansky student, had died. Reading the autopsy report on Kolletschka, Semmelweis had a sudden insight. The pathological findings on the corpse of this man who had been nicked by a knife while conducting an autopsy bore considerable resemblance to the pathological findings on the corpses of women who died in childbirth. Semmelweis realized there must be a common element that would explain why some (but not all) women died in childbirth, as well as why a healthy physician could, in death, exhibit similar symptoms: phlebitis, peritonitis, multiple abscesses, pyemia. Perhaps, since Kolletschka had died from a wound (which became septic) incurred during an autopsy, medical students and doctors who moved directly from dissecting victims of puerperal fever to delivering other women might themselves be the vehicles of transmission.

Many physicians prior to Semmelweis had thought and written about puerperal fever; some had anticipated him in realizing that puerperal fever (with its all too frequently fatal consequences) was not an inevitable risk of childbirth. But the idea that doctors themselves might be implicated was horrifying, and required a bold leap of imagination that few wanted (and fewer had dared) to make. There was nothing to be seen on the hands of the practitioners, and many other theories (dirty hospital walls or foul air) seemed at least as plausible. Among the pioneers who were on the right path were Charles White in Manchester, England (1773); Alexander Gordon in Aberdeen, Scotland (1795); Robert Collins in Dublin, Ireland (1835); and Oliver Wendell Holmes in Boston, Massachusetts (1843).

Semmelweis's conclusion—that since midwives did not conduct autopsies and medical students did, the lower rate of death in the midwives' clinic could be explained by the absence of 'cadaveric particles' on the midwives' hands to be conveyed to their lying-in patients—did not please Johann Klein. This hypothesis amounted to an indictment of practices Klein had overseen and authorized, and the damning statistics Semmelweis had produced put the First Clinic in a very bad light. (Semmelweis had also once publicly contradicted Klein in a meeting before the commission appointed to investigate the distressing mortality rate, further irritating the older man.) When Semmelweis began requiring students and physicians alike to wash their hands thoroughly in chlorinated lime, it must have seemed to Klein a direct affront to his authority—although he accepted and complied with the new hand-washing routine.

Some features of Semmelweis's statistics and their analysis have been criticized (earnest though he was, neither he nor most other physicians at the time were in a position to use statistical methods in a sophisticated manner). But the precise accuracy of his calculations is less important than the clear picture that emerged from them. Semmelweis produced numerous tables—month-by-month reviews showing the number of patients, the number of deaths, and the resulting percentages, for both the First Clinic and the Second Clinic—that revealed just how striking the discrepancies were. His strict hand-washing policies for medical attendants in the First Clinic resulted in a precipitous drop in the death rate. The significantly different rates in the two clinics in the years 1840–46, for example, became negligible in the years 1847–61 (after handwashing had begun). This, of course, vastly oversimplifies what happened. Semmelweis himself did not understand the nature of the cadaveric particles he cited. And only slowly did he come to the realization (missed by most contagionists) that those particles were not the sole noxious agents. Whereas only smallpox can cause smallpox, for example, puerperal fever could be caused by any putrid or decaying organic matter. Puerperal fever was thus not a specific contagious disease.

Semmelweis's discovery was by no means the end of the story. The number of deaths did not plummet to zero, and on occasion the death count spiked for no apparent reason. As Semmelweis became increasingly convinced that he had found not only how to explain the cause of childbed fever, but also how to stop its spread, he became less and less patient with those who disagreed with him. Yet he was slow to put his discovery into print. His friend, Ferdinand von Hebra, was the first to publish word of Semmelweis's findings (1847-48 and 1849); not until 1861 did Semmelweis himself publish a serious, full-scale report of his theory and his findings—his magnum opus. When that tome of more than 500 pages (written in German) did appear, it contained a detailed account of his discovery. Unfortunately, portions of it were quite confused, and pages of invective directed at those who dared to disagree with him meant it was not easy reading. The sharp contrast with the short lecture in passionate and elegant English (published in 1843 and then republished with a long introduction in 1855) by Oliver Wendell Holmes, which reached the same conclusion—that doctors were unwittingly carrying the infection of puerperal fever to their patients—has frequently been remarked.

Today Semmelweis is generally acknowledged to have made a discovery of monumental importance. Although some individuals accepted his theory, not until almost the end of the nineteenth century did a large number of physicians in Hungary and in England (including the obstetrician Sir Spencer Wells and the Hungarian-born Theodor Duka) actively promote greater recognition for Semmelweis. Subsequent debates over whether Semmelweis or Joseph Lister was the true father of antisepsis are beside the point; both played important roles. In its own way, the earlier work done by Semmelweis (he was a few years older than Lister) could be seen as the more impressive, precisely because he did not have at his disposal the benefits Lister derived from living in the age of bacteriology (after Louis Pasteur's work on fermentation). Semmelweis worked empirically, using pathology and statistics to deduce what could not be seen or even surmised in a period prior to the emergence of germ theory.

In October 1850 Semmelweis alienated friends and supporters in Vienna (where he had done his seminal work) when he abruptly left that city without saying a proper farewell. He returned to Hungary, seemingly quite disheartened that his great discovery had received less publicity and acceptance than he thought it warranted. In 1851 he was appointed head of the gynecological department at St Rochus Hospital in Pest. There he again produced a stunning reduction in mortality rates among women in childbirth, although he was not always able to keep the rates down. In 1855 he was promoted to professor of obstetrics at the university in Pest; there he began also to do gynecological surgery. (In 1863 he performed the first ovariotomy in Hungary; although the patient died, this initial operation was influential). In June 1857, however, Ignác Rott—a general practitioner—persuaded the ministry in Vienna that no one should be allowed to hold both a municipal and a state post. Semmelweis was removed from the hospital post, and Rott was appointed in his place.

In the end Semmelweis himself incurred a minor wound that turned septic and led to his death at the age of forty-seven (in the Mental Asylum of Lower-Austria, outside Vienna). Thus he, like his friend Kolletschka (and countless postpartum women), was a victim of an infection caused by putrid organic matter. Exactly how he died (septicemia-induced insanity? maltreatment in the asylum?) has been a subject of much debate. What cannot be

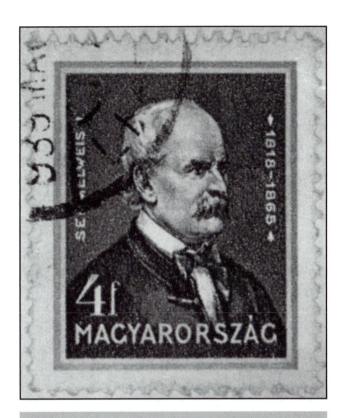

Postage stamp commemorating Ignaz Philipp Semmelweis. Wellcome Library, London.

denied is that Semmelweis, now often sentimentally referred to as 'The Savior of Mothers'—*Az Anyak Megmentóje*—contributed in a major way to medical progress: He figured out the etiology of a terrifying disease, and identified ways to prevent it. Furthermore, his etiological characterization of puerperal fever may have had more influence on the methodology of subsequent medical science than is normally recognized.

Bibliography

Primary: 1905. (Győry, Tiberius von, ed.) *Semmelweis' Gesammelte Werke* (Jena); 1861. *Die Aetiologie, der Begriff und die Prophylaxis des Kindbettfiebers* (Pest, Vienna, and Leipzig); 1983. (Carter, K. C., ed. and trans.) *The Aetiology, Concept, and Prophylaxis of Childbed Fever* (Madison, WI).

Secondary: Carter, K. Codell, 2003. 'Etiological Characterizations' in Carter, K. Codell, *The Rise of Causal Concepts of Disease: Case Histories* (Aldershot) pp. 38–61; Carter, K. Codell, and Barbara R. Carter, 1994. *Childbed Fever: A Scientific Biography of Ignaz Semmelweis* (Westport, CT); Benedek, István, 1983. *Ignaz Philipp Semmelweis, 1818–1865* (Vienna); Silló-Seidl, Georg, 1978. *Die Wahrheit über Semmelweis* (Geneva); Gortvay, György, and Imre Zoltán (Éva Róna, trans.), 1968. *Semmelweis: His Life and Work* (Budapest); Lesky, Erna, 1964. *Ignaz Philipp Semmelweis und die Wiener Medizinische Schule* (Vienna); *DSB*.

Constance Putnam

SEN, GANGA PRASAD (PANDIT) (b. Vikrampore, India [now Bangladesh], 1824; d. ?, 1896), *kavirajes, ayurvedic medicine.*

Ganga Prasad Sen was one of the most influential *kavirajes* or ayurvedic practitioners of the eastern province of Bengal, India in the nineteenth century. Born into an illustrious family of ayurvedic practitioners, Sen grew up in an age when Western medicine was being institutionalized in medical colleges in India, as the colonial education policy prioritized the diffusion of Western knowledge.

Sen moved to Calcutta at age nineteen, recognizing its potential market and its growth as a center of administrative and cultural power. Here he set up an ayurvedic practice based on consultation fees, founded a commercial pharmacy, and employed his journal, the *Ayurvedic Sanjivani,* to market his preparations. In this journal he addressed an emerging market of clients and readers with articles on disease prevention and hygiene in the immediate family as well as in the community, and offered medical advice on the etiology and treatment of prevalent diseases. Among his illustrious patients he treated the reformist ascetic and founder of the Ramakrishna Mission, Swami Ramakrishna Paramahansa.

Sen, along with contemporaries such as Pandit Gangadhar Ray, was one of the pioneers reforming and adapting ayurvedic learning and practice as it encountered Western knowledge. His ideas and writing therefore form part of the broader movement of cultural renaissance in Bengal, which spread to other parts of India in the late nineteenth century. His teaching, writing, and innovative practice in an emerging market for medicines in Calcutta—he is known to have initiated consultation fees and exported ayurvedic medicines to Europe—inspired a remarkable generation of students including Bijoy Ratna Sen and Jamini Bhushan Roy, and influenced *kavirajes* such as Gannath Sen. They produced translations of ayurvedic works in the vernacular—e.g., Bijoy Sen's Bengali translation of the Sanskrit classic, the *Ashtanghridaya of Baghbhatt.* Gannath Sen, leader of corporate bodies such as the Ayurved Sammelan, founded the Vishwanatha Ayurveda University in 1932 which taught a 'scientific' curriculum for Ayurveda. Toward the end of his career (1877), Ganga Prasad Sen was awarded a distinguished service medal by the British Colonial government.

Bibliography

Primary: Sen, Girijaprasana, and Jyotiprasanna Sen, (n.d.). *Svarigiya Kaviraj Gangaprasad Sen Mahasayer chikitsalaya: Catalogue of the Dispensary* (Calcutta); Chatterjee, Prabhakar, 1960. 'Contents of Ayurvedic Encyclopaedia-IV.' *Nagarjun* 8 May (Calcutta); *Vaidya Sanjivani Patrika* (Calcutta) (a journal although the precise years and series are not known).

Secondary: Gupta, Brahmananda, 1976. 'Indigenous Medicine in Nineteenth and Twentieth Century Bengal' in Leslie, Charles, ed., *Asian Medical Systems, A Comparative Study* (Berkeley) pp. 368–377; Mukhopadhyaya, Girindranath, 1926. *History of Indian Medicine* 2 vols. (Calcutta).

Kavita Sivaramakrishnan

SEN, PRAFULLA KUMAR (b. Calcutta [now Kolkata], India, 7 December 1915; d. Calcutta, 22 July 1982), *cardiothoracic surgery.*

Sen, son of Parijat Sen and Civil Surgeon Pramatha Nath Sen, attended Victoria College, Nagpur, and later Seth G. S. Medical College, Bombay (now Mumbai) (1933–38). In 1940 he completed his MS with distinction from Bombay University. After spending a year as a junior resident (1938), he rapidly rose in position: resident anesthetist (1939), surgical registrar (1939–42), and surgical tutor (1942) at the King Edward Memorial (KEM) Hospital, Bombay. He became assistant surgeon and lecturer at the same hospital (1943–49). During this period, Sen demonstrated an interest in developing collaborations among different specializations by involving the departments of pharmacology and pathology in experimental surgery dealing with shocks and burns. Soon after, he was awarded a visiting fellowship by the Rockefeller Foundation to study experimental surgery at the Harrison Department of Surgical Research at Philadelphia, Pennsylvania. In Philadelphia he met and married Marie Barnes; they had no children.

Upon his return to India in 1951, he combined private practice with an honorary teaching position at Seth G. S. Medical College. In order to combat rheumatic heart disease, a fairly common affliction in India, Sen developed an innovative snare to occlude the atrial appendage to control bleeding, and soon perfected the technique of closed mitral valvotomy. He went on to standardize and refine procedures for open-heart surgery under hypothermia. His lifelong interest in academic research gained precedence over a lucrative practice when, in 1956, he took charge, with support from the Rockefeller Foundation, as director of surgery in the newly established departments of medicine and surgery at KEM Hospital.

In 1957, following Arthur Vineberg, Sen experimented with internal mammary artery ligation to treat ischemic myocardia—with no significant success. Sen then went on to study the circulation system in reptiles, and pioneered the technique of transmyocardial acupuncture with notable success in dogs in 1964. Although his clinical trials at the time showed no significant difference, the technique has now been widely recognized as effective for the treatment of ischemic heart disease.

Sen's desire to be on the front line of medicine and surgery was demonstrated by his attempt to perform a heart transplant in February 1968, within two months of Christiaan Barnard's groundbreaking operation. Constrained by the lack of laws on organ donation, or legal definitions of brain death in India, Sen had to use the heart of a recently dead patient. Unsurprisingly this, and his second transplant (carried out in September 1968), were unsuccessful: his first patient died of respiratory failure, and the second of anuria.

Along with his student, Sharad Panday, he developed a simplified technique of the aortic arch replacement that became his most successful surgical procedure. By creating a right subclavian to left carotid bypass a few days before the surgery, they reduced dramatically the time required for such operations. Sen published a monograph on nonspecific aorta-arteritis. He also contributed to cardiac radiology by experimenting with nuclear isotopes. Elected president of the Association of Surgeons in India for two terms (1970 and 1971), he was one of the few Indian surgeons honored by both the Soviet Academy of Medical Sciences and the American College of Surgeons.

Sen was an inspiring teacher. Moreover, he actively promoted teamwork at a time when medical research in India focused on individual achievements.

Bibliography

Primary: 1953. 'The Use of Snare Tourniquet in Mitral Valvotomy—A Suggested Modification of Techniques.' *Indian Journal of Surgery* 15(1): 15; 1965. (et al.) 'Transmyocardial Acupuncture.' *Journal of Thoracic Cardiovascular Surgery* 50: 181–189; 1972. (et al.) *Non-Specific Aorto-Arteritis: A Monograph Based on a Study of 101 Cases* (Bombay).

Secondary: Mittal, Chander Mohan, 2002. 'Profulla Kumar Sen: His Contributions to Cardio-vascular Surgery.' *Texas Heart Institute Journal* 29: 17–25; 1991. 'P.K. Sen Commemorative Issue.' *Journal of Postgraduate Medicine* 37 (Supplement 1).

Indira Chowdhury

SENNERT, DANIEL   (b. Breslau, Germany, 25 November 1572; d. Wittenberg, Germany, 21 July 1637), *medicine, chemistry.*

Initially, this son of a shoemaker studied the *artes liberales* at Wittenberg from 1593 (MA 1598). This was followed by medical studies at Leipzig, Jena, Frankfurt an der Oder, and again Wittenberg. For a short period he worked as a medical doctor in Berlin. After a stay at Basel, he received his MD in 1601 and a professorship of medicine in 1602, both at Wittenberg. Working as a personal physician to the elector, he died from the plague in 1637. Sennert esteemed Aristotle, but was no dogmatic adherent, in his works of natural science. His *Epitome naturalis scientiae* of 1618 shows that even at the beginning of his academic career, Sennert was willing to accept the teaching of the *novatores* (renovators) whenever he encountered 'probable' evidence against the truth of Peripatetic doctrines.

Of particular interest is his acquaintance with Giordano Bruno's works, of which Sennert owned several volumes. Sennert quoted and paraphrased Giordano Bruno in a disputation of 1599 and in the same year also imitated his *De imaginum compositione* (1591) in his own *Templum Mnemosynes*. He was characterized by his open ecclesiasticism, which he applied to the field of medicine. Accordingly, he tried to revive atomism in physics in order to give a mechanistic explanation of nature, although he did not always apply it. As to medicine, the effort to reconcile Aristotle, Galen, and the young chemical medicine, especially in *De*

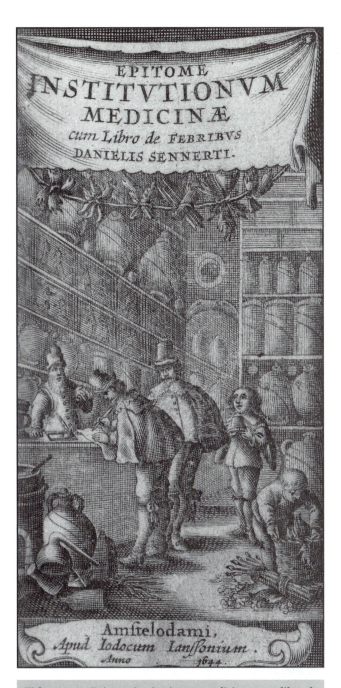

Title page to *Epitome institutionum medicinae cum libro de febribus*, Amsterdam, 1644. Rare Books, Wellcome Library, London.

chymicorum (1619), represented this attitude. This was an important contribution to the introduction of the chymiatric discourse in the academic sphere. For this, but also for his theory that animals have a soul as man does, Sennert was vehemently criticized and attacked by Johannes Freitag (1581–1641) from Groningen, who called him a heretical founder of a *Nova secta Sennerto-Paracelsica* (1637). But he was acquitted from the charge of heresy by medical faculties of most Protestant universities.

Medieval alchemists had a form of corpuscular theory that found its most influential exponent in the *Summa perfectionis* of Geber, probably written in the late thirteenth century. Sennert combined Geber's theory with contemporary natural philosophy in order to arrive at a comprehensive theory that the world is composed of atoms. Unlike the atomists of antiquity, such as Democritus and Leucippus, Sennert based his claims on laboratory processes of analysis and synthesis. He was able to show that the dissolution of silver in nitric acid and its recapture upon precipitation could not be adequately explained according to the reigning scholastic theories of mixture. Sennert's atoms also differed from those of the ancients in that his were endowed with substantial forms that accounted for the sensible qualities of the atoms. Especially because of his atomism, Sennert's *Hypomnemata physica* (1636) was censored and put on the *Index librorum prohibitorum* (1667). Sennert's work was silently appropriated and reworked after his death by Robert Boyle, the famous popularizer of the mechanical philosophy.

In his soul theory there is an interesting parallel between Sennert and Leibniz. Sennert and Leibniz upheld the orthodox Lutheran account of the propagation of souls through the medium of the parents' seeds (*traducianism*), and both posited an indivisible core in individual substances in which such souls were contained. In each case, also, the soul or active principle within each substance was what accounted for the law-like development from a seed to a full-grown animal, a fact that both authors believed was inexplicable in a purely materialist version of classical atomism.

Sennert's medical conceptions tended mostly toward humoral pathology, and his pathophysiology, semiotics, and therapy, classically orientated toward Galen's ideas, were obligatory subjects for European medicine until the 1680s. Even for Roman Catholic physicians, Sennert's work was indispensable. Claude Bonnet, a professor at Avignon, produced an expurgated edition of his works suitable for use by Roman Catholics in 1654.

Bibliography

Primary: 1641. *Opera omnia* (Paris and Venice) [many other later edns., including the most complete, 1676 (Leiden)]; 1599. *Templum Mnemosynes* (Wittenberg); 1618. *Epitome naturalis scientiae* (Wittenberg); 1619. *De chymicorum cum Aristotelicis et Galenicis consensu et dissensu* (Wittenberg); 1619. *De febribus libri IV* (Wittenberg); 1620. *Institutionum medicinae libri v* (Wittenberg); 1624. *De scorbuto tractatus* (Wittenberg); 1628. *Practicae medicinae libri VI* (Wittenberg); 1636. *Hypomnemata physica* (Frankfurt).

Secondary: Lüthy, Christoph, 2005. 'Daniel Sennert's Slow Conversion from Hylemorphism to Atomism.' *Graduate Faculty Philosophy Journal* 35(4): 99–121; Eckart, W. U., 2005. 'Daniel Sennert' in *Enzyklopädie der Medizingeschichte* (Berlin) p. 1320; Lüthy, C., and W. R. Newman, 2000. 'Daniel Sennert's Earliest Writings (1599–1600) and Their Debt to Giordano Bruno.' *Bruniana & Campanelliana* 6(2); Emily, Michael, 1997. 'Daniel Sennert on Matter and Form: At the Juncture of the Old and the New.' *Early Science and Medicine* 2: 272–300; Lohr, Ch. H., 1980. 'Renaissance Latin Aristotle Commentaries.' *Renaissance Quarterly* 33: 724–725; Eckart, W. U., 1978. *Grundlagen des medizinisch-wissenschaftl. Erkennens bei Daniel Sennert*. Medical dissertation (Münster); Lasswitz, K., 1890. *Geschichte der Atomistik*, vol.1 (Leipzig) pp. 436–454; Bonnet(i)us, Claudius, 1654. *Epitome Universam Dan. Sennerti Doctrinam summa fide complectens* (Avignon); Freitag, Johannes, 1637. *Novae Sectae Sennerto-Paracelsicae* (Amsterdam); *DSB*.

Wolfgang U. Eckart

SEVERINO, MARCO AURELIO

SEVERINO, MARCO AURELIO (b. Tarsia, Cosenza, Italy, 2 November 1580; d. Naples, Italy, 12 July 1656), *anatomy, surgery.*

Severino, the son of Jacopo Severino, a successful lawyer, and Beatrice Orangia, was only seven when his father died. He started his education in Calabria, and then went to Naples where he met Tommaso Campanella (1568–1639) from whom he learned the rudiments of Telesio's philosophical system; this formed the basis of his critical anti-Aristotelianism. After graduating from Salerno (1606), Severino practiced medicine in Tarsia, but after three years he returned to Naples to study surgery with Giulio Jasolino (1538–1622). From 1610 he taught surgery and anatomy privately, and thereafter, from 1615, at the University of Naples. Shortly afterward he was nominated first surgeon at the Ospedale degli Incurabili.

His fame as a surgeon spread quickly, and soon many students, who later became well-known scientists, came to Naples from all parts of Europe to study under him. Among these were Thomas Bartholin (1616–80) in 1643–44, and Johann Georg Volkamer (or Volckamer, 1616–93) from Nuremberg, who later became president of the famous *Academia Cesareo-Leopoldina Naturae Curiosorum*. Volkamer was particularly close to Severino, who offered him hospitality at Naples for about six months in 1641 and 1642. So close were the men that Severino entrusted Volkamer with the publication of his celebrated *Zootomia Democritaea*, published in Nuremberg in 1645. Severino corresponded with many of the important physicians and scientists of his time, including William Harvey.

Severino's printed works dealt above all with surgery and anatomy. He published both comprehensive treatises and specific detailed monographs on these subjects. His most famous surgical work was the treatise on abscesses (1632). His position regarding surgery was illustrated in his *De efficaci medicina* (1646), in which he championed surgery as a legitimate medical technique in opposition to the iatrochemical approach of some contemporaries.

Severino's most important work was the *Zootomia Democritaea, id est anatome generalis totius animantium opifici* (1645), not only because it is the earliest comprehensive treatise on comparative anatomy, but more importantly because it constituted the manifesto of a new anatomy, conceived as a convergence of experiences achieved in every class of living beings. This new anatomy, influenced by atomism and inspired by iatromechanics, proposed to break down the machines of our organism into their most minute parts, pinpointing the seat of that local motion in which must reside the functions of the organs. Some years later, this new conception of anatomy would reach its full development with Marcello Malpighi (1628–94).

Severino was also interested in the anatomy of serpents (1651) and the respiration of fish. In *Antiperipatias* (1655–59), he argued against the Peripatetic view that fish do not breathe air, by trying to demonstrate, following the atomistic philosophy of Democritus, that fish actually utilized the air that is dissolved in water.

Bibliography

Primary: 1632. *De recondita abscessuum natura libri VIII* (Naples) [2nd edn., 1643 (Frankfurt)]; 1645. *Zootomia Democritaea, id est, anatome generalis totius animantium opificii* (Nuremberg); 1646. *De efficaci medicina* (Frankfurt); 1651. *Vipera Pythia. Id est, de viperae natura, veneno, medicina, demonstrationes, et experimenta nova* (Padua); 1654. *Seilo-phlebotome castigata, sive de venae salvatellae usu et abusu* (Hanau); 1655–59. *Antiperipatias. Hoc est adversus Aristoteleos de respiratione piscium diatriba* (Naples).

Secondary: Schmitt, Charles B., and Charles Webster, 1971. 'Harvey and M. A. Severino. A Neglected Medical Relationship.' *Bulletin of the History of Medicine* 45: 49–75; Torrini, Maurizio, 1970. 'Lettere inedite di Tommaso Cornelio a Marco Aurelio Severino.' *Atti e memorie Accademia toscana di Scienze e Lettere La Colombaria* (n.s.) 20: 139–155; Belloni, Luigi, 1963. 'Severinus als Vorläufer Malpighis.' *Nova Acta Leopoldina* (n.f.) 27: 213–224; Ducceschi, Virgilio, 1923. 'L'epistolario di Marco Aurelio Severino (1580–1656).' *Rivista di storia delle scienze mediche e naturali* 14: 213–223; DSB.

Giuseppe Ongaro

SEVERINUS, PETRUS (aka PEDER SØRENSEN)

(b. Ribe, Denmark, 1540 or 1542; d. Copenhagen, Denmark, 28 July 1602), *chemical medicine.*

Sørensen, better known by the Latin version of his name, Petrus Severinus, was the son of Søren Jessen and Bodil Sørensdatter of Ribe, an important provincial town in southern Jutland astride the major land route to Germany. He attended Ribe Latin School, which had come under the liberalizing influence of Philipp Melanchthon's (1497–1560) humanist pedagogy as a consequence of Denmark's Reformation after 1537. His love for classical letters flourished at the University of Copenhagen, where he reportedly lectured on Latin poetry before reaching twenty years of age, leading to speculation that he attained the bachelor's degree in 1561.

The following year, owing to the deficiency of faculty at Copenhagen, Severinus went to France to study medicine, but soon returned, probably for financial reasons, and was promoted to the master's degree in 1564 along with another aspiring Danish medical student, Johannes Pratensis. The two became fast friends, and shared a royal stipend to study abroad; they matriculated at Padua in 1566. Severinus also traveled to France, presumably studying at Paris in 1567 and, after a brief stay in Denmark, returned to Italy via Germany and Switzerland in 1569 and 1570. Pratensis was awarded the MD at Padua; when and where Severinus was promoted is not known, but he styled himself 'doctor of philosophy and medicine' in the preface to his book, *Idea medicinæ philosophicæ* [An Ideal for Philosophical Medicine], which was dated Florence, 1 November 1570. During their travels, both students were taken with the 'new' medical ideas of the Swiss-German reformer Paracelsus, and sought to incorporate these into a systematic theoretical and practical medicine. They returned to Copenhagen in 1571 as known adherents to Paracelsus's innovations.

Copenhagen in the 1570s was amenable to new philosophical and medical ideas. Frederik II was eager to establish Denmark as a Lutheran kingdom along the lines of Philipp Melanchthon's humanism, developing the arts and sciences. His government sponsored the educational grand tour of Severinus and Pratensis to become medical scholars, and upon their return, the king appointed Severinus his personal physician, while making Pratensis professor of medicine at the University of Copenhagen. Beyond the formal requirements of sticking to Galenic and Hippocratic medicine, Pratensis also taught chemical methods, until his death in 1576. Frederik also patronized the important nobleman and astronomer, Tycho Brahe, during these years, and the foundation stone for Uraniborg, Tycho's observatory and chemical laboratory, was laid that same year. Tycho, Pratensis, and Severinus were friends, sharing common intellectual interests as well as the pursuit of Paracelsian medicine. Tycho's own patronage must also be reckoned into the flourishing of chemical philosophy and iatrochemical preparation in Denmark during this period.

Paracelsus had died in 1541, leaving behind several books and many more manuscript treatises that were completed, edited, and published by his followers. Paracelsian texts were beginning to circulate during the very years that Severinus and Pratensis were studying medicine, so it is no wonder that they took an interest in the latest ideas and their applications. Paracelsus did not hand down to posterity a well-articulated theory or method for using chemical drugs, so it was up to his followers to experiment with laboratory preparation of drugs, systematize the new therapeutics, and give chemical medicine a solid philosophical basis. Severinus's effort was directed toward the latter. He was so taken with Paracelsus's medicine that he composed an open letter to him, a paean praising him as the restorer of the ancient medicine of Hippocrates. This was printed in 1570; it served both to announce to the world that Severinus was a Paracelsian physician and to advertise his coming synthesis of Paracelsian theory, the *Idea medicinæ* (1571).

Little is known about Severinus's actual practice of medicine. Sparse references in correspondence somewhat ambiguously support his use of chemical drugs, and a posthumous comment by his colleague, Johannes Paludanus, indicates that he was eclectic, using Galenic treatments in ordinary circumstances and deploying stronger, chemically prepared drugs against more intractable diseases. No doubt this is how many 'Paracelsian' physicians operated on a daily basis. Paludanus also reported that Severinus had been seeking a panacea, a Paracelsian *arcanum*, or general cure, that could be used against many diseases.

Severinus retained his position as royal physician when King Frederik died in 1588, although he traveled with his new master, Christian IV, less frequently and became ever more active in the medical and administrative life of Copenhagen and its university. He was attempting to secure an appointment as professor of medicine there when he died in 1602, reportedly of plague. His wife survived him, and three of their children lived to adulthood, one of whom married the mayor of Copenhagen. Another daughter married a prominent diplomat, and the son, Frederik Severinus, became a physician. Severinus's reputation in Denmark as a chemical physician also lived on, as is evident in Caspar Bartholin's recommendations for a course of medical study, which was addressed to Severinus's grandson and printed in 1628. But it was Severinus's book, renowned as an eloquent explanation of Paracelsian theory, that conferred on him an international reputation equal to that of his contemporary, Tycho.

The *Idea medicinæ* is not a Paracelsian manual for healing, and offers no practical instruction in the preparation or use of chemical drugs. It is a philosophical treatise, expounding a metaphysical underpinning for Paracelsian ideas about the normal and pathological function of living beings, as well as the operation of drugs. Indeed, it is a new metaphysics for a biological understanding of nature that is based on Paracelsus's chemical medicine and cosmological ideas, but interpreted in terms of Aristotelian, Galenic and, more especially, Hippocratic and Neoplatonic concepts. The core of this organic philosophy is Severinus's assumption that all physical activity in nature is intrinsically spiritual; that the coming into being of bodies, their interactions, and their return to states of potential are governed by *rationes seminales*—rational agencies that were disseminated in the material world at its creation. This was a Stoic and Plotinian concept that was given Christian scope and application by St Augustine as an explanation for the temporal action of divinity in a providential cosmos.

Severinus hypothesized that being flowed forth from each seed-like spiritual center in the course of development, and in this way the spiritual center created a body, giving it characteristics and capacities that represented the predestined activity of the seed. When the seminal body had fulfilled its ordained function, it retreated to dormancy, becoming a spiritual potency once more. On this metaphysical basis, Severinus built an elaborate theoretical edifice that accounted for the natural appearance, reproduction, growth, senescence, and decay of animals, minerals, and vegetables as the temporal expressions of these predestined seeds, or *semina*. Pathology was also explained as an invasion of disease causing entities—*semina morborum*—which enter the healthy body with food and drink, or perhaps are latent within it as inherited *semina*, awaiting the appropriate times and conditions before sprouting into actual chemical pathogens. Normal, healthy *semina* might also be perverted by 'impressions', which were forms supervening on them from an exogenous source—for example, astral influences. Impressions could thus imprint on a seed and cause a transmutation of its seminal virtue from one set of characteristics to another, producing a pathological process in a healthy body, or else correcting a pathology by restoring normal function. Severinus called this 'transplantation', and it encompassed a wide range of causal activities, including the curative action of drugs, astrological influences, and the spontaneous appearance of diverse biological forms from pure lineages: i.e., some wild darnel (a weed seed) will always appear in a farmer's wheat field, he explained, because no matter how carefully the seed is selected for purity, some potential for transplantation into darnel exists within it, and will eventually become actualized as darnel.

This elaborate biological theory, which can be conveniently labeled '*semina* doctrine', is clearly quite different from the Galenic accounting of health and disease on the basis of qualitative balances and their physical manifestations in mixtures of the four basic body fluids (blood, phlegm, yellow bile, and black bile). Likewise, although Severinus's basic scheme of seminal development from potency to actuality has roots in Aristotelian biology, the idea is fundamentally Neoplatonist, embracing the constant emanation of material body from a spiritual primeval reality. And because Severinus envisioned the expressed characteristics of *semina* as chemicals, his theory provided a solid basis for Paracelsian therapeutics as well. The thorough elaboration of this *semina* doctrine, which was flexible and based on Christian philosophical principles, made the *Idea medicinæ* attractive to a wide readership during the one hundred years following its publication in 1571. A second, smaller-format (and somewhat corrupt) edition was printed at Erfurt in 1616, and a third was published in 1660 at the Hague, along with the first of two lengthy commentaries by William Davidson.

The historical importance of Severinus's work must be understood in the general context of the reception and integration of chemical philosophy and therapeutics. The book hit the market in the early stages of a period of confrontation between traditional Galenic medicine and various heterodoxies that were issuing from the printing press, the most salient of which contained Paracelsian medical, cosmological, and religious ideas. The Paris faculty of medicine, which controlled medical practice within Paris and was *de facto* a standard for the kingdom, proscribed the use of antimony internally in 1566, an act designed to discourage empirical practitioners in general, but targeted Paracelsians in particular. Beyond professional disputes, however, loomed a collision of world views between the Paracelsians and the university-trained Galenists and Aristotelians that embraced moral and religious elements as well as medical and pedagogical concerns, and this dispute was not confined to France. Beginning with the criticisms of Johan Wier and especially with Thomas Erastus's four-part censure of Paracelsian medicine on therapeutic, philosophical, and religious grounds (1572–74), a polarization between orthodox medicine and Paracelsian medicine gradually but steadily radicalized the latter along a path of separatist and mystical Protestant teaching, resulting in the Rosicrucian synthesis of the early seventeenth century.

When Erastus singled out particular passages, lifted anonymously from the *Idea medicinæ*, for attack as Manichæan heresy, he was tacitly labeling the Dane's work as part of the Paracelsian world view that needed to be suppressed. Although most physicians and philosophers who subsequently referred to Severinus's ideas were interested mainly in his *semina* theory, Erastus's criticism remained cogent enough to elicit a defense in Ambrosius Rhodius's 1643 commentary on the *Idea medicinæ*. Rhodius was a student of the chemical physician and Paracelsian critic, Daniel Sennert, but was moved to take up Severinus's ideas after moving to Denmark and marrying Severinus's granddaughter.

The *Idea medicinæ* was widely read on the continent and in England in the last decades of the sixteenth century, finding favor with prominent Paracelsian physicians including Joseph Duschesne (Quercetanus) and Thomas Moffett. Moffett, an exponent of Paracelsian chemical therapy in England, beseeched Severinus to take up his pen against Erastus and other anti-Paracelsians, but the Dane never again published. Among those of that generation who read the *Idea medicinæ* most carefully were Oswald Croll, Johannes Hartmann, and their vituperous antagonist, Andreas Libavius. The theoretical portion of Croll's *Basilica chemica*, an important early vehicle for the dissemination of iatrochemical preparations, clearly reveals the influence of Severinus's *semina* doctrine. Hartmann's influence on chemical education at Marburg, which was the center for expression of Paracelsian-Rosicrucian heresy, is well documented; in the laboratory he expanded on Croll's methods, and his theoretical formulations were so dependent on Severinus that Andreas Libavius identified him as a mouthpiece for Severinus's ideas when he attacked his 'vital philosophy' in *Examen philosophiæ novæ* (1615). Libavius

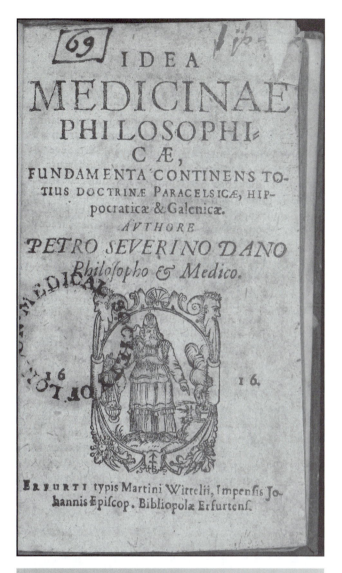

Title page of *Idea medicinae philosophicae . . .* Erfurt, 1616. Rare Books, Wellcome Library, London.

regarded Severinus as a greater influence on Croll, Hartmann, and contemporary Paracelsians than were the writings of Paracelsus himself; just four years later, Daniel Sennert judged Severinus's interpretation of Paracelsian ideas to be sufficiently influential to warrant the term '*secta Severiana*'—a Severinian school (*De chymicorum cum Aristotelicis et Galenicis consensu ac dissensu*, 1619). But *semina* doctrine was also studied and in many cases adopted by less ardent followers such as Gregor Horst and Guy de la Brosse, who variously saw it as a way of accommodating chemical theory to Galenic medicine, or else as a foundation for a new theory of chemical therapeutics. Thus, by the time the Thirty Years' War was heating up, Severinus's book had won widespread recognition as a major source for Paracelsian theory. This fact explains why it was also read outside strictly medical circles, mentioned by Francis Bacon, Edward Herbert, and John Donne, and also how *semina* theory came to serve as a general explanation for both the heat and differing medicinal characteristics of spa waters in Edward Jorden's study of mineral baths. In the second half of the century, Severinus was still identified as a Paracelsian author, but increasingly readers were turning to more recent sources for chemical medicine, especially the works of Sennert and J. B. van Helmont. *Semina* doctrine continued to inform the theories of Robert Boyle in England, Urban Hiärne in Sweden, and William Davidson in France and Poland, but the formulation of these ideas took on a more Helmontian character, described in terms of ferments and ebullitions, and Severinus came to be viewed in historical context as a bygone stage in the continuing development of chemical medicine, as expressed by his compatriot Olaus Borrichius in his 1660 *De ortu et progressu chemiæ*.

Bibliography

Primary: 1570?. *Epistola scripta Theophrasto Paracelso, in qua ratio ordinis et nominum, adeoque totius Philosophiæ Adeptæ methodus compendiose et erudite ostenditur a Petro Severino Dano Philosophiæ et Medicinæ Doctore* (Basel); Reprinted in Paracelsus, *Opera omnia* (1658); 1571. *Idea medicinæ philosophicæ fundamenta continens totius doctrinæ Paracelsicæ Hippocraticæ et Galenicæ* (Basel). [2nd edn., 1616 (Erfurt); 3rd edn., 1660 (The Hague)]: 1979. Bastholm, Eyvind, and Hans Skov. *Petrus Severinus og hans Idea medicinae philosophicae. Acta historica scientiarum naturalium et medicinalium*, vol. 32. [Danish translation of the *Idea medicinæ*] (Odense).

Secondary: Shackelford, Jole, 2004. *A Philosophical Path for Paracelsian Medicine. The Ideas, Intellectual Context, and Influence of Petrus Severinus (1540/2–1602), Acta historica scientiarum naturalium et medicinalium* 46. (Copenhagen); Shackelford, Jole, 2002. 'The Chemical Hippocrates: Paracelsian and Hippocratic Theory in Petrus Severinus' Medical Philosophy' in Cantor, David, ed., *Reinventing Hippocrates* (Aldershot) pp. 59–88; Shackelford, Jole, 1998. 'Seeds with a Mechanical Purpose: Severinus' *Semina* and Seventeenth-Century Matter Theory' in Debus, Allen G., and Michael T. Walton, eds., *Reading the Book of Nature: The Other Side of the Scientific Revolution, Sixteenth Century Essays and Studies*, vol. 41.(Kirksville, MO) pp. 15–44.

Jole Shackelford

SHARMA, PANDIT SHIV (Patiala, Patiala [now Punjab] India, 1906; d. Bombay [now Mumbai], India, 1982), *vaid, ayurvedic medicine.*

Eldest son of the royal physician to the Maharajah of Patiala, Pandit Ram Prasad Sharma, Sharma was arguably the most influential face of revived and professionalized ayurvedic practice in independent India. Shiv Sharma gained his initial training in ayurveda from his illustrious father, after which in 1928 he joined the faculty of the newly founded Ayurvedic Section of the Hindu reformist D. A. V. College in Lahore, the capital city of Punjab.

In 1938 Sharma became the youngest head of the All India Ayurvedic Sammelan, or Congress, an organization he headed and controlled for nearly seventeen years, transferring the Ayurvedic Congress office to Lahore and expanding its membership. In the 1940s, when boards of indigenous medicine were being established in various provinces, to frame norms for registered indigenous medical practice, Sharma inducted large numbers of practitioners without institutional education into the Ayurvedic Congress. Sharma's prolonged control over the leadership of corporate bodies such as the Ayurvedic Congress and the Provincial Punjab Vaid Congress sometimes sparked resistance and criticism from vaid leaders like Swami Harisharananand, editor of the journal *Ayurved Vigyan*.

Hailing from a family with important networks in the nationalist Congress, Sharma's influence in the Ayurvedic Congress went side by side with political networks and the ability to influence policy among the highest ranks of the nationalist Congress party, even in the decades after India's independence. In post-independence India, he presided over all notable enquiries and policy debates regarding government support for ayurvedic education and practice.

Sharma was also able to persuasively address through his writings both a constituency of lay people—patients and patrons—as well as ayurvedic physicians by means of his writings for newspapers. He also authored an erudite commentary on the classical treatise called *Ashtanga Hridaya* by Baghbhatt.

In particular, Sharma demonstrated his polemical skills in his advocacy of 'shuddha', or pure ayurveda, on the grounds of a Hindu nationalist self-sufficiency, propounding an ayurveda with a pure curriculum whose integrity was untouched by the therapeutics and technology of cosmopolitan medicine. His support of shuddha and its contents brought him into conflict with leading vaid practitioners like Pandit Yadavji Trikhamji and Kaviraj Gannath Sen.

In 1960 Sharma framed a plan for an Asian Health Organization with the help of the Sri Lankan government based on his ideals of ayurveda, later abandoned with the outbreak of the Sino-Indian conflict. By means of heading government bodies like the Central Council for Indigenous Medicine, Sharma continued until the 1970s to exercise influence over the Indian government's policy on indigenous systems of medicine.

Bibliography

Primary: 1929. *The System of Ayurveda* (Bombay); 1940–55. 'Presidential Addresses.' [Delivered at the annual meetings of the All India *Ayurved Sammelan* held at various locations across India. These speeches consisted of an account of the corporate body's activities and often delineated Sharma's agenda for ayurvedic reform and professionalization. They were printed by the *Ayurved Sammellan* in the Mahasammelan Patrika—the official journal of this body, available at its office in Delhi].

Secondary: Sivaramakrishnan, Kavita, 2006. *Old Potions New Bottles: Recasting Indigenous Medicine in Colonial Punjab* (Delhi);

Leslie, Charles, 1992. 'Interpretations of Illness: Syncretism in Modern Ayurveda' in Leslie, Charles, ed., *Paths to Asian Medical Knowledge* (Berkeley) pp. 177–208.

Kavita Sivaramakrishnan

SHARMA, THAKUR DUTT (PANDIT) (b. Ajnala district, Punjab, India, *c.* 1880; d. ?, 1950), *vaid, ayurvedic medicine.*

Born in a small-town family of revenue officials in the colonial Punjab, Thakur Dutt (Sharma is as much a family name as a caste name for Brahmins; Pandit is a title) was attracted to the clientele and medical market of Lahore. Here he established Amritdhara, one of the most renowned and effectively marketed commercial pharmacies in India. Amritdhara pharmacy's patented medicines were publicized in an emerging vernacular press, including Thakur Dutt's own Urdu and Hindi publications, such as his journal, *Desh Upkarak.* Of all his patent medicines, the Amritdhara balm—believed to cure all manner of ailments ranging from stomach ailments, skin afflictions, injuries and other aches and pains—was to become a household name as an all purpose ayurvedic medicine that was exported to Burma (Myanmar), Sri Lanka, and parts of Western Europe.

Thakur Dutt's *Desh Upkarak* enjoyed a readership among the lay people and medical practitioners in urban centers in North India. In an accessible and engaging style, the journal addressed a range of health issues, guiding readers on community health, considering subjects relating to the health of children and women in the family, discussing the causes and symptoms of common and chronic diseases, and also sharing drug remedies. It also served Thakur Dutt as a platform for disseminating ideas relating to Hindu social reform, and helped consolidate his leadership in both vaid corporate bodies and caste associations.

His leadership of the provincial Ayurvedic Congress, and his representation of Punjab's provincial interests in the All India Ayurved Congress, matched Thakur Dutt's commercial success. He was also an important leader of the Lahore faction of the Arya Samaj, a Hindu reformist body. He simultaneously presided over other caste and kinship bodies, such as the Brahmin Congress. His support of Hindu reformist politics earned him enduring patrons within the provincial and nationalist political parties. He emerged as an adept fundraiser for projects such as the proposed Central Ayurvedic University, supported by Jagannath Prasad Shukla of the Ayurved Congress. He also participated in fundraising for nationalist Congress funds.

Although from 1911 he was an early member of the Delhi-based All India Ayurvedic and Tibb Conference, in later years he increasingly extended his sympathies to the All India Ayurvedic Congress and its interests. He therefore supported campaigns to propagate Ayurveda in Hindi in Punjab, with the understanding that Hindi, as the mother tongue of Hindus and representing Hindu nationalist interests, would shore up Hindu minority interests in Punjab and earn the minorities greater support from other provinces with Hindu majority populations.

After Indian independence (1947) and the partition of Punjab Province between India and Pakistan, Thakur Dutt shifted his pharmacy to the hill town of Simla in India. With the loss of frontier markets west of Punjab, and the reduced volume of the trade in raw drugs via towns in Punjab, his pharmacy trade was much reduced.

Bibliography

Primary: *Desh Upkarak* (Lahore) (see especially, Plague Issue, October 1905) [in Urdu]; 1905. *Plague Pratibhandhak Upay* [Remedies to Eradicate the Plague] (Lahore); Kaviraj, Pratap Singh, 1958. *Kavi Vinod Vaidya Bhushan Shriman Thakur Dutt Sharma Vaidji Ki Heerak Jayanti Par Abhinandan Granth.* (Dehra Dun) (a Commemoration volume for Pandit Thakur Dutt Sharma on his diamond jubilee).

Secondary: Sivaramakrishnan, Kavita 2006. *Old Potions New Bottles: Recasting Indigenous Medicine in Colonial Punjab* (Delhi); Neville, Pran, 1997. *Lahore: A Sentimental Journey* (Delhi).

Kavita Sivaramakrishnan

SHARP, JANE (fl. *c.* 1641–1671), *midwifery.*

The little that is known of the life and work of Jane Sharp is derived almost entirely from her book *The Midwives Book, or, the whole art of midwifery discovered. Directing childbearing women how to behave themselves in their conception, breeding and nursing of children etc.* Her textbook or manual was advertised in the Stationers' Company *Term Catalogue* in May 1671 and offered for sale by Simon Miller at St Paul's. The existence of effective contacts within the publishing world of London might suggest that her life and career were associated entirely with the capital. However, the dedication of her book was to her 'ever honoured friend the Lady Ellenour Talbutt'. Lady Talbutt, a sister of the tenth Earl of Shrewsbury, probably lived in Shropshire or Gloucestershire, and this may indicate Sharp's association with that area of England. Extensive searches by scholars have failed to find unquestioned evidence of Sharp's life. However, recent feminist scholars emphasize the difficulty of tracing seventeenth-century women's identity.

Sharp's book was probably the most well-known midwifery manual written by a woman that was published in English. It appeared as a small octavo volume that was sold for two shillings and sixpence (twelve and a half new pence, or £0.125), and it went through four editions by 1725. Her work does not rival the publications of contemporary European midwives.

In her book Sharp describes herself as a 'Practitioner in the Art of Midwifery above thirty years', so she can probably best be pictured as representative of a large group of female midwives of her time. In seventeenth-century England, almost all women delivered their infants at home while being cared for by a female practitioner selected by the mother or her family and were attended through the traditional ceremonies of the birthing chamber by female gossips or friends. In practice, midwives worked within a tradition that accepted the importance of a role learned experientially and that respected the female secrets of childbirth. The skills and level of education of midwives varied. At the top were those who served long apprentice-ships with established practitioners, some of these women purchasing a Bishop's license. Poorer women might be supported through a less rigorous preparation by their congregations as a means of earning their living and serving their parish.

Sharp's decision to write her book appears to have resulted, at least in part, from an awareness of the threat to female practitioners posed by 'man midwives'. The seventeenth century had witnessed failed attempts by the Chamberlen family to create and manage a midwifery college. The position of male practitioners was problematic. They aspired to a scientific role, and midwifery manuals were predominantly written by men who had access to anatomical and scientific knowledge but who frequently lacked the practical knowledge of an experienced midwife. It was difficult for men to acquire skills of normal delivery, and Nicholas Culpeper (1616–64) admitted in *A directory for midwives* (1651) that he had no practical experience with normal childbirth. Study of midwifery manuals demonstrates the derivative nature of much of their contents. Commentators have pointed to the straightforward translation and lifting of earlier material in many of these works. Sharp's book did borrow from earlier sources; indeed, she claimed to 'have been at Great Cost in Translations' in preparing her text. It was, however, shaped and informed by her female view, which filtered the selection, integration, and editing of the material from her sources.

Significantly, Sharp's book, addressed to her fellow midwives, underlines the tensions surrounding the traditional roles of midwives in the contemporary world.

Bibliography

Primary: Hobby, Elaine, ed., 1999. *The Midwives Book or the Whole Art of Midwifery Discovered* (Oxford).

Secondary: Evenden, Doreen, 2000. *The Midwives of Seventeenth-Century London* (Cambridge); Hess, Ann Giardina, 1993. 'Midwifery Practice among the Quakers in Southern Rural England in the Late Seventeenth Century' in Marland, Hilary, ed., *The Art of Midwifery: Early Modern Midwives in Europe* (London) pp. 49–76; *Oxford DNB*.

Barbara Mortimer

SHATTUCK, GEORGE CHEYNE, SR (b. Templeton, Massachusetts, USA, 17 July 1783; d. Boston, Massachusetts, USA, 18 March 1854), *medicine, philanthropy*.

Shattuck was the son of a pioneer physician and was the father, grandfather, and great-grandfather of distinguished members of the profession who graced the medical scene in Boston, Massachusetts, for generations. He earned his AB in 1803 at Dartmouth College and his MB in 1806 as a much-cherished student of Nathan Smith at the medical school Smith had founded in Hanover, New Hampshire, in 1797. Further medical training in Boston (with Samuel Danforth) was followed by study under Benjamin Rush at the University of Pennsylvania, where Shattuck earned an MD in 1807.

A measure of Shattuck's character is the range of significant roles he played in the lives of the many individuals and institutions to which he gave financial support. His account books for the 1830s, for example, have frequent entries of 'defer' and 'null' next to patients' names; seldom was an amount given and marked 'settled'. His impoverished students often received gifts of clothing from him. In 1854 Shattuck endowed the professorship of morbid (later pathological) anatomy at Harvard Medical School, and he provided Harvard with many scholarships. He made bequests to fifteen or more benevolent institutions.

Shattuck married Eliza Cheever Davis in 1811. Of their six children, the only one to survive was George Cheyne, Jr., whose own impressive career continued along the medical and philanthropic paths his father had paved so well. Eliza Shattuck died in 1828; Amelia Bigelow became Shattuck's second wife in 1835 (she died eight years later).

Shattuck's importance in American medical history rests on far more than his family's medical lineage, his friendship with Nathan Smith, and his philanthropy. He early developed a large practice, at times earning as much as $10,000 a year. Living in a fashionable section of Boston and having a socially prominent wife helped, but his medical skills and personal concern were key.

Lyman Spalding—another Nathan Smith protégé and first president of the College of Physicians and Surgeons in Fairfield, New York—convinced Shattuck to lecture there for two terms. But it was in Boston that Shattuck made his mark, among other things as consulting physician to the city and as a private instructor. He was president of the Massachusetts Medical Society (1836–39) and of the American Statistical Society (1845–51), and he was a cofounder with Oliver Wendell Holmes and others of the Boston Society of Medical Observation.

As a young man, Shattuck contributed a winning paper to the prestigious annual Boylston Prize Medal essay contest sponsored by Harvard Medical School; the following year, he submitted papers on both contest topics and won both prizes. He published his three essays the next year (1808). Neither a scientist nor a committed scholar, he published almost nothing else, although—characteristically—he underwrote publications for others more than once (e.g., James Thacher's *American New Dispensary* and *American Medical Biography* and John James Audubon's *Birds of America*), thus helping shape Boston's medical and cultural landscape. Shattuck's 'Dissertation on the Uncertainty of the Healing Art', read before the Massachusetts Medical Association in 1828, deserves to be better known. His emphasis on the need to adapt treatments to particular patients and his understanding that no physician can know everything are still important lessons today. As he commented, 'The selection, and adaptation of the force of the remedy to the severity of the disease involve nicety in the skill and judgment beyond the reach of human power' (1829, p. 156).

Bibliography

Primary: 1808. *Three Dissertations on Boylston Prize Questions for the Years 1806 and 1807* (Boston); 1829. 'A Dissertation on the Uncertainty of the Healing Art' in *Medical Dissertations Read at the Annual Meetings of the Massachusetts Medical Society,* vol. 4 (Boston).

Secondary: Smith, Emily A., 1914. *The Life and Letters of Nathan Smith, M.B., M.D.* (New Haven); Bartol, C. A., 1854. *The relation of the medical profession to the ministry: a discourse preached in the West Church, on occasion of the death of Dr. George C. Shattuck* (Boston); Jarvis, Edward, 1854. *Memoir of the Life and Character of George Cheyne Shattuck, M.D.* (Boston); *DAMB.*

Constance Putnam

SHATTUCK, LEMUEL   (b. Ashby, Massachusetts, USA, 15 October 1793; d. Boston, Massachusetts, USA, 17 January 1859), *statistics, public health.*

Shattuck, fifth child of John and Betsy Miles Shattuck, grew up on his parents' farm as an avid reader despite meager formal schooling. He left home in 1816 to earn his way as a schoolteacher, first in Albany and then in Troy, New York, migrating eventually to Detroit, Michigan. After returning to Massachusetts in 1823, Shattuck settled in Concord for ten years before moving to Cambridge and then to Boston, where he spent the rest of his life. He married Clarissa Baxter in 1825, and they raised five children.

His 100-year anniversary history of Concord (1831), derived from church, town, and school records, included statistical data that opened a new view of history to Shattuck, prompting him to collect and analyze vital and institutional records. Concord teachers were instructed to record all pupils' progress in the School Committee Annual Report, a practice eventually required throughout Massachusetts.

When Shattuck moved to Boston in 1835, he was elected to the City Council (1837), and a decade later, he was elected to the General Court (Massachusetts State Legislature). As one of the principal founders and first secretary of the American Statistical Association (1839), Shattuck became a significant force among citizens interested in gathering reliable data to improve social knowledge and order. His correspondence with William Farr encouraged him to sponsor legislation establishing the Massachusetts Registration Act (1842), the first state government in the United States to require records of births, deaths, and marriages. This achievement was recognized by the Massachu-

setts Medical Society and the American Academy of Arts and Sciences and assured his reputation as a statistician.

Shattuck's special concern with public health stemmed from the collection and analyses of vital data. His recognition of potentially dangerous differences between recent immigrants and more prosperous citizens underscored deteriorating conditions in Boston between 1810 and 1841 and the value of statistics in revealing the consequences of changing social and physical environment. Shattuck had earlier emphasized personal responsibility for poor health, but in the 1840s, he reminded the Boston City Council that conditions where immigrants lived required the city to provide public water and other services to reduce the spread of contagions.

Shattuck, twice elected to the General Court, was present when the Massachusetts Medical Society and the American Statistical Association petitioned for a sanitary survey designed to identify threats to public health. Epidemics of cholera in other American cities (1849) heightened public interest in Boston's sanitary conditions, and Shattuck took responsibility for providing an assessment supported by statistical evidence. His analyses of data reflected the impact of changes in the social characteristics of the population as well as conditions in which people lived. Immigration from Ireland in the previous decade inevitably produced crowding and filth that were understood as precursors of disease outbreaks. Shattuck, not always free of prejudice, nonetheless argued forcefully in the *Report of the Sanitary Commission of Massachusetts* (1850) that although social conditions did indeed increase the risk of epidemics, personal responsibility could not be exercised without the support of community services, above all public water. Over the next decade, Shattuck's pioneering document garnered significant support in Massachusetts, leading to the first effective State Board of Health in the United States (1869).

Bibliography

Primary: 1850. *Report of a general Plan . . . relating to a Sanitary Survey of the State* (Boston) [The 'Shattuck Report', facsimile edn., 1948, (Cambridge, MA)].

Secondary: Rosenkrantz, Barbara Gutmann, 1972. *Public Health and the State. Changing Views in Massachusetts, 1842–1936* (Cambridge, MA); Willcox, William F., 1940. 'Lemuel Shattuck, Statist, Founder of the American Statistical Association.' *Journal of the American Statistical Association* 35: 224–235 (1940); Jarvis, Edward, 1851. 'Review of the Report of the Massachusetts Sanitary Commission.' *American Journal of Medical Sciences,* n.s., 21: 391–409; *DAMB.*

Barbara Guttman Rosenkrantz

SHERLOCK, SHEILA PATRICIA VIOLET   (b. Dublin, Ireland, 31 March 1918; d. London, England, 30 December 2001), *medicine, hepatology.*

Sherlock was the only daughter of Samuel Philip Sherlock, a Captain in the Green Jackets, and his wife, Violet Beckett. The family moved to London and then to Sandgate, Kent, in 1929. Sherlock was educated at the Folkestone County School for Girls. In August 1936, she was accepted as a medical student by the University of Edinburgh. She graduated (1941) top of her year (summa cum laude). After a year as an assistant lecturer to James Learmonth, professor of surgery, she went to work with John McMichael (1904–93) at the British Postgraduate Medical School at Hammersmith Hospital. McMichael had introduced the techniques of cardiac catheterization and liver biopsy for the first time in this country at Hammersmith. Sherlock used liver biopsy for an important study of hepatitis, published in 1943. Her MD thesis, which in 1945 earned a gold medal from the University of Edinburgh, was based on this work.

In 1947 she was awarded a Rockefeller traveling fellowship for study at Yale University. Not only was her year at Yale important to her scientific career, but she also met the leading hepatologists in the United States. She was one of the founders of the American Liver Association, whose meetings she attended for fifty years.

Sherlock was appointed lecturer in medicine and consultant physician to Hammersmith Hospital in 1948. She was one of the youngest consultants in the country, a remarkable achievement for a woman at that time. She spent the next eleven years establishing her unit as a leading international center for the investigation and treatment of liver disease. A year later, she was the youngest woman to be elected FRCP.

Her research through those years was to be dominated by the use of hepatic biopsy and of catheterization of the blood vessels of the liver, techniques that were controversial in those early days. In later years, Maurice Pappworth (1910–94), in his book *Human Guinea Pigs* (1967), castigated the research activities at Hammersmith as being unethical, lacking informed consent, and being carried out for the benefit of research rather than being in the interest of the patient.

Sherlock's major achievement, however, was her book *Diseases of the Liver and Biliary System* (1955). It was reprinted twice within a year. She went on to write ten new editions, and the book was translated into German, Greek, Italian, Japanese, Russian, Portuguese, and Spanish.

In 1959 Sherlock became professor of medicine at the Royal Free Hospital School of Medicine, London, as the first clinical professor at that School and the first woman in Britain to be appointed to a chair of medicine. Her work now became more orientated to clinical studies of liver disease, in particular new methods of diagnosis and treatment, rather than to the physiological studies that had characterized her Hammersmith work and which had attracted such criticism on ethical grounds.

In 1974 the Royal Free Hospital moved to a new building in Hampstead. Here she was given facilities that were vastly superior to those she had previously enjoyed. The new Medical Unit occupied the tenth floor. The wards for her patients were now close to the offices and research laboratories.

Sherlock's increasing distinction through those years was recognized by her election as president of the British Association for the Study of the Liver and, also, in 1973, her election as president of the British Society of Gastroenterology, whose journal *Gut* she edited from 1967 to 1975. Other presidencies included the European Association for the Study of the Liver.

At the RCP, she was the first woman to be elected vice president (1976). She gave the Harveian Oration in 1985. In 1978 she was made a Dame Commander of the British Empire. Sherlock retired in 1983 but continued to work until the beginning of 2001. At the Royal Free Hospital, she became, between 1990 and 1998, president of the School of Medicine. In 1994 the new postgraduate center was named the Sheila Sherlock Education Centre. Her eighteen honorary degrees from universities around the world, including from her own, Edinburgh, as well as from Cambridge and Yale, attested to her international distinction. In 2001, the year of her death, she was elected FRS. But her abiding accomplishments were two—her book *Diseases of the Liver and Biliary System* and her demonstration that, as a woman, it was possible to become one of the leading medical scientists of her day.

She was cremated at Golders Green Crematorium on 8 January 2002.

Bibliography

Primary: 1955. *Diseases of the Liver and Biliary System* (Oxford).

Secondary: Pepys, Mark, 2003. 'Dame Sheila Patricia Violet Sherlock.' *Biographical Memoirs of Fellows of the Royal Society* 49: 476–493; *Oxford DNB*.

Christopher Booth

SHIGA, KIYOSHI (b. Sendai, Miyagi Prefecture, Japan, 18 December 1870; d. Isohama, Miyagi Prefecture, Japan, 25 January 1954), *bacteriology*.

Shiga Kiyoshi, the discoverer of the dysentery bacillus, was born in the city of Sendai, Miyagi Prefecture, in the northeastern region of Japan. He was the fifth child of Satō Shin, a *samurai* serving the local feudal lord. Having lost his position due to the abolition of the feudal province (*han*) system in 1871, Satō supported his family by running a private learning class for local children. The Satōs' livelihood was not always easy, and his uncle, Shiga Risn, a practitioner of traditional Kanpō medicine, adopted Kiyoshi. Under his foster father's influence, Kiyoshi naturally determined to be a medical doctor, and the more affluent Shigas could afford his higher education. He proceeded to the School of Medicine at the University of Tokyo in 1892.

Unlike his foster father, Shiga was trained in Western medicine. Under its Westernizing policy after the Meiji Revolution of 1868, the Japanese government had officially

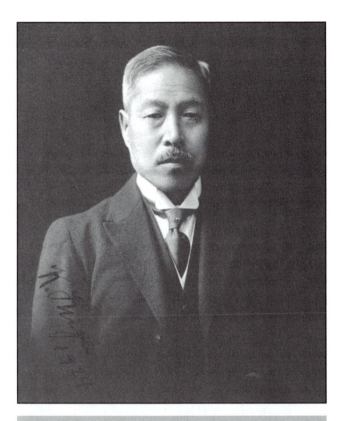

Kiyoshi Shiga. Photograph, Wellcome Library, London.

decided in 1874 that the country's medical education should be based on Western medical sciences. Traditional medical education and practices were thereby made 'irregular', if not illegal. At the University, Shiga was taught by eminent professors such as Ogata Masanori (1853–1919) and Aoyama Tanemichi (1859–1917), both of whom had studied in Germany.

It was, however, not these professors, but Kitasato Shibasaburō, the director of the Institute for Infectious Disease (IID), who impressed Shiga most during his university years. In November 1894, Shiga was fascinated by Kitasato's special lecture held at the University, in which Kitasato talked about how he had discovered the plague bacillus in Hong Kong earlier that year. Shiga dreamed of being a bacteriologist like Kitasato. In January 1897, Shiga entered the IID after his graduation.

Dysentery

Shiga spent his first few months at the IID acquiring basic bacteriological skills under Kitasato. Shiga later recalled that Kitasato was a strict teacher, and often raised his voice at his pupils' negligence. But from Kitasato's point of view, Shiga was a hopeful pupil. He soon came to acknowledge Shiga's diligence and reliability. This can be inferred from the fact that Kitasato assigned important research on dysentery to Shiga, still a newcomer.

Dysentery was a generic term describing diarrheal disturbances with blood and mucus in the feces. Its Japanese word, *sekiri*, signifies 'red diarrhea'. From the 1870s onward, the disease had seriously affected Japan. At first severe outbreaks occurred mainly in the southwestern part of the country; then the core of prevalence shifted to the northeast. It reached Tokyo in 1897. In that year, the number of patients amounted to about 7,000 in the Tokyo Prefecture, of whom more than 2,000 died. Dysentery's infectiousness was now clear from the diffusive feature, and the task of identifying its causative agent devolved on Shiga.

Under Kitasato's guidance, Shiga conducted staining tests, and microscopic examination, one by one, of various organisms taken from patients' feces, eventually isolating a suspicious rod. Yet Shiga had to mark time for months, as he had no final means for identification. An inspiration came from France. In the previous year, G. F. I. Widal (1862–1929) had established a diagnostic method for typhoid fever by utilizing the agglutination of the typhoid bacillus with the serum of typhoid patients. Shiga applied the Widal method to dysentery. Having succeeded in observing an agglutination of the suspected organism with the serum of dysentery patients, he became confident that it was the bacillus causing dysentery. The findings were published in a Japanese journal in December 1897.

In addition to the discovery, Shiga reported the results of his experiments with dysentery vaccine. He had injected a dose of sterilized culture solution into himself. While suffering a severe suppuration around the site of the injection, he was optimistic about its immunological efficacy in his first report. The suppuration needed an incision, and its scar remained on his back for life; Shiga was proud of his 'honorable scar'. He subsequently developed a serum-based vaccine, and then an oral vaccine. The latter was refined and administered to many people in Japan from the mid-1920s. Nevertheless, Shiga had by this time lost his initial optimism; the epidemic was still fierce in the 1930s in Japan, and he pointed out the danger of relying too much on vaccines in the control of dysentery.

The German version of Shiga's report was published in a German journal in 1898. In 1899, on his way to the Philippines, Simon Flexner (1863–1946) of Johns Hopkins University called at the IID in Tokyo, where he was shown cultures of Shiga's bacillus. In the following year, Flexner endorsed Shiga's discovery in Manila by himself isolating the same bacillus. But not everyone easily accepted the discovery that had taken place in the Far East. Walther Kruse (1864–1943) of Bonn University insisted in 1900 that he himself should be the true discoverer of the dysentery bacillus. He denied Shiga's achievement, arguing that Shiga's descriptions did not match the bacillus he isolated, with regard to its motility, the form of colonization, and the degree of Widal reactions. Shiga confronted Kruse face to face at an international conference held in Hamburg in

1901, but they failed to settle their disagreements. In 1902 an international investigation committee was organized under the initiative of Robert Koch (1843–1910) to settle the controversy, which concluded that Shiga and Kruse had described the same bacillus, and therefore that Shiga should be regarded as the first discoverer of the dysentery bacillus. It is now commonly called *Shigella dysenteriae*, but sometimes the Shiga-Kruse bacillus.

While leaving an emotional discord between the two, the Shiga-Kruse controversy prompted further research leading to the knowledge that the dysentery bacillus could take more than one form. Apart from *S. dysenteriae* (Group A, by modern classification), different types of *Shigella* were identified in the early twentieth century by Kruse (the Kruse-Sonne bacillus, or *Shigella sonnei*, Group D), Flexner (*Shigella flexneri*, Group B) and some other researchers.

Chemotherapy

When Shiga met Kruse in Hamburg, he was on his way to the Institute for Experimental Therapy in Frankfurt to study under its director, Paul Ehrlich (1854–1915). Ehrlich and Kitasato had been colleagues at the Koch Institute in Berlin, and the choice of Frankfurt indicates that Shiga, and Kitasato who advised him, were aware that bacteriology needed new innovations. The golden age of bacteria hunting was winding down. It was also becoming clear that serotherapy had its limits. Shiga, guided by Kitasato, shifted his attention to the application of chemistry to biological sciences that Ehrlich had been pursuing.

Shiga arrived in Ehrlich's Institute in November 1901, when Ehrlich set about the development of chemotherapy. Ehrlich at first instructed Shiga to list the microbicidal effects of aniline dyes on bacteria. Shiga later confessed that, while repeating the testing of various dyes on different bacteria day by day, he was, at this stage, not quite sure how these simple experiments were relevant to chemotherapy. Only Ehrlich knew what he was doing. Then, in December 1902, Shiga was instructed to test anilines on *Trypanosoma*, the parasite causing African sleeping sickness, or trypanosomiasis, which had been discovered earlier that year. Now Shiga realized that tests on bacteria were preparations for those on protozoa, which had compositions that are more complex.

He examined the effect of hundreds of dyes on *Trypanosomes*, first in test tubes and then in mice. After nearly a year of diligent work, he finally found a dye that eliminated the parasite without affecting the host. The dye was named trypan-red. In April 1904 the findings were published under the joint names of Ehrlich and Shiga. Trypan-red was developed into a medicine for clinical use in 1906.

During his stay in Frankfurt (1902–04), Shiga thus made remarkable contributions by assisting Ehrlich in marking the first step toward the establishment of chemotherapy. He was followed by Hata Sahachirō (1873–1938), a fellow member of the Kitasato school, who assisted Ehrlich

in developing Salvarsan in 1909. Shiga had an opportunity to study again at Ehrlich's Institute from 1911 to 1912. He looked up to Ehrlich as his other lifelong mentor alongside Kitasato, and published a biography (in Japanese) of Ehrlich in 1940.

Later Life

Shiga returned to Tokyo from Frankfurt in January 1905. At the IID, he was the chief officer of its serum division. He was in charge not only of research, but also of the production of sera and vaccines. Nationalized in 1899, the IID had a monopoly on serum and vaccine products in the country. In addition to its main products such as smallpox vaccine, tuberculin, and diphtheria and tetanus sera, Shiga and his colleagues also developed several other products, including those for dysentery.

Right after his return Shiga undertook a study on beri-beri, or *kakke*, in view of the high incidence of the disease among soldiers during the Russo-Japanese War (1904–05). The protracted controversy since the 1880s over the causes of *kakke* had not yet reached a conclusion. While naval medical officers suspected an unbalanced intake of nutriments, army and Tokyo University doctors insisted on beri-beri's infectiousness. Shiga started his research from a neutral standpoint, but later advocated a nutriment theory based on his own experiments. In the meantime, his pursuit of chemotherapy was suspended, partly because chemical materials were not freely available in Japan at that time. During his second visit to Ehrlich's Institute (1911–12), he started working on chemotherapy for tuberculosis, but did not see much success.

Shiga knew that research was his forte, but circumstances did not allow him to stick only to research. In 1914, when the government forced an organizational restructuring of the IID, Kitasato, in protest, resigned as its director. Behind this was a factional conflict between the medical faculty of the University of Tokyo and the Kitasato school. Shiga was inevitably involved in the turmoil, and although the government expected him to lead the Institute after Kitasato's resignation, he chose to follow his mentor. Shiga joined the establishment of the Kitasato Institute, and took charge of its serum and vaccine division as he had at the IID.

Kitasato tried to secure the influence of his school not only within Japan, but also in Japan's colonial territories. In 1920 Shiga, complying with Kitasato's request, went to Korea to serve as the director of the (Japanese) Colonial Government Hospital of Korea. When the Keijō (Seoul) Imperial University was founded in 1926, Shiga became the dean of its medical school. In 1929 he was appointed president of the University and became swamped by administrative work, which was not his forte. In October 1931, he resigned before the term of his office expired. This came four months after the death of Kitasato, toward whom

Shiga never lost his feelings of gratitude. Shiga returned to his research life in the Kitasato Institute.

Shiga and his wife, Ichiko, were blessed with four sons and four daughters. But the family experienced great sorrow during the war years. In 1944 Ichiko died of stomach cancer. As he was en route to his mother's funeral, the boat of Shiga's eldest son, Naoshi, was sunk by a torpedo attack. Naoshi was a professor of medicine at the Taihoku (Taipei) Imperial University. Torn by grief, Shiga evacuated to a village called Isohama near Sendai City, his birthplace, as Tokyo was threatened by increasingly fierce air raid attacks.

After the war, Shiga stayed in Isohama and lived quietly in retirement, while maintaining his keen interest in, and keeping his observant eyes on, infectious disease research and policies. He died at his home in Isohama in January 1957.

Bibliography

Primary: 1936. 'The Trend of Prevention, Therapy, and Epidemiology of Dysentery since the Discovery of Its Causative Organism.' *New England Journal of Medicine* 215: 1205–1211; 1966. *Aru saikingakusha no kaiso* [A memoir of a bacteriologist] (Tokyo).

Secondary: Trofa, Andrew F., H. Ueno-Olsen, R. Oiwa, and M. Yoshikawa, 1999. 'Dr. Kiyoshi Shiga: Discoverer of the Dysentery Bacillus.' *Clinical Infectious Diseases* 29: 1303–1306; Nagaki, Taizo, 1989. *Kitasato Shibasaburo to sono ichimon* [Kitazato Shibasaburo and his disciples] (Tokyo); Takahashi, Isao, 1957. *Shiga Kiyoshi* (Tokyo).

Takeshi Nagashima

SHIPPEN, WILLIAM, Jr (b. Philadelphia, Pennsylvania, USA, 21 October 1736, d. Philadelphia, 11 July 1808), *anatomy, medical education, surgery.*

Shippen was the son of William Shippen, Sr., a distinguished Philadelphia physician, and Susannah Harrison, both Presbyterians. He was the great grandson of the first mayor of Philadelphia (founded in 1681) and the nephew of the Chief Justice of Philadelphia. Shippen prepared at West Nottingham Academy, in Colora, Maryland, for the College of New Jersey (later, Princeton University), receiving his BA in 1754. For the next four years, he was apprenticed in medicine to his father.

In 1758 Shippen sailed for Great Britain to further his medical education, as did many of the other sons of the Philadelphia establishment. In London, he studied anatomy under John and William Hunter, even living in their home for eight months. For midwifery, he attended the lectures of Colin Mackenzie. Shippen also 'walked the wards' at St Thomas's, Guy's, and St George's hospitals and observed Percival Pott perform surgical procedures at St Bartholomew's Hospital. During these two years, he became friends with John Fothergill, a great friend of the Colonies. Fothergill later provided him with anatomical specimens for Pennsylvania Hospital, upon his return to

Philadelphia. Possibly, there were discussions about the sorry state of medical education in the colonies.

By 1760 Shippen had gone to Edinburgh to take the course in medicine, where he heard the lectures of Alexander Monro *primus* on anatomy and William Cullen on the principles of medicine. Shippen received his MD degree in September 1761 with his dissertation 'An Anatomico-Medical Dissertation on the Connection of the Placenta with the Uterus'. He then returned briefly to London, before wintering in France, and was back in Philadelphia in May 1762.

On 16 November 1762 he initiated a course of lectures on anatomy at the State House (now Independence Hall). Fothergill's plaster models and drawings had just arrived at Pennsylvania Hospital, and Shippen set to work, utilizing them in his lectures both in his private anatomy school and at the hospital. In addition to anatomy, Shippen also taught midwifery.

By 1765 John Morgan, who also had been studying in London and Edinburgh (MD, 1763), had returned home. On 3 May 1765 Morgan was named professor of theory and practice of medicine at the College of Philadelphia. Shippen was visibly disturbed because he thought he had earlier conceived of the idea of a medical school. Jealousy would continue between the two for many years until Morgan's death in 1789, and often Benjamin Rush entered into the fray. In September 1765 Shippen petitioned the Board of Trustees and on 23 September was named professor of anatomy and surgery at the College of Philadelphia. He delivered the inaugural lecture on anatomy on 14 November 1765. Shippen's course seems to have been almost identical to the lectures he had heard in Europe, with Shippen apparently adding very little if anything to them of his own experience.

Over the next decade, the school seemed to have grown, and Morgan and Shippen tolerated one another. Shippen had been chosen to give the charge (speech) to the first graduating class of eight in June 1768. With war almost imminent, Morgan resigned from the faculty in 1775 to take up the post of director general and chief physician of the medical department of the American army. By the time war was declared in 1776, Shippen had been appointed on July 15 to the Flying Camp in New Jersey under Morgan. The following year, Morgan was removed from office, and Shippen was named director general. Equanimity was short-lived: Shippen himself was accused of impropriety during the next four years, with Benjamin Rush being involved. Shippen was acquitted of all charges in two court-martials.

Most educational endeavors, like other activities in Philadelphia, were abruptly halted during the war. When the British troops finally left Philadelphia, the College of Philadelphia was reorganized in 1780 as the University of the State of Pennsylvania, later becoming the University of Pennsylvania. Shippen was once again appointed professor of anatomy and surgery and continued in this capacity in active teaching until 1806, even adding the chair of midwifery to his charge. He seems also to have been responsible for some of the design of Surgeons' Hall, the first medical school building in the United States.

Shippen was a prominent physician in Philadelphia, serving on the staff of the Pennsylvania Hospital from 1778 to 1802. He was elected to the American Philosophical Society in 1777 and was one of the founders of the College of Physicians of Philadelphia in 1787, for which he served as president from 1805 until his death.

During the 1790s Philadelphia was the capital of the new United States of America. George Washington and John Adams were among the prominent people to dine and even lodge at Shippen's home. In 1798 he gave up his practice and began spending most of his time in his country home in Germantown. His first love was likely teaching, which he continued to do for another ten years. His later life was much quieter, as his wife and their remaining daughter (there were eight children) withdrew from society. Shippen may be remembered for his teaching skills, but he wrote little for the fledgling scientific press.

Bibliography

Secondary: Blake, J. B., 1974. 'The Anatomical Lectures of William Shippen, 1766.' *Trans. Stud. Coll. Physicians Philadelphia* 42: 61–66; Parish, L. C., and T. N. Haviland, 1965. 'Surgeons' Hall: the Story of the First Medical-school Building in the United States.' *New England Journal of Medicine* 273: 1021–1024; Olch, P. D., 1965. 'The Morgan-Shippen Controversy: A Commentary on the Birth of Medical Education in America.' *Review of Surgery* 22: 1–8; Corner, George W., 1965. *Two Centuries of Medicine: A History of the School of Medicine, University of Pennsylvania* (Philadelphia); Corner, George W., 1951. *William Shippen, Jr., Pioneer in American Medical Education: A Biographical Essay. With Notes and the Original Text of Shippen's Student Diary, London, 1759–60; Together with a Translation of His Edinburgh Dissertation, 1761* (Philadelphia); *DAMB*.

Lawrence Charles Parish

SHUKLA, JAGANNATH PRASAD (PANDIT) (b. Allahabad, India, *c.* 1885; d. ?, *c.* 1945), *vaid, ayurvedic medicine.*

Shukla was an ayurvedic practitioner born into a family of upper caste and reputed *pandits*, or traditional intellectuals. He was almost single-handedly responsible for initiating the revival of the Ayurved Sammelan, or Congress, in North India, a largely moribund corporate body of ayurvedic practitioners. After 1910 Shukla and a coterie of North Indian ayurvedic practitioners initiated an aggressive campaign that projected the role of the Ayurved Sammelan among a Hindi-speaking middle class in the North Indian heartland of the British United Provinces. They secured the Sammelan's influence in regulating institutionalized ayurvedic education and practice, and negotiated its claims to speak on behalf of their community with the British colonial government.

Shukla, in his polemical writings (in Hindi), responded to the introduction of the Medical Registration Act of 1911, which he perceived as indirectly affecting the status and practice of ayurvedic medicine. He campaigned to give the Ayurved Sammelan a distinct, Hindu identity, and cultivated wealthy urban Hindu patrons so as to make it a force independent from the All India Vaid and Yunani Tibb Conference, a group of Hindu/Muslim practitioners led by the renowned unani practitioner and nationalist leader, Hakīm Ajmal Khān.

Shukla was also closely associated with movements supporting Hindi revival, and was well known among Hindi literary figures and publicists of his era. Deploying many of these networks to sustain the Ayurved Sammelan, he pioneered a campaign that publicized ayurvedic professional interests by mobilizing an emerging Hindi-language vernacular press, and associating ayurvedic revival with Hindu nationalist concerns. For his contribution to the cause of Hindi through his writings, and his support for projects to print ayurvedic texts in popular forms, he received the title of Hindi Kesari. His contribution allowed a later generation of practitioners such as Pandit Shiv Sharma to project ayurveda as a unified, Hindu cultural-political tradition.

Bibliography

Primary: [References to Jagannath Prasad Shukla and his ayurvedic writings are available in the form of articles and editorials in issues of the Hindi journal *Sudhanidhi* (Allahabad), 1912–1935. See especially *Sudhanidhi*, 1912, 2: 169; 1928, 19: 8–14].

Secondary: Sivaramakrishnan, Kavita, 2006. *Old Potions New Bottles: Recasting Indigenous Medicine in Colonial Punjab* (Delhi).

Kavita Sivaramakrishnan

SHUTTLEWORTH, JAMES PHILLIP KAY- (b. Rochdale, Lancashire, England, 20 July 1804; d. London, England, 26 May 1877), *public health.*

Born as James Phillip Kay into a devout Calvinistic family, Shuttleworth was intended for a career in the cotton trade. Yet, after education at a private grammar school in Salford and a period in banking, he eventually gained permission to study medicine at Edinburgh, where he completed his MD thesis on asphyxia in warm-blooded animals in 1827. This challenged the work of the French anatomist and physiologist Marie-François-Xavier Bichat (1771–1802) and won him the attention of the physician William Pulteney Alison (1790–1859), for whom he worked as clerk. Alison publicized Kay's research in his own papers and helped to secure him a position at Edinburgh's New Town Dispensary—his first insight into the lives and health of the poor.

Kay was increasingly interested in social, economic, and political issues and came to see poverty and illness as determined by these factors rather than individual personal failings. After his early training in Edinburgh, he moved to Manchester, by 1828 already an overcrowded town in which it proved hard to make a medical living. He lacked personal contacts and capital, but managed to establish a reputation based partly on his literary skills (he was a founding editor of the *North of England Medical and Surgical Journal*, 1830). He was one of the founders of the Ardwick and Ancoats Dispensary (1828) and served on the local board of health and at Knott Hill Cholera Hospital during the 1832 cholera outbreak.

Kay began to document his experiences of working with the poor, publishing a widely read pamphlet, *The Moral and Physical Condition of the Working Classes Employed in the Cotton Manufacture in Manchester* (1832). In the development of theories on sanitary reform, he was a proponent of the use of new social science techniques. He helped to establish the Manchester Statistical Society (1833), the first such society in England. However, he was not fully accepted into Manchester's social or medical elite: a marriage proposal to the daughter of a wealthy cotton merchant was rejected, and both his attempts to be elected as an honorary physician to the Manchester Infirmary failed, despite the publication of his work *The Physiology, Pathology and Treatment of Asphyxia* (1834), for which he was later awarded the Fothergillian medal by the Royal Humane Society.

Kay left Manchester, never to practice medicine again, but found employment in East Anglia as a Poor Law commissioner. Here he developed his interest in education, which was recognized nationally by his appointment in 1839 as assistant secretary to the Privy Council's education committee. He was a consummate civil servant, and he used his base to progress his own interests in both public health and education. He worked closely with Edwin Chadwick (1800–90) and established a successful inspectorial partnership with Neil Arnott (1788–1874) and Thomas Southwood Smith (1788–1861) on the Royal Sanitary Commission (1839).

In 1839 Kay became a key member of the team, which steered the course of sanitary reform in Britain for the next decade. His medical and literary skills were useful to Chadwick in preparing the seminal 1842 *Report on the Sanitary Condition of the Labouring Population of Great Britain*. He had also progressed socially, marrying into the titled Shuttleworth family of Gawthorpe Hall, Lancashire (1842), on the condition that he add Shuttleworth to his own family name of Kay.

However, the stress of civil service work and his failure to be fully accepted into the intellectual and political circles in London affected his health. Following an epileptic fit while at work (1848), he was effectively marginalized, and he resigned with a baronetcy (1849). He was subsequently estranged from his wife, and although he attempted to develop a political career and to enter Parliament, his last years were devoted to managing his estate and writing.

Bibliography

Primary: 1832. *The Moral and Physical Condition of the Working Classes Employed in the Cotton Manufacture in Manchester* (Manchester); 1963. (Bloomfield, B. C., ed.) *Autobiography of Sir James Kay-Shuttleworth* (London).

Secondary: Selleck, R. J. W., 1994. *James Kay-Shuttleworth: Journey of an Outsider* (Woburn); Smith, F., 1923. *The Life and Work of Sir James Kay-Shuttleworth* (London); *Oxford DNB*.

Sally Sheard

SIEBOLD, PHILLIP FRANZ BALTHASAR VON   (b. Würzburg, Germany, 17 February 1796; d. Munich, Germany, 18 October 1866), *parasitology, medical education.*

Phillip Franz Balthasar von Siebold was the first son of Johan George Christoph von Siebold (1767–98), a professor of medicine at the University of Würzburg, and his wife Maria. Because of the early death of his father in 1798, young Siebold was cared for by a maternal uncle. In 1815 Siebold entered the University of Würzburg to study medicine. Here he studied natural history and ethnology under the influence of Ignaz Doellinger (1770–1841), a professor of anatomy, and developed a romantic yearning for exploring the natural history of little-known regions. In 1820 he graduated from the university with an MD, and had himself appointed as a naval surgeon to the Dutch East India Company. He started to work in Batavia in 1822, from where he was appointed a doctor in Dejima, or the Dutch factory in Nagasaki. For Siebold, this appointment was a fulfillment of his ambition. For the Dutch government, this highly motivated German doctor fit very well with its new diplomatic strategy of promoting medical, scientific, and natural history exchanges with Japan in order to boost trade, which had gone through a serious decline during the turmoil of the Napoleonic Wars.

Siebold arrived in Nagasaki in August 1823 at the age of twenty-eight. During the following eight years of his stay, he established a lasting influence upon the Japanese medical and natural scientific community. At the request of the Dutch government, the Japanese governor at Nagasaki granted Siebold special permission to go beyond Dejima, to collect medicinal plants outside the factory and to treat patients at the houses of Japanese interpreters in Nagasaki. Admittedly, these were few openings for exchanging scientific ideas, but both Siebold and the Japanese voraciously exploited the occasions. Patients flocked to Siebold for treatment, especially for surgical and ophthalmologic ailments. Medical practitioners, whose appetite for Western medicine had been whetted by Sugita Genpaku's *Kaitai shinsho* [A New Book on Anatomy] (1774) and other works, were attracted to the chance of observing Siebold's bold operations on difficult cases.

High demand encouraged Siebold to open his own private medical school in 1824 at Narutaki in Nagasaki, known as Narutaki-juku. In this and other places, Siebold taught in total around sixty individuals, among whom Takano Chōei (1804–50), Mima Junzō (1807–37), Kō Ryōkai (1799–1839), and Oka Kenkai (1799–1839) were most famous. In return for lessons in medicine and the Dutch language, the students collected material for Siebold's natural history research of Japan. Siebold's journey to Edo in 1826 stirred a chain reaction of excitement among Japanese scholars, who brought information, specimens, and artifacts to the German natural historian. In return, Siebold gave them medicines, instruments and other curiosities. Siebold's voracious passion for collecting cost him dearly, however. A naval accident revealed that he attempted to bring back maps of Japan, which was strictly prohibited under the seclusion policy. Under house arrest for more than a year in Dejima, Siebold was tried, found guilty, and sentenced to forced repatriation in 1830. Many individuals who had contact with him were also tried and punished.

Upon Siebold's return, the government of the Netherlands provided him with ample facilities to work on his collection. Major works on Japan soon started to appear, such as *Nippon* (1832–58), *Fauna Japonica* (1833–50), and *Flora Japonica* (1835–44). They established Siebold's place as the first and greatest Japanologist in Europe. Between 1859 and 1863, Siebold made his second stay in Japan, first as an adviser to the newly founded Dutch Trading Company, and later as an adviser to the Shogunate on political and diplomatic matters. Although he wished for a third visit through the influence of Napoleon III of France, Siebold died in Munich in 1864.

Bibliography

Primary: 1832–1858. *Nippon* 5 vols. (Leiden).

Secondary: Kure, Shūzō, 1926. *Siebold sensei: sono shōgai oyobi kōgyō* (*Doctor Siebold: His Life and Works*) [German trans., 1996 *Philipp Franz von Siebold—Leben und Werk* (Munich)].

Akihito Suzuki

SIMON, JOHN (b. City of London, England, 10 October 1816; d. Kensington, London, England, 23 July 1904), *pathology, surgery, public health.*

Simon was the sixth child of Louis Michael Simon and Mathilde Nonnet. He was educated in Pentonville and Greenwich and spent some time in Germany before being apprenticed to Joseph Henry Green (1791–1863), who was surgeon at St Thomas's Hospital and King's College. In 1838 he became MRCS, and he became demonstrator in anatomy at King's College in the following year and then senior assistant surgeon at King's College Hospital when it opened (1840). He held the post at King's until 1853 and remained at St Thomas's until 1876, becoming a surgeon in 1863. In the 1840s Simon built up a private practice and enjoyed a reputation as a pathological investigator. He was awarded the first Astley-Cooper prize (1844) for an essay on the thymus gland (published 1845) and was elected FRS (1847) at only thirty-one years of age for his work on the thyroid gland. In 1850 he published his lectures on pathology, the same year in which he was a founding member of

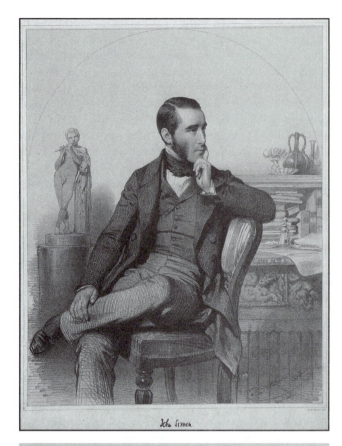

Sir John Simon. Lithograph by C. Baugniet, 1848. Iconographic Collection, Wellcome Library, London.

the Epidemiological Society of London. As well as being active in metropolitan medical and scientific circles, Simon was also interested in philosophic and artistic subjects and mixed in that company, numbering among his friends John Ruskin (1819–1900), Charles Kingsley (1819–75) and the pre-Raphaelites.

Although he remained a distinguished surgeon and pathologist, it was for his work in public health that Simon was and is best known. He was appointed to the post of Medical Officer of Health for the City of London in 1848 and in 1854 became Medical Officer to the Privy Council—effectively the chief medical officer for England and Wales and one of the most powerful positions ever held by a medical man in Britain. In the latter role, which he held until 1876, he was head of a small but influential government department, a leading advocate of public health reform, and in effect the sanitary conscience of the nation. The reports that came from his department defined and exposed sanitary deficiencies and set out what could and should be done to improve the nation's health. He became a leading authority on all aspects of public health and its leading theorist between the eras of Chadwickian sanitarianism of the early Victorian period and the bacteriologically informed preventive medicine of the late nineteenth century.

It appears that Simon gained the position of Medical Officer to the City of London in 1848 through family connections (his father was a stockbroker), rather than because of any qualifications in sanitary science, though he was already a member of the Health of Towns Association. It may be that he was seen as an insider who could be trusted to resist the centralizing impulses of Edwin Chadwick (1800–90) and the recently formed General Board of Health (GBH). There was no brief for the post, so Simon defined his own role and quickly deployed one of the trademarks of sanitarianism—the shaming report of poor local conditions, which were linked to ignorance and neglect at all levels of society. One of his first initiatives was to develop systems to collect and collate mortality data and then to publish information on overcrowding, water supply, waste and sewage disposal, burials, and food adulterations. The press picked up his reports and he used the existing legislation on nuisances to provide services to homes and businesses, and to improve the condition of streets. He became the first president of the Association of Metropolitan Medical Officers of Health (1855).

Simon's new expertise was recognized when he was appointed by the government to report on the national cholera epidemic of 1853–54 and when he was offered the post of medical officer to the new, sans-Chadwick GBH in 1854. At first this was a temporary position, but it was made permanent (1858) when responsibility for sanitary affairs was transferred to the Privy Council. The following year, he published a report summarizing all of the GBH inquiries into the cholera epidemics of 1848–49 and 1853–54, in which he gave prominence to John Snow's (1813–58) water-borne theory. However, Simon resisted any exclusive explanation of the epidemics and saw polluted water as one factor among many in allowing the spread of the disease. In 1857 he published a volume on smallpox vaccination detailing the value of the practice, which his department had oversight of, but which was administered locally by Poor Law Guardians. In the following year, Simon introduced Edward Greenhow's *Report on the Sanitary State of the People of England*, which focused on the environmental factors that produced 'excess' mortalities in particular areas and among specific social groups.

The new Privy Council Department had relatively limited powers given that sanitary legislation tended to be enabling, with local authorities and local boards of health left to be responsible for voluntary implementation. It was also relatively small, and hence much depended on Simon's energy, initiatives, and political maneuvering. Simon was an effective lobbyist internally and externally, with influential friends and the means, through the press and his reports, to get his views into the public domain. His department had specific statutory responsibilities for vaccination, the control of epidemics and quarantines, and the Medical Act of 1858, but also had a wider brief to respond to health issues as they arose. Simon worked first to strengthen the position of public vaccinators and to tighten the vaccination legislation, with improvements in administrative and technical procedures and with greater compulsion introduced in successive Acts. However, it was the inquiries into local epidemics and specific disease problems between 1859 and 1872 for which the Department became best known. Simon used his metropolitan connections to attract a cadre of part-time investigators who were sent around the country to research and report on issues raised by the public, the politicians, or the medical profession. Many of these reports enjoyed a high political profile—for example, the inquiries into dangerous trades (1862–63), hospitals (1863), and housing (1865)—whereas others dealt with specific epidemics such as cholera in 1865–66 and smallpox in 1871. The Department also steered through the Sanitary Act 1866 and the Pharmacy Act 1868. In 1867 Simon initiated scientific investigations, commissioning laboratory work on the pathology and etiology of infectious diseases, employing John Burdon Sanderson (1828–1905), J. L. W. Thudicum (1829–1901), and E. E. Klein (1844–1925) among others. Simon promoted the new ideas on specific contagia and the narrowing of the etiological focus of sanitary interventions, but he had doubts about their practical value. His continuing commitment to sanitarianism was evident in reservations he expressed about the new ideas in 1867: 'Nowhere out of Laputa could there be serious thought of differentiating excremental performances into groups of diarrheal and healthy, or of using the highest powers of the microscope to identify the cylindro-taenium for extermination. It is excrement, indiscriminately, which must be kept from fouling us with its decay.'

The continued weakness of central departments and diversity of local provision in all manner of public services led the government to establish a Royal Commission to report on the local government in the late 1860s. The result was the creation of the Local Government Board (1872), which effectively merged the Medical Department with the national Poor Law Board. Simon was very unhappy with the proposal, feeling that what was needed was a national 'Ministry of Health' separate from the local structures, concerns, and mentality of the Poor Law. His fears were realized by the operation of the Local Government Board under James Stansfield, and relations between the two men became increasingly difficult. Simon soldiered on for four years but resigned in 1876. He remained bitter about this turn of events and at what he considered had been a missed opportunity to create institutions that would have improved the health of the nation; indeed, in his book *English Sanitary Institutions* (1890), ostensibly a survey of English public health but in fact a sustained attack on recent reforms, he wrote that the creation of the LGB had been 'virtually a policy of retreat'.

In retirement Simon continued to be active in metropolitan medical institutions and continued commenting and publishing on various aspects of public health. He was elected president of the RCS (1878), having been previously a council member and vice president. He also became the Crown member of the General Medical Council, serving from 1879 to 1895. He was awarded the Harben Medal of the Royal Institute of Public Health (1896) and the Buchanan Medal of the Royal Society (1897). He was elected CB on his retirement and knighted (1887). He died at home in Kensington Square and was buried at Ladywell Cemetery, Lewisham, London.

Bibliography

Primary: 1845. *A Physiological Essay on the Thymus Gland* (London); 1850. *General pathology as conducive to the establishment of rational principles for the diagnosis and treatment of disease* (London); 1858. *Papers relating to the Sanitary State of the People of England* (London); 1887. (Seaton, E., ed.) *John Simon, public health reports* (London); 1890. *English Sanitary Institutions* (London); 1894. *Personal Recollections of Sir John Simon* (London).

Secondary: Lambert, R., 1963. *Sir John Simon, 1816–1904, and English Social Administration* (London); Sanderson, J. Burdon, 1905. 'Sir John Simon, 1816–1904' *Proceedings of the Royal Society of London* 75: 336–346; *Oxford DNB*.

Michael Worboys

SIMOND, PAUL-LOUIS (b. Beaufort-sur-Gervanne, Drôme, France, 30 July 1858; d. Valence, Drôme, France, 3 March 1947), *medicine, bacteriology.*

Simond, the son of a French Protestant clergyman, completed secondary studies at Tournon, then became a laboratory technician at the Bordeaux Faculty of Medicine and Pharmacy (1878–82) before entering the French Navy's School of Medicine there in 1882. He wrote a prizewinning medical thesis in 1887 on leprosy in French Guyana, where he had been posted for two years. Until 1894, as a Naval physician, he attended to colonial troops in postings ranging from French Guyana to Indochina to the Chinese coast. Simond's career changed dramatically after he took the Pasteur Institute of Paris's course in bacteriology (1895–96) where he was assigned to the laboratory of Elie Mechnikov.

In 1897–98 the Pasteur Institute sent him to India to relieve Alexandre Yersin and continue the latter's program of administering the Pasteur antiplague serum to Indian patients. In 1898 Simond developed his flea transmission theory after he noticed that a small blisterlike lesion, called a phlyctena, was usually found on the foot or leg of Indian plague patients. In his makeshift laboratory he found organisms resembling *Y. pestis* in the stomach of fleas that had fed on infected rats. Simond next sought to transmit the disease by feeding fleas on infected rats and then healthy ones. Using a small number of laboratory animals at his disposal, he succeeded in four trials and failed in two. The *Annales de l'Institut Pasteur* published his article in 1898, stating boldly that the bite of rat fleas constituted the mode of infection for both rats and humans. Elated at his discovery, he could not resist remarking that he 'had uncovered a secret that had tortured man since the appearance of plague in the world' (1898, p. 83).

Luminaries such as Robert Koch and Patrick Manson were partial to Simond's theory but wanted more evidence. They formed a small minority. Experts on the German and Indian plague commissions disregarded the flea theory and held that, while rats were important for initial outbreaks, thereafter human agency played the greater role in spreading disease. Not until the second Indian Plague Commission of 1905 conducted its own field and laboratory experiments did Simond begin to receive scientific credit. It took a further three years before the conservative Indian Medical Service finally accepted the flea's role in plague transmission.

From India Simond went to Indochina where he was named director of the Pasteur Institute's branch in Saigon, a post he held from 1898 to 1900. His next Pasteurian assignment took him to Brazil (1901–05) with Emile Marchoux and Alexandre Salimbeni as a three-man team assigned to study the yellow fever control methods of Oswaldo Cruz in Rio de Janeiro. Simond was also able to apply these methods between 1908 and 1909 in Martinique, one of France's possessions in the Caribbean.

Simond's next foreign secondment was Constantinople (1911–13), where he served as director of the Ottoman Imperial Institute of Bacteriology. During World War I Simond was director of Health Services for the French Colonial Army in Indochina, but in 1917 a falling-out with military authorities caused him to resign his military commission.

In retirement Simond returned to his native department of Drôme, serving in the town of Valence as the mayor's advisor on tuberculosis. He remained there until his death in 1947. Too often neglected in general medical histories, Simond deserves a place beside his fellow Pastorian Alexandre Yersin in the history of bubonic plague.

Bibliography

Primary: 1898. 'La propagation de la peste.' *Annales de l'Institut Pasteur* 12: 625–687.

Secondary: Crawford, Edward A., 1996. 'Paul-Louis Simond and His Work on Plague.' *Perspectives in Biology and Medicine* 39: 446–458.

Myron Echenberg

SIMPSON, JAMES YOUNG (b. Bathgate, Scotland, 7 June 1811; d. Edinburgh, Scotland, 6 May 1870), *obstetrics, anesthesia.*

Simpson was the youngest son of David Simpson and Mary Jarvey, bakers in the village of Bathgate. He attended the local parish school and was sent to Edinburgh University at the age of fourteen (1825), entering the faculty of medicine in 1827. In addition to the official teaching, Simpson attended the lectures given by the surgeon Robert Liston (1794–1847). His MD thesis on the process of inflammation, submitted in 1832, got Simpson a job as assistant to the professor of pathology, John Thomson. He spent three years teaching pathology to medical students and, after a tour of the Paris hospitals (1835), was appointed to the Edinburgh City Lying-In Hospital. Here he began to research and, from 1839, to teach obstetrics. In the summer of 1839, he was appointed professor of midwifery, and in December he married Jessie Grindlay, his cousin.

In December 1846 Liston demonstrated ether anesthesia for surgery at University College Hospital, London. Simpson, already interested in the problem of obstetric pain, began to experiment with ether and in January 1847 used it for the first time in labor. During the summer of 1847, he used ether frequently and designed an inhaler. By the autumn, however, he had begun to realize the toxicity of ether, and in November he used chloroform for the first time. In 1850, at the age of thirty-nine, he was elected president of the RCPEdin. Simpson became the public proponent of anesthesia in labor and defended the technique against religious and traditionalist opposition. Much of this opposition was quieted when John Snow (1813–58) administered chloroform to Queen Victoria during the birth of her eighth child in 1853.

Simpson continued to develop his obstetric practice throughout the 1840s and 1850s, making many technical innovations. In *Accupressure* (1864) he described a way of preventing surgical hemorrhage by pressure on ruptured blood vessels. His method was not itself a success, but the book was praised for its discussion of the role of blood flow in wound healing.

Simpson's later career was dominated by his work on hospital infection. He came to the problem through his work on puerperal sepsis, and in 1850 he proposed that both surgical and puerperal sepsis were caused by 'materia morbi' carried on the hands of physicians. Transmission of sepsis could be prevented by regular hand-washing, but on a broader level, Simpson believed that the prevalence of hospital infections reflected the poor design of large hospitals—a problem he termed 'hospitalism'. He argued for the breaking down of metropolitan hospitals into smaller units, where hygiene could be maintained more easily. For this reason he opposed Joseph Lister's (1827–1912) antiseptic method, arguing that the problem of hospital infection was better solved by improving the design of wards. He put some of his ideas into practice when he was involved in planning the medical services for the Crimean War: through this he came to influence Florence Nightingale (1820–1910) in her campaign for improvements in hospital conditions. In 1866 Simpson was created baronet, one of the first physicians to receive this honor.

Accounts of Simpson's career are frequently dominated by his work on obstetric anesthesia, and it was this that made him famous. His innovations as an obstetrician and his campaign for hospital reform, though they received less publicity, were central to the improvement of hospital conditions and the status of hospital medicine.

Bibliography

Primary: 1850. 'On the analogy between puerperal fever and surgical fever.' *Monthly Journal of Medical Science* 10: 414; 1864. *Acupressure* (Edinburgh).

Secondary: Moscucci, Ornella, 1990. *The Science of Woman: Gynaecology and Gender in England, 1800–1929* (Oxford); Duncum, Barbara M., 1994. *The Development of Inhalation Anaesthesia* (London); Simpson, Myrtle, 1972. *Simpson the Obstetrician: A Biography* (London); *Oxford DNB*.

Richard Barnett

SIMS, J(AMES) MARION   (b. Lancaster County, South Carolina, USA, 25 January 1813; d. New York, New York, USA, 13 November 1883), *gynecology.*

Sims was the son of Jack Sims, semiliterate farmer and storekeeper, and Mahala Mackey. He received a BA from South Carolina College (1832), spent one year at the Medical College of South Carolina, and graduated MD (1835) from Jefferson Medical College.

After a disappointing general practice in his hometown, he moved to Mount Meigs, Alabama, but remained dissatisfied with his professional progress. In 1840 he settled in Montgomery.

Sims's reputation as the 'father of gynecology' derives from his operation for vesicovaginal fistulae, a horrendous condition for women who had suffered severe damage in prolonged or badly managed childbirth. The condition came to his attention when three young slave women, known only as Ararcha, Betsey, and Lucy, were referred to him by masters who wanted their slaves restored to plantation labor. Initially dismayed by what seemed an impossible task, Sims recognized that a metal spoon fashioned as a speculum would enable him to see the upper part of the vagina and perhaps to repair the torn bladder.

For the next four years he experimented on the three women and several other slaves whom he maintained in a so-called hospital. Despite repeated failures and the agony of his patients, he refused to quit. Success came when Sims began using silver wire sutures tightened with perforated lead shot, thereby eliminating disintegration of silk sutures.

Sims believed he had made one of the most important discoveries of the age for relief of suffering humanity, and most of his biographers agreed. He has since been criticized for exploiting slave women who had no say in their treatment and who were forced to endure pain and humiliation in multiple operations conducted without anesthesia.

For the next three years, Sims was unwell. He stopped work but published an account of the vesicovaginal fistula operation in the *American Journal of Medical Sciences* in January 1852. In 1853 he moved to New York. Two years later, he opened a small hospital where poor women received gynecological treatment. Several wealthy New York women helped promote his plans. The charter for the Woman's Hospital of the State of New York was obtained in 1857, and within a few years, construction of a larger hospital was necessary. Anesthesia and newer surgical techniques permitted gynecological operations in addition to fistulae.

Disheartened by the sectionalism leading to the Civil War and conflicted by his southern loyalties, Sims spent much of the 1860s in Europe. He was widely acclaimed, especially in Britain and France, where he demonstrated his surgical skills and developed a lucrative practice that attracted several famous women, including Empress Eugénie. In Belgium he was named Knight of the Order of Leopold I. During the Franco-Prussian War, he helped organize the Anglo-American Ambulance Corps and served as surgeon-in-chief. The French made him Commander of the Légion d'Honneur.

Under the direction of Thomas Addis Emmet, the Woman's Hospital had thrived in his absence. Sims joined the board of surgeons in 1872 but resigned two years later, protesting a ruling that limited the number of spectators allowed to witness his operations. In 1876 he was president of the American Medical Association and in 1880 of the American Gynecological Society.

In addition to treatment of vesicovaginal fistulae, Sims is remembered for the Sims speculum and Sims position, which remain part of gynecological practice. Much of his later practice was devoted to treatments for sterility and development of pessaries. He supported Battey's ovariotomy, believing it helped many female disorders.

Sims married his childhood sweetheart, Eliza Theresa Jones, who shared his early years of poverty and discouragement and later years of glory and satisfaction. Several monuments commemorate his accomplishments, including one in Central Park, New York.

Bibliography

Primary: 1866. *Clinical Notes on Uterine Surgery* (London); 1884. (Sims, H. M., ed.) *Story of My Life* (New York).

Secondary: McGregor, Deborah Kuhn, 1998. *From Midwives to Medicine* (New Brunswick, NJ); Harris, Seale, 1950. *Woman's Surgeon* (New York); *DAMB*.

Amalie M. Kass

IBN SĪNĀ, ABŪ ʿALĪ AL-ḤUSAYN B. ʿABD ALLĀH B. SĪNĀ (aka AVICENNA) (b. Afshana, near Bukhara, Uzbekistan, 980; d. Hamadan, Iran, 18 June 1037), *medicine, philosophy.*

We know about Ibn Sīnā's life from his autobiography and works by his disciple and friend, Abū ʿUbayd al-Juzjānī. These sources do not contain exhaustive personal details. An autobiography was an unusual genre in classical Arabic and Persian texts. It was more a *sira* (biography), which comprised official information, strongly connected to an individual's occupation. For a scholar and intellectual such as Ibn Sīnā, the information would include accounts of his studies, his teachers, and the books he composed. The comparison of Ibn Sīnā's autobiography and its con-

tinuation, written by Abū ʿUbayd al-Juzjānī, reveals that Ibn Sīnā tried to portray himself as a scholar-ascetic whose time and efforts were completely devoted to study. He supplied only a minimum of personal information, which is self-congratulatory. Abū ʿUbayd al-Juzjānī provided a slightly different picture. We learn that Ibn Sīnā was motivated by money and personal security. He appreciated good research facilities and considered himself to be primarily a scholar. He was not a good statesman, but had to participate in court life—even at the cost of his own. Finally, he was sexually voracious, which probably contributed to the deterioration of his health.

Ibn Sīnā informed us that he was born into a family originally from Balkh (modern Afghanistan) of an official of the Samanid administration (a Persian dynasty ruling in Transoxiana from 395 to1005). He was married to a woman called Sitara. Ibn Sīnā's native tongue was Persian. His parents had another male child, Ibn Sīnā's younger brother, who accompanied him all his life and is mentioned with regard to Ibn Sīnā's moving to service in Isfahan (*c.* 1024). According to a notice left by an anonymous commentator in Ibn Sīnā's autobiography, in his youth the Shaykh (i.e., Ibn Sīnā) 'was one of the handsomest people of his time. On Friday when he left his house to go to the mosque, the people used to crowd together in the streets and roads in order to catch a glimpse of his perfection and beauty.' Being well-educated (according to some biographers, he was a tax collector and specialist in money exchange), Ibn Sīnā's father had a solid knowledge of mathematics, geometry, and algebra, as well as philosophy. All these topics were frequently discussed in his home. He and his younger son were influenced by the *Ismaʿīlī* propaganda. The *Ismaʿīlīs*, who constituted the major branch of the *Shiʿa*, were famous for their dialectical methods and teachings. Ibn Sīnā, although well informed in this subject, refused to become an adherent of this movement.

Ibn Sīnā's autobiography deals primarily with his achievements in science and philosophy, but still provides an interesting insight into his personality: he obviously possessed extraordinary intellectual abilities and was no doubt aware of them. He never missed a chance to mention the number of books he had read and boasted of the thoroughness with which he mastered new, previously unknown material. His instructors, at least those he mentioned, were reputable teachers. He stressed his superiority over them and showed that to a very significant degree his achievements and discoveries were due to his own experiences in autodidactic methods.

Ibn Sīnā received his primary education in Bukhara (a major cultural center in the ninth to eleventh centuries) after his family moved there from Afshana. He studied Qurʾān and Arabic literature, excelling in these subjects. Later a grocer called al-Maḥmūd al-Massāḥī instructed him in Indian calculation; his intellectual independence was well served by an extraordinary intelligence and memory, which allowed him to overtake his teachers at the age of fourteen. When the famous physician, logician, and *Isma'īlī* scholar Abū 'Abd Allāh an-Nātilī arrived in Bukhara, Ibn Sīnā's father offered him a place in his house and hospitality in exchange for teaching. It is not known whether Ibn Sīnā's brother attended an-Nātilī's sessions, as Ibn Sīnā listed only himself among the pupils. At that time Ibn Sīnā was already learned in law, having received instruction from Isma'il az-Zāhid, and had a good knowledge of logic. He recorded that an-Nātilī's comprehension of logic proved to be limited: he could explain to his pupil only simple parts of this science. He did not understand Euclid or Ptolemy, so Ibn Sīnā explained these theorems to him. Ibn Sīnā was an avid learner, mentioning that during his study of philosophy 'he did not sleep a single night nor devote [himself] to anything else during the day'. If he was overwhelmed with sleep, he drank a goblet of wine and continued his studies. He did, however, find difficulty in understanding Aristotle's Metaphysics. He committed it to memory but could not grasp the meaning until he read al-Fārābī's commentary.

Ibn Sīnā's subsequent life became an uninterrupted struggle for the attention and benevolence of the rulers he served. In order to win this attention, he had to grasp large amounts of information previously unknown to him and use it freely. Thus, at the latter stage of his life, serving the ruler of Isfahan, he was accused of not being a grammarian. Ibn Sīnā spent three years studying philology. He did it so successfully, that he was able to compose three books, imitating the famous stylists. The person who accused him could not detect the forgery.

In his autobiography Ibn Sīnā mentioned that he taught himself the art of medicine, although other sources inform us that Abū Manṣūr al-Qamarī, an eminent practitioner from Bukhara, taught him. Ibn Sīnā proved to be so successful that distinguished physicians began to read medicine under him when he was only sixteen. At this time, the ruler of Bukhara, sultan Nūḥ ibn Manṣūr, contracted a severe illness, baffling his doctors. Having heard of Ibn Sīnā, he ordered him to join his medical staff. Ibn Sīnā successfully treated the sultan and was rewarded with access to his splendid library. He writes that it comprised a number of rooms, full of rare books of the ancient sages, who along with their works, were not widely known. By the age of eighteen he had mastered all the scientific knowledge contained in the library's books. The autobiography has an interesting marginalia: 'a fire broke out in this library and the books were totally destroyed. Some of the opponents of Ibn Sīnā said that he set fire to those books in order to appropriate these sciences and precious knowledge for himself and cut off the sources of these useful sciences from their adherents; but God knows best.'

Ibn Sīnā started to commit his thoughts to paper in an early age. For his neighbor Abū 'l-Ḥasan al-Arūdhī (The Prosodist) he composed a digest, which comprised all the sciences he had learned, with the exception of mathematics. For another neighbor, 'a lawyer by inclination', Abū Bakr al-Barakī, he composed a digest on jurisprudence, Qur'ān commentary, and asceticism and a book on ethics. This period of his life was marked by intensive astronomical observations. He wrote a treatise about meteorites and the trajectories of Mercury and Venus.

At the age of twenty-two his life changed. The Samanid dynasty lost its power to the Qarakhanid dynasty and was subsequently conquered by Maḥmūd of Ghazna (971?–1030). In the same year Ibn Sīnā's father died and he had to earn his own living. He moved from one place to another, looking for a decent livelihood and a superior *amir* who would be able to appreciate his knowledge. He left Bukhara for Gurganj and the court of Abū l-'Abbās Ma'mūn II b. Ma'mūn (r. 1009–17). This ruler accumulated brilliant scholars at his court, some of whom, like Ibn Sīnā, moved from their hometowns, impelled by the unsettled conditions following the Samanids' fall. Among them were the philologist Abū Manṣūr Abd al-Mālik ath-Tha'ālibī, the physician Abū 'l-Khayr al-Ḥasan b. al-Khammār, the philosopher Abū Sahl al-Masīḥī and the mathematician Abū Naṣr al-Arrāq. The intellectual atmosphere was benign. Ibn Sīnā received a 'monthly salary which provided enough for someone like him' and was able to work. His results of activities are found in two of his major works: the *Canon* and the '*Kitāb ash-Shifā*'. Although Ibn Sīnā described the art of medicine as easy to learn and considered himself to be a philosopher, it is his medical book, *Kitāb al-Qānūn fī-ṭ-Ṭibb* [The Canon. [Book] on Medicine], that made his name famous for posterity. The whole work belongs to the genre named by the Greek word *kanon* (canon), i.e., a model. In fact, it was a model of systematic description of the medical knowledge of his time. It comprises five books; each of these books is subdivided into divisions (*fann*), parts (*djumla*), treatises (*maqāla*), and paragraphs (*faṣl*). The first book deals with the theory of medicine and comprises the following parts: anatomy, physiology, causation of diseases, symptoms, dietetics, principles of treatment, and prophylactics. The chapters that deal with the preservation of health can be considered as the most important medieval work on hygiene. The second book deals with simple remedies. The third book comprises descriptions of various diseases 'from head to toe', methods of their diagnoses, and subsequent treatment. The fourth book deals with methods of treatment of various contagious diseases, tumors, etc. The fifth book describes composite remedies and antidotes. Altogether, the *Canon* mentions 811 remedies; modern medicine uses only 150 from this total. The *Canon* was translated into Latin by the twelfth century, and it was first printed in 1473. In the Latin West Ibn Sīnā was known as Avicenna. The second translation into Latin, made at the beginning of the sixteenth century, became a standard teaching manual in Italian universities.

In his autobiography, Ibn Sīnā mentioned 'necessities' that led him to leave the court of Ma'mūn II b. Ma'mūn. In fact, it was a demanding letter, sent to Maʾmūn II b. Maʾmūn in 1012 by Maḥmūd of Ghazna, who was gradually conquering Gurganj. He insisted that Ibn Sīnā and the other scholars had to be dispatched to his court so he could 'enjoy their company'.

Maʾmūn II b. Maʾmūn offered the scholars a free hand, and many of them had moved to his court. Ibn Sīnā and his friend Abū Sahl al-Masīhī escaped to Iran through the desert of Qārā-Qum dressed as *derwishes*, but Abū Sahl died en route. Trying to escape Maḥmūd of Ghazna, who ordered him to be found, apparently sending his portrait everywhere, Ibn Sīnā moved to Nasa and on to Baward, Tus, Samarqand, Jajarm, and Jurjan. He said his destination (*qasad*) was *amir* Qābūs, i.e. Shams al-Maʿālī Qābūs ibn Wushmagīr, a poet and a patron of poets and scholars, who took part in the dynastic struggles between the Buyids and Samanids for control of Khurāsān and Jurjān, usually on the side of Samanids. But *amir* Qābūs was at that time imprisoned in a castle and died there. Ibn Sīnā had to go to Dihistān, where he became ill, and he later returned to Jurjān. In Dihistān, Abū ʿUbayd al-Juzjānī joined Ibn Sīnā and stayed with him until his death.

According to some sources, Maḥmūd of Ghazna wanted the rulers of Rayy and Jurjān to send Ibn Sīnā to his court. Ibn Sīnā left for Qazwīn and from there to Hamadhan, where he became a statesman (*vizier*) at the court of Buʿid *amir* Shams ad-Dawla, whom he cured of colic. Here he almost died when the army rioted, accusing him of not paying the agreed salary. Shams ad-Dawla refused to execute Ibn Sīnā, but had to banish him from the state to satisfy the army. Ibn Sīnā went into hiding for forty days, but the colic seized Shams ad-Dawla again and he summoned Ibn Sīnā to treat him and restored his rank of *vizier* (literally 'bearer of burdens', a title of a government official). Around 1024 Ibn Sīnā was secretly corresponding with the ruler of Iṣfahān, ʿAlā ad-Dawla Abū Jaʿfar Muḥammad ibn Dushmānziyār (d. 1041), whose service he wanted to join. When this wish became clear, Ibn Sīnā was imprisoned for four months. When he was freed, he fled to Iṣfahān, where he was accepted by ʿAlā ad-Dawla and given a house. He also had Friday nights designated for learned assemblies in his presence: 'All of the different classes of learned men attended, the Master among them, he was not outclassed in any of the sciences.' ʿAlā ad-Dawla made him a member of the court and one of his companions. Here he was involved in solving astrological problems, correcting mistakes in various calculations and inventing astronomical instruments. He also devoted himself to medicine, conducting many experiments that he recorded in the *Canon*. Abū ʿUbayd al-Juzjānī mentioned that Ibn Sīnā 'was vigorous in all his facilities, the sexual facility being the most vigorous and dominant of his concupiscible facilities and he exercised it often. It affected his constitution upon whose strength it depended to the point, that . . . he was afflicted with colic.' He decided to cure himself and self-administered an enema

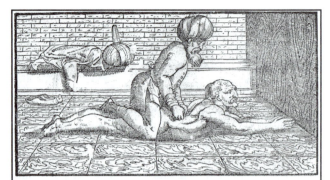

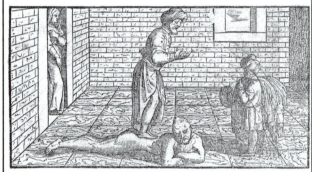

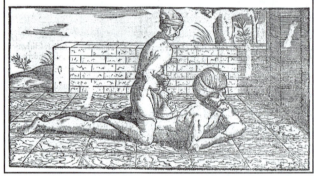

Methods of spinal manipulation. Woodcut from *Canon medicinae* . . . Venice, 1595. Rare Books, Wellcome Library, London.

eight times in one day 'to the point that some intestines ulcerated and an abrasion broke out on him'. The colic was followed by seizures. He continued his treatment administering enemas for the abrasion and the residue of the colic. Then one day, wishing to deal with the flatulence, he ordered two *danaqs* of celery seed be included in the enema. But one of the doctors administered five *danaqs*, and the sharpness of the seed aggravated the abrasion. 'I do not know', wrote al-Juzjānī, 'whether he did it intentionally or by mistake because I was not present'. Ibn Sīnā also took *mithridate* for the seizures. However, one of his slaves threw a great quantity of opium into it. The slaves, having stolen a great deal of Ibn Sīnā's money, desired his death in order to be free from the consequence of their actions. Even in this poor state of health, he continued to attend ʿAlā ad-Dawla's court and indulged himself in sexual intercourse. He had not recovered from his illness and had intermittent relapses and recoveries. He set off for Hamadhan with Abū ad-Dawla; by the time they reached their destination, however, he knew his strength had wasted away. He stopped his treatment, died, and was buried in Hamadhan.

Ibn Sīnā's career was heavily dependent on the tastes and mercy of his patrons, who surrounded themselves with scholars, poets, astrologers, mathematicians, and medical men. A constant struggle for the patron's benevolence was inevitably connected with eliminating various competitors. Ibn Sīnā's magnificent memory was a great advantage. He composed around 300 works in his lifetime; obsessed with their production, he labored through the night on his great works, which were written with astonishing rapidity. Being frequently compelled to move, he would write on horseback, and sometimes in prison, his only resource for reference being his memory. It has been found surprising that he differs from Aristotle in his works, but he quoted him without re-reading him, and, above all, his independence of mind inclined him to present his own ideas, rather than repeating those of others. Aristotle's logic seemed to him insufficient because it could not be applied in a way that was sufficiently close to life. Many recent controversies have followed an increasing interest in his work, but the most plausible view of his personality is still that he was a scientific man who attempted to bring Greek theories to a more rigorous level.

Bibliography

Primary: 1981. *Kanon Vrachebnoi nauki* 6 vols. (Tashkent).

Secondary: Rosenfeld, B. A., and E. Ihsanoglu, 2003. *Mathematicians, Astronomers and other Scholars of Islamic Civilisation and their Works (7th–19th c.)* no. 317 (Istanbul); Gohlman, W. E., 1974. *The Life of Ibn Sīnā. A Critical Edition and Annotated Translation* (Albany, NY); *DSB.*

Nikolaj Serikoff

SKIRVING, ROBERT SCOT   (b. East Lothian, Scotland, 18 December 1859; d. Bellevue Hill, Australia, 15 July 1956), *medicine, surgery.*

Skirving was the son of a farmer of the same name and his Irish-born wife, Elizabeth Owen. They were an austere Calvinist family. Their son attended Edinburgh Academy and Eastman's Royal Naval Academy at Portsmouth, but he was several weeks too old to join the navy as a cadet officer, so he became an apprentice in the merchant service. After taking ill on a voyage from Australia, he decided to study medicine, graduating MB CM from the University of Edinburgh in 1881. Still too young for a hospital position, he continued study in Dublin and Vienna before appointment as a house physician at the Royal Infirmary, Edinburgh.

In 1883 he sailed for Australia as ship's surgeon on an emigrant ship. Skirving initially worked in Queensland until offered the position of medical superintendent at the (Royal) Prince Alfred Hospital later that year. He soon left

for private practice but remained at the hospital as an honorary physician from 1884 to 1911; after that he was a consultant physician until his death. He was also honorary physician at the Hospital for Sick Children (1884–89). He lectured in clinical medicine at the University of Sydney for many years (1889–1911) and became known as a dynamic, popular teacher who valued practical experience above theoretical knowledge.

Although Skirving was admired for his diagnostic skills, he was also an accomplished surgeon. During much of the time that he was a specialist physician at one hospital, he was a specialist honorary surgeon at another, St Vincent's (1889–1923). Patients remarked on his warmth and compassion, with a few continuing to consult him until shortly before his death at the age of ninety-six. He kept abreast of professional developments until the end.

Skirving served in both the South African War and World War I. For a time he was a surgeon specialist at Queen Alexandra Military Hospital in London. In 1918 he was asked to report on Australian medical units in France. His broad medical experience resulted in his achieving the rare distinction of becoming a Foundation Fellow of both the nascent Royal Australasian College of Surgeons (1927) and the Royal Australasian College of Physicians (1938). Even at that time this was an unusual combination, but it was consistent with his distaste for the trend toward narrow compartmentalization of medicine. Later he was elected FRCS London (1953). Like most of his senior colleagues, he served a term as president of the New South Wales Branch of the British Medical Association (1891–92). Despite numerous other commitments, he still found time between 1911 and 1936 to be chief medical referee for the Australian Mutual Provident Society, a life assurance company.

Skirving believed doctors should be broadly educated, and he disparaged those who did not share his passion for English literature. He wrote prolifically about his medical and other interests. Some were clinical articles, but a large number were personal reminiscences of his career and the people or hospitals where he worked. A colleague wrote that 'Skirving had a vast system of prejudices' (Moran, 1939, p. 114). These included art, the Irish, 'games with little balls', and many of his peers, whom he described in colorful language reflecting both the Bible and his years before the mast in the merchant marine. He wrote a novel (1901) and a manual for yachtsmen (1931). He always said that the sea was his greatest love, continuing to sail his own yacht when he was over eighty.

Bibliography

Primary: 1901. *Love and Longitude* (Sydney); 1901. *Our Army in South Africa* (Sydney); 1936. 'Surgery at Sea in the Eighties.' *Medical Journal of Australia* 1: 783–785; 1998. Macintosh, A., ed., *Memoirs of Robert Scot Skirving* (Sydney).

Secondary: Obituary, 1956. *Medical Journal of Australia* 2: 734–736; Moran, H. M., 1939. *Viewless Winds* (London); *AuDB*.

Peter J. Tyler

SKLIFOSOVSKII, NIKOLAI VASIL'EVICH (b. near Dubossary, Russia, 25 March [6 April] 1836; d. near Poltava, Russia, 30 November [13 December] 1904), *surgery.*

Sklifosovskii, renowned for his expertise in military and academic surgery, championed the introduction of antisepsis and then asepsis into academic practice during a turbulent era of medical professionalization in Russia. He was born to an impoverished aristocratic family. He attended the Odessa gymnasium and then the Medical Department of Moscow University (1854–59). He began his career as the director of the surgical department of the Odessa City Hospital. In 1863 at Khar'kov University he defended his doctoral dissertation on tumors of the parametrium. In 1866–68 he traveled abroad for further training, studying first at Virchow's Pathological Anatomical Institute and then at the surgical clinics of Bernhard von Langenbeck in Berlin and James Young Simpson in Edinburgh, among others, before returning to Odessa to become the head doctor of the City Hospital. After one year at Kiev University (1870–71), he moved to the preeminent Military-Medical Academy in St Petersburg as head of the Department of Surgical Pathology and Treatment (1871–78).

In 1880 Sklifosovskii was invited to be a professor in the Faculty Surgical Clinics at Moscow University, where he immediately pioneered the use of Lister's antisepsis, dramatically decreasing the rate of postsurgical infection. During his tenure in Moscow, the number of major operations performed at the clinics increased from eighty in 1880 to 376 in 1893. While serving an eight-year term as dean of the Medical Department, he oversaw the construction of the new 'medical village', a medical campus for the university. From 1893 to 1900, he was the director of the Great Princess Elena Pavlovna Clinical Institute for Advanced Medical Education in St Petersburg, the only such institution in Russia at the time. In 1900 his health faltered and he moved to his estate near Poltava.

A contemporary of Billroth, Mikulicz-Radecki, and Lister, Sklifosovskii was a leader in the golden era of surgery following the introduction of infection control methods and anesthesia. Among other innovations in orthopedic surgery, he developed a technique known as the 'Russian lock' for the repair of femur fractures. In 1879 he was among the first Russian surgeons successfully to undertake gastrostomy as a palliative procedure when he performed the surgery in two patients with advanced stomach cancer, and in 1885 he was among the first in the world to use local cocaine anesthesia. He operated on seven patients to remove echinococcal cysts of the liver, of whom six survived (reported 1893).

Sklifosovskii first experienced military surgery in 1866 during the Seven Weeks' War when he served in the Prussian Army; then during the Franco-German War of 1870 he observed the operations of military hospitals. During the Balkan Crisis (1876) he worked in Montenegro with the Russian Red Cross, and he served the Russian Army during the Russo-Turkish War between 1877 and 1878. Following N. I. Pirogov, Sklifosovskii advocated the use of medical tents and careful triage of wounded soldiers near the front prior to their evacuation by train to many dispersed sites for definitive care.

Sklifosovskii contributed to the growing prominence of both professional medical associations and specialized journals in Russia in the aftermath of the Great Reforms of the 1860s. Not only was he active in surgical societies; he was also among the founders of the Pirogov Society in 1883, the largest organization of Russian physicians before 1918 and a rare public platform for liberal discourse surrounding issues of health in the Empire. He was a prolific writer and was an editor of two Russian surgical journals, *Khirurgicheskaia letopis'* [The Surgical Chronicle] in Moscow (1891–96) and *Letopis' russkoi khirurgii* [The Chronicle of Russian Surgery] in St Petersburg (beginning in 1896). In 1897 he was elected chair of the Twelfth International Congress of Physicians in Moscow.

Bibliography

Primary: 1953. *Izbrannye trudy* [Selected Works] (Moscow).

Secondary: Kovanov, V. V., 1952. *N. V. Sklifosovskii* (Moscow); [Anon.], 1905. 'Prof. Nikolai Vasilevich Sklifosovskii skonchalsia.' *Khirurgiia* 17: 82–87.

Michael Z. David

SKODA, JOSEPH (b. Pilsen, Bohemia [now Czech Republic], 10 December 1805; d. Vienna, Austria, 13 June 1881), *medicine.*

Skoda studied medicine at Vienna (1825–31), where he received his MD in 1831. He first worked as a general physician in Bohemia, then returned to Vienna to the Allgemeines Krankenhaus [general hospital] as a Sekundararzt. During this time he had close working relations with the leading pathologist of the New Vienna School of Clinical Medicine, Carl v. Rokitansky (1804–78). In 1841 he became Primararzt [principal physician] and head of the department for thorax patients there. Study trips led him to France and England to learn about the clinical medicine in those countries.

Returning with multiple ideas from the leading centers of European medicine, he received the professorship of the Medical Clinic in Vienna in 1846. Following the French example, Skoda completely devoted himself to the diseases of the thorax. He published an extensive book on percussion and auscultation (inaugurated by L. Auenbrugger and R. T. H. Laennec), placing it in a position of clinical and scientific maturity by basing it on natural science, pathology, and anatomy. His systematization of the individual acoustic phenomena opened these physical methods of diagnosis to scientific objectivity; they could thus better be taught and learned. Skoda was first to differentiate normal physiological heart sounds from pathological cardiac murmurs, and he described vesicular and bronchial respiratory sounds. He enriched the clinical diagnostics of acoustic phenomena by a plausible system of categories and nomenclature with understandable terminology. The progress for the clinical diagnostics of thoracic diseases was considerable, for it made it easier to register the pathophysiological processes of internal diseases, an essential contribution to going beyond the ontological conception of disease, still prevailing at that time. More important was the fact that Skoda was able to reveal multiple pathological changes of the lung and heart by his 'method of resonance', even if no therapeutic measures existed yet, a fact that always depressed him. After all, Skoda's highly differentiated clinical diagnostics meant the end to 'rapid diagnosis', commonly applied at that time in Vienna. It has to be mentioned that Skoda was one of the first medical professors in Vienna to lecture in German and not in Latin. Skoda, together with Joseph Dietl, belonged to the most famous representatives of 'therapeutic nihilism'.

Bibliography

Primary: 1839. *Abhandlung über Percussion u. Auscultation* (Vienna) (English edn., 1853).

Secondary: Lesky, Erna, 1976. *The Vienna Medical School of the 19th Century* (Baltimore); Sternberg, M., 1924. *Josef Skoda* (Vienna); *DSB*.

Wolfgang U. Eckart

SMELLIE, WILLIAM (b. Lesmahagow, Lanarkshire, Scotland, 5 February 1697; d. Lanark, Scotland, 5 March 1763), *obstetrics, midwifery*.

Smellie was the only son of Archibald Smellie, probably a schoolteacher, and Sara Kennedy. He was educated at the grammar school in Lanark and was apprenticed there to William Inglis, apothecary (1714). He seems also to have been a pupil of John Gordon, a Glasgow surgeon. Smellie served briefly as a naval surgeon before establishing his own apothecary's shop in Lanark (1722). For the next fifteen years, he practiced as a surgeon-apothecary and was often summoned to assist with obstetric emergencies. When faced with a labor obstructed by the head, Smellie would try to turn the baby to the feet. If unsuccessful, his only alternative was craniotomy, which, he said, 'gave me great uneasiness'. Learning of the invention of the obstetric forceps and its potential for delivering a live child under such circumstances, Smellie traveled first to London and then to Paris, where he attended Grégoire's forceps classes. Returning to London (1740), Smellie set himself up as a male midwife and a teacher of midwifery.

Smellie lectured on pregnancy and labor and conducted practical demonstrations on 'machines' of his own construction that simulated the maternal pelvis and the unborn child. His courses, which were relatively cheap, attracted a large number of students. Soon Smellie complemented his academic classes with visits to the confinements of poor women in their own homes. The patients were not charged for Smellie's services under these circumstances, and his students received clinical instruction in the management of both normal and difficult labor, with the latter being the main focus of his bedside teaching.

Despite his earlier interest in the forceps, it seems that as a teacher, Smellie initially stressed the importance of managing obstructed labor without instruments. He felt that forceful use of the forceps, in the manner of Grégoire, carried an unacceptable risk of injury to the mother. Sometime in 1745, however, Smellie realized that the forceps might be used to assist the rotation of the head of the fetus in its passage along the birth canal. If the blades were carefully positioned and sensitively deployed in this manner, the baby could often be delivered safely, with only moderate traction and without damage to the maternal parts. From then on, Smellie used the forceps regularly in cases of obstructed labor by the head. He experimented with various modifications to the design of the blades and handles, both to improve the instrument's utility and to render it less intimidating to the mother.

Throughout his career as a man-midwife, Smellie kept detailed records of his cases. He drew on this material to produce his magisterial *A Treatise on the Theory and Practice of Midwifery*, the first part being published in 1752; the second in 1754, with an accompanying volume of illustrations; and the third, posthumously (1764). The appearance of the first volume established Smellie as the major British authority on midwifery. His accounts of the mechanisms of both normal and abnormal labor were more precise and better observed than any previously available. Smellie outlined how the shape of the maternal pelvis affected the course of labor. Problematic presentations were described, and reliable and detailed recommendations made for their management. The *Treatise* was a summation of a vast amount of clinical experience and intelligent inquiry.

Despite his success at the bedside and as a teacher, Smellie was never a fashionable London accoucher. He lacked the necessary social polish. But his skill and resourcefulness in the traditional surgeon's sphere of emergency obstetrics gained him fame and a substantial income. In 1759 he retired to Lanark, where he died.

Bibliography

Primary: 1752–1764. *A Treatise on the Theory and Practice of Midwifery* 3 vols. (London).

Secondary: Wilson, Adrian, 1995. *The Making of Man-Midwifery* (London); Butterton, J., 1986. 'The Education, Naval Service and Early Career of William Smellie.' *Bulletin of the History of Medicine* 60: 1–18; *Oxford DNB.*

Malcolm Nicolson

SMIRK, FREDERICK HORACE (b. Accrington, England, 12 December 1902; d. Dunedin, New Zealand, 18 May 1991), *medicine, clinical pharmacology.*

Smirk, the son of Betsy Ann Cunliffe and Thomas Smirk, was educated at Haslingden Grammar School, where his father was headmaster. From there he went to the Victoria University of Manchester with a University Entrance Scholarship and Gaskill Mathematical Scholarship—no doubt to the delight of his father. Other honors soon came his way. He achieved the MB ChB with first class honors (1925), the MD with a British Medical Association gold medal in 1927, a graduate research scholarship, and a Medical Research Council grant. The award of the MRC's Dickenson Traveling Scholarship enabled Smirk to go to Vienna and continue the work on tissue osmotic pressure he had begun as a medical registrar at the Manchester Royal Infirmary.

After World War II a research career would have been wide open to a physician who had shown such early promise, but it was different during the 1920s. Smirk is one of that outstanding group of medical scientists who became established investigators mainly because they were awarded a Beit Memorial Medical Research Fellowship (established in 1909). Comparable posts in Britain were almost nonexistent. During those years of depressed economic activity—Smirk was appointed in 1930—a Beit Fellow could feel passing rich on £1,500 a year. One happy result of the award was that Smirk met Aileen Bamforth, an almoner at the University College Hospital, and married her. Theirs was to be a long and happy marriage blessed with three sons and a daughter.

Smirk took up his Beit Fellowship at the University College Hospital (UCH) Medical School, where T. R. Elliot became his chief and Sir Thomas Lewis one of his mentors. Teaching appointments at UCH followed. By 1935, when the chair of pharmacology at the Egyptian University in Cairo became vacant through the appointment of J. H. Gaddum to the Edinburgh chair, Smirk became his well-qualified successor. Four years later, as the successful applicant for the Mary Glendining Chair of Medicine at New Zealand's Otago University, he could claim proven administrative as well as research ability.

In the 1940 edition of their *Digest*, the Otago medical students officially greeted the new professor, 'whose lean, energetic figure is already a familiar sight striding about the school at a furious pace and with incredible purpose'. Smirk had much to do. His department lacked laboratories, equipment, and technicians. The outbreak of war had brought supply problems that were soon to be made worse

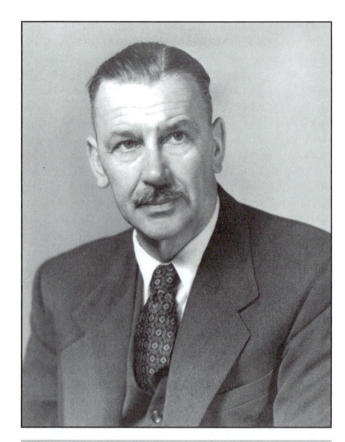

Frederick H. Smirk. Photograph, 1960s. Hocken Collections, Uare Taoka o Hkena, University of Otago, Dunedin.

by the fall of France. At one point textbooks were in such short supply that providing stenciled notes was a major task. Yet within ten years of his coming to Dunedin, Smirk published a paper that 'represents the beginning of the modern era of antihypertensive treatment' (Dollery, Colin, 1987. *British Heart Journal* 58: 181).

When he obtained the Cairo chair, Smirk was able to diversify his research. Until then he had been concerned mainly with investigating water diuresis and the production of edema. Work in this field established his skill as an investigator, but it was not a field in which one was likely to make a therapeutic breakthrough. Smirk therefore became increasingly interested in essential hypertension. Although it was realized that about 20 percent of adults in Western countries are hypertensive, the search for drugs to lower elevated blood pressure had been carried out halfheartedly because of the prevailing belief that one was dealing with an irreversible process. Smirk did not hold this view. He thought it important to lower the blood pressure when it was abnormally high, because that would lessen the chance of an outcome such as stroke or heart failure. Moreover, he did not consider the odds against finding an effective drug to be so high as to preclude looking for it himself. He began the search in 1935 at Cairo and continued it at Otago from 1940 on.

Most of the 3,000 compounds screened were the seeming oddities that abound in chemical catalogues and could in most cases be purchased cheaply in the small amounts needed for pharmacological study. Chemical relatives of interesting compounds were synthesized in his department at Otago. Some of these drugs were sufficiently promising to be tested on patients with severe hypertension—a procedure that could be easily justified at a time when the so-called 'malignant' form of hypertension was likely to kill patients within a few months. None of these compounds proved sufficiently useful to deserve further trial, but testing them gave Smirk invaluable experience from which he eventually profited. While on study leave in 1949 as a visiting professor at the Postgraduate Medical School at Hammersmith in London, he learned about the recently discovered ganglion-blocking action of hexamethonium. Soon after his return to Otago, Smirk was able to demonstrate its therapeutic value. Before 1950 it was a matter for conjecture whether a sustained lowering of the blood pressure of hypertensive patients would be harmless *per se*, let alone beneficial. With hexamethonium, Smirk and P. A. Restall were able to perform a conclusive investigation.

Once the value of antihypertensive treatment was widely appreciated, the Cardiovascular Clinic at Dunedin Public Hospital became a major site for the therapeutic trial of promising drugs. Patients were referred to it in increasing numbers. Before long, records were available for hundreds of patients. Geographical isolation, so disadvantageous in many other respects, greatly aided long-term studies. Several major drug firms were quick to recognize Smirk's outstanding judgment as a clinical pharmacologist. They provided a wealth of interesting new drugs as well as *ex gratia* payments. Smirk's views about the treatment of hypertension became widely known through the publication of his 768-page monograph, *High Arterial Pressure* (1957).

The search for antihypertensive drugs had other benefits. Thus the study of a chemical called amarin led to the recognition of the 'R on T' phenomenon that commonly precedes ventricular fibrillation and of the intermediate condition now known as *torsades de pointes*. S-methylisothiourea sulphate, another compound that had until then been of interest only to chemists, was found to be useful for treating the severe hypotension that may develop in spinal anesthesia. The investigation of various related compounds revealed a new pharmacological group made up of small amidinium cations with a characteristic excitatory action on neuromuscular systems. Their effects are now known to be due mainly to inhibition of NO synthesis. Among Smirk's other major contributions to experimental medicine was the development of a strain of rat with genetic hypertension, the first of several hypertensive strains now known.

During the early 1940s research had to take a back seat while Smirk strengthened his teaching. By the 1960s he had obtained enviable research facilities for the Department of Medicine. His expert services were frequently sought overseas, and international recognition came with his election as a councillor of the International Cardiology Society and of its Hypertension Council. However, the department's other facilities left much to be desired. There were hardly any fulltime university posts. Most of the ninety people then under his direction were on 'soft' money. As further success in obtaining research funds from various sources could not be guaranteed, it gradually became clear that unless more financial support could be obtained through the university, the department's activities would have to be severely curtailed. Shedding much of the research might have been easy, but the dean of the Medical School, Sir Edward Sayers, persuaded the Wellcome Trust in London to fund the building in Dunedin of a Wellcome Medical Research Institute. Smirk could then give all his time to research, especially after becoming research professor of medicine in 1961.

Smirk's influence on research at the Otago Medical School was remarkably broad. He played a major part in the diversification of research. Smirk was not one of those who merely deplored the 'brain drain'; he also realized that the situation could be greatly improved by adopting such measures as convincing local benefactors that it was in the national interest to support postgraduate work in New Zealand rather than to provide scholarships for sending the best graduates abroad on what so often proved to be a one-way trip. Another enlightened policy was to encourage junior physicians to seek membership in the Royal Australasian College of Physicians, which could be obtained locally, in lieu of the London or Edinburgh memberships. Smirk did not underestimate the value of overseas experience. What he sought to impress on ambitious young graduates was that they were less likely to benefit from overseas experience by going abroad immediately than if they would begin such experience with their 'membership' and examination worries behind them.

Shortly after his arrival in New Zealand, Smirk had been made both a fellow and a censor of the RACP. He was elected its New Zealand vice president for 1958–59. Among other honors to come his way was a knighthood (1958) and honorary doctorates of science from the Hahnemann Medical College in Philadelphia (1961) and Otago University (1975). In 1965 he went to Canada to receive a Gairdner International Award for outstanding achievement in biomedical research worldwide. The *New Zealand Medical Journal* marked his retirement in 1968 with a large commemorative issue, a rare distinction.

Smirk drove himself at a pace that matched that set at the school a few years earlier by (Sir) John Eccles, professor of physiology 1944–51, in his successful pursuit of a Nobel Prize. Colleagues who thought that they were making an early start upon reaching the medical school by 8:00 A.M. would see Smirk just about to drive home for breakfast after having worked for several hours on his book. Throughout the twenty-eight years at Otago that preceded his retirement, Smirk retained a superb vitality. Sadly, it was not to last. Long before his death Sir Horace had become an obvious victim of Alzheimer's disease. Thus in 1987 he was unable to receive personally the silver medal of the Medical Research Council of New Zealand, on which he had served from 1944 until 1960. The gradual destruction of that fine mind deprived him of what he would probably have regarded as his greatest reward, namely receiving the praise and admiration of those many pupils whose subsequent success was owed in such great part to him.

Bibliography

Primary: 1948. (with Fastier, F. N.) 'Some Properties of Amarin, with Special Reference to Its Use in Conjunction with Adrenaline for the Production of Idioventricular Rhythms.' *Journal of Physiology* 107: 318–331; 1957. *High Arterial Pressure* (Oxford); 1958. (with Hall, W. H.) 'Inherited Hypertension in Rats.' *Nature* 182: 727–728.

Secondary: Fastier, F. N., 1968. 'Sir Horace Smirk; Professor Emeritus.' *New Zealand Medical Journal* 67: 258–265; Doyle, A. E., and C. I. Johnston, 1988. 'Australasian Contributions to Research into Hypertension.' *Australian & New Zealand Journal of Medicine* 18: 245–249.

F. N. Fastier

SMITH, NATHAN (b. Rehoboth, Massachusetts, USA, 12 September 1762; d. New Haven, Connecticut, USA, 26 January 1829), *medicine, surgery, medical education.*

Praised long after his death as one of the most important physicians and surgeons in postcolonial New England, Smith is less well-known today than some more dogmatic or prolific physicians, but his far-reaching influence is undeniable. He single-handedly founded the fourth-oldest medical school in the United States, at Dartmouth College (1797), and he was instrumental in putting three other medical schools on a solid footing: at Yale University (1813), Bowdoin College (Medical School of Maine), and the University of Vermont (both in 1821).

Smith's medical career began in Chester, Vermont, where the family had moved when Nathan was ten. In 1784 a surgeon named Josiah Goodhue arrived to perform an amputation and called for an assistant; Smith—then a twenty-two-year-old farmer—volunteered. Thrilled by the experience, he abruptly decided to become a doctor. Goodhue accepted him as an apprentice after he had undergone six months of tutoring.

Following a three-year apprenticeship, Smith started his own practice in Cornish, New Hampshire. He quickly earned a reputation as an observant and knowledgeable physician. He nonetheless enrolled in 1789 in the new medical school founded by John Warren, becoming Harvard Medical School's fifth graduate when he received his MB in 1790. Smith's first apprentices in Cornish, Lyman Spalding and Jo Gallup, subsequently distinguished themselves as physicians and medical educators. Smith married Elizabeth Chase of Cornish in 1791. After her death two years later, he married her younger half-sister, Sally, in 1794; Sally bore his ten children, of whom nine lived to adulthood. All four sons became physicians, and the subsequent five generations have each included at least one physician.

In 1796 Smith began negotiations with the Trustees at Dartmouth, urging them to enhance the institution's prestige by letting him offer medical lectures there. In anticipation of doing so, Smith spent several months in Edinburgh, Glasgow, and London. He returned in late 1797, having been elected a Corresponding Member of the Medical Society of London, and gave the first medical lecture at Dartmouth that November. Smiths' performance as a teacher, first at Dartmouth (where he did virtually all the lecturing for more than a decade) and then at Yale, proved that he was a masterful medical educator. Many of his students became medical school professors themselves; others stayed to practice in rural New England, directly impacting the quality of medicine in that region.

Smith was much admired for his diagnostic skills. Firmly believing in the *vis medicatrix naturae*, he avoided 'heroic' therapies. But surgery, also conservatively practiced, was Smith's forte. One example is his treatment of the young Joseph Smith (no relation), future founder of the Church of the Latter Day Saints (Mormons). Instead of amputating the boy's leg (the then-standard means of dealing with osteomyelitis), Smith drilled the bone, removed the diseased portions, and thereby saved the limb. He performed an early ovariotomy (unaware that Ephraim McDowell had previously done so). He devised operations to repair harelip and imperforate anus, inserted a metal plate for traumatic skull defect, and used the 'Bigelow Method' (before Henry Jacob Bigelow) for reducing a dislocated hip.

Smith published several short accounts of cases; his unpublished 'Dissertation on Scirrhous & Cancerous Affections' (*c.* 1808) is evidence he had more to offer. In his most influential work, *A Practical Essay on Typhous Fever*, he identified the disease (actually typhoid) as self-limiting and as 'a disease *sui generis*'.

Bibliography

Primary: 1824. *A Practical Essay on Typhous Fever* (New York); 1827. 'Observations on the Pathology and Treatment of Necrosis.' *Philadelphia Monthly Journal of Medicine* 1: 11–19, 66–75; 1831. (Smith, Nathan R., ed.) *Medical and Surgical Memoirs* (Baltimore).

Secondary: Hayward, Oliver S., and Constance E. Putnam, 1998. *Improve, Perfect, & Perpetuate: Dr. Nathan Smith and Early American Medical Education* (Hanover, NH); Smith, Emily A., 1914. *The Life and Letters of Nathan Smith, M.B., M.D.* (New Haven); *DAMB.*

Constance Putnam

SMITH, THEOBALD   (b. Albany, New York, USA, 31 July 1859; d. New York, New York, USA, 10 December 1934), *bacteriology, pathology*.

Smith was the son of German immigrants Philip Schmitt and Theresia Kexel. Upon settling in Albany, Philip changed his last name to 'Smith' and became a tailor. Young Theobald had a talent for mathematics and music, later supplementing his income by playing church organ. He attended public schools and then won a scholarship to Cornell, where he was particularly interested in zoology and evolutionary theory. Afterward, Smith entered Albany Medical School (1881). He completed his medical education, which included a brief period at Johns Hopkins, and received his MD from Albany (1883).

Later that year, D. E. Salmon, director of the Veterinary Division of the U.S. Department of Agriculture (USDA), brought Smith to Washington to work on diseases in (largely farm) animals. In 1884 the Division became the Bureau of Animal Industry (BAI). Many of the diseases Smith studied there promised to be illuminated by the new bacteriological methods being pioneered in Europe. He taught himself these methods and used them to differentiate hog cholera from swine plague in American pig populations. In 1889 he turned to the disease for which he is best known: Texas Cattle Fever. It was unclear how the costly disease was transmitted from sick to healthy cattle populations: the tick was a likely but unproven suspect. Testing a variety of animal and arthropod permutations at the BAI fields, Smith, with Fredrick Kilborne, demonstrated the tick's role as disease vector and elucidated the complete cycle of transmission. Bacteriologist Hans Zinsser later described Smith's pioneering report as 'one of the classics of medical literature' (Zinsser, p. 271). While in Washington, Smith married Lilian Egleston (1888). The couple had two daughters: Dorothea and Lilian.

In 1896 the Smiths left Washington for Massachusetts, where Theobald was named director of the State Antitoxin Laboratory and professor of comparative medicine at Harvard. Smith made significant contributions to both his appointed fields. While working on antitoxins, he noted a strange phenomenon: guinea pigs injected with horse serum would, when injected again later, suffer respiratory distress and even death. Although he did not pursue the observation experimentally, he did discuss it with German immunologist Paul Ehrlich. Ehrlich's colleague, Richard Otto, studied the phenomenon and, in publications on what would come to be called 'anaphylaxis', dubbed it the 'Theobald Smith Phenomenon'. In comparative medicine, Smith upended conventional wisdom that traced the origins of human tuberculosis to cows. Although the bovine form was *capable* of producing tuberculosis in humans, it was not, as a rule, responsible for human cases. This study at the intersection of human and veterinary medicine was important to Robert Koch's work on tuberculosis. It also fuelled Smith's interest in a host's ability to produce permanent variations in resident microbial parasites.

Although not an administrator by nature, Smith was appointed director of the Rockefeller's new Department of Animal Pathology at Princeton in 1915. Holding the position until he retired in 1929, he influenced a generation of bacteriologists with his evolutionary understanding of disease. The approach informed his classic treatise, *Parasitism and Disease*. Appearing just months before his death, the book articulated Smith's interpretation of infectious diseases as 'incidents in a developing parasitism' (1934, p. 3). Such parasitism thus was not so much 'pathological' as 'a normal condition having its roots in the interdependence of all living organisms' (1934, p. 2). Smith's vision helped shape future studies of disease ecology.

Bibliography

Primary: 1893. (with Kilborne, F. L.) 'Investigations into the Nature, Causation, and Prevention of Texas or Southern Cattle Fever.' USDA, BAI, Bulletin No. 1 (Washington, DC); 1898. 'A Comparative Study of Bovine Tubercle Bacilli and of Human Bacilli from Sputum.' *J. Exp. Med.* 3: 451–511; 1934. *Parasitism and Disease* (Princeton).

Secondary: Dolman, Claude E., and Richard J. Wolfe, 2003. *Suppressing the Diseases of Animals and Man: Theobald Smith, Microbiologist* (Boston); Clark, P. F., 1959. 'Theobald Smith, Student of Disease (1859–1934).' *Journal of the History of Medicine and Allied Sciences* 14: 490–514; Zinsser, Hans, 1936. 'Theobald Smith, 1859–1934.' *National Academy of Sciences Biographical Memoirs* 17: 261–393; *DSB; DAMB.*

Kim Pelis

SMITH, THOMAS SOUTHWOOD   (b. Martock, Somerset, England, 21 December 1788; d. Florence, Italy, 10 December 1861), *public health*.

Smith's parents, strict Baptists, intended their son to become a preacher, but after some years training for this vocation in the west of England, including a scholarship to Bristol Baptist College (1802) at the early age of fourteen, he decided to train for medicine. He attended Edinburgh Medical School beginning in October 1812, where he also took charge of a local Unitarian congregation. He graduated MD (1816) and returned to the West Country to Yeovil to practice as a preacher and part-time physician. However, in 1820 he moved to London, determined to make medicine his primary career. He obtained his MRCP (1821), and from 1824 he worked as a physician at the London Fever Hospital and later at the Eastern Dispensary and the Jews' Hospital. He continued to preach and also wrote for the new *Westminster Review* (founded 1824), contributing an article on Jeremy Bentham's (1748–1832) system of education to the first issue, through which his close connection with the philosopher was established. Smith also researched and published on fever, anatomy, medicine, and physiology. His most significant early publications expounded his theory that epidemic fever was the cause of much poverty in Britain and that it was preventable. In his *Treatise on Fever* (1830), he reported on the nature of contagious and epidemic disease and concluded that quarantine was largely ineffective for epidemic disease.

When Bentham died, he left his body in his will for public anatomical dissection, a controversial issue at this time, as the supply of legitimate bodies was limited until the passing of the 1832 Anatomy Act, which Smith was instrumental in getting through Parliament. Smith lectured at the dissection of Bentham's body at the Anatomy School, Webb Street, London, on 9 June 1832. He kept the skeleton, with a replacement wax head, in his consulting rooms, until it was transferred to University College London (1850).

Smith was instrumental in the development of health and safety legislation. He was a member of the 1832 Board of Inquiry into the condition of children working in factories, which preceded the Factory Acts. He was also closely involved with Edwin Chadwick (1800–90) in the development of sanitary reform in Britain. Smith researched and reported on sanitary improvement from 1838 until his retirement. He was a founder member (1839) of the Health of Towns Association, which acted as a pressure group for national public health legislation, and was closely involved with the Metropolitan Association for Improving the Dwellings of the Working Classes (founded 1842). He also gave evidence to the 1844 Parliamentary Inquiry on the Health of Towns and the 1847 Metropolitan Sanitary Commission. In 1848 he was appointed as medical member of the General Board of Health, initially in a voluntary part-time capacity. His appointment was made salaried and full-time in 1850, and he produced a number of valuable reports on quarantine (1845), cholera (1850), yellow fever (1852), and the results of sanitary improvement (1854). When the Board was abolished (1854), Smith failed to secure another civil service appointment. In mark of his significant contributions to health, a public subscription was raised (1856), and he was belatedly awarded a pension (1858). He ranks alongside Chadwick as one of the pioneers of sanitary reform and preventive medicine in Britain.

Bibliography

Primary: 1830. *A Treatise on Fever* (London); 1832. *The Use of the Dead to the Living* (London); 1835–37. *The Philosophy of Health* 2 vols. (London); 1856. *Epidemics Considered with Relation to Their Common Nature, and to Climate and Civilisation* (London).

Secondary: Webb, R. K., 1993. 'Southwood Smith: The Intellectual Sources of Public Service' in Porter, Dorothy, and Roy Porter, eds., *Doctors, Politics and Society: Historical Essays* (London) pp. 46–80; Pelling, Margaret, 1978. *Cholera, Fever and English Medicine, 1825–1865* (Oxford); Poynter, F. N. L., 1962. 'Thomas Southwood Smith—the Man (1788–1861).' *Proceedings of the Royal Society of Medicine* 55: 381–392; *Oxford DNB*.

Sally Sheard

ŚNIADECKI, JĘDRZEJ (ANDREW) (b. Żnicz [now Wielkopolska], Poland, 30 October 1768; d. near Wilno, Poland [now Vilnius, Lithuania], 29 April 1838), *medicine, chemistry.*

Śniadecki was one of the most prominent European physicians and certainly the most famous Polish professor of medicine of his time. His *Theory of Organic Beings* presented a new vision of disease as a form of life in altered condition, among other findings. He and his mathematician brother Jan (1756–1830) are considered the most outstanding figures of the Polish Enlightenment. Together they revolutionized the Polish sciences.

Śniadecki was brought up largely by his older brother and attended secondary school in Cracow. He began his university studies in mathematics but quickly chose to devote himself to medicine. In 1791 he traveled to Padua, where he studied under various prominent physicians, including Spallanzani and the public health specialist J. P. Frank. In Italy Śniadecki's work focused primarily on John Brown's theory, which was not yet widely accepted. He completed his doctorate in medicine and philosophy in 1793 and pursued his studies in Edinburgh under the direction of Gregory, Monroe, and Duncan. He became a follower of the Scottish Philosophy of Common Sense.

In 1795 he turned down a promising position in the British colonies in order to return to his homeland. He spent a year traveling through Europe but was thwarted in his plans to visit Paris by the French Revolution. He undoubtedly had hoped to meet with Lavoisier, whose theory of combustion he ardently defended.

Śniadecki went back to Poland in 1796 and participated in fighting a major plague epidemic. A year later he was named professor of chemistry and pharmacy at the Polish University of Wilno. For the first time he abandoned Latin as the language of instruction and taught exclusively in Polish. When Napoleon Bonaparte visited the university, he inquired of Śniadecki 'Quelle chimie enseigne-t-on ici? to which the Polish professor responded 'La chimie qu'on enseigne à Paris'.

In 1800 Śniadecki published *The origins of chemistry*, the first Polish textbook on chemistry. In the book he developed a Polish medical terminology based on the *Méthodes de nomenclature chimique* (1787) by Lavoisier, Morveau, Berthollet, and Fourcroy.

In 1804 Śniadecki became famous throughout Europe with the publication of the first volume of his *Theory of Organic Beings*, a treatise in physiology and biochemistry presenting an original concept of nature based on the most recent findings in science. According to Johannes Müller, Berlin professor of physiology, Śniadecki's work offered 'the first philosophical basis for a scientific system in medicine'. The theory of general pathology which Śniadecki developed in his *Theory of Organic Beings* brought about major changes in clinical medicine in Poland. Śniadecki also came close to the etiology of infectious diseases. He believed that the causal factor of such diseases could be transmitted by air and living matter, and that inadequate nourishment, promiscuity, and poor living conditions favored the appearance of infectious diseases.

In 1805 Śniadecki founded the first scientific journal in Wilno and brought out the second volume of the *Theory of Organic Beings*, this time devoted to the human organism and stressing organic individuality.

In 1812–13, with the outbreak of the Napoleonic wars, Śniadecki returned to hospital work. Until his death he remained one of the most popular university lecturers. In 1821–22 his course was attended by no fewer than 282 auditors. Śniadecki's funeral was held on 3 May, the anniversary of the Polish Constitution, and attracted over 20,000 mourners.

Besides chemistry and physiology, Śniadecki's interests also included public health. 'The health and life of the citizen', he wrote in *The origins of chemistry*, 'constitute his dearest property as well as the most important object of governmental protection.' He was equally interested in child rearing and devised a theory of education that inspired one of the most prominent specialists of the twentieth century, Janusz Korczak.

Śniadecki was a staunch believer in the application of science to social ends: 'Scientific knowledge becomes purposeful only when the truths which it has discovered and precisely recognized can be applied to serve the social good.'

Bibliography

Primary: 1840. Balinski, M., ed., *Complete Works* [in Polish] (Warsaw); 1800. *Pocztki chemii* (Vilna); 1804. *Teoria jestestw organicznych* (Warsaw); 1810. *Theorie des organischen Wesen* (Königsberg); 1825. *Théorie des êtres organiques* (Paris).

Secondary: Stasiewicz, I, ed., 1970. *Rzecz o Jędrzeju Śniadeckim* (Warsaw); 1969. *Archiwum Historii Medycyny* 321: 1–73 (Special issue devoted to Jędrzej Śniadecki); Balinski, M., 1840. 'Życie Jędrzeja Śniadeckiego' in Balinski, M., ed., *Dzieła Jędrzeja Śniadeckiego* vol. 1 (Warsaw) pp. 13–88.

Marta Aleksandra Balinska

SNOW, JOHN (b. York, England, 15 March 1813; d. London, England, 16 June 1858), *general practice, anesthesia, epidemiology.*

Snow was the eldest child of William Snow, an unskilled laborer, and Frances Askham. The family's financial situation improved over the next fifteen years as Snow's siblings were born (three sisters and five brothers). At the age of fourteen (1827), he began his apothecary's apprenticeship with William Hardcastle, a surgeon-apothecary (general practitioner) of Newcastle-upon-Tyne. Snow briefly attended Newcastle's new medical school (1832) and 'walked the wards' at the Infirmary. During the first cholera epidemic (1831–32), he helped with Hardcastle's patients.

A year later (1833), his apprenticeship over, Snow became an assistant to John Watson, apothecary of Burnop Field, County Durham.

After less than a year, Snow found work with Joseph Warburton in Pateley Bridge, West Yorkshire, where he stayed until early summer in 1836. In August, after visiting his family in York and his maternal Uncle Charles Empson in Bristol, he went to London to study for the LSA and MRCS, probably with financial help from Empson. This period is noteworthy for Snow's conversion to vegetarianism, temperance, and teetotalism.

Already familiar with John Frank Newton's *The Return to Nature: A Defence of the Vegetable Regimen* (1811) from his reading as an apprentice, Snow adopted a vegetarian diet and where possible drank only distilled water, chemically tested for purity. This reputed cure for digestive problems and maintaining the health of the stomach and intestines could be difficult if living as part of another's household, but Warburton was sympathetic and supported the temperance movement. By the time he left Pateley Bridge, Snow had become teetotal and spent his summer participating in abstinence meetings, sometimes with his family.

London

Snow signed up for a two-year course of lectures at the Hunterian School of Medicine and lodged nearby in Bateman Street. After medical school, he remained in the Soho district, moving to better living and consulting accommodation as his finances permitted. After qualification (MRCS, May 1838; LSA, October 1838), he opened his first practice at 54 Frith Street.

While still a student (October 1837), Snow joined the Westminster Medical Society (merged with the Medical Society of London, 1849). Characterized by free debate, society meetings provided Snow with opportunities for discussion, even if other members were unimpressed by his enthusiastic championing of nascent laboratory medical sciences to support his bedside observations. Responding to reports of society meetings in *Lancet* and *London Medical Gazette* formed the basis for some early publications.

Snow began his life as a general practitioner without significant advantage (a pre-qualification application as apothecary to the Westminster Hospital was unsuccessful), but from the start, he pursued and published independent research. An early, fundamental interest was the physiology and pathology of respiration, with special reference to the chemistry and physics of inhaled gases. Snow studied the effects of inhaled toxins on respiratory physiology as part of a wider concern with factors responsible for stimulating or depressing respiration. Similarly, his investigations of gaseous exchange also fed inquiries into what supported or interfered with this process in the body's tissues. Frequently attending difficult midwifery cases, he developed an apparatus to help resuscitate stillborn babies.

Besides his research, Snow continued to improve his professional standing, gaining the MB (1843) and MD (1844) of the University of London. He served as lecturer in forensic medicine at the Medical School, Aldersgate Street, in the east end of London from 1846 to 1849. The year 1846 proved to be auspicious for another reason: on 19 December, the dentist James Robinson demonstrated the anesthetic gas ether for the first time in Britain, two months after its initial American use. Nine days later, Snow witnessed a similar operation.

Anesthesia

Ether could free surgery from its attendant agony. For the doctor who administered this drug—even crudely dropping a little ether onto a folded handkerchief, held over the patient's face—it offered the potential for increased earnings. Still struggling financially, Snow was not adverse to either benefit. In his thorough, scientific style, he was not content merely to scramble for business and set out to establish the best and safest method of ether anesthesia. Already familiar with the nuances of respiratory physiology and the effects of a range of inhaled substances, Snow similarly studied the effects of ether, including auto-experimentation. Over time, this research formed part of a larger study of the effects of a related family of substances, all of which he considered narcotics. He came to regard painlessness as a local epiphenomenon of narcotic drugs. On the basis of his close observations, he described the signs of increasing etherization as the five degrees of 'narcotism' (1847, pp. 3–13). Aware of the need for precision in dosage, he developed a special apparatus for administering ether, so that he could exactly control the amount inhaled, mixed with ordinary air, at a given temperature. Snow did not patent his device, and four instrument makers quickly began its manufacture. A greatly increased and more lucrative consulting practice rewarded his expertise.

No sooner had Snow determined the nuances of ether anesthesia than the Edinburgh obstetrician James Young Simpson championed a purportedly safer drug, chloroform (November 1847). Snow repeated his earlier research, now using chloroform and thereby widening the scope of his narcotic research program. Despite its troubled reputation, chloroform quickly became the anesthetic of choice.

By April 1853, chloroform and Snow were sufficiently popular for Queen Victoria to request that he administer anesthesia during the delivery of her eighth child, Prince Leopold. The Church of England may have thought that women should continue to suffer in childbirth, but the British Monarch and many doctors and obstetricians, including Snow, did not.

Unlikely as it may seem, Snow's extensive researches into respiration and anesthesia and his concern with intestinal health and personal pursuit of acceptable sources of pure drinking water would prove useful in tackling a very different problem: unraveling the epidemiology of cholera.

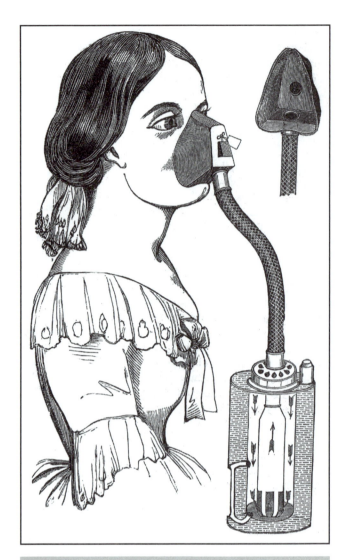

Snow's chloroform inhaler. Lithograph from *On Chloroform and Other Anaesthetics . . .* London, 1858. Wellcome Library, London.

Epidemiology

In autumn 1848, epidemic cholera returned to Britain, and its reappearance reinvigorated debates over the etiology and mode of transmission. Broadly speaking, there were three camps: miasmatists, contagionists, and contingent contagionists. Miasmatists blamed cholera on the offensive smells emanating from rotting human and vegetable waste, which spread through the air and was inhaled by its victims. Contagionists required contact with a cholera patient or perhaps their close personal possessions—e.g., clothing and bed linen. In certain circumstances or contingencies, within the same outbreak, cholera could change from a miasmatic to a contagious disease. Medical theories had important sociopolitical ramifications. Quarantine restrictions disrupted international trade, crucial to the British economy, and were only effective against a contagious disease. Miasmatists such as Edwin Chadwick attempted to combat infectious (literally inhaled) diseases and improve public health by prioritizing the removal of human waste with flush toilets and underground sewers, instead of cesspits. Often sewage passed untreated into rivers that were also used as sources of drinking water. Far from improving health, this imperiled the lives of those living downstream from the sewer outlet.

An apothecary's apprentice during the first cholera epidemic, Snow the mature practitioner moved beyond the range of orthodox opinion on cholera's etiology and transmission during the second epidemic, perhaps prompted to its study by attempts to use chloroform therapeutically. By August 1848, he had abandoned his initial idea that cholera was an asphyxia-like condition and published *On the Mode of Communication of Cholera.* Cholera was not a miasmatic disease. His understanding of respiratory physiology indicated that an infectious agent (he remained guarded on its precise identity) was not inhaled but swallowed—'the disease is communicated by something that acts directly on the alimentary canal' (1849a, pp. 8–9)—and he used intestinal worms as an analogous example. The local poison attacked the mucous membrane of the alimentary canal, the region initially affected. Much of the characteristic pathology— e.g. turgid, thickened blood—was secondary, resulting from fluid loss caused by diarrhea and vomiting. Snow reasoned that if the etiological agent was present in the alimentary canal, it would also be found in cholera patients' evacuations. Should this material pass into a source of drinking water, those served by this supply would be at risk of ingesting it and contracting cholera. He published supporting evidence for a water-borne theory in October in the *London Medical Gazette*, but as the epidemic died down, Snow laid aside his epidemiological research. When cholera returned a third time in the summer of 1853, he was ready to refine his theory and thereby establish new standards in epidemiological research.

The Broad Street Pump

Snow is perhaps best remembered as the doctor whose advice in September 1854 to remove the handle of a water pump in Broad Street, Soho, London, ended the epidemic's most severe local outbreak. Thereafter, discovery of the cholera vibrio awaited Robert Koch's researches in 1883, but a model of water-borne transmission had been explicated. The Broad Street pump adds drama to the history of Snow's epidemiological research, but it built upon his previous work described as a 'grand experiment' in south London in the winter of 1853 and the summer of 1854. With the help of William Farr's clerks at the Registrar General's Office and his own assistant, John Whiting, Snow correlated cholera mortality and morbidity incidence with the source of water supplied. His investiga-

tions involved establishing maps following door-to-door inquiries and the chemical testing of water to determine its source. Houses with water supplied by the Lambeth Water Company, taken from the Thames above London and uncontaminated with fecal material, remained relatively free of cholera. In contrast, homes supplied by the Southwark and Vauxhall Company, with water drawn from the Thames' tidal reaches contaminated with sewage, suffered greatly from the disease. There were too many other differences between these two areas to incriminate the water supply alone, but the crucial test lay in those districts where 'the mixing of the supply is of the most intimate kind . . . A few houses are supplied by one Company and a few by the other . . . In many cases a single house has supply different from that on either side. Each company supplies both rich and poor, both large houses and small; there is no difference either in the condition or occupation of the persons receiving the water of the different Companies' (1855, pp. 74–75). Based on this house-by-house study and additional contact tracing, where cholera was brought into neighborhoods by an infected person, Snow established that cholera victims contracted the disease by the fecal-oral route and that epidemics were transmitted through contaminated water supplies—hence his advice to remove the pump handle of the contaminated water source in Broad Street, after a period of careful mapping of the outbreak, which included correlating cholera statistics with the distance to this pump and the nearby alternatives. Such a map is known now as a Voronoi diagram.

This dramatic incident has become an apocryphal moment in the history of public health and epidemiology, but Snow converted few people during what remained of his life, and his successes were posthumous applications of his methods and ideas—e.g., mapping, statistical correlations, and predictions. By 1858, when he died of a stroke, he was once again researching chloroform anesthesia.

Bibliography

Primary: 1841–42. 'On asphyxia, and on the resuscitation of still-born children.' *London Medical Gazette* 29: 222–227; 1847. *On the Inhalation of the Vapour of Ether in Surgical Operations* (London); 1849a. *On the Mode of Communication of Cholera* (London) (2nd edn., 1855); 1849b. 'On the pathology and mode of communication of cholera.' *London Medical Gazette* 44: 745–752, 923–929; 1858. (Richardson, Benjamin Ward, ed.) *On Chloroform and Other Anaesthetics* (London).

Secondary: Vinten-Johansen, Peter, Howard Brody, Nigel Paneth, Stephen Rachman, and Michael Rip, 2003. *Cholera, Chloroform, and the Science of Medicine: A Life of John Snow* (New York); Ellis, Richard H., 1994. *The Case Books of Dr. John Snow. Medical History Supplement* 14; *DSB*; *Oxford DNB*.

Helen Bynum

SOEDARMO, POORWO (b. Malang, Java, Indonesia, 20 February 1904; d. Malang, 13 March 2003), *medicine, public health, nutrition.*

Soedarmo was the second son of the Soedirjo family. He graduated in 1927 as an Indonesian doctor during the Dutch colonial period and as a western doctor during the Japanese occupation of the islands. He studied nutrition at the Harvard School of Public Health (1954–55) and the Institute of Nutritional Science at Columbia University (1960).

From January 1928 until 1941, he worked for the Indonesian government as a local medical doctor. His assignments at government hospitals included several Indonesian cities, such as Jakarta, Toboali, Malang, Cirebon, and Cianjur on the island of Java. In 1943 he was appointed public health doctor at Banten, West Java, and worked from 1948 to 1949 as a health inspector for West Java. Beginning on 1 January 1950, at his own request, he worked at the Food Institute for People. On 5 March 1952 he was appointed director of the Food Institute for People, a position he held until 1959. In 1955 he was also selected as special lecturer on hygiene at the Faculty of Medicine, University of Indonesia, Jakarta; and in January 1958 he became special professor on nutrition at the Faculty of Medicine. In June 1959 he was appointed chairman of the Department of Nutrition of the Faculty of Medicine. In January 1971 he resigned with honor.

In Indonesia, Soedarmo was well known as the expert who initiated nutrition education for the people and who introduced several popular slogans to the public, including 'Four health, five excellent' and 'Four is enough, five comprehensive', which meant that to be healthy a person should include these four or five main categories in his or her diet: (1) a staple food consisting of rice or corn and containing mainly carbohydrates, (2) meat and poultry as sources of protein, (3) vegetables, (4) fruit, and (5) milk to be complete.

Another slogan he coined was 'Not sick and not healthy'. This referred to the many people who are not sick or ill but who are not healthy and do not experience life to its full potential. He applied this idea to two groups of people. The first were people who did not complain and had no signs or symptoms of sickness but were inactive and often felt tired. Usually these people were anemic and borderline malnourished. The second group consisted of people who were obese and hyperactive, took no time to rest and had a high concentration of blood cholesterol. In an effort to overcome the popularity and advertising campaigns of modern snack or junk foods such as Kentucky Fried Chicken, Soedarmo advised the public to diversify their food intake and to seek to enjoy nutritious, good quality food at a reasonable price.

Bibliography

Primary: 1995. *Nutrition and Me.*

Charles Suradji

SOLOV'EV, ZINOVII PETROVICH (b. Grodno, Russia [now Belarus], 10 November [2 November] 1876; d. Moscow, Russia, 6 November 1928), *epidemiology, public health, social hygiene, military medicine.*

An icon of Soviet public health, Solov'ev had a political career that was more important than his medical one, but as he was the most articulate proponent of the principles and organization of early Soviet medicine, he is a significant figure in the history of health care. He was born into the family of a poor provincial land surveyor and entered the Simbirsk classical gymnasium in 1886. He began studies at the medical faculty of Kazan University in 1897. After finishing at Kazan in 1904, Solov'ev worked during the Russo-Japanese War for the Red Cross on the front in Manchuria.

Already long a political radical, Solov'ev escaped the crackdown after the 1905 Revolution to become a district doctor in the vicinity of Saratov. An epidemiologist with a particular interest in tuberculosis and occupational illnesses, Solov'ev's energy and his writing and organizational abilities were quickly noticed, and he was promoted to assist N. I. Teziakov in the *gubernia* (province) sanitary bureau. He published a number of articles on epidemiology at the regional level.

Arrested in 1909, Solov'ev moved to Moscow in 1912 after three years of internal exile. He became heavily involved in the Pirogov Society and the All-Russian League for the Struggle with Tuberculosis, raising the profile and authority of the latter and publishing a number of articles on tuberculosis. During World War I he worked as the secretary of the Medical-Sanitary Department of the *Zemstvo* Union (Union of Councils).

After the Bolsheviks took power, a large part of Solov'ev's career was devoted to military medicine, as he headed the main military-sanitary management of the Red Army. He energetically led the fight against typhus in the Red Army over the latter part of the Civil War in 1920–21. Solov'ev also headed the medical section of the People's Commissariat of the Interior, becoming Deputy Commissar for Health once the post was created in 1918. As such, he was instrumental in integrating Soviet medicine and building public health services.

Along with Nikolai Semashko, Solov'ev appropriated preventive medicine as distinctively Soviet. For him, preventive medicine combined the close study of the everyday life and work of the patient with agitational and organizational initiatives from the state. Clinical medicine was also to be bound very closely to the organization and program of prevention. Because of the influence of social hygiene, environmental factors and social illnesses were singled out for special attention, while enormous significance was attached to the statistical identification and analysis of public health problems.

At the time of the Bolshevik Revolution, the prevailing orientation of Russian doctors and their Pirogov Society was toward decentralized 'community medicine'. Solov'ev attacked this and 'reoriented' Soviet medical practitioners in post-Revolutionary conditions toward a highly centralized, statist ethos. With the pre-Revolutionary Rein Plan as a starting point, Solov'ev developed the idea and practice of the state planning of public health throughout the 1920s.

Soviet medicine in the 1920s was strategic and ambitious. It was also potentially very intrusive but, as it was almost entirely lacking in resources, the intrusions were rather limited in practice. Solov'ev was one of the strongest proponents of the ambition and potential sweep of early Soviet medicine.

Bibliography

Primary: 1928. *Krasnyi krest i sanitarnaia oborona. Doklad na I Moskovskoi gubernskoi konferentsii O-va Krasnogo Kresta RSFSR 27 oktiabria 1927 goda* [The Red Cross and Sanitary Defense. Speech at the First Moscow Provincial Conference of the Society of the RSFSR Red Cross of 27 October 1927] (Moscow); 1932. *Stroitel'stvo sovetskogo zdravookhraneniia* [The Construction of Soviet Public Health] (Moscow); 1970. *Voprosy sotsial'noi gigieny i zdravookhraneniia. Izbrannye proizvedeniia* [Problems of Social Hygiene and Public Health] (Moscow).

Secondary: Hutchinson, John F. 1990. *Politics and Public Health in Revolutionary Russia, 1890–1918* (Baltimore); Solov'eva, V. A., ed., 1980. *Zhizn' i deiatelnost' Z. P. Solov'eva (po vospominaniiam sovremennikov)* [Life and Work of Z. P. Solov'ev (the reminiscences of contemporaries)] (Moscow); Golubkova, A. P., and N. A. Kosta, eds., 1929. *Pamiati Z. P. Solov'eva. Sbornik* [Recollections of Z. P. Solov'ev. Collection] (Moscow).

Chris Burton

SOPER, FRED LOWE (b. Hutchinson, Kansas, USA, 13 December 1893; d. Wichita, Kansas, USA, 9 February 1977), *malaria eradication, international health.*

First Years

Fred Lowe Soper was born into a middle class family of British origin, the third of eight children. His father was a pharmacist and his mother a schoolteacher. After receiving a bachelor's degree in 1914 from the University of Arkansas, he became interested in embryology and pursued a master of science degree. In 1918 Soper graduated as a medical doctor from Rush Medical College, which was then part of the University of Chicago. During his medical studies he also spent a year as an intern at Chicago's Cook County Hospital.

Shortly after his graduation he was recruited by the International Health Board (later Division) of the Rockefeller Foundation to conduct hookworm surveys and campaigns in Brazil. Before departing for South America he married Juliet Snider, who would be at his side in many of his travels around the world for the rest of his career. In the early 1920s he felt that the hands-on education in public health he had acquired was insufficient and he went to Baltimore to study at the School of Public Health and Hygiene of Johns Hopkins University, where in 1923 he obtained a certificate in public health (a precursor to the present Master of Public Health or MPH). Two years later Johns Hopkins also awarded him a doctorate *in absentia*. At the end of 1923, he returned to the Rockefeller Foundation and was sent for three years to Paraguay to organize hookworm control and demonstration programs. Thanks to his experiences in Brazil and Paraguay, Soper learned Portuguese and Spanish. Moreover, he was exposed to different cultural and institutional idiosyncrasies and learned how to wrestle with local bureaucracies.

Brazil

In 1927 Soper was appointed the Rockefeller Foundation's representative in Brazil and moved with his wife to Rio de Janeiro, then the capital of the country. This was at a time when the Foundation's emphasis on international public health had changed from hookworm to yellow fever and malaria. He would remain in Brazil in this position until 1942. A year after his arrival he participated in an important medical campaign: the reemergence of yellow fever in Rio, a city which had been free of the disease for twenty years. From a scientific perspective the event was also relevant because it confirmed what some experts suspected: the Amazon areas could reinfect coastal cities, and the disease was transmitted not just by the mosquito *Aedes aegypti*, as originally established in the early twentieth century. It is important to underscore that it was only in 1927 that the etiological origin of the fever was discovered, and only in 1935 that an effective vaccine to prevent yellow fever was developed in the Rockefeller Foundation's New York laboratories.

In Brazil, and throughout Latin America in the late 1920s and early 1930s, Soper encouraged the definition of 'jungle yellow fever' as distinct from 'urban yellow fever', although both were caused by the same virus. He also promoted the use of the new technique of viscerotomy, which involved the postmortem collection and laboratory examination of liver tissue within eleven days of illness from every person who died. He considered it a more reliable diagnosis for yellow fever than clinical diagnosis. Soper was confident that sufficient political backing and medical determination could overcome any family resistance in rural areas to the necessity of puncturing bodies for this examination. During his stay in Brazil, Soper also represented the Rockefeller Foundation at Pan American Sanitary Conferences held in Buenos Aires in 1934, Bogotá in 1938, and Rio de Janeiro in 1942.

A major campaign headed by Soper in Brazil brought about the successful eradication of the *Anopheles gambiae*. In the early 1930s this dangerous African malaria vector, considered the most lethal and efficient of its kind, appeared in the northeast region of Ceara. Nothing was done until the dramatic epidemic of malaria of 1938 that killed thousands of people in this area. Thanks to Soper's insistence, the necessary resources and political will sprang up to support a sort of military control of the area. For about two years Soper, who became director of northeast Brazil's malaria service, used meticulous planning, scrupulous supervision, detailed recordkeeping, and the Paris green larvicide to combat the epidemic. As a result, he and his staff wiped out the vector from the region.

Some of the main features of his leadership developed during the campaign would reappear in later years: to be certain that all subordinates check, recheck, and crosscheck field work. His impatience with inefficient subordinates gave him a reputation among Brazilian health workers, who called him 'comandante', a term usually reserved for military leaders. The experience also reinforced his belief that hard work, integrity, and careful administration were the keystones of a successful health campaign and thus could succeed in any cultural setting.

World War II

Shortly after the entry of the United States into World War II, Soper left Brazil. Beginning in 1942 he actively participated in the medical support of the Allies; technically he was 'on loan' from the Rockefeller Foundation to the U.S. Secretary of War. He worked mainly in Egypt, Algiers, and Sardinia against malaria and louse-borne typhus fever. The latter resulted from refugee movements, overcrowding in prisons, lack of bathing facilities, and misery. In Egypt he presented a proposal for an *Anopheles gambiae* eradication program inspired by his Brazilian experience; however, the proposal was not immediately followed by British and Egyptian authorities. Local congressmen shouting 'We Want Soper!' chastened the authorities, who, with a little help from the Rockefeller Foundation, finally provided Soper his antimalaria program. He spearheaded a successful campaign in Egypt which eliminated the mosquito from the Nile.

In Sardinia he became acquainted with and fascinated by the new and powerful insecticide DDT, which would later be widely used in malaria eradication campaigns. Between 1943 and 1944 he was a member of the U.S. Typhus Commission in North Africa and Italy and used DDT to delouse people and eliminate the human louse that transmits the disease. This work enabled Allied forces to put an end to epidemics in Europe by the end of the war. After the war he returned again to the Rockefeller Foundation. His experience in the war created a conviction that would grow in later years: disease control, and even disease eradication, was possible without major public health improvements.

Pan American Sanitary Bureau

At the Twelfth Pan American Sanitary Conference, which took place in Caracas in early 1947, Soper was elected director of the Pan American Sanitary Bureau (PASB), the executive agency of the Pan American Sanitary Organization (an organization that in 1958 changed its name to the Pan American Health Organization). PASB's headquarters in Washington, D.C., served twenty-one republics of the Americas, and its meetings included representatives of Canada and the European colonies located in the Caribbean and in northern South America. The origins of this institution could be traced to the International Sanitary Conference of the American Republics held in 1902, and its main document was the 1924 Sanitary Code, one of the first international treaties that supported the concept of health as a right of citizens. From 1920 to 1947 its director was Hugh Cummings, who for some years was also U.S. Surgeon General and head of the U.S. Public Health Service. Soper was later reelected for two more four-year terms, remaining as PASB's director until 1959.

Two years after Soper's first election, an agreement was signed between PASB and the World Health Organization (WHO), a multilateral organization created in 1948. The agreement made the former the first regional office of WHO and was perceived as a victory by many Latin American medical leaders, since originally WHO insisted on the absorption of PASB. Initially Soper was not on very good personal terms with Canadian Brock Chisholm, WHO's first Director General. However, after the election in 1953 of the Brazilian Marcolino Candau as WHO's second Director General, relations between the two agencies were friendly and fluid. This is partly explained by the fact that Candau had worked under Soper before. The Brazilian was familiar with and believed in the promise of disease-oriented projects such as those implemented by the Rockefeller Foundation during the interwar period.

Although Soper's activities in PASB were supported by the Rockefeller Foundation, his move to a multilateral agency can be seen in the broader and more complex perspective of the emergence of the field of international health, which arrived through the creation of a series of bilateral, multilateral and donor agencies. Some of these, such as the International Cooperation Administration created in the early 1950s (the predecessor of USAID), were part of a more active role by the U.S. Department of State linking health and foreign policy. Others, such as WHO and UNICEF, were part of the specialized agencies of the United Nations system that in its early years counted on full support of the U.S. government. New donor agencies such as the Kellogg Foundation were willing to fund the training of medical personnel and the purchasing of equipment for Latin American hospitals. In addition, major U.S. universities began to create departments of international health that emphasized the use of international medical programs to raise the standards of living of poor and newly-decolonized nations. In addition, by the beginning of the 1950s the Rockefeller Foundation was losing interest in international health, even though it had been one of the main players during the interwar period, and began to emphasize technological improvements in agriculture and the Green Revolution in poor countries. As a result, the International Health Division of the Rockefeller was officially terminated in 1951, opening the field to new donors and agencies. A byproduct of this trend was the move of a significant number of Rockefeller health experts to international health agencies in the years after World War II.

One aim of Soper's work was to continue the Rockefeller Foundation's traditions in disease control and eradication. He rapidly adapted to the Cold War context and motivations of the period, promoting, for example, disease control and eradication as a means to encourage capitalist development in backward countries. As with many Cold War warriors, he believed in technical interventions not only for humanitarian reasons but also for raising the standards of living and containing social upheaval. Soper even resorted to Cold War euphemisms to make his point, writing of 'enslaving' conditions for developing malaria, seen as a metaphor for communism, and the 'liberating' eradication of malaria, seen as a metaphor for 'modernization'.

In one of the most popular photographs of Soper, he appears receiving a donation from John Foster Dulles, the assertive and controversial anticommunist U.S. Secretary of State for most of the 1950s. Soper's leadership of PASB facilitated the support of this agency by the U.S. government. The U.S. perceived PASB, other inter-American agencies such as the Organization of American States (OAS), and even the United Nations, as a part of its tools in its Cold War against the Soviet Union and a necessary element of containment of communism's expansionist ideology. The support proved crucial. By 1956 PASB received from the U.S. government an annual contribution of about $1.3 million, which was more than any other inter-American agency except the OAS.

Soper was also a shrewd negotiator and was convinced of the merit of multilateral agencies such as PASB over bilateral agencies. Despite any apparent contradiction, he believed that bilateral organizations were inevitably nationalistic political enterprises, had to maintain a low profile, and as such had limited acceptability and utility in the receiving countries. According to Soper, international health and its practitioners could maintain an independent technical role, acting as neutral experts and making decisions that would be validated in any political setting. Soper believed multilateral organizations such as PASB had greater leverage and technical effectiveness and were not simple followers of individual governments. Soper's aspirations for a greater role for multilateral agencies as leaders in national, regional, and global programs were reinforced with the development of an international staff at PASB and WHO.

During Soper's tenure PASB acquired more independent finances, expanded its staff (from eighty-eight in 1947 to 750 in 1959), and established 'zone' (subregional) and field offices in El Paso (Texas), Lima, and Guatemala. It also established specialized research centers such as the Institute of Nutrition of Central America and Panama located in Guatemala, the Pan American Foot and Mouth Disease Center in Brazil and the Pan American Zoonoses Center in Argentina—all in existence to this day. In addition, it was partly thanks to Soper and PASB's grants that new health professions such as sanitary engineering, nutrition, and nursing developed. Nursing in Latin America was transformed from an occupation of untrained older women concentrated in hospitals to one of ambitious young female professionals with higher education degrees who worked in different institutional settings and who used symbols of respect like crisp white uniforms.

The development of these professions intensified the process of Americanization of Latin American medicine and medical science that can be traced to the interwar period and to the fellowships and grants of the Rockefeller Foundation. At the beginning of the twentieth century the medical Mecca for many Latin American students was Paris, and it was common to find a large number of French textbooks in local medical libraries. During the second half of the twentieth century, U.S. universities became the favorite choice for Latin American medical students pursuing postgraduate education, and a reading command of English became a requirement for medical training.

According to several testimonies, Soper inspired among his staff and disciples devotion, discipline, *esprit de corps*, loyalty, zeal, sometimes fear, and always respect. He also developed unique diplomatic skills to deal directly with bloody Cold War dictators such as Rafael Trujillo of the Dominican Republic and François 'Papa Doc' Duvalier of Haiti. He sincerely believed that while negotiating with them he engendered full political support without interference so as to ensure the success of international health interventions.

Soper traveled extensively to confer with political and health authorities, with deans and professors of medical schools, and with prominent local physicians and surgeons of the Americas. According to one testimonial, when Soper entered a room everybody knew who the boss was. During his period as director of PASB he also traveled to Asia and India to compare malaria eradication programs.

Disease Eradication

By the mid-1950s Soper acquired a remarkable reputation as an international public health administrator who knew how to get things done. He also made a significant contribution to the concept and implementation of infectious disease eradication on a worldwide basis, an idea previously entertained by important medical doctors and agencies such as the Rockefeller. The concept reinforced the credibility of vertical disease-oriented campaigns as the health priority in developing countries. The motivation for controlling these diseases included humanitarianism, a fear of reinfection of developed countries, and the protection of international commerce and of Americans and U.S.

investments abroad. In addition, a number of new medical technologies promised the possibility of a zero incidence of diseases under attack.

Soper's promotion of eradication was also based on the assumption that the window of political opportunity for public health usually did not last very long. According to Soper, short term interventions were the best option to find full political support because people expected the solution of their urgent problems in the quickest possible manner. Eradication, a single clear-cut definable objective, also appeared in Soper's mind as a clear target for politicians, public health field officers, and the public.

The vertical approach was considered superior to unspecific, multipurpose, and long-term programs with broad objectives. He dismissed these programs as vague and ineffective. According to Soper, eradication had additional advantages because it dealt with economic obstacles to development. Malaria, for example, was frequently portrayed as an 'economic disease': a burden on the economies of every malarious country. First, it would cause a permanent drain on medical care, drugs and hospitalization. Second, the disease led to losses in manpower from premature death and the decline of available worktime, especially in agriculture. Moreover, malaria eradication demonstrated that international collaboration was important and beneficial, setting the pattern for global responsibility of the health conditions of any nation. Soper believed eradication made necessary the coordination of all the agencies that emerged in the postwar period.

PASB's first major internationally coordinated eradication campaign was in Haiti in 1951 against yaws, a crippling and disfiguring disease. The work included the valuable effort of UNICEF—not as an operating but as a supply agency—which provided medicines, equipment and supplies, and U.S. bilateral assistance to provide additional funds. PASB was responsible for technical advice and codirection. The government of Haiti arranged for local personnel and buildings and shared with PASB the campaign's direction. The work consisted of a massive house-to-house visit of about 50 percent of the population in order to inject the ill and their contacts with penicillin (rather than arsenicals and bismuth, previously available). Eventually the antiyaws campaign included the Dominican Republic, Venezuela, and other countries in the region.

Soper would also promote the eradication of *Aedes aegypti* and in his later years envisioned a program to eradicate tuberculosis in the United States. He also pointed to the menace of *Aedes aegypti*, advocated for its continental elimination, and complained about the United States relaxing rules put in place to control the mosquito.

Malaria Eradication

In 1954 the Fourteenth Conference of PASB, held in Santiago, Chile, approved Soper's ambitious scheme for continental eradication of malaria, which involved using indoor spraying of DDT and new synthetic antimalaria drugs. At the time it was estimated that about 143 million people in the Americas, or 36 percent of the total population of the region, lived in malarious areas. The decision was fully endorsed by most experts of the time (including Arnoldo Gabaldón of Venezuela, Emilio Pampana of Italy, and Paul Russell of the United States) and led to the organization of autonomous national malaria eradication services in all Latin American countries. In order to be effective, insecticide spraying had to be applied thoroughly, nationally, and in two annual cycles before the mosquito developed resistance. Starting in 1951 there had been reports on the resistance to insecticides of some species of *Anopheles*.

During the second half of the 1950s, WHO, UNICEF, and U.S. bilateral assistance organizations joined enthusiastically in malaria eradication. UNICEF usually provided the insecticides, spraying equipment, and vehicles for the antimalaria campaigns. But by the late 1960s, because of technical, social, and political considerations the target was not accomplished. By the early 1970s, malaria eradication suffered serious setbacks. The disease slowly increased in South and Central America, where the number of cases had been reduced in prior years to low levels. Important factors that undermined the campaign were unexpected rural migration, the deterioration of the socioeconomic conditions of Latin American countries, and the growing concern about the polluting effects of DDT. Moreover, the whole concept of 'vertical' campaigns came into question, and the political Cold War assumption, namely, that modernization following capitalist lines would improve the living conditions of backward countries, never came to fruition. This was the beginning of a process that led to community-oriented public health efforts and to Primary Health Care. Soper did not care much for these new trends. He supported the urgency of eradication and the relevance of vertical campaigns against a growing international critique in medical circles. Soper's followers believed that his retirement from PASB in 1959 dampened the spark that had engendered eradication.

Final Years

Upon his retirement Soper became director emeritus of the PASB, a consultant on malaria eradication to the International Cooperation Administration (the predecessor of USAID), and a visiting lecturer at the Harvard School of Public Health. Early in 1959 he embarked on a tour of India, Thailand, Taiwan, and other countries, assessing malaria eradication programs for the Rockefeller Foundation. From 1960 to 1962 he was the first director of the Pakistan-SEATO Cholera Research Laboratory in Dacca. (The acronym SEATO stands for the countries of the South East Asia Treaty Organization.) His appointment was a result of concern with the reemergence of cholera in Thailand a few years before. The laboratory was to implement U.S. assistance by sending staff and equipment. Because of unexpected tensions between U.S. and Pakistani personnel, Soper resigned from his position in 1962 and returned to the United States. Shortly after his return he was appointed special consultant in the Office of National Health of the U.S. Public Health Service and was made Secretary of the Gorgas Memorial Institute, a laboratory facility with establishments in Panama and Washington, D.C.

The death of his wife and companion in 1968 was a tragic blow. During his final years Soper organized his papers and books (over 120 publications), wrote his memoirs, and worked on manuscripts (including a history of public health in Latin America that he never finished). These activities were carried out at the National Library of Medicine in Bethesda, MD. Thanks to the assistance of J. Austin Kerr, he published a selection of his works, and thanks to John Duffy he published his memoirs before his death; the work was entitled *Ventures in World Health*. His papers are kept at the History of Medicine Division of the National Library of Medicine. Among the decorations he received were the Lasker Award for his work against malaria in Brazil, the WHO Leon Bernard Foundation Medal, the PAHO Gold Medal, the American Society of Tropical Medicine and Hygiene Walter Reed Medal, and the Grand Cross of the Brazilian Order of Medical Merit.

When Soper reached eighty years, Mirón Wegman wrote a poem that reflects the admiration he elicited among his coworkers. A partial transcription follows (Wegman, 1973):

> Scientific papers tell
> That friend and foe shed ne'er a tear,
> As *Ankylostoma* heard the knell
> When Soper's entourage drew near.
>
> On *Aedes* he cast a spell;
> *Anopheles* soon quaked with fear.
> "Eradicate!" we leaned to yell
> As Soper's couriers sped like deer,
> O'er land and sea his creed to sell.
>
> *Ricketssia* turned a frightened ear,
> The lice were quiet as they fell.
> Polioviruses proved no peer
> As Fred L. Soper gave them hell
> Until they had to disappear.
>
> Triumphant he in public health,
> We rightly call him sage and seer.
> For none can measure all the wealth,
> The joy that he has made appear.
>
> So, proudly, it's abandon stealth,
> For Fred, our hero—Cheer, Cheer, Cheer!!

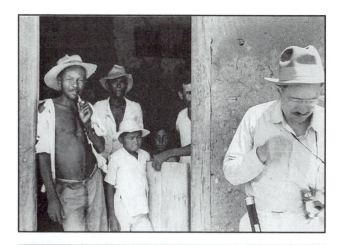

Fred Lowe Soper (far right) during the campaigns against yellow fever and malaria, Brazil, 1930s. Photograph, Oswaldo Cruz Foundation Historical Archives.

Bibliography

Primary: 1943. (with Wilson, D. Bruce) Anopheles gambiae *in Brazil, 1930 to 1940* (New York); 1965. 'Rehabilitation of the Eradication Concept in Prevention of Communicable Diseases.' *Public Health Reports* 80(10): 855–869; 1970. (Kerr, J. Austin, ed.) *Building the Health Bridge: Selections from the Works of Fred L. Soper* (Bloomington, IN); 1972. *Hacia la conquista de la salud; obra de solidaridad entre los pueblos* (Washington, DC); Wegman, M., 1973. Myron E. Wegman to Fred L. Soper [Letter entitled 'For Fred L. Soper at 80']. 13 December 1973. Folder 'Eightieth Birthday Celebration'. Box 5. Soper Papers, National Library of Medicine; 1977. (Duffy, John, ed.) *Ventures in World Health: The Memoirs of Fred Lowe Soper* (Washington, DC).

Secondary: Cueto, Marcos, 2004. *El Valor de la Salud: Historia de la Organización Panamericana de la Salud* (Washington, DC); Gladwell, M., 2002. 'Fred Soper and the Global Malaria Eradication Programme.' *Journal of Public Health Policy* 23(4): 479–497; Litsios, Socrates, 1997. 'René J. Dubos and Fred L. Soper: Their Contrasting Views on Vector and Disease Eradication.' *Perspectives in Biology and Medicine* 41(1): 138–149; Packard, Randall M., and Paulo Gadehla, 1997. 'A Land Filled with Mosquitoes: Fred L. Soper, the Rockefeller Foundation, and the *Anopheles gambiae* Invasion of Brazil.' *Medical Anthropology* 17(3): 215–238; Vaccarezza, Raul F., 1981. 'Devoción a la causa de la salud: Fred Lowe Soper.' *Medicina* [Buenos Aires] 41: 101–106; Waserman, M., 1975. 'Fred L. Soper, Ambassador of Good Health.' *Americas* 27: 10, 30–37.

Marcos Cueto

SORANUS OF EPHESUS (b. Ephesus, Asia Minor [now near modern Selcuk, Turkey]; fl. 100), *gynecology, obstetrics, nosology, pharmacology, philosophy, medicine, surgery.*

There are few extant details of the life of Soranus, and these come from a tenth-century Byzantine source, the *Suda* Lexicon. Soranus, son of Menander and Phoebe, was

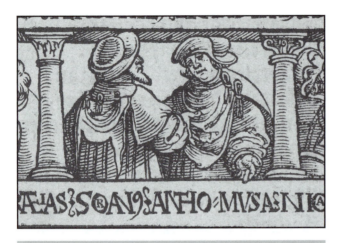

Soranus (left) and Antonius Musa. Detail of a woodcut depicting classical herbalists and medical scholars, from the title page to Lorenz Fries, *Spiegel der Artzney . . .* , 1532. Iconographic Collection, Wellcome Library, London.

born in Ephesus, by then the administrative and economic center of the province of Asia. Like Galen some fifty years later, Soranus traveled to Alexandria, a key medical center, where he would have encountered the teachings of the major medical sects, and he was influenced by the works of Herophilus on uterine anatomy and midwifery. Soranus, again like Galen, then moved to Rome, where he practiced medicine under Trajan and Hadrian (98–138). Soranus's name apparently derives from Quintus Marcius Barea Soranus, the popular proconsul of Asia *c.* 61–63. The story of Soranus as court physician to Cleopatra VII is apocryphal, but his visit to the province of Aquitania to cure 200 people affected by the skin disease *mentagra* (sycosis) is perhaps tenable.

Soranus wrote over twenty books on a variety of topics, which attests to his range as a doctor. Most are now lost, including *On the soul*, used by the Church Father Tertullian in his discussion of the immortality of the soul. Although *Lives of the physicians* is lost, elements may have survived in later Hippocratic biographies. If authentic, these show that Soranus had little interest in fostering a cult of Hippocrates or creating an image of him, as Galen was later successful in doing. The roll of lost works continues with *Etymologies of the Body of Man*, apparently a work on medical names, and *Seed and Generation*, where Soranus described how the female seed did not contribute to reproduction, and that, in contrast to the traditional view, the female uterus lacked cotyledons. In *Causes of Diseases* he delineated the Methodist theory of disease causation, while in *Commonalities* he discussed this central tenet of Methodism, and would doubtless have taken the opportunity to correct prior Methodic inexactitude, a characteristic feature noted in his extant work. His *Fevers* also probably incorporated correctives to earlier Methodist work on the subject. His *Hygiene* was likely to have been a general work and not devoted

exclusively to sexual hygiene. The lost *Remedies* appears to have given a detailed discussion of Methodic metasynkrisis, by which the therapeutic potency of drugs and related treatments was tailored according to the patient's condition. *Doctor's Friend* was probably a layman's compendium of medical knowledge and therapeutic lore.

Soranus also wrote *Drugs* and *Handbook of Pharmaceuticals*; the first was the more comprehensive, the second a summary. *The Eye(s)* was a specialized text that probably illustrated not only Soranus's debt to Herophilus on this subject, but also his willingness to use anatomical knowledge commensurate with the therapeutic priorities of the Methodist School. Of the lost treatise *Surgery*, a fragment is extant under the sixty illustrations in the two principal works of Soranus that have come down to us, which consist of the Latinized *Acute Diseases* and *Chronic Diseases* of Caelius Aurelianus, and the Greek text of *Gynecology* which, like his other major treatises, would originally have been illustrated.

If not in Alexandria, then certainly in Rome, Soranus would have encountered the Methodist medical sect, allegedly founded by a pupil of Asclepiades of Bithynia, Themison of Laodicea (fl. end of the first century BCE), and brought to its pitch of fame and alleged notoriety in Rome by Thessalus of Tralles (fl. 50 BCE). Subject to gross distortion and defamation, especially by Galen, Methodism and its practitioners nevertheless advocated a form of medical practice that was not only popular but, by the second century, was arguably a dominant medical sect in the Roman world. Outside the biased purview of Galen, what is known of Methodism is due in large part to Soranus, its most erudite spokesman. Disease was explained by recourse to the notion of excess of two basic qualities or 'commonalities', constriction and laxity or fluidity. Treatment was based on observation of the patient, which permitted a determination to be made of what was required to counter either excess (or a combination of both in contiguous or separate parts of the body). There was no place here for the popular doctrine of the four humors, and indeed Methodism never carried heavy theoretical baggage (thus Soranus argued that, in dealing with morning sickness, humoral considerations did not apply, only the particular state of the woman's body and what could be done to treat it). The pursuit of anatomical knowledge was regarded as a waste of time, but this did not mean that such knowledge should be altogether ignored; for example, Soranus made full use of Herophilus's advances in uterine anatomy, since these could increase treatment efficacy, and allowed him to argue forcefully against the prevalent Hippocratic notion of the wandering womb. Methodist medicine was thus therapeutically oriented. Soranus also criticized his Methodist predecessors if the occasion warranted, condemning Asclepiades' doctrine of uterine suffocation, and noting that Themison had been led astray in his treatments because of mistakes made by Asclepiades himself, but this was due to insufficient knowledge at that time. Soranus presented Methodism in a mature form, showing a rather subtle medical sect capable of change and development within the framework of its broad tenets, and commensurate with its therapeutic priorities.

This is well demonstrated in Soranus's four-volume work, the *Gynaecology* (*Gynaikeia*), which also dealt with obstetrics. Soranus was as much a gynecologist as Galen. However, the survival of this work, virtually alone of his oeuvre, tends to lead to the conclusion that Soranus was an ancient specialist in this field. He was certainly as competent in this subject as he seems to have been in other topics, to judge from Caelius Aurelianus and the titles of the lost works. The first volume of the *Gynaecology* dealt with the criteria necessary for a good midwife, then examined female anatomy and contraception. Soranus was in favor of contraception, as he regarded it as safer than abortion. He opposed abortion for the sake of vanity or convenience (in cases of adultery). The purpose of coitus was procreation, and permanent virginity for both sexes was the most beneficial for health. Volume two was concerned with birth and neonatal care. The third volume examined pathological states and began with a discussion as to whether women have conditions peculiarly their own. According to Soranus, some, such as the Empiricists and Diocles of Carystus, held that there were special diseases of women. Others maintained the opposite; these included Herophilus, Erasistratus, Asclepiades, Themison, and Thessalus. Soranus's position was in accord with broad Methodist teaching. He maintained that there existed natural conditions peculiar to women, such as conception, birth and lactation. But, in accord with Methodist orthodoxy, conditions contrary to nature were not generically different, for in both sexes the causes were due either to constriction or laxity. The difference lay in the particulars, such as where in the female body the problem arose, and the nature of the symptoms. This was well brought out in Soranus's examination of the menstrual flux, dysmenorrhea and amenorrhea. Treatment of these disorders was metasyncritic, with venesection, a Hippocratic staple in uterine bleeding, being used only as a last resort, and Soranus took Themison to task for advocating it as a mainstay in treating this condition. The fourth and final volume was devoted to labor, surgery, and drugs.

Latinized versions of parts of the *Gynaecology* began in the second century. Subsequent Latin versions were produced by Caelius Aurelianus in the fourth century and by Muscio (probably another North African physician) a century later. Oribasius, the physician and compiler, incorporated Soranus's gynecological anatomy as part of his seventy-volume medical compendium. Aëtius of Amida made use of parts of it in his encyclopedia in the sixth century, as did Paul of Aegina in the seventh, each version increasingly attenuating the text's Methodic content. Moreover, from Muscio onwards, Soranus's strictures against the concept of a wandering womb were effectively reversed in the Latin west. Saint Augustine referred to Soranus as 'the most famous medical author', and Tertullian described him as 'the most learned of the Methodist physicians'. But by the twelfth century, Soranus was now cited as the dominant authority from antiquity in obstetrics and gynecology, while Soranus the Methodist had long since disappeared. The Greek text of Soranus's *Gynaecology* survived as a fifteenth-century Parisian manuscript. The discovery of the wider significance of this document occurred in 1830, but a critical edition did not appear until 1882. This was superseded in 1927 and a further revised version was produced in 2000.

Caelius Aurelianus fittingly described Soranus as *Methodicorum princeps*, the 'prince of physicians'. There is much that is attractive in Soranus or rather, in the medical persona displayed in his writings. It is of immense regret that no more of his works have survived. Possession of his *Gynaecology* meant that Soranus has been viewed primarily as the foremost gynecologist of antiquity. This is unavoidable. But Soranus should be seen as a multifaceted practitioner of the medical art, a worthy adversary to Galen, a doctor interested in both the history and philosophical issues of his calling, and as perhaps the best representative of an unjustly vilified medical sect.

Bibliography

Primary: Ilberg, Johanes, 1927. *Sorani Gynaeciorum Libri IV; de signis fracturarum; de fasciis; vita Hippocratis secundum Soranum*, CMG IV (Leipzig and Berlin); Temkin, Owsei, 1956. *Soranus' Gynecology* (Baltimore); Burguière, Paul, Danielle Gourevitch, and Yves Malinas, 1988–2000. *Soranos d'Éphèse: maladies des femmes* 4 vols. (Paris).

Secondary: King, Helen, 1998. *Hippocrates' Woman. Reading the Female Body in Ancient Greece* (London and New York); Hanson, Ann, and Monica Green, 1994. 'Soranus of Ephesus: *Methodicorum princeps*' in Haase, Wolfgang, and Hildegard Temporini, eds., *Aufstieg und Niedergang der Römischen Welt* (ANRW) 37(2): 968–1075 (Berlin and New York).

Julius Rocca

SORIANO FISCHER, ELISA (b. Madrid, Spain, 22 October 1891; d. Madrid, 1964) *ophthalmology, education, women's rights.*

Soriano was the eldest daughter of José Soriano Surroca (1865–1939), a Madrid gynecologist, academic, and author of several medical papers. In 1910, coinciding with a new regulation on equal university entry requirements for males and females, Elisa simultaneously undertook baccalaureate and teaching studies, and two years later entered the Medical School of the Central University (Madrid), where only half a dozen women had previously studied. At a time of uncertainty for women with university degrees, the first female graduates in medicine usually attained an additional teaching qualification to ensure their future employment in the less hostile field of education. This was not without reason, since none of the students preceding Soriano at the Madrid School of Medicine had gone on to practice as a physician.

During her time at university she became committed to the suffragist movement and the struggle for women's rights, and she was president of the Juventud Universitaria Femenina. She was the only female student in her year but enjoyed the support and encouragement of the dean of medicine and professor of gynecology, Sebastián Recasens (1863–1933). She dedicated herself to ophthalmology, a specialty of Trinidad Arroyo Villaverde, one of the three women in Madrid practicing medicine by this time. Many other women subsequently chose this specialty, which became one of the most feminized in Spain during the first half of the twentieth century.

After gaining her PhD with a thesis on ocular tumors in 1920, she embarked on the dual professional career maintained throughout her life: as ophthalmologist and as professor at the Escuela Normal Central de Maestras [Women Teachers' Preparatory College], where she taught hygiene, physiology, and anatomy. Her clinical work was carried out in numerous public institutions as well as in her own private office. Throughout the 1920s and 1930s she maintained a frenetic level of activity. She belonged to numerous medical, educational, cultural, and feminist associations and regularly contributed to the journals *La Medicina Social Española* (1918–20) and *El Siglo Médico*, in which she wrote about health education, eye diseases, and women's rights.

In 1928 she won a public competition for a position as physician of the Merchant Marine, and for one year she worked as medical inspector on board two passenger liners that traveled to South America. In the same year she founded the Asociación de Médicas Españolas (AME) with a group of colleagues, including some of the female pioneers in Spanish medicine such as Trinidad Arroyo (honorary president) and Concepción Aleixandre (1862–1952, president). The AME was linked to the international movement of female physicians that had been spreading throughout the world since its launch in 1919 by women doctors in North America. Indeed, during her visit to Europe in 1927, Soriano met the president of the Medical Women's International Association (MWIA), the physician and historian Kate Hurd-Mead (1888–1949). The AME and MWIA shared the objectives of professional defense of female physicians and the improvement of the health of women and children. The association ceased to exist after the Spanish Civil War but was reestablished by new colleagues in the last phase of the Franco regime (1965–78).

After the Civil War, Soriano continued her work as professor and pediatric ophthalmologist and actively promoted cultural and literary meetings. In 1962 she was awarded the Medal of the City of Madrid.

Bibliography

Primary: 1918. '¿Por qué no se extiende más en España el estudiar la mujer medicina?' *La Medicina Social Española* 3: 624–628; 1953. 'La ceguera en la infancia.' *Archivos de la Sociedad Oftalmológica Hispano-Americana*, 13(9): 1073–1085.

Secondary: Cabré i Pairet, Montserrat, 2001. 'Autoridad e historia. El proyecto historiográfico de las médicas norteamericanas, 1925–1940.' *Asparkía* (12): 113–124; Ortiz Gómez, Teresa, 1988. 'Asociacionismo médico femenino en España: La Asociación de Médicas Españolas (1928–36) y su fundadora, Elisa Soriano' in *Actas del VIII Congreso Nacional de Historia de la Medicina* (Murcia) pp. 595–604.

Teresa Ortiz-Gómez

SOURNIA, JEAN-CHARLES

SOURNIA, JEAN-CHARLES (b. Bourges, France, 24 November 1917; d. Paris, France, 8 June 2000), *medicine, history of medicine, oriental studies.*

Sournia, the son of an artillery officer, studied medicine at the Ecole du Service de Santé des Armées in Lyon. He was interned in 1940 and spent eighteen months as a POW. During this period the Service de Santé des Armées had to reduce its activities and decommissioned some of its members. Sournia was among them and in 1943 became a resident student at Lyon. In 1948 he became the director of the surgical hospital of the medical faculty. Sournia studied under P. Santy and specialized in surgery of the thorax. He worked in Sweden (where he met his wife) for a short time and was also a surgeon-in-chief for those involved in maintaining the Suez Canal.

Beginning in 1953 Sournia worked in Aleppo, Syria, and subsequently in Damascus for the public health service. In 1956 he moved to Beirut to take up the position as professor at the university. Three years later he returned to France to become a pediatric surgeon at the medical centre at Rennes, and he stayed there for a decade. His professional contacts with P. Huard resulted in a deep interest in the history of medicine, particularly the history of hospitals. He was elected a member of the Societé Française d'Histoire de la Médecine in 1965 and later became general secretary and the vice-president of this society. He also edited the society's journal, the *Histoire des Sciences Médicales*. As a historian of medicine, Sournia laid methodological foundations of this branch of historical studies. He contributed immensely to medical lexicography and was responsible for editing and publishing the *Dictionnaire de medicine*. He was also a founder of *Le Service Médica* and *La Revue de l'Assurance Maladie*.

During his career in the Middle East, he developed a strong interest in the history of Islamic medicine. Together with a French Orientalist, G. Trupeau, he contributed significantly to the work of Ibn Māsawayh (Mesue), a Nestorian Christian, the first doctor who wrote in Arabic. He produced an anthology with a commentary of the works of Arabic medicine and supervised numerous PhD theses on

Ibn Māsawayh, Ibn Sīnā, and others. He also spent his time at archeological excavations with a particular emphasis on the history of the Byzantine Middle East (fourth to seventh centuries). Together with his wife, who taught languages and literature at the University of Rennes, he authored an important study on the Early Christian history of the Middle East.

Bibliography

Primary: 1984. (with Ruffié, J.) *Les épidémies dans l'histoire de l'homme: essai d'anthropologie médicale* (Paris).

Secondary: 2002. 'Eloges du Professeur Jean-Charles Sournia. 24 novembre 1927 [*sic*]—8 juin 2000.' *Histoire des sciences médicales* 36(2): 195–238.

Nikolaj Serikoff

SOUZA, GERALDO HORÁTIO DE PAULA   (b. Itu, São Paulo, Brazil, 5 May 1889; d. São Paulo, 2 May 1951), *public health.*

Souza was a crucial figure in the movement to modernize sanitation and public health in São Paulo, Brazil. Throughout his career he worked to build new institutions and infrastructure as well as new understandings of public health. Based on the recollections of those who knew him, he was a strong, driven, sometimes rigid advocate of modern sanitation methods.

Souza was educated, as suited the son of Antônio Francisco de Paula Souza, engineer, founder, and first director of the Escola Politécnica de São Paulo, in the finest educational institutions that Brazil and Europe offered at the beginning of the twentieth century. He received his MD from Rio de Janeiro in 1913; however, he harbored some ill will toward the Rio medical establishment, possibly because of his inability to build a career there. After the completion of his medical education, he began an ambitious rise in the academic ranks in São Paulo. It was there that he met and impressed Rockefeller Foundation physicians who were working in Brazil with the Rockefeller International Health Board. Those physicians recommended him for a fellowship to the United States. Rockefeller records indicate that he was single in 1918 when he began his fellowship to study public health at Johns Hopkins University. He was given a renewal after receiving glowing recommendations from his professors and remained in Baltimore until 1920.

In 1920 hygienists condemned the general condition of the city of São Paulo. In reaction to this situation, Souza, upon the completion of his education, directed his considerable talent, learning, and connections to this situation. Quoting a Rockefeller Foundation officer who knew him well: '[Souza] returned from America in an extremely radio-active state, emitting concentrated energy in all directions and difficult to handle without getting burnt' (Hackett, October 11, 1921: Hackett Rockefeller Archive,

Rockefeller Foundation, record group 1.1, series 305, box 18, folder 152; Rockefeller Archive, Box 4, Record Group 1.1, Series 305).

His number of scientific publications, future scientists trained, and success in institution building were considerable, notwithstanding the enemies he made among the powerful, traditional physicians and clinical doctors in São Paulo and Rio de Janeiro who were unsupportive of his ideas. He reorganized, in 1925, the sanitary service of the State of São Paulo and introduced the Centro de Saúde [health center] and a sanitary education service which included home visits and public health education.

Souza had a long, varied, and illustrious career. He labored long to establish the Institute of Hygiene of São Paulo and maintained the position of director from 1922 until his death almost thirty years later. He was director of the São Paulo Sanitary Service from 1922–1927 and delegate to the League of Nations. In his capacity as international representative of Brazil, he participated in the meetings in the mid 1940s that created the United Nations system and its specialized agencies, such as the World Health Organization (WHO). He is recognized for making a joint proposal, with the delegate of China, for the creation of WHO, the main health multilateral agency of the post–World War II period.

Bibliography

Primary: 1923. *Algumas considerações sobre a mortalidade infantil em São Paulo* (São Paulo); 1923. *O estado de São Paulo e alguns dos seus serviços de saude publica* (São Paulo).

Secondary: Kemp, Amy, 2004. 'The Rockefeller Foundation and the Faculdade de Medicina de São Paulo: A Case Study in Philanthropy as Policy.' PhD thesis, Indiana University; Mascarenhas, Rodolfo dos Santos, 1973. 'História Da Saúde Pública No Estado De São Paulo.' *Revista de Saúde Pública de São Paulo* 7: 433–446.

Amy Kemp

SPALLANZANI, LAZZARO   (b. Scandiano, Italy, 12 January 1729; d. Pavia, Italy, 11 February 1799), *natural sciences, embryology, physiology.*

The Training and Apprenticeship of a Naturalist

Spallanzani carried out research on an enormous range of subjects, from chemistry to mineralogy, volcanology to physics, but his main interests lay in the field of the life sciences.

He received a basic education in the classics at the Jesuit school of Reggio Emilia. His father, Giannicolò, decided that Spallanzani should study jurisprudence, so he went to Bologna University (1749) and was captivated by Laura Bassi's classes in physics and mathematics—far more than he was by the lectures in law. With the support of Bassi, Spallanzani succeeded in abandoning the faculty of law in

1753 in order to devote himself to these new scientific interests. In 1755 he graduated in philosophy and two years later he was appointed professor of physics and mathematics at the University of Reggio Emilia.

This early period of a still generic scientific vocation ended in 1761, when Spallanzani finally identified his 'ruling passion' as the natural sciences and began his apprenticeship as a microscopist, repeating the observations of George-Louis Leclerc de Buffon (1707–88) and John Tuberville Needham (1713–81) on the generation of infusoria (now Ciliates). He began his investigations in Reggio and then continued (1763) at the University of Modena, where he was a reader in philosophy. Since all teaching staff at this university were required to take holy orders, he was quickly ordained as a priest, thanks to a special dispensation from the Pope.

Spallanzani's initial indifference towards epigenesis and preformation developed into a generic approval of the former (as attested to by his laboratory notebooks), but he subsequently opted for the latter. His refutation of Buffon's and Needham's spontaneous generation theories was expressed in the work which announced Spallanzani's debut on the stage of European science, his *Saggio di osservazioni microscopiche* (1765).

Fame

Spallanzani began his correspondence with the Genevan naturalist Charles Bonnet (1720–93) by sending him the *Saggio*; he also accepted the guidance of Bonnet and established an association that after some years became a true intellectual symbiosis. At the same time, he turned his attention to animal regeneration. After four years of experimental activity, he announced a treatise but published only the *Prodromo di un'opera da imprimersi sopra le riproduzioni animali*. In the same year (1768) his work *Dell'azione del cuore ne' vasi sanguigni* was printed; that work was a treatise in which he dared to correct the results obtained by Albrecht von Haller (1708–77) on the physiology of the cardiocirculatory system.

The *Prodromo* was a great success and won Spallanzani an appointment (1769) as professor of natural history at the prestigious university of Pavia. The *Prodromo* found room not only for an exposition on regeneration in various animal species (including the famous decapitated snails), but also for a new 'proof' of ovist pre-existence, drawn from his contemporaneous research on frogspawn and tadpoles. However, the need to return to his experiments on *infusoria*, in order to silence Needham's new criticism, interrupted this program of studies on generation. Spallanzani refrained from publishing even the promised treatise on regeneration.

During the 1770s, he returned to the physiology of blood circulation (*Dei fenomeni della circolazione*, 1773) and confirmed for the first time Malpighi's discovery of capillaries in warm-blooded animals. His published protocols on phenomena relating to the arterial pulse and languid circulation brought him into a lively argument with Haller. He continued

his research on *infusoria* and, in his *Opuscoli di fisica animale, e vegetabile* (1776), he launched his final attack on spontaneous generation and also set out an array of new research plans, tackling the study of 'spermatic worms' (spermatozoa), the 'resurrection' of rotifers, 'little mould plants', animals and vegetables 'closed within air', and tissue respiration.

In 1780 *Dissertazioni di fisica animale, e vegetabile* communicated the results of experiments on digestion conducted on animals and even on himself. He ingested containers with portions of food in them and caused them to be regurgitated, both in order to study the stages of the digestive process and to analyze the gastric juice, whose decisive role he understood, ascertaining this *in vitro*. Despite the exemplary structure of his experimentation and the significance of the results achieved, his findings were violently attacked by the Scottish physician John Hunter. In the *Dissertazioni* he also returned to his research on generation, now focusing on systematic interference in the natural processes of fecundation. Spallanzani set forth the results he had obtained with artificial insemination—with which he succeeded for the first time in amphibians—but he did not understand the true function of spermatozoa. Having experimentally ascertained that the traditional *aura spermatica* did not exist, he connected fecundation primarily with the 'concrete' part of the semen and carried out sophisticated selections to isolate, quantify, and preserve the powers of the active fraction. Since spermatic liquids apparently devoid of 'little worms' seemed to be effective, he concluded that the latter were definitely extraneous to the process of generation and successfully extended his experiments to mammals.

Spallanzani's failure to comprehend the role of spermatozoa remains to be explained, as this so strongly contrasts with the exceptional ability he developed in microscopic and micromanipulation techniques. What he noted, as one reads in his laboratory diaries, was not actually the absence of spermatozoa, but that of spermatozoa which were 'at least alive', or moving. In his printed work, the absence of moving spermatozoa turned into total absence. Spallanzani concluded that sperm acted as an activator that was not biological but physical, and so he did not go back to the idea that fecundation was also possible by means of the intervention of various chemical substances. Indeed, in his laboratory diaries he reported putting into practice a daring project, in which the stimulating action of semen was replaced with that of various liquids: dishomogeneous, dried, or colored sperm; and varieties impregnated with odors, pollen, or even with electrical fluid.

His Travels and Natural History Collections

From the very first years of his scientific career, Spallanzani associated experimentation in the laboratory with observations in nature. He went on trips to explore natural phenomena, some of which coincided with his contemporary investigations or were undertaken as a new interest and led to completely novel spheres of research. From his excursion into the Reggian Appennines (1761) to his travels in the Lombard Alps (1772), Switzerland (1779), the Ligurian Riviera (1780, 1781), the upper part of the Adriatic coast (1782), or to Portovenere, Apuane, and Garfagnana (1783), the results were set down in notebooks crammed with observations on flora and fauna found on the land and in the waters he explored. In 1785–86 he undertook a journey to Constantinople during which he carried out geological and mineralogical research, studied the marine fauna, and collected precious *specimina*. His expedition to the kingdom of the two Sicilies in 1788 was prompted primarily by volcanological interests.

During his travel to Constantinople, G. A. Scopoli took advantage of Spallanzani's absence and together with other teaching staff from Pavia University hatched a plot against his colleague. At that time Spallanzani was not much liked because of his prickly personality, and he was much envied because of the wide favor in which he was held by the Hapsburg authorities, engaged in carrying out a reform of the university. The plotters had him accused of taking some *specimina* from the university's Museum of Natural History (of which he was the curator) to enrich his personal collection. Spallanzani was subjected to a full investigation, but eventually an Imperial decree was issued declaring him innocent.

A scientist at the hub of a vast web of intellectual exchanges, translated into the most widely spoken European languages, a member of the most important academies, Spallanzani never held any specifically political position during the period of Hapsburg domination, nor did he take part in the civil ferment which inflamed even the Italian states immediately following the French Revolution. He preferred to spend the last years of his life studying the blind flight of bats and the chemistry of gas. Indeed, in the wake of Lavoisier's discoveries, between 1794 and 1799 Spallanzani devoted himself to an intense series of studies regarding the physiological and biological aspects of respiration, focusing on the parenchyma. The diary relating this investigation closes with an interrupted experiment; his death following uremic coma deriving from prostatic hypertrophy and chronic bladder infection prevented him from consigning the results of these 10,000 experiments to print. The experiments, some of which were published posthumously, are available in the recent edition of *Giornali* and give us a picture of the author immersed in the living process of research.

His Method

Spallanzani's scientific method produced a model for sequential experimentation. His procedures systematically associated a main experiment with a successive series of repetitions destined to consolidate the facts established, to

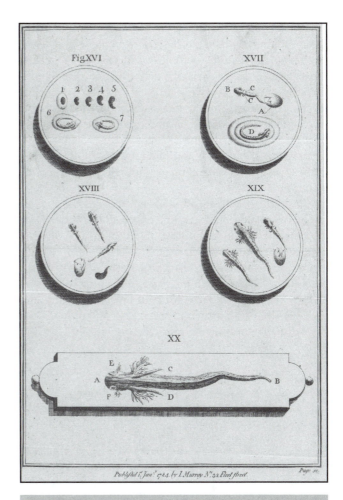

Development of the salamander. Engraving from *Dissertations Relative to the Natural History of Animals and Vegetables*, London, 1789. Rare Books, Wellcome Library, London.

analyze how extensively they might be applied (or, even better, their limits) in different places and circumstances, and to perfect the experimental processes and equipment on a daily basis. He thus advanced slowly and tortuously, using a process of crystallizing partial results; nothing was more alien to him than stark refutations or dazzling proof. All this must have seemed to him to be an insult to the patience and daily toil of a serious scientific method, which was, as he wrote, made up of 'cautious and well-designed experiments'.

The exceptional nature of Spallanzani's research consisted in his ingeniousness and rigor, and the perseverance by which he did not seek to destroy others' hypotheses, but tested them, refining and varying experimental procedures and devices beyond all expectations, solving technical problems, and going to extreme lengths to elaborate the experimental process. In a totally original way, he took methods and procedures assimilated to their utmost limits until he rendered them unrecognizable.

His theoretical originality was confirmed in the mirage of finding a '*canone universalissimo*' of life that would establish the irreducible nature of the vital factor but would at the same time program its expression in mathematical terms and be obtained solely by means of varying and repeating the experiments. This idea of a definitive and entirely universal law (which had very little to do with the normal standards of science of the times) could have impeded the development of his experimentation, but instead it gave Spallanzani a case of indomitable intellectual bulimia and a limitless ambition to do more and better than the others—and a very high consideration for the method used and the results obtained.

Until not so long ago, Spallanzani suffered the curious fate of being judged an *ante litteram* positivist. Instead, for his part, he would have been horrified to hear himself defined as a 'purely mechanical . . . observer'. A science project conceived as a fundamental investigation into the confines of life and death was surely something completely different: this was the true focus of his plan of work and this was what he pursued in forty years of study via the most disparate branches of research.

Bibliography

Primary: 1984–2004. *Edizione nazionale delle opere di Lazzaro Spallanzani . . . a cura di Pericle Di Pietro* 24 vols. (Modena); 1994. *I Giornali delle Sperienze e Osservazioni. A cura di Carlo Castellani* 6 vols. (Florence).

Secondary: Monti, Maria Teresa, 2005. *Spallanzani e il programma delle rigenerazioni animali. L'inchiesta, la comunicazione la rete* (Florence); Castellani, Carlo, 2001. *Un itinerario culturale: Lazzaro Spallanzani* (Florence); Bernardi, Walter and Marta Stefani, eds., 2000. *La sfida della modernità* (Florence); Bernardi, Walter, 1986. *Le metafisiche dell'embrione. Scienze della vita e filosofia da Malpighi a Spallanzani (1672–1793)* (Florence); Montalenti, Giuseppe, and Paolo Rossi, eds., 1982. *Lazzaro Spallanzani e la biologia del Settecento. Teorie, esperimenti, istituzioni scientifiche* (Florence); Rostand, Jean, 1951. *Les origines de la biologie expérimentale et l'Abbé Spallanzani* (Paris); *DSB*.

Maria Teresa Monti

SPOCK, BENJAMIN MCLANE (b. New Haven, Connecticut, USA, 2 May 1903; d. San Diego, California, USA, 15 March 1998), *medicine, pediatrics, politics, popular medicine.*

Spock was the eldest of six children of Benjamin Ives Spock, Yale-trained lawyer to the New Haven Railroad, and Mildred Stoughton, whom he described as devoted but strict parents. He attended Hamden Hall, New Haven (1915–19), Phillips Academy, Andover, Massachusetts (1919–21), and Yale University, where he rowed with the gold medal varsity crew in the Paris Olympics (1924). Work experience at a home for disabled children sidetracked him into medicine. After Yale Medical School (1925–27), he transferred to Columbia University's College of Physicians and Surgeons, New York, graduating top of his class (1929). He married

Jane Cheney (1927), and they had two sons. Following internships at Presbyterian Hospital (1929–31) and Cornell Medical College (pediatrics, 1931), plus a psychiatry residency at Cornell's Payne Whitney Clinic (1933), Spock studied psychoanalysis at the New York Psychoanalytic Institute, believing this would help him give psychologically correct advice to mothers. He opened a New York pediatric practice (1933), struggling through the economic depression (during which he briefly flirted with socialism) to emerge with an expanding reputation and part-time consultancy at the City Health Department.

Approached by Pocket Books (1943) to write a twenty-five-cent child-care manual, he worked with Jane on the manuscript while serving as a psychiatrist in the U.S. Naval Reserve Medical Corps (1944–46) during World War II. *The Common Sense Book of Baby and Child Care* (1946) aimed to empower parents as the real experts in raising their children and was the first text to discuss children's emotional problems. It was reassuring and readable and caught the mood of a fecund postwar generation seeking to jettison the rigid domestic routines of the past for a relaxed, flexible family life. An instant best seller, the book's sales reached one million copies annually within three years. Spock was offered a teaching and research post at the Mayo Clinic's Child Health Institute, Rochester (1947). He moved to Pittsburgh University (1951) before becoming professor of child development, Western Reserve University, Cleveland (1955–67), where he launched a Child Rearing Study (1958). Columns in magazines such as *Ladies Home Journal* (1954), *American Weekly* (1954), and *Redbook* (1963), plus a nationwide television show, *Doctor Spock* (1955), made him a household name, and he was filmed with the Kennedy family during John F. Kennedy's presidential campaign (1960). He cut an impressive figure, being tall and slim with a loud authoritative voice. Professional colleagues were nevertheless critical of his academic underachievement. Others blamed his 'permissiveness' for producing a 'Spock-marked' generation of undisciplined antiestablishment protestors.

Spock himself became active in the peace movement, first publicly demonstrating in Cleveland with the National Committee for a Sane Nuclear Policy (SANE, 1962). Later, he opposed the Vietnam War and was given a two-year sentence for conspiracy to aid resistance to the draft (1968), which was quashed on appeal. As the People's Party candidate in the 1972 presidential election, polling 75,000 votes, he supported withdrawal of American troops from abroad, a minimum family income, free medical care, and legalization of abortion and marijuana. Following his divorce from Jane (1975), he married Mary Morgan (1976), a young divorced mother whom he had met on the peace campaign circuit and with whom he collaborated and traveled. Spock had always enjoyed sailing.

While participating in nonviolent civil disobedience on behalf of peace or humanitarian organizations and giving between seventy-five and 100 talks a year around the country, he continued to update *Baby and Child Care*. It was revised seven times in response to feminist criticism about stay-at-home motherhood and to changing ideas about child care, single parenthood, teenage pregnancy, and other emerging social issues. In 1990 *Life* magazine named him one of the 100 most important people of the twentieth century. By the year of his death, *Baby and Child Care* had sold over fifty million copies in thirty-one countries and thirty-nine languages. Spock wanted to be remembered both for the book and for working toward disarmament and peace, but he guessed that his epitaph was already written.

Bibliography

Primary: 1946. *The Common Sense Book of Baby and Child Care* (New York); 1955. (with Lowenberg, Miriam E.) *Feeding Your Baby and Child* (New York); 1956. (with Reinhart, John, and Wayne Miller) *A Baby's First Year* (New York); 1962. *Dr Spock Talks with Mothers: Growth and Guidance* (London); 1971. *A Young Person's Guide to Life and Love* (London); 1989. (with Morgan, Mary) *Spock on Spock: A Memoir of Growing up with the Century.* (New York).

Secondary: Maier, Thomas, 1998. *Dr Spock: An American Life* (New York and London); Bloom, Lynn Z., 1972. *Doctor Spock: Biography of a Conservative Radical* (Indianapolis).

Carole Reeves

SPOERRY, ANNE (b. Cannes, France, 13 May 1918; d. Nairobi, Kenya, 2 February 1999), *medicine, flying doctor service.*

Despite a relatively privileged upbringing, Spoerry was determined from a young age to practice medicine. Born in Cannes to an affluent family descended from prestigious Swiss stock, Spoerry took her baccalaureate at the Lycée of Mulhouse in France (1926–37), then entered the Faculty of Medicine in Paris (MD, 1941) and practiced for a short time in a Parisian hospital. During the French occupation she and her brother, architect François (Henry) Spoerry, joined the Resistance. Her duties during this time included sheltering the persecuted and helping them to obtain new papers and ration cards. Unfortunately, in 1943 she and her brother were captured by the Germans. She was interrogated by the Gestapo and interred in Ravensbrück for one and one-half years.

After her release, Spoerry made plans to leave Europe. With an eye to a career overseas, she went to Basel, Switzerland, and took the Diploma of Tropical Medicine in 1948, subsequently obtaining her first government overseas posting at Aden in 1949. Her heart was set on working in Ethiopia, however—supposedly inspired by the adventures of Henri de Monfried. She traveled there only to be told that there was no suitable medical work for a lone woman. Undeterred, Spoerry traveled onto British East Africa (now Kenya), settling there in 1950 after quickly succumbing to its charms.

Spoerry initially established herself as part of a farming cooperative and was a general practitioner at Ol Kalou (between Lake Navaisha and Thomson Falls), but her attentions soon grew more widely focused and she became interested in the widespread problem of delivering medical care to extremely isolated rural areas. One of her first tasks was to establish several small local clinics offering remote indigenous communities basic contraception and child and maternal health care facilities. This gradually turned into larger outreach schemes that fed into wider national initiatives.

Of stable independent means, Spoerry channeled her financial assets into the local communities, famously purchasing her own airplane and learning to fly it at forty-five years of age. She became one of the pioneers of the East Africa Flying Doctor Service, joining its founder, Michael Woods, during the early years of its operation. She was to be an essential part of their 'medicine by air' program from the time she joined it in 1964 until her death some thirty-five years later.

Nicknamed affectionately as 'Mama Daktari' (Kiswahili for Mother Doctor), Spoerry was an important figurehead for the flying doctor service in Kenya and was committed to establishing community-based health projects run by local people. The success of the African Medical and Research Foundation—an organization run by Africans for Africans—was due largely to her work. A prominent local figure, Spoerry served as a member of the Navaisha County Council (1958–62); was Medical Officer of Health of Nyandarua Country Council (1964–65); and was Chairman of the Health and Social Affairs Committee of Navaisha. She was also a member of the Kenya Medical Association and the Kenya Branch of the British Red Cross. Working tirelessly until the end of her life, and remaining unmarried, she died of a stroke in Nairobi at the age of eighty and was buried in Shela cemetery on the island of Lamu.

Bibliography

Primary: 1997. *They Call Me Mama Daktari* (Norval, Ontario).

Secondary: Woods, Michael, 1987. *Different Drums, Reflections on a Changing Africa* (London); Wynne, Barry, 1968. *Angels on Runway Zero: The Story of the East African Flying Doctor Service* (London).

Anna Crozier

SQUIBB, EDWARD ROBINSON (b. Wilmington, Delaware, USA, 5 July 1819; d. Brooklyn, New York, USA, 25 October 1900), *medicine, medicinal chemistry, pharmaceutical manufacturing.*

Squibb was the first of five children of James Robinson Squibb and his wife, Catherine Harrison Bonsall. Squibb's mother died shortly after the death of her three daughters in 1831. James and the two boys moved to the Philadelphia region to be close to relatives. Edward went to live with his grandmother in the suburb of Darby.

During his teens, Squibb resolved to become a doctor. In 1837 he took a part-time job to earn money toward the tuition fees for his medical education. He became apprenticed to Warder Morris, a Philadelphia pharmacist, from whom he learned to mix elixirs and compound powders. He then went to work for a pharmaceutical manufacturer, J. H. Sprague.

He entered Jefferson Medical College in 1842, receiving his MD degree in 1845. He then practiced medicine in Philadelphia for two years before accepting an appointment as assistant surgeon with the United States navy. He served as medical officer on the U.S. frigate *Perry* in the Caribbean, later being assigned to the *Cumberland* in the Mediterranean.

While in the navy, he noted the poor quality of many of the medical supplies, which were bought under contract 'from the lowest bidder'. He and others lobbied Congress for action, and in 1851 he obtained an appointment at Brooklyn Naval Yard. There he established a pharmaceutical laboratory to make and test drugs for the Navy. The rule was later changed to 'quality first and price second'.

Squibb set up his own drug company in 1858, based initially on the manufacture of ether. He took a lease on a building in Brooklyn, but in December 1858 there was a disastrous fire. He attempted to save his books and diaries, but his face and hands were severely burned. He recovered but was badly scarred.

His experience with the fire led him to look at safer ways of manufacturing ether. His solution was to invent a distillation apparatus using steam, a process that was eventually adopted by the United States Pharmacopoeia (USP). His success with the ether apparatus led him to look at other processes. He invented a range of equipment and instruments including percolators and separation funnels.

His interest in drug quality brought him into contact with the USP Commission. He commented on the preparation and assay of many drugs. He had a particular interest in opium and worked on improving its assay. His method was adopted by the USP in 1870. Squibb was active in both the American Medical and Pharmaceutical Associations, and he published over one hundred papers.

He made a number of proposals concerning the functioning and organization of the pharmacopoeia. He lobbied for the appointment of a full-time director and for regular updates between publications of the pharmacopoeia itself. He also proposed the development of an International Pharmacopoeia.

He was an active and outspoken proponent for legislation relating to the purity of food and drugs. He drafted the bill that was enacted in the states of New York and New Jersey in 1880. The Federal Food and Drug Act was enacted in 1906.

The drugs supplied by Squibb's laboratory were mostly of plant or mineral origin. As well as ether, it supplied chloroform and chloral. The company grew steadily over the next few decades. By 1887 it had about one hundred employees.

Later in his life, Squibb turned the company over to his two sons. He continued to participate actively in its affairs, despite his failing health. He died at his home in Brooklyn in 1900. After his death, his sons could not agree on how to develop the business, and it was sold in 1905.

Bibliography

Primary: 1930. *The Journal of Edward Robinson Squibb M.D. Parts I and II* (printed privately).

Secondary: Florey, Klaus, 1989. 'Edward Robinson Squibb: The Man and His Company.' *Pharmaceutical Historian* 19(3): 2–8; Blochman, Lawrence Goldtree, 1958. *Doctor Squibb: The Life and Times of a Rugged Idealist* (New York); *DAMB*.

Stuart Anderson

STAHL, GEORG ERNST (b. Ansbach, Germany, 21 October 1659; d. Berlin, Germany, 4 May 1734), *medicine, chemistry.*

Georg Stahl was born in Ansbach in Franconia, the son of a Protestant church official there. From 1679 to 1684 he studied medicine at the University of Jena, where he became especially familiar with the teachings of the well-known iatrochemist Georg Wolfgang Wedel. In 1684 Stahl received his doctorate in medicine. After teaching for a short time in Jena, in 1687 he was summoned to Weimar and appointed the personal physician of Duke John Ernest II of Saxony-Weimar.

In 1694 Stahl accepted appointment by the Elector of Brandenburg Frederick III (later Prussia's king Frederick I) to the second chair in medicine at the newly founded University of Halle. Stahl lectured on botany, chemistry, anatomy, physiology, and pathology. Together with his medical colleague Friedrich Hoffmann, he helped make the fledgling medical faculty in Halle into the leading German center for the training of academic doctors at the beginning of the eighteenth century. In 1715 Stahl was appointed by the Prussian king Frederick William I as his personal physician and the president of the Royal Medical College in Berlin. Stahl thereupon left Halle and remained in these functions in Berlin until he died. He played a major role in changes in the Prussian health care system in the first third of the eighteenth century and to the Prussian Edict on Medicine, promulgated in 1725.

Medical Theory

The point of departure for Stahl's ideas was the observation that the living body, despite its highly perishable composition of viscous, oily and, aqueous substances, shows an astonishing degree of permanence. Consequently, there must be processes in the body which can account for the maintenance of this complicated and sensitive mixture.

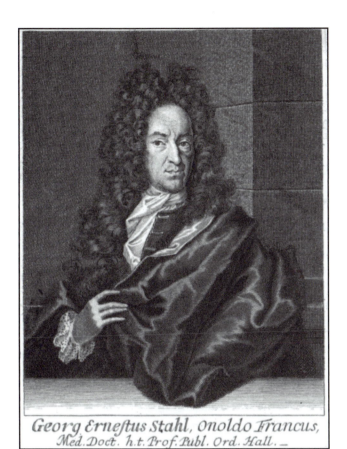

Georg Ernst Stahl. Line engraving, 1715. Iconographic Collection, Wellcome Library, London.

These processes were mechanical in terms of form, Stahl reasoned, because they consisted of constant movements which preserved the body from decomposition by the secretion and excretion of putrefactive substances. The most important of these bodily movements were blood circulation, secretion, and excretion. The undisturbed functioning of these processes is termed health.

Even though the preservation of the body is tantamount to life and is directly dependent on mechanical and physicochemical processes, the cause behind these processes cannot be deduced solely from material elements. Rather, Stahl argued, the evident preservation of the living body from the constant threat of decay was proof for the existence of an immaterial principle which the ancients had called nature or the soul. This principle counteracted decay by purposive and targeted movements. For this reason, that principle had to be acting 'reasonably': it had to be ready to adapt its movements to the varying and changing conditions of the bodily mechanism. Via the so-called *motus tonicus vitalis*, the principle had an impact on the tissues and organs of the body and directed blood circulation, secretion, and excretion.

Stahl chose the notion of 'soul' for the life principle grounded on reason, but he expressly pointed out that it was

irrelevant for medical theory whether this equation was in keeping with the truth. Stahl tended to avoid fixing the use of the terms, calling the principle 'anima', 'natura', 'physis', 'principium vitale', or other concepts with no differentiation. For that reason the frequently asked question regarding Stahl's medical theory as to the essence of the *anima* or *natura* also tends to overlook Stahl's intentions. Stahl did not at all seek to define that nature of the soul. In his view, it was only important to recognize that the phenomenon of life was fully inconceivable without the assumption of a guiding or governing nonmaterial principle.

In Stahl's eyes, the cause for disease was harmful materials or mechanical disturbances to the circulation of blood and to secretion and excretion. The direct cause of all perceived phenomena of sickness was, however, the nonmaterial principle, which reacted to the changed conditions or the harmful substance with movements manifested as disease. Thus, the symptoms of a disease were not the passive consequences of errors that had appeared in the bodily mechanism but were an expression of the changed preservative activity of nature, which was counteracting the threat of harm. This oftenincreased activity to maintain the body could, in Stahl's view, lead to complaints, as the example of fever showed.

As a result of this enhanced stimulation of blood circulation, secretion, and excretion, nature generally succeeded in removing harmful substances as soon as possible from the body, even without the aid of a physician. To recognize this self-healing power of nature was for Stahl the fundamental basis of wise medical treatment. Often, when a doctor could see that nature was proceeding in a well-regulated and purposive manner, it was sufficient for the physician to stand by and simply observe its activities. Medical intervention was superfluous and even harbored the danger that it could disturb nature in its movement of healing. It was better to do nothing than to act falsely.

But if the physician understood that nature was not strong enough to stimulate the movements to the necessary degree, the physician should try to assist nature. Although he could not influence the movements of nature, he could, through measures that stimulated excretion or by the removal of blood, attempt to support the natural movement of the blood and the movements of excretion and secretion. But in this case as well, healing ultimately was effected by the power of nature—not by the art of the physician. Stahl strictly rejected the use of opium because it acted to paralyze the movements of nature.

In his medical theory, in which the bodily processes were subject to 'intelligent' guidance, he fought against the iatromechanical and iatrochemical concepts derived from mechanical natural philosophy and championed by his colleague Friedrich Hoffmann, among others. Stahl counterpoised his conception of the living organism to a purely mechanical physiology and pathology. In the living organism, functions of the body and the soul formed an integral unity.

Pietism

In medical/historical research, Stahl is often viewed as an adherent of Pietism, the Protestant movement of religious renewal in the seventeenth and eighteenth century. Pietism and its theology, based on the personal experience of faith, penitence, and conversion, had a shaping impact on teaching in the divinity school at the young university. In addition, as a result of the schools founded by August Hermann Francke, who was active in Halle from 1692 as a minister of the church and a professor of Greek and Oriental languages, Pietism developed an influential institutional center in Halle.

Pietism of the eighteenth century regarded physical symptoms and diseases as intentional intervention by God. They were meant to call the afflicted person's attention to the condition of his own soul and the necessity for penitence and conversion. Illness was thus not viewed as an accident but rather as a meaningful event in the individual religious biography of a person. Pietist doctors adopted this interpretation and combined it with the medical theories of Georg Ernst Stahl. But in contrast with Stahl, who had avoided an authoritative definition about the nature and function of the nonmaterial principle governing the organism, Pietism identified the *natura* or *anima* from Stahl's theory as the religious core of the individual. This notion made it possible for Pietist physicians such as Christian Friedrich Richter and Michael Alberti to explain the reconciliation with God that occurred in conversion as a therapeutic factor. In the Pietist view, the soul quieted by conversion was far more able to stimulate the movements of the bodily organs and fluids necessary in illness. For that reason the sick should be treated by physicians, but they should also be given spiritual treatment so that the meaning of the illness could be grasped and the necessary quiet for the soul to overcome the disease could be created.

Stahl's concept provided Pietist authors the theoretical foundations for medicine associated with religious zeal. However, Stahl's own writings do not contain any religious statements that can be clearly interpreted in the context of Pietism. For that reason, it should not be hastily concluded on the basis of the popularity of Stahl's medical ideas among Pietists that Stahl's theory had itself been decisively influenced by Pietism.

Chemistry

As a chemist, Stahl espoused the view that a simple mechanical philosophy could not adequately explain the phenomena observed. The atoms combined in molecules had to have certain qualities, which Stahl attempted to explain as the properties of three elementary substances—air, water, and earth. For its part, the substance earth was composed of three subgroups, of which the second, 'phlogiston', did not enter into any stable compounds but rather was released by solid bodies in combustion. Substances that contained no phlogiston were noncombustible, while substances with large amounts of phlogiston were highly flammable.

Impact

Stahl's medical theory sparked vehement controversies that spilled outside the boundaries of medical discourse. Well known is his dispute with Gottfried Wilhelm Leibniz, who in 1709 had attacked Stahl's concept of the living organism. Initially, Stahl's ideas were recognized almost exclusively by Pietists. Later in the eighteenth and in the early nineteenth century, his thinking influenced anthropological discourse in the German Enlightenment; in the French vitalists, such as François Boissier de la Croix de Sauvages, Théophile de Bordeu, and Paul Joseph Barthez; as well as in German medical thinkers in the age of Romanticism. Stahl's theory of phlogiston was replaced in the 1770s by Antoine L. de Lavoisier's theory of oxidation.

Bibliography

Primary: 1697. *Zymotechnia fundamentalis* (Halle); 1708. *Theoria medica vera* (Halle); 1720. *Negotium otiosum seu skiamachia* (Halle).

Secondary: Chang, Ku-Ming (Kevin), 2004. 'Motus Tonicus: Georg Ernst Stahl's Formulation of Tonic Motion and Early Modern Thought.' *Bulletin of the History of Medicine* 78: 767–803; Geyer-Kordesch, Johanna, 2000. *Pietismus, Medizin und Aufklärung in Preußen im 18. Jahrhundert* (Tübingen); Engelhardt, Dietrich von, and Alfred Gierer, eds., 2000. *Georg Ernst Stahl in wissenschaftshistorischer Sicht* (Heidelberg); Helm, Jürgen, 2000. 'Das Medizinkonzept Georg Ernst Stahls und seine Rezeption im Halleschen Pietismus und in der Zeit der Romantik.' *Berichte zur Wissenschaftsgeschichte* 23: 167–190; DSB.

Jürgen Helm and
Karin Stukenbrock

ŠTAMPAR, ANDRIJA (b. Drenovac, Croatia, 1 September 1888; d. Zagreb, Yugoslavia [now Croatia], 26 June 1958), *medicine, social hygiene, public health.*

Štampar was born in the Croatian village of Drenovac when it was still part of the Austro-Hungarian Empire. His father, Ambroz, had been a village schoolteacher and political activist for the nationalist cause. In high school Štampar published a literary work before moving to Vienna to pursue medical studies in 1906. His main interests focused on social medicine, medical institutions, and medical insurance for laborers. Štampar was much inspired by Professor Julius Tandler's lectures on the right of every human to be healthy. Summering at home, he became familiar with the problems facing Croatian farmers and often asserted that the common people were his teachers.

As a medical student Štampar published popular articles on alcoholism, tuberculosis, venereal diseases, and acute contagious diseases. It was during this time that the basic concepts underlying his sociomedical practice took shape, influenced by Tandler, Teleky, and Milan Jovanović Batut. Štampar advocated a reduction in working hours, improvements to living conditions for the poor, special care for mothers and children, paid maternity leave, and free treatment for contagious diseases. Returning to Croatia upon graduation in 1911, he engaged in general practice as well as educational work. After the formation of the Yugoslav state in 1918, Štampar was appointed as the head of the Hygienic Department at the Ministry of Health, a post he held until 1930.

Štampar believed strongly that health care for the people was not only the duty of doctors, but also an obligation of the entire society. Physicians, he maintained, must not be economically dependent on their patients, and every person, rich or poor, has an equal right to be healthy. He argued that ideally, health therapies should be applied socially rather than individually; physicians should seek out patients, not vice-versa. In line with such ideals, Štampar organized a public medical service in the newly formed Yugoslavia, including a network of over 500 hygiene establishments, and contributed to the establishment of legal regulations concerning social medicine and public health.

Štampar founded the School of People's Health, in Zagreb, now part of Zagreb University, where he also taught as professor of social medicine and hygiene. He later served as dean of the Medical Faculty and was also eventually University Rector, emphasizing a curriculum that focused on social and preventive measures. Between the two world wars, Štampar lectured widely as a visiting professor in Czechoslovakia, Germany, Greece, Hungary, the Netherlands, Poland, Spain, and Turkey. As an expert on hygiene organization, he was sent by the League of Nations to China, where he helped reorganize the public medical service between 1932 and 1936. Visiting the United States in 1938, Štampar taught social medicine and hygiene courses at Columbia, Cornell, Harvard, and Yale universities. He continued to work closely with his former mentor, Tandler, who described Štampar as his disciple in Europe, his collaborator in America, and his teacher in Asia. Štampar's experiences are summarized in the book *Zdravlje I Društvo* [Health and Society], published in 1939. A synthesis of his sociomedical thought may be found in his 1940 textbook, *Higijena I Socijalna Medicina* [Hygiene and Social Medicine].

Štampar played an active part in the formation of the World Health Organization (WHO). At the United Nations London Conference in 1946, he was elected first vice president of the Economic and Social Council, and as a member of the Preparatory Committee for the Creation of WHO. Later that year, Štampar was appointed president of the Interim Commission that served until the WHO Constitution was finalized in 1948; he then presided over the first World Health Assembly in Geneva. Starting in 1947, Štampar served as president of the Zagreb-based Yugoslav Academy of Sciences and Art. A member of the New York Medical Academy, Štampar was decorated with the Léon Bernard medal in 1955.

Bibliography

Primary: 1919. *O zdravstvenoj politici* [About Health Politics]; 1939. *Zdravlje I drustvo* [Health and Society]; 1966. (Grmek, M. D., ed.) *Serving the Cause of Public Health: Selected Papers of Andrija Stampar* (Zagreb).

Secondary: Zylberman, P., 2004. 'Fewer Parallels than Antitheses: René Sand and Andrija Stampar on Social Medicine, 1919–1955.' *Social History of Medicine* 17: 77–92; 1964. *Medicinska enciklopedija*, 9 Shiz-Tul (Zagreb); Grmek, Mirko Dražen, 1958. 'O životu i delima Andrije Štampara' in *Andrija Štampar (1.IX.1888-26.VI.1958)* (Zagreb).

Jelena Jovanovic Simic and
Predrag J. Markovic

STARLING, ERNEST HENRY (b. London, England, 17 April 1866; d. Kingston, Jamaica, 2 May 1927), *physiology, endocrinology.*

Starling's father, Matthew Henry Starling, was Clerk to the Crown in Bombay, and the seven children were brought up by their mother in London. In 1882 Starling entered Guy's Hospital Medical School and spent much of 1885–86 in Heidelberg working with Willy Kühne (1837–1900), a pioneer in the physiology of digestion. After qualifying (1889), he abandoned his earlier ambition of becoming a Harley Street physician and embarked on a career in physiology. In addition to a post at Guy's, he also worked part-time in Edward Schäfer's (1850–1935, later Sharpey-Schafer) laboratory at UCL. When Schäfer left for Edinburgh (1899), Starling was elected to his chair, at age thirty-three. University College was where he started a lifelong association with his brother-in-law, William Maddock Bayliss (1860–1924). Bayliss was 'gentle, retiring and kindly', whereas Starling was 'brisk, ambitious, a bit quixotic, serious, generous, highly strung'.

In 1892 Starling returned to Germany to work in Breslau with Rudolf Heidenhain (1834–97) who was researching the formation of lymph. On his return, he formulated what came to be called the 'Starling equilibrium', the idea that equal and opposite forces move across the capillary wall—an outward (hydrostatic) force and an inward (osmotic) force from plasma proteins. The latter he measured with an osmometer of his own making.

In 1898 Bayliss and Starling described the peristaltic wave responsible for the movement of food through the intestine. Next they investigated pancreatic secretion. Pavlov had shown that gastric secretion was under the influence of the nervous system, and it was assumed that this was true for the pancreas. In 1902 Starling and Bayliss dissected away the nerves to the pancreas and duodenum, put acid into the duodenum, and found that pancreatic secretion occurred normally. Working on the hypothesis that acid caused the release of something from the duodenum into the blood, they made an extract of duodenal mucosa and injected it intravenously into a dog. Pancreatic secretion followed a few seconds later. They called this 'chemical messenger' secretin, but it was not until he gave the Croonian lectures in 1905 that Starling used the word 'hormone', from the Greek word meaning to stir up or arouse.

Between 1912 and 1914, Starling and his collaborators developed a heart-lung preparation with an artificial resistance, which mimicked normal arteriolar peripheral resistance. This meant that the effects of heart rate, venous flow, and arterial resistance on cardiac output could be studied. This led to the discovery of Starling's famous 'Law of the Heart'—that when heart muscle dilated, it was able to produce more energy for contraction.

Starling, more than anyone else, established physiology as an independent discipline in England and was responsible for the Institute of Physiology opened at UCL (1909). He was a great teacher, known worldwide through his books such as *Elements of Human Physiology* (1892) and its successor *Principles of Human Physiology* (1912). During World War I, he advised the British government on nutrition, advice that Lloyd George later said had decided the outcome of the war. This experience led him to deplore 'the disastrous ignorance of the most elementary scientific facts displayed by members of the government'.

Bibliography

Primary: 1897. 'The Arris and Gale Lectures on Some Points in the Pathology of Heart Disease.' *Lancet* i: 569–572, 652–655, 723–726; 1902. 'The Mechanism of Pancreatic Secretion.' *Journal of Physiology* 28: 325–353; 1905. 'Croonian Lecture: On the Chemical Correlation of the Functions of the Body.' *Lancet* ii: 339–341, 423–425, 501–503, 579–583; 1918. *The Linacre Lecture on the Law of the Heart* (London).

Secondary: Henderson, John, 2005. *A Life of Ernest Starling* (New York); O'Connor, W. J., 1991. *British Physiologists, 1885–1914. A Biographical Dictionary* (Manchester) pp. 139–149; Colp, R., 1952. 'Ernest H. Starling: His Contribution to Medicine.' *Journal of History of Medicine and Allied Sciences* 7: 280–294; *DSB*; *Oxford DNB*.

Robert Tattersall

STENSEN, NIELS (aka NICOLAI STENONIS, STENO)

(b. Copenhagen, Denmark, 1 January 1638 [new style]; d. Schwerin, Germany, 25 November 1686), *anatomy, natural science, theology.*

Stensen was the son of goldsmith and innkeeper Sten Pedersen; his mother was Anne Nielsdatter. As a boy he worked in his father's and stepfather's workshop, where the foundation of his later amazing skill and dexterity as a dissector was laid. He attended the University of Copenhagen between 1656 and 1659. Among his teachers was the anatomist Thomas Bartholin, a discoverer of the lymphatic system.

In 1659 Stensen left Copenhagen for Amsterdam. For the first time he dissected on his own, and on 7 April 1659 he discovered the excretory duct (later named *ductus Stenonis*) through which salvia passes from the parotid gland to the oral cavity. Soon after, Stensen left Amsterdam for Leiden.

In Leiden Stensen continued his research on glands. He published four anatomical studies on the glands of the nose, the sweat glands, the tear gland, and the lachrymal canal. Inspired by the posthumous publication in 1662 of Descartes' *Treatise of Man,* he also embarked on studies of muscles, the heart, and the brain. He left Leiden in 1664 for Copenhagen, returning to his home town as one of the foremost European anatomists. In Copenhagen he published *On muscles and glands* in which, in opposition to his teacher Thomas Bartholin, he defended the thesis that the heart is a muscle.

He had hoped to succeed Thomas Bartholin in Copenhagen, but another candidate was appointed, and the disappointed Stensen left Copenhagen for Paris in the winter of 1664. In spring 1665 in Paris he held a lecture on the anatomy of the brain (*Discours sur l'anatomie du cerveau,* 1669). In his lecture Stensen criticized Descartes' theory of the brain and the function of the pineal body (*glandula pinealis*) as the place for the interaction between soul and body.

In early 1666 Stensen received an invitation from the Grand Duke of Tuscany, Frederik II. Arriving in Florence, he was attached to the court as a scientist. In 1667 he published one of his major works on muscles, *Specimen of Element of Myology or Geometrical Descriptions of the Muscles,* which contained a geometrical description of the structure and function of muscle fibers. In an idealized model the fibers were depicted as parallelepipeds between parallel tendon plates. When the fibers contract, the tendon plates move in parallel planes and the muscle swells and shortens. The model predicted that the muscle swells without any change of volume. In this way he refuted the traditional theory that the rush of the so-called animal spirits caused the swelling and shortening of the muscle. On 7 November 1667 Stensen converted to Catholicism, but continued his scientific work.

Some time before the conversion, he had begun to study geological formations in Tuscany. In 1669 he argued in *Prodromus to a Dissertation on solids naturally contained within Solids* that the geological strata must have been deposited in horizontal layers, and that the tilted position in which they often were observed must be due to changes caused by water. In this way it was possible to reconstruct sequences of events in the history of the earth. With this study Stensen became one of the founders of modern geology.

In 1672 Stensen was recalled to Denmark as a royal anatomist, and in January 1673 he began a series of public dissections. In his introductory lecture he said the famous words, 'Beautiful is what appears to the senses without dissection, more beautiful what dissection draws forth from the hidden inside; yet by far the most beautiful is what, escaping the senses, is revealed by reasoning helped by what the senses perceive' (cited in Kardel, 1994b, p. 119).

With royal permission Stensen returned in 1674 to Florence. In 1675 he took holy orders which brought his scientific career to an end, and he was in 1677 appointed titular bishop in Germany. In 1988 Stensen was beatified by Pope John Paul II.

Bibliography

Primary: 1910. *Opera Philosophica* 2 vols. (Copenhagen).

Secondary: Kardel, Troels, 1994a. *Steno on Muscles. Introduction, Texts, Translations* (Philadelphia); Kardel, Troels, 1994b. *Steno. Life–Science–Philosophy* (Copenhagen).

Carl Henrik Koch

STEPHENSON, ELSIE (b. Bishop Auckland, England, 22 January 1916; d. Edinburgh, Scotland, 16 July 1967), *nursing, nurse education.*

Stephenson, the youngest child of Henry Walker Stephenson, a farmer, and Ethel Watson, completed general nurse education at the West Suffolk Hospital, studied midwifery at Queen Charlotte's Maternity Hospital, London, and completed health visiting in Newcastle.

In the closing years of World War II, Stephenson went as one of a British Red Cross Society (BRCS) team to assist refugees in various camps in Egypt, Italy, and Yugoslavia. For her services, she was awarded the Italian Star and the Defence Medal and was made a Serving Sister of the Order of St John of Jerusalem.

Postwar, Stephenson joined a mobile BRCS hospital and provided relief at Bad Münder, caring for patients, some of whom were from concentration camps or had been prisoners of war. Then, at the invitation of Civilian Relief Overseas, she was part of a child welfare team in postwar Berlin, where the accent was on rehabilitation.

Subsequently, the BRCS appointed Stephenson as senior nurse consultant to the Middle and Far East, advising on general hygiene, disease prevention, and welfare organization.

During 1947, with Rockefeller Foundation funding, the University of Edinburgh made a momentous decision in the history of nursing; it agreed to set up the first Unit (later Department of Nursing Studies) in the UK where nurses would be prepared in an academic setting. Stephenson was appointed as Director. Initially, programs were offered in the Faculty of Arts to nurse educators (1956) and nurse administrators (1958). Then, in 1964, the World Health Organization (WHO) funded The International School to operate within the Department, and it attracted qualified nurses mainly from Europe, Africa, and the Far East.

Meantime, in 1960, an undergraduate course was established, but when a new Faculty of Social Sciences was created in 1963, nursing was relocated as an autonomous department offering the degree of BSc (Soc Sc-nsg). It was the first in the UK, indeed the first in Europe, where nursing was recognized as a graduating subject.

In keeping with an academic setting, Stephenson immediately promoted research activities, and she also was determined to establish a chair of nursing. In fact, a Nursing Research Unit was created (1971), as was a chair of nursing (1972), although Stephenson did not live to enjoy the realization of these goals, dying of lung cancer in 1967.

Stephenson married William Henry Gardner (1895–1977), a retired assistant under secretary of state, in 1964. She had many interests, served on various national and international committees, and was editor of *The International Journal of Nursing Studies*, president of the Florence Nightingale International Foundation, and a member of the WHO expert committee on nursing and the WHO expert committee of midwifery. She was awarded an honorary MSc by the University of Edinburgh and was made a fellow of the Royal Society of Health (1956).

Her inimitable contribution to the nursing profession is celebrated in the Elsie Stephenson Memorial Lecture held at the University of Edinburgh.

Bibliography

Secondary: Allen, Sheila, 1990. *Fear Not to Sow: A Life of Elsie Stephenson* (Penzance); *Oxford DNB.*

Winifred Logan

STEPTOE, PATRICK CHRISTOPHER (b. Witney, Oxfordshire, England, 9 June 1913; d. Canterbury, Kent, England, 22 March 1988), *gynecology, reproductive medicine.*

Steptoe was the sixth boy (seventh child) of the eight children of Grace Maud (née Mimms) and Harry Arthur Steptoe, who was Witney's Registrar of births, deaths, and marriages. He read medicine at King's College, London, and qualified after his clinical training at St George's Hospital (1939). After spending World War II in the navy, he worked in obstetrics and gynecology in London at St George's (1947–49) and the Whittington Hospital (1948–51) before moving to Oldham and District General Hospital in 1951 as a consultant, with his wife Sheena (née Kennedy) and two children.

In Oldham, Steptoe initially concentrated on seeing a large back list of patients and gaining his Fellowship of the Royal College of Obstetrics and Gynaecology (1961). When time allowed, he began considering the technique of laparoscopy—internal visual examination of the abdomen using an illuminated tubular instrument, a laparoscope, passed through a small incision in the abdominal wall—and determining its potential for diagnosis of disorders of the reproductive organs, including infertility. After developing his diagnostic skills, using advances in laparoscope technology in collaboration with colleagues in Europe, he explored the operative prospects, initially focusing on sterilization. Steptoe's surgical use of the laparoscope effectively introduced the routine use of keyhole surgery, but not without much early skepticism, despite the success of his first book (1967).

In 1968 Steptoe met the reproductive physiologist Robert Edwards. Steptoe was aware of the distress among his patients caused by infertility and was keen to exploit laparoscopy's potential to assist in vitro fertilization (IVF). Edwards, although based in the physiology department at Cambridge, established a small laboratory in the pathology department at Oldham and District General Hospital. At Steptoe's clinic, referred volunteer couples provided the human eggs, harvested by him with a laparoscope after injections of stimulating hormones, to be mixed with their partner's sperm in sterile conditions outside the human body and grown to the blastocyst stage. With this procedure formalized and with consistent results obtained, the next stage was implantation of the embryo in the mother's womb.

The Medical Research Council rejected a program grant application, which would have brought Steptoe to Cambridge. Instead, he established a small IVF unit at Kershaw's Hospital, Royton (1971). Edwards continued commuting, usually accompanied by technician Jean Purdy. Implantation proved difficult to achieve. Edwards's experience with mammalian reproductive physiology in the laboratory proved less helpful than before, and the team's decision to reintroduce at most two embryos was also problematic. Wider ethical and media debate on human IVF caused difficulties. Careful assessment of each stage of the technique from 1971 to 1974 indicated that the use of Primulot, a hormone preparation given to prevent abortion, actually terminated embryo growth. Ceasing to use Primulot, in 1975 they achieved the first unfortunately ectopic pregnancy, terminated at three months. Further refinements of the overall program followed; for example, development of an improved hormone medication using a single oocyte that also is produced during a normal cycle and transfer of an eight-celled embryo during the next normal cycle. The first successful pregnancy for Lesley Brown resulted in the first 'test tube baby', Louise, born 26 July 1978 by caesarean section amid intense media coverage.

The successful partnership of Steptoe and Edwards continued at a private clinic (Steptoe was obliged by his age to retire from the National Health Service) at Bourn Hall, Cambridge (opened September 1980). From Bourn Hall, the world's largest IVF clinic in 1980s, they remained at the forefront of developments in IVF, in contact with groups in Australia, the United States, and France, as well as at centers in Manchester and London in Britain. The screening of embryos for genetic defects, although initially very limited at Oldham, is a further development of their work. Greater understanding of male reproductive medicine and the introduction of new techniques helped combat male infertility. Elected FRS (1987) and CBE (1988), Steptoe also received honors from professional organizations in his specialty.

Bibliography

Primary: 1967. *Laparoscopy in Gynaecology* (Edinburgh); 1969. (with Edwards, Robert G., and B. D. Bavister) 'Early Stages of Fertilization In Vitro of Human Oocytes.' *Nature* 221: 632–635; 1978. (with Edwards, Robert G.) [Letter to the editor] *Lancet* ii: 366; 1980. (with Edwards, Robert G., and J. M. Purdy) 'Clinical Aspects of Pregnancies Established with Cleaving Embryos Grown In Vitro.' *British Journal for Obstetrics and Gynaecology* 87: 737–756; 1980. (with Edwards, Robert) *A Matter of Life. The Story of a Medical Breakthrough* (London).

Secondary: Edwards, Robert G., 1996. 'Patrick Christopher Steptoe.' *Biographical Memoirs of Fellows of the Royal Society* 42: 435–452; *Oxford DNB*.

Helen Bynum

STILL, ANDREW TAYLOR   (b. Jonesville, Virginia, USA, 6 August 1828; d. Kirksville, Missouri, USA, 12 December 1917), *osteopathy, osteopathic medicine.*

Still was the third of nine children born to Abram Still, a Methodist minister and self-taught physician, and his wife, Martha. Still's father received successive frontier appointments until the family located in Baldwin, Kansas. During this time, Still received an intermittent formal education. As a young man, Still was an active participant in the anti-slavery movement and was elected to the quasi-legal Free Kansas Legislature in 1854, which sought admission of the Kansas Territory into the Union as a non–slave-holding state. During the subsequent armed and sometime violent conflict with slavery supporters, Still became a lieutenant to the abolitionist leader James Lane. During the Civil War, Still was appointed a 'hospital Steward', in the 9th Kansas Cavalry, and later organized his own command and ultimately achieved the rank of major, seeing action in the successful drive against Confederate forces advancing upon Kansas City.

Still began practicing medicine in the mid-1850s. His training consisted of learning at the side of his father, reading what textbooks were available to him, and disinterring and dissecting Indian corpses. His first patients were the Shawnee. 'I soon learned to speak their tongue' and 'gave them such drugs as white men used, cured most of the cases I met, and was well received'. Although his first appointment in the military was as a 'hospital steward', Still later stated that he actually held the office of 'surgeon'. He also later claimed that he had briefly attended a Kansas City medical school, right after the Civil War, but his self-reported dates of attendance are inconsistent, and there are no surviving school records to ascertain the facts.

Still became dissatisfied with the theory and practice of medicine in 1864 when, despite all the efforts of fellow physicians, three of his family members died of spinal meningitis. Though Still would not abandon orthodox medicine for another decade, this personal loss led him to evaluate various alternative systems, such as homeopathy and eclecticism. He ultimately concluded that 'all was a conglomerate mess of conjectures on the ignorant sick man', and he maintained that the central issue in medicine was not which drug to use and in what dosage, but whether drugging itself was a scientific form of therapy.

In investigating drugless substitutes, Still found considerable value in the principles and practices of 'magnetic healing'. An offshoot of Mesmerism, many magnetic healers conceived of the human body as a machine throughout which flowed a universal magnetic fluid, which if impeded or obstructed would cause disease. Some magnetic healers used touch to influence this flow, and a few focused their attention on the spine as a central place of neural influence. Also important to Still were the principles and practices of the art of bonesetting. In addition to reducing dislocations, lay bonesetters also manipulated painful and diseased joints, thinking these conditions were also caused by a 'bone out of place'. Nevertheless, some patients with restricted joint mobility who remained unrelieved after treatment by regular doctors apparently benefited from manipulative treatment administered by such unlettered empirics.

Still began using manipulative techniques in his practice and was amazed at the results he obtained around the state of Missouri, having moved to Kirksville in 1875. In employing bonesetting, Still made an important discovery, namely that the sudden flexion and extension procedures peculiar to this art were not limited to orthopedic problems and that they constituted a more reliable means of healing than simply rubbing the spine as some magnetic healers had done. He later recounted this story from 1880: 'An Irish lady had asthma in bad form, though she had only come to be treated for a pain in her shoulder. I found she had a section of upper vertebrae out of line, and I stopped the pain by adjusting the spine and a few ribs. In about a month, she came back to see me without any pain or trace of asthma. . . . This was my first case of asthma treated in the new way and it started me on a new train of thought.' Soon he was handling an increasing variety of other chronic ailments, all by manipulating vertebrae back into their 'proper position'.

In explaining his success, he developed a theory, fusing elements of magnetic healing and bonesetting into one unified doctrine. The effects of disease, as the former said, were due to the obstruction or imbalance of the fluids—principally the blood—but this in turn was caused by misplaced bones, particularly in the spinal column, which interfered with nerve supply regulating blood flow. By the 1880s, Still had given birth to his own distinctive system, which at the end of the decade he called 'osteopathy'.

Often, Still had a difficult time getting his ideas across to potential clients. He saturated his speeches with an odd collection of metaphors, parables, and allegories that left many listeners bewildered. His unusual attire—a rumpled suit, a slouch hat, his pants tucked inelegantly in his boots—caused some to look rather than listen. Many times, he could be seen on the streets clenching a long wooden staff he used as a walking stick while toting a sack full of bones over his shoulder. Not surprisingly, such behavior led people to decide he was an eccentric genius or a deranged old man. Nevertheless, his clientele grew, and by 1889, he had established a permanent infirmary in Kirksville that drew thousands of visitors and became 'a Mecca for healing'.

In 1892, to meet the demands of many patients and their family members to learn the new science, Still established the American School of Osteopathy (ASO) in Kirksville. The highlight of the curriculum was watching Still evaluate and treat patients. According to one, 'We would hold the patients in position while Dr. Still . . . worked upon them, explaining to us as he treated why he gave this movement in one place, and a different movement in another. He would tell us what it would mean to the nerves from that particular region if muscles were "tied up" or a bone was out of line.' In diagnosing these conditions, a student explained, Still taught 'that we should place the patient on his side and then pass our hands carefully over the spinal column from the base of the spine, noting temperature changes as we went along. Should there be a lesion along the spine, where nerves may be disturbed, it would easily be detected through an abnormal coldness or hotness of the tissue at that point.'

Osteopathy was being introduced at a time when the role of microorganisms in disease was becoming well-established. Early critics pointedly asked how the germ theory could be reconciled with the doctrine that anatomical misplacement was the major cause of disease. Similarly, what possible benefit could manipulating the spine have in treating infectious disorders? Still ignored the questions. 'I believe but little of the germ theory', he once declared, 'and care much less.' His early faculty, however, preferred to face the problem more directly, arguing that although bacteriology seemed to undermine part of Still's original theory, its sister field, immunology, clearly supported him. Germs, they hypothesized, might be the active cause of disease, but spinal displacements, or what were then being called spinal 'lesions', could be predisposing causes. If, as they believed, these structural lesions produced derangement of physiologic functions, it would follow that in their presence, the body would be put in a lowered state of resistance. Thus, correcting lesions shortly after they occurred would lessen the likelihood of germs gaining a foothold in the body. By correcting lesions after infection had struck, the body's natural defenses could then more effectively respond to the invaders. Under these assumptions, osteopathic procedures seemed entirely applicable and necessary.

Despite vigorous opposition of MDs in the state, the ASO grew rapidly, boasting some 700 students in attendance by the end of the century. Graduates of Still's program

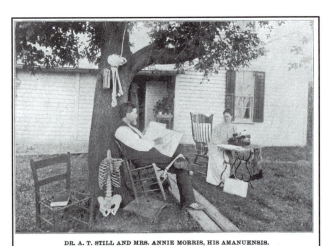

DR. A. T. STILL AND MRS. ANNIE MORRIS, HIS AMANUENSIS.

Mrs. Morris's residence in the background, where Dr. Still studied many of the problems of Osteopathy.

Andrew Taylor Still with skeletal specimens in the garden of his amanuensis, Mrs Annie Morris. Half-tone reproduction from Emmons Rutledge Booth, *History of Osteopathy . . .* Cincinnati, 1905. Wellcome Library, London.

were awarded Doctors of Osteopathy, or DO degrees, and they soon established other osteopathic schools, organized professional societies, lobbied for licensure laws, and combated imposters and imitators, the most significant of whom were the chiropractors. They also worked collectively to lengthen the college curriculum. In 1904 osteopathic schools that were members of the Associated Colleges of Osteopathy began instituting a mandatory three-year program, which was finally extended to the current four years in 1916.

Almost from the beginning, the early osteopathic curriculum encompassed the same basic science and clinical subjects—including surgery and obstetrics—as did allopathic medical schools. However, the American Osteopathic Association (AOA), established in 1901 and serving as the accrediting body for the colleges, forbade the teaching of materia medica and pharmacology in the standard curriculum. Still had argued that 'medicine and osteopathy as therapeutic agencies have nothing in common either theoretically or practically, and only an inconsistent physician will attempt to practice both'. Other osteopathic practitioners sharply disagreed, and shortly before Still died at the age of eighty-nine, they were successful at repealing a recently passed AOA policy that threatened the schools with a loss of accreditation should they incorporate these forbidden subjects. In 1929 the AOA formally approved the teaching of materia medica and pharmacology in osteopathic schools.

In the years since Still's death, osteopathy in the United States has fully evolved into what is more appropriately called 'osteopathic medicine'. In the 1930s, osteopathic medical colleges began to seriously address educational deficiencies in their programs, and as a result, DOs became

fully licensed—the same as MDs—as 'Physicians and Surgeons' in all states. In the same period, the AOA also began approving internship and residency programs and creating specialty certification boards. In the 1960s, the profession began to grow significantly, from five colleges to twenty-two by 2004, with more currently being developed. In 2005 there were more than 50,000 active DOs practicing in the United States, one in seven new U.S. medical school graduates was an osteopathic physician, and upwards of thirty million Americans relied on DOs for their health care needs. Relations between DOs and MDs, once marked by hostility, have become much more cooperative in the past several decades. Since the mid-1960s, osteopathic graduates have been eligible for and have made increasing use of residency programs approved by the American Council on Graduate Medical Education that were once reserved exclusively for MDs.

Though osteopathic principles and manipulative practices continue to be a standard feature of the osteopathic college curriculum (approximately 12 percent total hours in the first two years), the role these subjects play in overall DO practice in the United States has declined over the decades. This is not true internationally; in Europe, Asia, and Australia and elsewhere, growing interest in Still's ideas and methods have led to the establishment of many small colleges that do not teach medicine broadly and graduate practitioners who confine their intervention largely to manipulative medicine.

Bibliography

Primary: 1897. *Autobiography* (Kirksville, MO); 1899. *Philosophy of Osteopathy* (Kirksville, MO); 1902. *Philosophy and Mechanical Principles of Osteopathy* (Kirksville, MO); 1910. *Osteopathy: Research and Practice* (Kirksville, MO).

Secondary: Gevitz, Norman. 2004. *The DOs: Osteopathic Medicine in America* (Baltimore); Trowbridge, Carol. 1991. *Andrew Taylor Still, 1828–1917* (Kirksville); *DAMB*.

Norman Gevitz

STILL, GEORGE FREDERIC (b. Highbury, London, England, 27 February 1868; d. Harnham Croft, Salisbury, England, 28 June 1941), *pediatrics*.

Still was educated at the Merchant Taylor's School in London and at Gonville and Caius College, Cambridge. He matriculated (1885) and achieved first class honors in the classical tripos (1888). He studied medicine at Guy's Hospital Medical School and graduated MB, BChir (1893). Very early in his career, he became interested in diseases of childhood, having been appointed as house physician at Guy's Hospital to Sir James Goodhart (1845–1916), a professor of clinical medicine who had a particular interest in children's medicine. In 1894 Still was appointed as a clinical assistant at the Hospital for Sick Children, Great Ormond Street. In 1895 he was appointed registrar to Thomas (later Sir Thomas) Barlow (1845–1945) at Guy's Hospital. It is noteworthy that Barlow had in 1883 spoken at a meeting of the BMA section of diseases of children in a lecture entitled 'Notes on rheumatism and its allies in children' (Annual Meeting of the BMA, Section of Diseases of Children. 1883 *British Medical Journal* ii: 509–519). In the lecture he observed that 'rheumatoid arthritis is not without its examples in childhood'. In 1896 Still was awarded his MD by the University of Cambridge for a remarkable thesis entitled 'A special form of joint disease met with in children'. A paper based on this was published in 1897. This childhood type of rheumatoid arthritis later came to be called by the eponymous title 'Still's Disease'. Perhaps Still's teacher had generously 'collected together those 19 cases for him to review', as Bywaters (1977) has suggested.

Still was appointed physician (1899) at the Hospital for Sick Children and at the same time physician for diseases of children at King's College Hospital. In 1901 he became FRCP. In 1906 he became honorary professor of diseases of children at King's College London; this was the first time this title had been awarded in Great Britain, and King's College Hospital was the first of the London teaching hospitals to have a department specifically for diseases of children. During his career, Still studied the relationship between rickets and scurvy as well as the one between rickets and syphilis. He was also very interested in the problem of epidemic meningitis and wrote an influential account of celiac disease.

In 1928 he became the first president of the British Paediatric Association. In 1937 he was honored by his appointment as KCVO, having been pediatrician to Princesses Elizabeth and Margaret. He remained unmarried throughout his life, living with his mother. Both were regular devout worshippers at Salisbury Cathedral.

His chief relaxations were scholastic. He was fluent in ancient Greek and Latin and also was familiar with Hebrew and Arabic. He enjoyed reading the writings of figures of importance in the care of sick children from antiquity until the end of the eighteenth century. This resulted in his book *The History of Paediatrics* (1931). This influential book was the first on the topic to be written by an Englishman. It was written largely from a biographical perspective, concerning great men and their written works. It was a scholarly work with extensive quotations from the authors, often translated from the original language by Still and so made accessible to the English reader.

He published extensively in pediatrics, and his own textbook, *Common Diseases of Childhood* (1909), became an established text, with five editions, the last appearing in 1927.

Still was probably the chief pioneer in Britain for the emergence of pediatrics as a separate clinical discipline. There had been considerable resistance to this development from distinguished figures such as Samuel Gee (1839–1911) at St Bartholomew's Hospital and William Osler (1849–1919), Regius professor of medicine in Oxford. By the 1920s, however, there had emerged a general consensus that there was a role, albeit small, for pediatrics as a branch of medicine. Yet it was not until the establishment of the National Health Service (1948) that pediatricians were appointed throughout the nation.

Bibliography

Primary: 1897. 'On a form of chronic joint disease in children.' *Medico-Chirurgical Transactions* 80: 47—59; 1909. *Common Disorders and Diseases in Childhood* (London) (2nd edn. 1912, 3rd edn. 1915, 4th edn. 1924, 5th edn. 1927); 1931. *History of Paediatrics. The Progress of the Study of Diseases of Children up to the End of the XVIIIth Century* (London, reprinted 1965).

Secondary: Keen, J. H., 1998. 'George Frederic Still—Registrar, Great Ormond Street Children's Hospital.' *British Journal of Rheumatology* 37: 1247; Bywaters, E. G. L., 1977. 'The History of Paediatric Rheumatology.' *Arthritis Rheum* 20: 145–152; *Munk's Roll*; *Oxford DNB*.

John Walker-Smith

STILLÉ, ALFRED (b. Philadelphia, Pennsylvania, USA, 30 October 1813; d. Philadelphia, 24 September 1900), *medical education*.

Stillé, the son of John Stillé, a merchant, and Maria Wagner, graduated from the University of Pennsylvania in 1832 and from the medical school at the same university in 1836. In 1835 he was appointed resident physician at the Philadelphia Hospital, where he received further medical instruction according to the principles of the Paris medical school. The Parisian clinical researchers aimed to correlate the lesions found in the organs of their patients during postmortem examination with the disease symptoms that had been observed when the patient had been alive. Careful observation and medical statistics were also central to their approach. Applying these principles, Stillé's teachers conducted research that led to the distinction between typhus and typhoid fever. Inspired by this accomplishment, Stillé studied in Paris between 1836 and 1839. He returned as an outspoken promoter of the French approach to medical research and advocated the modernization of medical education in the United States to conform to the Parisian model.

Upon his return to Philadelphia, Stillé became resident physician at the Pennsylvania Hospital. In 1845 he was appointed as lecturer in pathology and the practice of medicine at the Philadelphia Association for Medical Instruction. He was prominently involved in the medical reform movement, which aimed to place medicine on a scientific footing, increase the requirements for medical education, and improve the medical curriculum. One of the outcomes of this movement was the establishment of the American Medical Association in 1847. As a recognition of his contributions, Stillé was elected secretary at its first meeting. In 1871 he served as president of the association.

From 1854 to 1859, Stillé was professor of the theory and practice of medicine at the Pennsylvania Medical College. After serving as president of the Pathological Society of Philadelphia and the Philadelphia Medical Society, he was appointed as professor of the theory and practice of medicine at the University of Pennsylvania in 1864, where he remained until his retirement in 1884. At the beginning of his tenure, Stillé advocated improvements to the medical school and the medical curriculum. During his tenure, the medical course was extended from two to three years, and the semester was extended from four to five months. At the same time, the University moved to its current site in Western Philadelphia, where a new university hospital was added to the medical school. At the end of the 1870s, the University of Pennsylvania was one of the leading medical schools in the United States.

Stillé was highly respected as a medical reformer and educator. He remained faithful to the principles of the Paris medical school during his whole career. He therefore rejected the germ theory, bacteriology, and the new laboratory medicine that had developed in the 1870s and 1880s in Germany. As a consequence, his importance diminished significantly at the end of his career.

Bibliography

Primary: 1848. *Elements of General Pathology: A Practical Treatise on the Causes, Forms, Symptoms, and Results of Disease* (Philadelphia); 1860. *Therapeutics and Materia Medica: A Systematic Treatise on the Action and Uses of Medicinal Agents, Including their Description and History* (Philadelphia); 1879. (with Maisch, John M.) *The National Dispensatory: Containing the Natural History, Chemistry, Pharmacy, Actions and Uses of Medicines, Including Those Recognized in the Pharmacopoeias of the United States and Great Britain* (Philadelphia).

Secondary: Warner, John Harley, 1998. *Against the Spirit of System: The French Impulse in Nineteenth-Century American Medicine* (Princeton); Osler, William, 1902. 'Alfred Stillé.' *University of Pennsylvania Medical Bulletin* 15: 126–132; Stillé, Katherine Blackiston, 1901. *Fragments: Being a Sketch of Dr. Alfred Stillé* (San Francisco); Burr, Charles W., 1901. 'A Sketch of Dr. Alfred Stillé.' *University Medical Magazine* 13: 759–765; DAMB.

Hans Pols

STOKES, WILLIAM (b. Dublin, Ireland, July 1804; d. Dublin, 7 January 1878), *medicine, cardiology, clinical teaching.*

Stokes was the son of the physician and surgeon Whitley Stokes (1763–1845), who was a Fellow and later regius professor of physic at Trinity College Dublin, a United Irishman and respected friend of Wolfe Tone, and an Irish language scholar and the translator of the New Testament into Irish. Whitley Stokes had abandoned the Church of Ireland (1815) for the Church of God, a nonjuring Calvinist sect founded by his former Trinity colleague, the classicist and mathematician John Walker. As a consequence of this, William Stokes was educated privately by Walker and thus was unable to matriculate at Trinity, though he did attend chemistry and anatomy classes there. Following this and with some clinical training at the Meath Hospital, he removed to Glasgow and then Edinburgh, taking his MD at the latter (1825), alongside his Catholic contemporary Dominic Corrigan (1802–80). At Edinburgh University, Stokes thrived under the tutelage of William Pulteney Alison (1790–1859), and as an undergraduate, he published the first work in English on Laennec's stethoscope (1825).

At twenty-two, he followed his father as physician to the Meath Hospital, where he and Robert Graves (1796–1853) revolutionized clinical teaching in the British Isles by introducing the central European practice of teaching students at the patient's bedside. They also foregrounded the diagnostic use of the stethoscope and the importance of attention to the physical symptoms of disease. Their work at the Meath reached a wider audience as *Clinical Reports of the Medical Cases in the Meath Hospital* (1827), part of a series of *Dublin Hospital Reports and Communications in Medicine and Surgery* published between 1818 and 1830. Stokes's research and teaching were also encapsulated in two works that quickly achieved classic status: *Diagnosis and Treatment of Diseases of the Chest* (1845, translated into German in 1846) and *Diseases of the Heart and Aorta* (1853, translated into German, French, and Italian).

In *Diseases of the Heart and Aorta*, Stokes expanded his 1846 article 'Observations of some cases of permanently slow pulse', drawing on the earlier work of Robert Adams (1791–1875) and John Cheyne (1777–1836) to describe what became known as Stokes-Adams syndrome (the foundational eponym of Irish cardiology) and Cheyne-Stokes respiration. The Slovenian Marcus Gerbezius (1658–1718) anticipated Stokes-Adams syndrome, which refers to a type of heartbeat wherein accelerated pulsation of the right jugular vein, accompanied by blackouts, is intermitted with extremely weak contractions. The American physiologist Joseph Erlanger (1874–1965) gave Stokes-Adams retrospective proof in 1904 when he demonstrated how it resulted from the impairment of conduction between the auricles and the ventricles. Cheyne-Stokes respiration refers to a type of respiration in which breathing becomes progressively weaker, ceasing completely for about fifteen seconds and then rising to a level of pronounced rapidity, the whole sequence lasting around a minute, after which similar sequences resume over the same duration.

Inspired in his Edinburgh days by Alison, Stokes regarded compassion and care for the sick poor as core to the clinician's vocation. During the typhus epidemic (1826–27) and again during the Great Famine (1845–49), Stokes labored long hours treating fever patients and attempting to alleviate their starvation diets. In *Lectures on Fever* (1874), he contributed to the contemporary debate on the nature of Irish epidemics, following his peers in seeing fevers as generically related but regarding individual epidemics as different manifestations of the same phenomenon. Whereas Graves fed fevers, Stokes advocated wine, port, and brandy punch as curative stimulants.

With his brother-in-law, the surgeon and anatomist Robert William Smith (1807–73), Stokes cofounded the Dublin Pathological Society (1838) as a forum where physicians and surgeons could discuss the pre- and postmortem manifestations of selected cases. The Dublin society inspired the founding of similar societies in London, Philadelphia, and elsewhere. Its ruminations were published in the *Dublin Journal of Medical Science*, edited by Stokes from 1834 and the home for many of his publications, including his 1846 paper on slow pulse. He also published papers in the *London Cyclopaedia of Practical Medicine* (1853–54) and contributed prolifically to the *London Medical and Surgical Journal*. A Francophile in medicine as in much else (like his father), Stokes sought to transcend the traditional distinction between physicians and surgeons, and the College of Physicians honored him by three times electing him president. He was also appointed physician-in-ordinary to Queen Victoria in Ireland (1861) and awarded the Prussian Order of Merit by the German Emperor in 1875.

Despite Stokes's own education, Stokes and Graves agreed that university training in classics and mathematics was the best precursor to a medical career. Much of his own education in the humanities, acquired in his father's Harcourt Street salon, he replicated in his Merrion Square home. There his social circle included the poet James Clarence Mangan (1803–49), the artist Frederick Burton (1816–1900), and the Trinity scholar John Pentland Mahaffey, as well as fellow savant and neighbor Sir William Wilde (1815–76). It is thought that the model for the epigrammatic exchanges between Oscar Wilde's characters was the conversational exchanges between Stokes and Mahaffey witnessed by Oscar at his parents' dinner table. Stokes shared Wilde's topographical interests and close friendship with the antiquarian George Petrie (1789–1866), whose biography Stokes published (1868). Stokes was elected president of the Royal Irish Academy in recognition of his prominence as a polymath in its Victorian golden age of that society.

Bibliography

Primary: 1825. *An Introduction to the Stethoscope; With its Application to the Diagnosis in Diseases of the Thoracic Viscera* (Edinburgh); 1837. *A Treatise on the Diagnosis and Treatment of Diseases of the Chest* (Dublin); 1853. *The Diseases of the Heart and Aorta* (Dublin).

Secondary: Snellen, H. A., 1984. *A History of Cardiology* (Rotterdam); O'Brien, Eoin, 1975. 'Dublin Masters of Clinical Expression IV. William Stokes (1804–1877).' *Journal of the Irish Colleges of Physicians and Surgeons* 4: 100–105; Stokes, William, 1898, *William Stokes: His Life and Work, 1804–1878* (London); *Oxford DNB*.

James McGeachie

STOPES, MARIE CHARLOTTE CARMICHAEL   (b. Edinburgh, Scotland, 15 October 1880; d. Dorking, Surrey, England, 2 October 1958), *sexology, birth control*.

Stopes began her career as a scientist, graduating with a double first in biology and geology from University College, London (1902). She completed doctoral work on fossil plants at the University of Munich (1904). She then returned to England and became the first woman to join the scientific staff of the University of Manchester, as assistant lecturer and demonstrator in botany (specializing in coal research), later that year. In 1911, after a whirlwind romance, she married fellow scientist Reginald Ruggles Gates. This marriage, although disastrous, led Stopes to her study of female sexuality, for ironically—and perhaps puzzling for a biologist—it was a marriage that was not sexual, as Stopes was to learn. A lack of sexual satisfaction encouraged Stopes to study the works of various sexual experts in the British Museum; this led her to discover that she was still a virgin and that her husband was impotent. Stopes's course of action was to file for an annulment on the grounds of nonconsummation (1916). Her experiences in the marital bed—or lack thereof—were exploited by Stopes in her first work, *Married Love* (1918), which was supported by her rather more potent second husband, Manchester manufacturing magnate Humphrey Roe. This work argued that women should enjoy sex as much as men and that such enjoyment should be based on sound knowledge about sex. This message was well-received by postwar women, and the run of 2,000 copies sold out in the first fortnight following release. Ensuing editions were circulated widely—Stopes even sent one to Queen Mary. As a result, thousands of letters, from men and women, poured through Stopes's letterbox, thanking her for the enlightenment she had provided, but also asking sundry other questions. Although *Married Love* was appreciated for its frankness in the quest for satisfying orgasms, it contained very little information about birth control. A remedy to this omission was forthcoming almost immediately with the publication of *Wise Parenthood* (1918). This text was a concise guide to birth-control methods, the field for which Stopes is remembered. Stopes was opposed to chemical methods of contraception, famously saying, 'Never put anything in your vagina that you would not put in your mouth!' Rather, she favored the use of rubber cervical caps.

On 17 March 1921 Stopes opened the first British family-planning clinic, at 61 Marlborough Road, Holloway, north London. This clinic, which employed female nurses and doctors, offered free birth-control advice for married women. Its dual aim was to provide family-planning advice to the poor and to gather data about contraception. By

1925 this service was in high demand and so moved premises to 108 Whitfield Street, central London, where the nurses continued their consultations, provided a mail-order contraception service, and gathered data. Throughout this period, Stopes had numerous troubles with her critics. She ended up in court in an (unsuccessful) attempt to sue Catholic doctor Halliday Sutherland (1882–1960) for libel for his criticisms of her book. Many in the medical profession did not like her encroaching on their domain, and Stopes seems to have had a difficult personality, which was an obstacle to her sustained collaboration with other birth controllers (of which there were many). By 1930 other family-planning organizations had appeared, and they joined forces with Stopes to form the National Birth Control Council, which later became the Family Planning Association. Stopes disagreed with how it should be run, and she resigned (1933).

On a personal front, Stopes offered her support to the progressive eugenics movement. She also furthered her pursuit of married love by engaging in extramarital affairs with younger men with the consent of her husband. This was agreed upon in a contract drawn up by Stopes and Roe. Stopes spent the rest of her life campaigning for her causes. Much of her time was spent writing articles for her newspaper *Birth Control News*. She also wrote novels, plays, and poetry, including *Love's Creation* (1928) and *Love Songs for Young Lovers* (1938); her collected poems were published in 1975. She died of cancer in 1958.

Bibliography

Primary: 1918. *Married Love: a new contribution to the solution of sex difficulties* (London) [reprint 2005, McKibbin, Ross, ed. (Oxford)]; 1918. *Wise Parenthood: a sequel to 'Married Love'* (London).

Secondary: Rose, June, 1992. *Marie Stopes and the Sexual Revolution* (London); Hall, Lesley, 1991. *Hidden Anxieties: Male Sexuality 1900–1950* (London); *Oxford DNB*.

Ivan Crozier

STUART, THOMAS PETER ANDERSON   (b. Dumfries, Scotland, 29 June 1856; d. Double Bay, Australia, 29 February 1920), *physiology, medical education.*

Anderson Stuart was the only child of his father's second marriage, to Jane Anderson, whose family name was adopted by the son. Alexander Stuart was a tailor and local magistrate whose first wife died of tuberculosis, as did three of her children. Thomas was educated at Dumfries Academy until the age of fourteen, when he was apprenticed to a pharmacist. When he found that regulations prevented him from completing the course until he was twenty-one, he passed the examinations for entry to medicine at the University of Edinburgh. Before commencing that course he spent a year in Germany improving his grasp of French and German. Returning to the university, he proved to be a brilliant student, topping his final year with first class honors and a gold medal (MB CM 1880). After graduation he returned to Germany to study biochemistry and pharmacology in Strasbourg. His research there formed the basis for his MD thesis (1882) and another gold medal. While working as chief demonstrator in physiology at Edinburgh, he applied for the foundation chair of anatomy and physiology in the new medical school being formed at the University of Sydney.

When he arrived in Australia in March 1883, Anderson Stuart found that he was expected to work in a cramped, unsuitable building. He asked the government for better premises and a mortuary, dissecting theater, and lecture room were soon built. Funds were allocated for a permanent medical school, which was ready by 1889; by then there were about seventy students. Determined to set a high standard of excellence, he failed all the students in the initial intake.

Anderson Stuart was made a fellow of the University Senate as soon as he arrived; by 1891 he was dean of the faculty of medicine. He recruited talented staff from overseas, mostly from Edinburgh, his old university. Several went on to have distinguished careers, but some proved disappointing. This Edinburgh influence on Sydney medical graduates persisted for decades; many subsequently undertook postgraduate study in Scotland.

Among his many extramural activities, Anderson Stuart was a member of the Board of Health from 1891 until his death. He was appointed president in 1893, but resigned in 1896 when the Public Service Board objected to him holding two salaried positions.

Although Anderson Stuart dabbled in medical research, this was not his true métier. His strengths lay in organizational management. In 1901 he was influential in the establishment of a school of dentistry, becoming the first president of the United Dental Hospital in 1905. He also played a part in creating a department of veterinary science at the university in 1909. After becoming chairman of the (Royal) Prince Alfred Hospital (1901), which adjoined the university and provided clinical teaching resources, he dominated the running of the hospital. Under his direction it embarked on an ambitious construction program which made it the largest hospital in Sydney.

Students found 'Andy' to be a concise, meticulous lecturer. The few female students appreciated his support for equal opportunity within the medical faculty. Yet he was a forceful, arrogant man, disliked by most of his colleagues. A biographer has written that he 'became the virtual dictator of things medical in Sydney' (Young, 1990, p. 131). An important ally for him in achieving this status was a fellow Edinburgh medical graduate, Sir Normand MacLaurin, who was chancellor of the university from 1896–1913.

The fine Gothic Revival buildings of the old medical school at the University of Sydney were named after Anderson Stuart in 1960, a fitting memorial to the founder.

Bibliography

Primary: 1902. 'The majority of the medical school.' *Australasian Medical Gazette* 21: 491–503.

Secondary: Serle, P., 1949. *Dictionary of Australian Biography* (Sydney); Moran, H. M., 1939. *Viewless Winds* (London); Epps, W., 1922. *Anderson Stuart M.D.* (Sydney); *AuDB*.

Peter J. Tyler

SUBBOTIĆ, VOJISLAV (b. Novi Sad, Vojvodina [now Serbia], 6 January 1859; d. Belgrade, Yugoslavia [now Serbia] 5 December 1923), *surgery, military surgery.*

Subbotić (Subbotich) was born in 1859 in Novi Sad, Vojvodina, at that time a center of Serbian culture under the rule of the Austro-Hungarian Emperor. His father was a well-known lawyer and poet, Jovan Subbotić, and his mother, Savka Polit-Desančić, was from a distinguished patrician family. Subbotić went to Vienna to pursue medical studies but left school to volunteer in the Serbian-Turkish wars of 1876–78. He later took up his medical studies again, first in Paris, before becoming a medical doctor in Vienna in 1881, where he specialized in pathology (under Rokitansky), and then surgery (with Edward Albert, a disciple of Billroth). Subbotić's first position was as chief of the city hospital in Zemun, then a border city of the Habsburg empire.

In 1889 Vladan Djordjević persuaded Subbotić to move to Belgrade and become head of the surgical ward of the General State Hospital. There he introduced the methods of Pasteur and Lister as obligatory methods. Subbotić was particularly insistent upon employee discipline and on precision in preoperative diagnostics. During the first year of his stay in Serbia, he gave sixty lectures. He also organized the first meeting of Serbian surgeons (1907), and the first Yugoslav conference of operative medicine (1911). In 1916 he devised a method for immobilizing fractured femur bones. Subbotić was one of the founding members of the Belgrade Medical Faculty, and established the first Surgical Hospital, which was responsible for producing many distinguished Serbian surgeons.

An active medical participant in four wars, Subbotić made important contributions to military surgery. His 'War Experiences of Traumatic Aneurisms', published in *Lancet*, was widely quoted and earned him election as a member of the American and British Association of Military Surgeons. Subbotić was also a member of the French and German surgical societies and of the Paris Medical Academy. During World War I Subbotić served as the Serbian representative to the International Sanitary Commission in Paris, holding several lectures on the Serbian typhoid epidemic of 1914–15 that claimed more than 300,000 lives, among the worst in Europe's history. Among his thirty-four published medical works, a report dealing with operations on pancreatic cysts, published in 1887, is particularly noteworthy.

Bibliography

Secondary: Čolović B, Radoje, 2000. *50 godina Hirurške sekcije Srpskog lekarskog društva*; 1972. *Spomenica Srpskog Lekarskog Društva* (Belgrade); 1964. *Medicinska enciklopedija*, 9 Shiz–Tul (Zagreb).

Jelena Jovanovic Simic and
Predrag J. Markovic

SUGITA, GENPAKU (b. Edo [now Tokyo], Japan, 20 October 1733; d. Edo, 1 June 1817), *anatomy, dissection, Rangaku (Dutch studies), translation.*

Sugita Genpaku was born into a medical family. His father, as his father before him, was a surgeon who had studied the 'Southern Barbarian' or Nanban School, as the early school of European-style medicine was called. It consisted mostly of various techniques for treating gunshot and blade wounds, dislocated joints, and skin diseases. With the rank of low ranking samurai, father and son served the lord of Obama domain, in present-day Fukui Prefecture.

Education

In his early youth Genpaku did not seem to attract special attention, but by the age of seventeen he had made it clear to his father that he wished to study medicine and follow in his father's footsteps. At that time, he began studying Confucian philosophy in the Kogakuha, or School of Ancient Learning, and the study of medicine under Nishi Gentetsu, a physician of the Nanban School who served the Tokugawa Shogun in Edo (now Tokyo). Under Nishi, Genpaku developed a strong interest in European medicine and did his best to examine any European texts he could find.

In 1754, not long after Genpaku had started his study of medicine, the Kyoto physician Yamawaki Tōyō (1705–62) undertook the first medical dissection of a human body in early modern Japan. Tōyō failed to achieve his goal of proving his nine-organ theory of human anatomy, but he did succeed in stimulating interest in anatomy throughout the country. Thereafter, numerous physicians conducted dissections with the goal of better understanding the structure of the human body. A debate ensued between those who believed that the living body could not be understood by dissecting a corpse and those who asserted that earlier Chinese theories of the body were incorrect.

From Dissection to Translation

This debate intrigued Genpaku, who was familiar with both schools of thought. In Edo, there were numerous opportunities to discuss this issue with other physicians, and a group of them arranged to witness the dissection of an executed criminal in the spring of 1771. This group included two other renowned physicians of the day, Maeno Ryōtaku (1723–1803) and Nakagawa Jun'an (1739–86), and they took with them to this dissection both a Dutch translation of the *Tabulae anatomicae* by Johann Adam Kulmus (1689–1745) and several Chinese anatomy texts.

Genpaku later wrote that he observed a number of organs in the body that none of the Chinese texts identified by name. He asked the man who was doing the dissection about them and was told that they were always found in a body but he did not know what they were. On the other hand, they discovered that the *Tabulae anatomicae* did include names for these parts of the body. This was the impetus that compelled Genpaku and this group, who were joined by Katsuragawa Hoshū (1751–1809), to undertake the translation of the book without the aid of dictionaries—since none existed. In doing so, they had to coin a number of words for the first time in Japanese, including terms for nerves, ligaments, the pancreas, and other parts of the body. They published the *Kaitai shinsho* [New Book of Anatomy] in 1774.

This translation was arguably more important than the medical accomplishments he and his group achieved. The translation led to the creation of the first Dutch-Japanese dictionaries and the flourishing of what was called 'Dutch Studies', or Rangaku in Japanese. It was not long before this allowed scholars to compile dictionaries from other European languages including English, German, French, and Russian; in the process, Dutch Studies became 'Western Studies', or Yōgaku in Japanese, and came to include a broad range of disciplines.

Bibliography

Primary: 1774. *Kaitai shinsho* [New Book of Anatomy] (Edo); 1969. *Dawn of Western Science in Japan: Rangaku kotohaiime*, trans. Matsumoto, Rōyōz (Tokyo).

Secondary: Katagiri, Kazuo, 1971. *Sugita Genpaku* (Tokyo).

William Johnston

SULLIVAN, HARRY STACK

SULLIVAN, HARRY STACK (b. Norwich, New York, USA, 21 February 1892; d. Paris, France, 14 January 1949), *psychiatry, schizophrenia, psychoanalysis.*

Sullivan was the only child in a Roman Catholic farming family of Irish descent in New York State. He initially intended to be a physicist and commenced studying at Cornell University in 1908. However, he was suspended from Cornell in 1910, after an incident involving mail tampering. His whereabouts during this period are unknown, and his biographers have speculated as to whether he might have been hospitalized. Sullivan dated his interest in schizophrenia to this period. He then went to the Chicago College of Medicine and Surgery, and his interests became orientated toward psychiatry. A reading of the works of Freud, Jung, and Ferenczi drew him to psychoanalysis, and he had his first experience of psychoanalysis in 1915. After finishing medical school, he took up various positions and in 1920 was appointed as liaisons officer for the Veteran's Bureau at St Elizabeth's Hospital in Washington, D.C. This brought him into contact with William Alonson White. White's approach to psychiatry and mental health, and his eclectic application of psychoanalysis to the treatment of psychotics, had a lasting impact on Sullivan. From White, Sullivan took the conception that psychiatry had a role in all human affairs.

In 1922 he obtained a position at Sheppard and Enoch Pratt Hospital, Baltimore, from 1925 to 1930 as research director. It was here that he commenced a lifelong friendship with Clara Thompson. Sullivan encouraged Clara Thompson to go to Europe to be analyzed by Sándor Ferenczi, and Sullivan later had a spell of analysis with her himself. Sullivan held that Freud was responsible for drawing attention to the discontinuities in the stream of consciousness, and although the concept of the unconscious did not feature in Sullivan's work, he took up Freud's notion of symbolism. In 1924 Sullivan became a member of the American Psychoanalytic Association, although he was highly critical of the orthodox analysts (and they of him). During this period, Sullivan came into contact with Adolf Meyer, from whom he took the view that mental disorders were dynamic patterns and types of reaction to the demands of life and that psychosis was a total psychobiological response to a life situation. Sullivan's interests were focused on schizophrenia, and he became renowned for his capacity to enter into communication with schizophrenic patients. He stressed the continuity between the normal and the schizophrenic and was opposed to organicist models. He considered schizophrenia a 'disorder of living'—the result of disturbed interpersonal relationships in childhood. He held that through psychotherapy these issues could be identified and resolved. He viewed psychotherapy as an educational process through an interpersonal relation.

In 1926 he met the linguist Edward Sapir, and it was through him that he came into contact with the Chicago school of sociology. Sullivan maintained that whereas Freud and Meyer had focused on the individual person, the Chicago sociologist George Herbert Mead had shown that the 'person' was constituted by their relations with others and hence that it was impossible to separate a person from his or her network of interpersonal relations. At the same time, Sullivan began to draw on the cultural anthropology of Ruth Benedict and Bronislaw Malinowski. From schizophrenia, Sullivan expanded his work into a general theory of personality. He came to see personality as the 'relatively enduring pattern of recurrent interpersonal situations which characterize a human life'. Sullivan's work demonstrates the manner in which psychoanalysis in the United

States could be reformulated in terms of the environmentalism and meliorism that characterized American social science during this period.

In 1930 he moved to New York City, where he established a private practice. However, in 1933 he was declared bankrupt. Sullivan sought to reformulate psychiatry itself as the study of interpersonal relations. In so doing, he attempted to establish an interdisciplinary linkage between psychiatry and social science. His institutional endeavors were orientated toward these goals. In 1933 he cofounded the William Alanson White Psychiatric Foundation and became its first president. In 1936 he founded the Washington School of Psychiatry, which established an eclectic training program. In 1938 he founded the journal *Psychiatry* and was its first editor. After World War II, he was involved in the formation of the World Federation for Mental Health. During his lifetime, Sullivan published his work in the form of essays, and these together with unpublished works were collected into volumes and published after his death in a Paris hotel room in 1949.

Bibliography

Primary: 1953. *Conceptions of Modern Psychiatry* (New York); 1953. *The Interpersonal Theory of Psychiatry* (New York); 1971. *The Fusion of Psychiatry and Social Science* (New York); 1974. *Schizophrenia as a Human Process* (New York).

Secondary: Perry, Helen Swick, 1982. *Psychiatrist of America: The Life of Harry Stack Sullivan* (Cambridge, MA); *DAMB*.

Sonu Shamdasani

SUN, SIMIAO 孫思邈 (b. Chang'an, Shaanxi Province, China, 581?; d. Mt Taibo [now Zhongnanshan], Shaanxi Province, China, 682), *Chinese medicine, Daoism, ethics, gynecology, pediatrics.*

Celebrated as the 'God of Medicine' in Chinese popular religion since at least the fifteenth century, Sun Simiao's life has been the source of many legends. Accompanied by a tiger and a dragon, he has become associated with the eremitic life of a true Daoist adept, with supreme medicinal and alchemical knowledge, supernatural powers, and longevity or even immortality. The historical biographies from closer to his own time have left a less colorful but more trustworthy record, which can be authenticated with the autobiographical statements interspersed in his own writings.

Details in Sun's biographies suggest a birth date of the early sixth century. Given the fairly certain death date of 682, this would bring his age to over 140 years. But most scholars now agree that Sun was most probably born in 581. Already at the young age of seven, his exceptional understanding of the Confucian, Daoist, and Buddhist literature caused a provincial governor to recognize him as a 'sagely youth'. During his young adulthood, Sun refused several imperial summonses to government service, preferring to seclude himself, it is alleged, during times he considered leadership to be corrupt.

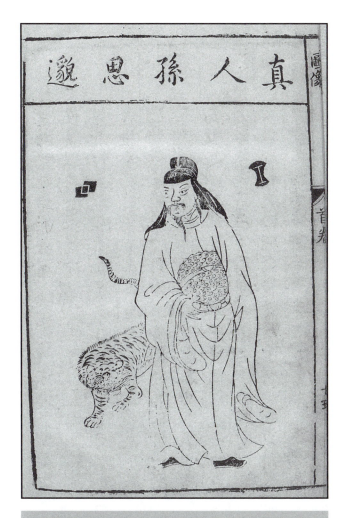

Sun Simiao. Lettering on this woodcut reads 'Zhenren Sun Simiao' [Daoist sage Sun Simiao]. From Chen Jiamo, *Bencao Mengquan* [Introduction to the Pharmacopoeia], 1573–1620. Library of Zhongguo zhongyi yanjiu yuan/Wellcome Library, London.

Medicine, Cosmology, and Politics

In 627, Emperor Taizong of the Tang dynasty ascended the throne. Some years earlier Sun had apparently predicted this event as heralding the arrival of a worthy ruler, so he responded to an imperial invitation to the capital. In contrast to the popular view of Sun Simiao as a secluded hermit, Sun remained in the service of the Tang government for a total of almost fifty years, either residing at the capital or accompanying the emperor on his travels. During his time at court, the emperor repeatedly attempted to bestow on him such official titles as 'Grand Master of Remonstrance' that illustrate the influential position and respect Sun held in the imperial retinue. Like a true sage, however, Sun persisted in refusing to accept any worldly honors. Further demonstrating his elevated status in the upper echelons of early Tang society, the biographies mention a number of eminent visitors who sought his counsel as a clairvoyant and sage advisor. For example, the vice director of the Chancellery presented his sons to him to have their future prognosticated. Imperial historians composing the official dynastic histories of the period before the Tang used his vivid recollection of past events as eye-witness accounts of unquestionable authenticity and recorded his political engagements advising the emperor and high-ranking members of the Tang elite. It is likely that he composed the bulk of his literary works during this period.

In contrast to his social activities recorded in the biographies, his own writings reveal a man deeply immersed in the study of medical, alchemical, cosmological, philosophical, and religious literature. These he applied in practice to the cultivation of his own material body in the pursuit of longevity and immortality, and to a religious cultivation influenced by both Daoist and Buddhist ideals. Although many of his works survive only as titles, they serve to show his broad range of interests. They span from collections of medical prescriptions to alchemical recipes, essays on the cultivation of *qi* and preservation of life, to commentaries on the philosophical classics *Laozi* and *Zhuangzi*, a *Fu lu lun* 福祿論 [Treatise on Happiness and Longevity], and a *Hui sanjiao lun* 會三教論 [Treatise on Uniting the Three Teachings (i.e. Confucianism, Daoism, and Buddhism)].

Sun's extant work, including quotations in texts by others, reflects much intellectual activity during this period in Chinese history in that it attempts to synthesize the three main philosophies and religions of China. In Sun's case this meant integrating the moral responsibilities and social and political engagement of secular Confucianism, Daoist practices of self-cultivation in pursuit of immortality and transcendence, and Buddhist metaphysical philosophy. In addition, his profound inquiry into the workings of the cosmos not only resulted in abstract cosmological musings, but was also directly related (in his own eyes as well as those of his contemporaries) to practical skills in the political, medical, and alchemical realms. The life and work of Sun Simiao can thus be seen in the light of correlative thinking; he successfully linked his understanding of the macrocosm, or cosmic body, with concrete applications to the political body on the one hand, and the individual human body on the other. As he purportedly stated himself, 'An excellent physician guides [*qi* and essence] with medicinal [i.e. lancing] stones and rescues them with needles and prescriptions. A sage [ruler] harmonizes them in order to perfect his power and uses them as support in order to manage the affairs of humanity. Thus, the human body has illnesses that can be cured and Heaven and Earth have calamities that can be dispersed' (my trans.). Here Sun equated the physician's activity of harmonizing the human body with the constancies of the universe by use of medicinal drugs, acupuncture, and lancing stones with the sage-king's activity of exercising political rule by patterning the affairs of human society after the heavenly cycles. Using different tools, both physician and sage-king shared the goal of ordering the microcosm and aligning it with the macrocosm.

The Essential Prescriptions Worth a Thousand Pieces of Gold

Although Sun Simiao is celebrated in China as one of China's greatest physicians, it is quite unlikely that he ever practiced medicine professionally. His official biographies contain only a single reference to practical medical activities in an account in which he cured an aristocrat and disciple of a 'malign condition which physicians were unable to treat'. In spite of this, Sun is undoubtedly one of China's greatest medical authors. His *Beiji qianjin yaofang* [Essential Prescriptions worth a Thousand Pieces of Gold for Every Emergency] is a monumental medical encyclopedia that is still referred to and cited frequently in contemporary Chinese texts on traditional Chinese medicine. In thirty scrolls, it covered over two hundred topics in more than five thousand entries of essays and prescriptions. It was organized into a preface; three scrolls on gynecology; one scroll each on pediatrics, on disorders of the seven orifices, on 'wind poison and leg qi', and on the various winds; two scrolls on cold damage; one scroll each on the ten major viscera and bowels, on dehydration and urinary problems, on abscesses, on hemorrhoids and fistulas, on resolving toxins and various other problems, on emergency treatment, on dietary therapy, on physical cultivation and lengthening life, and on vessel theory and pulse diagnostics; and two scrolls on acupuncture and moxibustion.

Taken as a whole, it is a gold mine of information on what was apparently the most sophisticated level of medical theory and practice in the early medieval period in China. The depth of Sun's medical knowledge was expressed in the theoretical essays, the conceptualization and organization of etiologies, and the complexities of the herbal prescriptions, many of which are still applied in clinical practice today. But perhaps even more important is its comprehensiveness, reflected particularly in the diversity of therapeutic techniques that include both internal applications—e.g., medicinal decoctions, powders, pills, pastes, jellies, and wines—and external applications such as ointments, hot compresses, suppositories, fumigations, baths, beauty treatments, physical manipulations, acupuncture and moxibustion, and such religious methods as talismans, exorcistic rituals, and spells.

To cite just one example of Sun's importance in the history of Chinese medicine, the *Essential Prescriptions* was instrumental in the formation of gynecology as a respected professional specialization from the Song period on. It was the first text to explicitly stress and explain the need for 'separate prescriptions' for women, containing the often-cited statement that 'women's disorders are ten times more difficult to treat than men's,' because of the cost of women's reproductive processes of menstruation, pregnancy, childbirth, and lactation. The categorization of prescriptions was still somewhat arbitrary, and treatment strategies occasionally contradicted each other, a consequence of the lack of an integrated and comprehensive theoretical basis from which to approach the female body in early medieval China. Only centuries later, however, was Sun's call for a specialized treatment of women answered by numerous gynecological authors who began to diagnose and treat women's disorders with much greater sophistication under the maxim that women's health is rooted in blood.

This text, and his accompanying work *Qianjin yi fang* 千金翼方 [Revised Prescriptions Worth a Thousand Pieces of Gold], were two of eleven medical texts that were meticulously revised and printed in the twelfth century by the Imperial Office for the Correction of Medical Texts. Since then, it has been reprinted regularly until the present day, when it is still found on the shelves of any well-stocked Chinese medical bookstore in Asia. It was also the most influential text in the transmission of Chinese medicine to Japan and therefore the foundational text in the creation of Japanese Kampo medicine.

Besides the clinical value of its prescriptions, it is recognized in China as the first text to address the question of medical ethics. Outlining the intellectual and moral requirements of a true 'Great Physician', the preface stressed that it is mandatory for the ideal physician to combine his clinical skills and practical experience with a solid literate education in the standard medical theory and prescription texts as well as the Confucian, Daoist, and Buddhist classics. In addition, he must have mastered such occult arts as divination and astrology and be familiar with religious taboos and calendrical prohibitions. He must follow an exemplary life style, maintain a dignified appearance, and devote himself wholeheartedly to alleviating the suffering of humanity by treating all patients equally regardless of their wealth, status, gender, or the nature of the ailment. Lastly, he must abstain from seeking personal gain and from criticizing his fellow physicians. In this essay, Sun's vision of the 'Great Physician' laid the foundations for the emergence of the 'literati-physicians', *ru yi*, several centuries later, when members of the literati class were finally able to engage in the professional practice of medicine without any loss of prestige. Sun thus proved to be instrumental in overcoming the traditional Confucian disdain for technical and specialized knowledge.

Retirement

In 674 Sun Simiao was finally permitted to withdraw from court life under the pretext of ill health. He was released in great honor and bestowed by the emperor with gifts that reflect the elevated position he held in the emperor's retinue. In his retirement, he continued to leave his mark by instructing a number of illustrious disciples, ranging from high officials in the Chancellery to alchemists and one of the greatest poets of the early Tang period. Posthumous hagiographical accounts depict Sun Simiao in the last few decades of his life as a recluse living in a cave on Mount Taibo in the company of only a dragon and a tiger, collecting medicinal substances and performing the supernatural feats associated with an advanced Daoist adept. The official biographies, on the other hand, recount his skills in such occult arts as physiognomy, astrology and calendrics, clairvoyance, alchemy, and longevity. The only fact about the end of his life that is reasonably certain is that Sun died in 682 after a long life full of political engagement alternating with reclusive episodes devoted to the individual cultivation of his spirit, mind, and body.

Bibliography

Primary: c. 652. *Beiji qianjin yaofang* 備急千金要方 [Prescriptions Worth a Thousand Pieces of Gold for Every Emergency]; (n.d.) *Qianjin yi fang* 千金翼方 [Revised Prescriptions Worth a Thousand Pieces of Gold]; (n.d.) *Sheyang zhenzhong fang* 攝養枕中方 [Pillow-Book of Prescriptions for Nourishing Life]; *Jiu Tang shu* 舊唐書 [Old Tang Histories] scroll 191, pp. 5094-5097 (completed in 945 CE).

Secondary: Unschuld, Paul U., 2000. *Medicine in China: Historical Artifacts and Images* (New York) pp. 88–95; Engelhardt, Ute, 1989. '*Qi* for Life: Longevity in the Tang' in Kohn, Livia, ed., *Taoist Meditation and Longevity Techniques* (Ann Arbor, MI) pp. 263–296; Unschuld, Paul U., 1979. *Medical Ethics in Imperial China* (Berkeley, CA) pp. 24–33; Sivin, Nathan, 1968. *Chinese Alchemy: Preliminary Studies* (Cambridge, MA) pp. 81–144.

Sabine Wilms

SUTTON, DANIEL   (b. Kenton, Suffolk, England, 4 May 1735; d. Bloomsbury Square, London, England, February 1819), *smallpox inoculation.*

Sutton, second son of eleven children (eight sons and three daughters) of surgeon, apothecary, and inoculator Robert Sutton (1708–88) and Sarah Barker of Debenham, Suffolk, trained with his father, served as an assistant to an Essex doctor between 1760 and 1762 or 1763, and thereafter briefly returned to working with his father. In October 1763 he set up his own inoculation practice in Ingatestone, Essex.

Sutton's father had pioneered a new approach to smallpox inoculation that resembled the method first observed in Constantinople, namely making a slight scratch on the skin and inserting a small amount of matter taken from a smallpox pustule. After inoculation had been introduced in England in the 1720s, the procedure had been modified so that surgeons made deep incisions and inserted a large amount of pocky material. This increased the chances of provoking a full-blown case of smallpox and hence made inoculation more risky. Robert Sutton's innovations helped reduce the mortality associated with smallpox inoculation.

Daniel Sutton diverged from his father's procedure in two ways: first, he reduced the amount of time to prepare patients for inoculation from one month to eight to ten days by modifying their diet. Second, he replaced indoor confinement following inoculation with an open-air regime.

Sutton's inoculation practice was remarkably successful. He earned 2,000 guineas in his first year of practice. Two years later, he opened three inoculation houses in Ingatest-one that catered to different classes of patients who paid six, four, or three guineas. Along with his father and brothers, he entered into partnerships with other physicians and surgeons to set up inoculation houses throughout England, including two in London. In 1765 Sutton earned £6,300.

In addition to promoting inexpensive, safer inoculations, Sutton played a central role in mass or general inoculations. He undertook his first general inoculation in Maldon, Essex, in May 1766, when he inoculated 487 inhabitants in one day. He carried out similar general inoculations in Maidstone, Kent, and Ewell, Surrey, in July and August of the same year. During the period 1764 through 1766, Sutton, his assistants, and his partners claimed to have inoculated approximately 20,000 individuals, without a single death. His practice was not without controversy, however. In 1766 he was charged with causing a smallpox epidemic in Chelmsford, but because all the physicians in Chelmsford also practiced inoculation, blame could not be placed on Sutton with certainty.

Sutton's inoculation method was publicized in other parts of Europe, especially by Sir John Pringle (1707–82). In recognition of his contributions, Sutton was awarded a coat of arms in 1767 with the motto 'Safely, quickly and pleasantly'. By 1768, the Sutton partnerships numbered forty-seven and were found in England, Ireland, Wales, the Netherlands, France, Jamaica, and Virginia. Sutton's method was widely adopted and greatly contributed to the struggle against smallpox. After 1769, the physician Thomas Dimsdale (1712–1800) replaced Sutton as the inoculator of choice among the English elite.

In 1767 Sutton married Rachel Westley, widow of William Westley of Shepton Mallet, Somerset. They had one son and one daughter. Sutton published *The Inoculator* (1796), in which he described his method. He lived long enough to see vaccination replace inoculation by 1800.

Bibliography

Primary: 1796. *The Inoculator* (London).

Secondary: Smith, J. R., 1987. *The Speckled Monster* (Chelmsford); *Oxford DNB*.

Andrea Rusnock

SUVANNAVONG, UDOM   (b. Viang Chan, Laos, 30 December 1917; d. ?, 1985?), *medicine.*

Udom Suvannavong was born in Viang Chan (Vientiane) as a member of one of Laos's two most preeminent families of the early twentieth century. The Suvannavongs began their social rise at the beginning of the period of French colonization with the French nomination of the family patriarch Khampha as Chao-muang (prefect) of Vientiane. Their family remained French after that and supplied various civil servants to the colonial administration.

Suvannavong first began his studies in Phnom Penh (Cambodia), and continued in Saigon (Vietnam) as well as at Hanoi medical faculty (Vietnam), and then went on to the medical faculty at Paris in 1946. In 1949 he became the first Laotian to attain the French degree of doctor of medicine; his thesis was on medicine in Laos. He began his practice in France as a doctor of internal medicine at the Puteaux hospital of Seine before returning to Laos.

Upon his return to Laos, Suvannavong occupied various posts in the health administration, propelling him into the contentious higher political spheres of his nation. Just as with Vietnam and Cambodia, Laos was also pulled into the maelstrom of the First Indochina War (1946–54) and the Second Indochina War, or 'Vietnam War' (1964–75).

In 1954 Suvannavong was nominated director of public health, then minister of public health and information in the Katāy Dōn Sasōrith government formed in the aftermath of the Geneva Accords. In 1956 he served as minister of health construction and urbanism under the government of Suvanna Phūmā.

Suvannavong finally retired from the political arena before the first coalition government in 1957, which was formed under international pressure and which temporarily united the country. This did not prevent him from achieving a full medical career—quite the contrary—but this part of his career occurred in the private rather than the public sector. He also assumed the function of president of the Laos Red Cross. In 1975 he became president of the Laos Red Cross in Vientiane as well as vice president for the Peace Committee.

As a product of a more modern medical training from the French colonial medical school, and for better or for worse as he tried to adapt this training to pathological, sociocultural, and economic Laotian realities, Suvannavong well represented the paradoxes of colonial medicalization.

Suvannavong also indirectly contributed to the renewal of traditional medical practices through his unwavering vision of a nation taking charge of its own sanitary concerns, using contributions from traditional medicine and biomedicine. Indeed, even though the French medical authorities fought against traditional indigenous medical practices throughout the period of colonization, there was an increasing open-mindedness toward traditional medicine in the 1920s and 1930s. This more positive outlook on the possible exchanges between western and traditional medicine was based on the idea that one must integrate traditional medicine to the colonial system and familiarize colonial and colonized physicians with the local sociocultural traditions and preferences. Certainly, Suvannavong and other Indochinese physicians who had been trained at the Hanoi medical school were primarily responsible for the efficiency of the movement.

Naturally, this open-mindedness toward traditional medicine was not only a moral obligation for the colonial authorities but a material one as well. The coexistence of both medical practices was considered essential on the theoretical level by physicians such as Suvannavong for the success of the French medico-social action in Indochina. Ultimately, for Suvannavong, 'the worst would be, by brutally opposing deep-rooted customs, to risk failure of a medico-social action, which in order to develop alongside traditional practices, does not remain any less efficient' (1956, p. 975).

Bibliography

Primary: 1956. 'Quelques pratiques de médecine traditionnelle.' *France-Asie* 12: 975–978.

Secondary: Souk-Aloun, Phou-ngeun, 2002. *Histoire du Laos moderne (1930–2000)* (Paris); Stuart-Fox, Martin, 2001. *Historical Dictionary of Laos* (London); Stuart-Fox, Martin, 1997. *A History of Laos* (Cambridge).

Frederic Roy

SWAMMERDAM, JAN   (b. Amsterdam, the Netherlands, 12 February 1637; d. Amsterdam, 17 February 1680), *anatomy, entomology.*

Swammerdam was born on 12 February 1637, the eldest son of Jan Jacobsz Swammerdam. The elder Swammerdam, an apothecary, possessed a cabinet of curiosities, one of the finest in the Dutch Republic, and this certainly fostered his son's interest in natural history. As a boy Swammerdam probably attended the lectures on anatomy and natural philosophy at the Amsterdam *Athenaeum Illustre.*

He matriculated at Leiden University on 11 October 1661 in order to study medicine under the supervision of Sylvius, and Johannes van Horne. Together with fellow student and lifelong friend Niels Stensen (Steno), he excelled in anatomical dissections, mostly of humans and dogs. Swammerdam also performed experiments on frogs that examined nerve function and muscle contraction, showing that movement could occur without connection between muscle and brain. During his lifetime, this experiment was elaborated upon and would become one of the classics in the history of physiology. Although Swammerdam's concluding description was not published until 1738, the results were well known to contemporaries such as Steno. During his student years, Swammerdam started to collect anatomical preparations and insects. Stimulated by the Amsterdam mathematician and *regent* Johannes Hudde and the female poet and alchemist Catrina Questiers, Swammerdam developed new techniques of anatomical

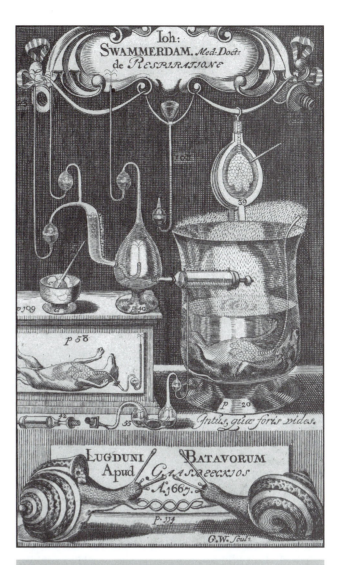

Title page of Jan Swammerdam's *De Respiratione* . . . Leiden, 1667. Rare Books, Wellcome Library, London.

preservation, including injections with colored wax, to make the vessels and other physiological details distinct. The early work of this promising student was mentioned in Sylvius's *Disputationum medicarum decas* (1663) and in a letter of Steno to Thomas Bartholin dated 5 March 1663.

Comparative Anatomy

After qualifying as a candidate in October 1663, Swammerdam spent about a year in France. In June 1664, within the academic circles in Saumur, he demonstrated the valves of the lymphatic vessels. This discovery was published a year later by Frederik Ruysch, possibly not coincidentally: a letter to Melchisedec Thévenot Swammerdam suggested that his father had shown the drawings he had sent him to Amsterdam physicians, including Ruysch. From September 1664 to the spring of 1665, Swammerdam lived in Paris. Together with Steno, he attended the weekly meetings of the scientific academy of Thévenot, one of the forerunners of the Académie Royal des Sciences. Here, Swammerdam performed experiments on living animals and appears to have dissected insects. Back in Amsterdam in September 1665, Swammerdam joined the Collegium privatum Amstelodamense. This informal research group is usually considered to be one of the pioneers of comparative anatomy. The Collegium was a private enterprise and had no access to human corpses. Instead, the members performed sections on fish, frogs, and domestic animals, jointly publishing the results in two volumes (*Observationum anatomicarum Collegii private Amstelodamensis*, 1666 and 1673). Its members included Gerardus Blasius and Matheus Sladus, a lifelong friend of Swammerdam.

Evidence suggests that Swammerdam was one of the leading members of the Collegium, responsible not only for some of the discoveries but also for the drawings made. On 24 October 1666 Swammerdam matriculated for the second time at Leiden University, this time to obtain his doctorate. The results of his previous research were summarized in a short *Disputatio medica inauguralis, continens selectas de respiratione positiones*, which earned him the MD on 22 February 1667. Some months later Swammerdam published a more voluminous *Tractatus de respiratione*, which was dedicated to Thévenot and which attracted the attention of Henry Oldenburg and Marcello Malphighi, among others. The *Tractatus* betrays much influence of Cartesian mechanism, not only on the problem of respiration, but on other anatomical and physiological themes as well. Swammerdam also elaborated further on one of Sylvius's favorite themes, iatrochemistry. Although an interesting work when seen from the perspective of contemporary notions on the motions of the lungs and the function of breathing, it was more a conclusion of an intellectual period than a starting point of a new one.

Insects

After his graduation in 1667 Swammerdam took up residence with his father. This was to become a constant source of irritation for the apothecary, who wanted his son to set up medical practice. Swammerdam, now suffering from malaria, devoted most of the rest of his short life to research, financially maintained by his reluctant father. Initially, Swammerdam often collaborated with his mentor Van Horne in nearby Leiden. At Van Horne's home Swammerdam made two important discoveries. First, while working on the human uterus, Swammerdam observed the female human 'eggs' (later known as follicles of De Graaf) as early as 21 January 1667. Second, in 1668 Swammerdam observed that the 'king' bee was actually a queen when he discovered egg masses in its intestines. This discovery greatly stimulated his pioneering research on the anatomy and generation of insects. When the Florentine prince Cosimo de' Medici visited Swammerdam (in about

June 1669), Swammerdam showed him that rudiments of limbs and wings of the future butterfly could be discerned in the entrails of a caterpillar. This was a revolutionary discovery since it was commonly assumed that the caterpillar died first in order to resurrect as a butterfly by some mystical process of metamorphosis.

Swammerdam's general theory of the generation of insects was published some months later. In November 1669 Swammerdam published his pioneering *Historia insectorum generalis, ofte algemeene verhandeling van de bloedeloose dierkens* (translated into French in 1682, Latin in 1685). It is worth quoting the title in full: *General account of the bloodless animals, in which will be clearly set forward the true basis of their slow growth of limbs, the vulgar errors of the transformation, also erroneously called metamorphosis, will be effectually washed away, and comprehended concisely in four distinct orders of changes, or natural budding forth of limbs.* Swammerdam stated self-consciously that he had solved a mystery that had puzzled mankind since the days of Aristotle. He refuted three traditional assumptions concerning insects. First, that they lack internal anatomy; second, that they originate from spontaneous generation; and third, that they develop by metamorphosis. Swammerdam demonstrated that all insects come from eggs and that what was usually considered to be a sudden transformation was in fact a slow growth of limbs. In other words, there was no fundamental distinction between insects and the so called higher animals; all belonged to the order of nature. All creatures had their origin ex ovo. Later, Swammerdam would state that it was his research on the female uterus which led him to the hypothesis that all other creatures originate from eggs.

Chance and contingency were excluded from Swammerdam's natural philosophy as being incompatible with the power of God, the Almighty Architect. This conviction, which Swammerdam derived from Descartes' natural philosophy, was the *leitmotif* of all of his investigations. The religiously sensible Swammerdam even went so far as to call the theory of spontaneous generation heretical and atheistic. Moreover, he ridiculed insect symbolism, an example of which was the image of the beehive as a model for human society. In this phase of his career Swammerdam was a convinced and radical rationalist who not only had contacts with Holland's leading Cartesians, but who appears to have known Spinoza personally.

In the *Historia* Swammerdam presented a new taxonomy of insects based on the four different life cycles he discerned. The first 'order' consisted of insects such as spiders—creatures that were then considered to be insects—and lice, in which the adult form hatches directly out of the egg. The second 'order' consisted of those insects in which nymphs hatch out of an egg, gradually developing into the adult form, and included locusts and mayflies. The third and fourth 'orders' were holometabolic insects with a pupal stage and included butterflies, bees, and flies. This scheme provided the framework for all of Swammerdam's future research.

Human Anatomy

After the programmatic *Historia* Swammerdam focused mainly on insects, although he remained active in the field of human anatomy and science in general. He clearly manifested himself in the scientific world, frequently visiting the Utrecht Collegie der Scavanten, an 'academy' not unlike Thévenot's and known for its Cartesian sympathies. Swammerdam was on friendly terms with Cartesians such as Burchardus de Volder and the Amsterdam professor Johannes de Raey. Swammerdam may have been the driving force behind the resuscitating of the Amsterdam Collegium Privatum in 1671. Just one year before, on 23 January 1670, Swammerdam had been granted the privilege to dissect corpses in the Amsterdam municipal hospital. He kept some of his anatomical preparations in his own cabinet of natural specimens and sent some of them as a gift to the Royal Society's 'repository'.

Swammerdam's observations on the human womb, which he had made with Van Horne in 1667, were published as a sole plate in 1671 and dedicated to the Amsterdam physician and burgomaster Tulp. The Royal Society was honored with some of his anatomical specimens and letters, which were eventually discussed and published in the *Philosophical Transactions* (examples include 'An unusual Rupture of the Mesentery', vol. X, 1674–75). In 1672 Swammerdam dedicated his anatomical work *Miraculum naturae sive uteri muliebris fabrica* to the Society. This polemical work was actually a response to De Graaf's *De mulierum organis* (1672), in which the Delft physician described the mammalian egg. Swammerdam felt deeply offended because he believed that De Graaf must have been aware of the fact that Steno, Van Horne, and Swammerdam himself had the priority for this discovery and did not mention it. Swammerdam invited the Society to give their judgment in this contention. By the time the Society tried to settle the dispute in a diplomatic manner—taking no sides in the debate between the two Dutchmen—De Graaf had already died. The question of priority has puzzled scholars ever since.

Microscopy

In the *Historia* Swammerdam had announced further research on insects. His work until 1669 was based on *a priori* reasoning and the meticulous observations of the external parts of insects, done mostly with the naked eye. Since his student years Swammerdam had owned a microscope and had knowledge of optical theories, thanks to Johannes Hudde, who provided both the microscope and the knowledge. Swammerdam knew and highly praised Robert Hooke's *Micrographia* (1665), but for unknown reasons he used this new instrument only rarely at first. After 1670 he started to use the microscope passionately and developed highly refined dissecting techniques, perhaps inspired by Malpighi's *De Bombyce* (1669), which was published while the *Historia* was in print. Although Swammerdam praised Malpighi's pioneering microscopic work, he felt the urge to replicate it—and found some errors. In his *Miraculum naturae* Swammerdam not only attacked De Graaf, but also corrected Malpighi. 'In questions of anatomy, I speak like I think, I do not believe anybody (I barely believe my own eyes) and there is nobody with whom I will blindly agree in matters of experiment', he stated.

Aware of his talents, Swammerdam now started a series of dissections of several insects, including the silkworm, the bee, and the ephemeron (mayfly). Using extremely small scissors, highly refined techniques of preparation, and both single-lens and compound microscopes, Swammerdam was the first to describe the entrails of insects and other small creatures in a systematic way. Although guided by theological and philosophical concepts, Swammerdam is remembered as a mere empiricist. Although he had some reservations on the humans senses (he once compared the results of his microscopic researches with 'a drawing of the sun with charcoal'), Swammerdam kept strictly to the idea that he would not believe anything until he had seen it with his own eyes. Now he made stunning observations of the internal anatomy of insects: lungs, nervous system, reproductive organs, and so on. Swammerdam performed all the dissections himself, made extremely detailed drawings of what he saw, and kept the microscopic sections in his cabinet. This collection was maintained with the explicit aim of being the testimony to Swammerdam's writings. Although Swammerdam's cabinet was not a public 'museum' (like Ruysch's collection of curiosities), it was visited by contemporaries such as Holger Jacobaeus, Christiaan Huygens, and Gottfried Wilhelm Leibniz. In 1674 (not in 1669, as is usually assumed) Cosimo de' Medici offered 12,000 guilders for it. In 1678 the Royal Society showed interest, but for unknown reasons did not acquire the cabinet.

Crisis

During 1673 Swammerdam fell prey to a religious crisis. The young and very self-confident Swammerdam had believed initially that his research brought him closer to God the Creator; but he now feared that he was worshipping an idol called *Curiositas*. In April 1673 Swammerdam wrote to the mystical prophetess Antoinette Bourignon (1616–80) for spiritual comfort. Bourignon claimed she was the mouthpiece of God and preached a life of inner devotion based on the idea of *imitatio Christi*. Bourignon strongly advised Swammerdam to renounce science and to devote himself to a life of religious contemplation. For two years after that Swammerdam experienced such an inner conflict that, as he stated, 'I shed tears of distress. For it was as if a warring host was there within my spirit, the one party compelling me to cling to God, the other, with infinite arguments, to continue my pursuits of curiosities'. Indeed, days of ceaseless research on the anatomy of the bee alternated with nights of prayer and writing religious poetry.

Swammerdam was also engaged in the translation of Bourignon's work. Swammerdam is therefore usually depicted as her willing victim, but recent research has shown that he was less passive than is assumed and that he played an important role in propagating her teachings in Amsterdam. In the spring of 1674, while Bourignon repeatedly urged Swammerdam to renounce the material world and follow Christ, Steno tried to convert Swammerdam to Catholicism. Later Swammerdam commented, 'I am more catholic than reformed, but I do not despise anybody for that and I would not like to change religion, for only he who loves God and his neighbors like himself may become blessed by Christ, even if he were a Turk by birth . . . But Steno is all too partial, he only thinks of making someone catholic.'

In July 1675, after repeated letters from Bourignon, Swammerdam claimed he was ready to reject his research, his 'only and beloved son, like another Ishmael'. In a letter to Bourignon, he pretended to have burnt all his manuscripts. In fact, he destroyed only his anatomy on the silkworm (but saved the drawings, sending them to Malphighi via Steno). As a farewell to the material world, Swammerdam published the *Ephemeri vita* in 1675. With a preface dated 12 July 1675, this curious book contained not only extremely detailed descriptions of the anatomy of the mayfly but also long lamentations on the miseries of human life and calls to imitate Christ. It also included some letters by Bourignon. On 23 August Bourignon granted Swammerdam permission to come to her small community of 'true Christians' in Schleswig-Holstein. The next week, Swammerdam sailed off and joined Bourignon's sect, where he was charged with her correspondence. He was also sent on a secret mission to the King of Denmark in order to obtain a privilege for Bourignon's community. The mission failed, but Swammerdam had the opportunity to visit Steno's sister in Copenhagen.

Swammerdam's leaving science turned out to be temporary. Presumably due to domestic troubles within Bourignon's community, Swammerdam traveled back to Amsterdam in the spring of 1676. Contrary to what is often maintained, he was still influenced by Bourignon. Back at his father's house, he continued to correspond with her, and he translated some more of her writings. Another misunderstanding still repeated in recent literature is that Swammerdam never resumed his research after his return from Schleswig-Holstein. By considering his research as an acceptable form of worship, Swammerdam was now able to reconcile science and religion, and to continue his pursuits. 'You do well, my good friend Oldenburg', he wrote to the secretary of the Royal Society in 1677, 'when by repeated letters you recall

me to the contemplation of nature. But to confess what is true, I have more need of the bridle than the spur . . . I was never at any other time busier than in these days, and the chief of all architects has blessed my endeavors.'

When Swammerdam's demanding father died in 1678, his inheritance was sufficient to enable him to continue his career as an independent scholar. He moved to a house owned by Debora Blaeu, the wife of his friend Johannes Hudde. Mentally more stable, he now underlined that man could serve God best by limiting himself to a mere *description* of nature. As he wrote to Oldenburg, '. . . this inquiry into natural things that we are concerned with takes up a great deal of that time which we owe wholly to God . . . at one and the same time it clearly brings before our eyes the immense wisdom of omnipotent God, and our weakness not to say imbecility.' The 'argument from design', which had already played a considerable role in the *Historia*, was now elaborated upon much further. Using the *Historia* as a framework, Swammerdam reworked previously published material and carried out new research. For example, the section on the ant, half a page in the *Historia*, was now expanded to over twelve pages, including microscopic observations. The minute dissections of these insects and other small creatures such as the viviparous snail revealed whole new worlds and offered absolute proof of the existence of God, the almighty creator, according to Swammerdam.

Swammerdam's lyrical outburst on the anatomy of the louse (1677) would become a *locus classicus* in apologetic literature: 'Herewith I offer you the Omnipotent Finger of God in the anatomy of a louse; wherein you will find miracles heaped on miracles and will see the wisdom of God clearly manifested in a minute point.' Likewise, Swammerdam described the delicate anatomy of bees, nose-horned beetles, gnats, cheese mites, fleas, etc. Tormented by continuous attacks of malaria, he was able to finish what he called his 'great work' in December 1679, two months before his death.

Postmortem

Swammerdam's manuscript, actually a hugely expanded copy of the *Historia* including splendid drawings, was bequeathed to Thévenot. According to Swammerdam's will, Thévenot was to publish the book. However, the Frenchman had a reputation for being negligent and died before he could prepare Swammerdam's notes for the press. Half a century later, Herman Boerhaave traced and bought the papers in France, then published a bilingual edition as *Bybel der nature / Biblia naturae* (1737–38). The manuscript was bestowed to the University library of Leiden, including Swammerdam's original drawings.

Starting with Boerhaave, biographers have usually portrayed Swammerdam as a brilliant but erratic and isolated figure; however, there is little evidence for this somewhat romantic perception. Swammerdam was an active member of the scientific community and played an important role in several scholarly and scientific societies, making sure that his stunning discoveries were known to the learned world. He knew Antoni van Leeuwenhoek very well, although the two pioneers of microscopic science did not like each other: Swammerdam noted that van Leeuwenhoek 'reasons in a very barbaric way, having no academic education'. Swammerdam was on friendly terms with and sometimes enjoyed the patronage of leading scientists such as Christiaan Huygens, Johannes Hudde, and *virtuosi* such as the Amsterdam burgomaster Nicolaas Witsen, who as early as 1671 had access to Swammerdam's microscopic drawings, he told Oldenburg.

Swammerdam's unpublished research was also known abroad. Steno was Swammerdam's intermediary in his contacts with Malpighi and Cosimo de' Medici. Moreover, Swammerdam kept a lively correspondence with the Royal Society, which in 1678 was interested in acquiring Swammerdam's cabinet. He also exchanged letters and ideas with Nicolas Malebranche and with Thévenot. Swammerdam was credited for being one of the pioneers of microscopic science and microbiology and for being the founder of scientific entomology. Many of his observations have not been surpassed until the twentieth century. The 'argument from design' as advocated by Swammerdam was to play an enormous role in eighteenth-century natural theology.

Bibliography

Primary: 1667. *Disputatio medica inauguralis, continens de respiratione positiones* (Leiden); 1667. *Tractatus physico-anatomico-medicus de respiratione usuque pulmonum* (Leiden); 1669. *Historia insectorum generalis, ofte algemeene verhandeling van de bloedeloose dierkens* (Utrecht); 1672. *Miraculum naturae sive uteri muliebris fabrica* (Leiden); 1675. *Ephemeri vita of afbeeldingh van 's menschen leven, vertoont in de wonderbaarelijcke en nooyt gehoorde historie van het vliegent ende een-dagh-levent haft of oever-aas* (Amsterdam); 1737–38. *Bybel der natuure of historie der insecten / Bibliae naturae; sive historia insectorum* (Leiden) (English trans. 1758).

Secondary: Baar, M. de, 2004. '*Ik moet spreken*'. *Het spiritueel leiderschap van Antoinette Bourignon (1616–80)* (Zutphen); Jorink, E., 2003. '"Outside God There Is Nothing". Swammerdam, Spinoza and the Janus-face of the Early Dutch Enlightenment' in Bunge, W. van, ed., *The Early Dutch Enlightenment* (Leiden) pp. 81–108; Cobb, M., 2002. 'Malpighi, Swammerdam and the Colourful Silkworm: Replication and Visual Representation in Early Modern Science.' *Annals of Science* 59: 111–147; Cook, H. J., 1996. 'Natural History and Seventeenth-Century Dutch and English Medicine' in Marland, Hilary, and Margaret Pelling, eds., *The Task of Healing. Medicine, Religion and Gender in England and the Netherlands, 1450–1800* (Rotterdam) pp. 253–270; Ruestow, E., 1996. *The Microscope in the Dutch Republic: The Shaping of Discovery* (Cambridge); Schierbeek, A., 1967. *Jan Swammerdam, 12 February 1637–17 February 1680: His Life and Works* (Amsterdam); *DSB*.

Eric Jorink

SWELLENGREBEL, NICOLAAS HENDRIK (b. Amsterdam, the Netherlands, 12 August 1885; d. Aerdenhout, the Netherlands, 1 January 1970), *parasitology, malariology.*

Swellengrebel was born into a notable protestant family. Trained as biologist, he wrote a PhD thesis on potato disease at Zurich University (1908). Shortly afterward, he was appointed as lecturer in parasitology at the Amsterdam University. In 1912 he left for the Netherlands East Indies to research plague, rats, and fleas and to collect teaching materials. He developed an interest in malaria after an encounter with Malcolm Watson, who had interesting views about malaria control. Watson's idea of detecting vector species, studying their behavior, and taking appropriate measures, leaving all other mosquitoes undisturbed, was taken up by Swellengrebel and called 'species sanitation'. It proved a useful tool in reducing the burden of malaria. He produced a monograph on Anophelines in the Dutch Indies.

During a second period from 1917, Swellengrebel's young wife, Meta de Graaf, accompanied him, assisting with his malaria surveys in Java and Sumatra. He collaborated with Schüffner (epidemiology of malaria) and Kuenen (life cycle of *Entamoeba histolytica*), two medical men who were to become his colleagues in Amsterdam.

His return to the Netherlands coincided with an epidemic of tertian malaria in the north of Amsterdam (1920). As a professor of parasitology, based at the Institute for Tropical Hygiene, he took the lead in research and control. After the epidemic had eased down, malaria was no longer considered a major public health problem. However, there were so many interesting biological phenomena to be unraveled that he pursued his research as a model for countries with more severe burdens. The Swellengrebels and several collaborators exposed themselves to infected mosquitoes to prove the peculiar course of local *Plasmodium vivax*. His experiments with the larvicide Paris green were supported by the Rockefeller Foundation, as were his spraying experiments of houses with parasite carriers and infected anophelines. He also made historical analyses of the meaning of 'malaria', before the disease became known as plasmodiosis.

Swellengrebel was a member of the League of Nations' malaria commission. He traveled through the United States and visited virtually all European countries with malaria, advising governments. Three trips were particularly impressive: six months through British India (1929); nine months in South Africa (with his wife and five children, 1930–31), and some months in Surinam to investigate the suitability of a safe haven for German Jews (1939).

In 1938 Swellengrebel hosted the Congress of Tropical Medicine and Malaria in Amsterdam. In the same year, he published *Malaria in the Netherlands*. After World War II, in which he lost his coauthor Abraham de Buck, he became director of the Institute for Tropical Hygiene and continued his battle against Dutch malaria with DDT. He was also visiting professor in the East Indies, where he studied malaria and other parasites in New Guinea. He was one of the few who voted against the idea of malaria eradication, particularly in highly endemic areas, an opinion firmly based on his global experience (Kampala, 1950). He wrote several editions of a Dutch book on parasitology, the seventh being rewritten in English. He was an excellent teacher, mastering many languages, and taught medical students and colleagues to think as a worm, a mosquito, or a malaria parasite. He was awarded many medals and an honorary degree in medicine. He died just before the WHO declared the Netherlands to be free of malaria.

Bibliography

Primary: 1916, 1921. *De Anophelinen van Nederlandsch Oost-Indië* (Amsterdam). [3rd edn. 1932 (with Rodenwald, E.) in German (Jena)]; 1938. (with de Buck, A.) *Malaria in the Netherlands* (Amsterdam); 1960. (with Sterman, M. M.) *Animal Parasites in Man* (Princeton).

Secondary: Verhave, J. P., 2000. 'The Disappearance of Dutch Malaria and the Rockefeller Foundation.' *Parassitologia* 42: 111–115; Verhave, J. P., 1991. 'Swellengrebel and Species Sanitation: The Design of an Idea' in Takken, W., et al., eds., *Environmental Measures for Malaria Control in Indonesia* (Wageningen) pp. 63–80; Verhave, J. P., 1989. 'Malaria: Epidemiology and Immunity' in Heteren, Godelieve van, et al., eds., *Dutch Medicine in the Malay Archipelago 1816–1942* (Amsterdam and Atlanta) pp. 86–104.

Jan Peter Verhave

SWIETEN, GERARD VAN (b. Leiden, the Netherlands, 7 May 1700; d. Vienna, Austria, 18 June 1772), *medicine, public health, medical education.*

Van Swieten was the only one out of seven children of Thomas van Swieten and Elisabeth Loo who survived early childhood. His mother died in 1708 and his father four years later, leaving Gerard a solitary orphan at the age of twelve. Thomas van Swieten, who had been a notary and a prominent member of the Catholic minority in Leiden, had taken care of the future of his surviving son, preventing admission to the municipal orphanage. Not long after his father's death in 1712, Van Swieten went to Louvain University, where he—probably—obtained a bachelor's degree in the arts faculty. In the beginning of 1715, he returned to the Dutch Republic, where he was registered as an apprentice to an Amsterdam pharmacist. A year later, he suddenly returned to Leiden, where he completed his training as an apothecary. At the age of twenty, he opened a shop in this town.

In 1717 he matriculated at Leiden University, where he faithfully attended the lessons by Herman Boerhaave (other teachers included H. Oosterdijk Schacht and B. S. Albinus). He trained himself in shorthand in order to be able to write down the exact words of his much-admired teacher. Even after he obtained his MD degree in 1725,

when he had settled as a physician in his hometown, he continued to attend Boerhaave's lectures for another thirteen years. Van Swieten seems to have been a popular practitioner, especially within the Catholic community. In addition to these activities, he also held a yearly course in materia medica, which was popular among the many foreign medical students. However, because this activity was considered an infringement on the privileges of the university teachers, it was discontinued by order of the university senate in 1734.

Soon after Boerhaave's death in 1738, Van Swieten decided to publish an annotated edition of his teacher's aphorisms concerning practical medicine. The extensive commentaries written by Van Swieten were based on Boerhaave's lectures, on the old and modern medical literature, and on Van Swieten's own experience. This work became much larger than Van Swieten had anticipated. The first volume appeared in 1742, the fifth—and final—volume thirty years later. It was published in several editions and translations all over the civilized world, remaining the standard reference work of practical medicine for many years.

After the first volume of the *Commentaries* had been published, Van Swieten was invited by Maria Theresa, ruler of the Habsburg Empire, to join her court in Vienna as her first physician-in-ordinary and to become prefect of the famous court library as well. Soon after his arrival in 1745, he discovered the dismal state of medical education in Vienna. With royal approval, he soon started lecturing on theoretical medicine in one of the rooms of the court library. Invited by the queen, he drafted a plan for drastic reforms of the medical faculty in Vienna, which was approved. Van Swieten became director of medical studies and permanent president of medical faculty, for which he attracted able men like Antonius de Haen and Nicolaas Jacquin.

The way Van Swieten took care of the thorough reform of medical education in Vienna strengthened Maria Theresa's confidence in his organizational capacities. She entrusted him with the highly necessary overhaul of the civil and military medical services in Austria. However, the most prominent and lasting contribution of Van Swieten was the foundation he had laid for the famous Viennese Medical School of the nineteenth century.

Bibliography

Primary: 1742–76. *Commentaria in Hermanni Boerhaave Aphorismos de cognoscendis et curandis morbis* 5 vols. (Leiden) [English trans., 1771–73 18 vols. (London)].

Secondary: Korst, J. K. van der, 2003. *Een dokter van formaat. Gerard van Swieten lijfarts van keizerin Maria Theresia* (Amsterdam); Brechka, Frank T., 1970. *Gerard van Swieten and His World 1700–1772* (the Hague); *DSB*.

Jan K. van der Korst

SYDENHAM, THOMAS

SYDENHAM, THOMAS   (baptized Wynford Eagle, Dorset, England, 10 September 1624; d. London, England, 29 December 1689), *medicine, nosography.*

Background and Education

Sydenham was the third surviving son of William Sydenham (1593–1661), a Puritan gentleman, and his wife, Mary Jeffrey (d. 1644). There were fourteen children, nine boys (four died young) and five daughters. He was probably first tutored at home and had a Latin education, possibly at Dorchester Grammar School. On 1 July 1642, at age seventeen, Sydenham went up to Oxford, residing at Magdalen Hall, at this time separate from Magdalen College. Magdalen Hall was a Puritan institution. Shortly after arriving at Oxford, Sydenham left to join his father and brother, who were fighting in the parliamentary militia for Dorset in the Civil War. Sydenham held the rank of cornet and served under his brother William (bap. 1615–61), a colonel. His two other brothers, Francis and John, also served. Royalist forces overran much of Dorset in 1643 (Sydenham's father was held prisoner), but in 1644 the Earl of Essex restored parliamen-

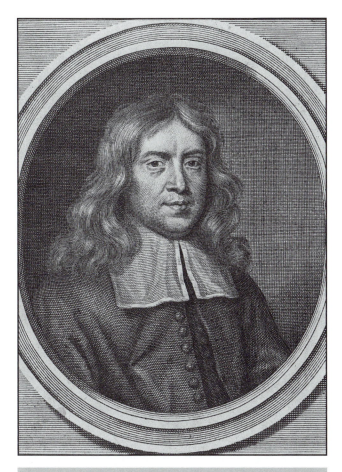

Thomas Sydenham. Engraving by A. Blooteling after Mary Beale, 1672. Iconographic Collection, Wellcome Library, London.

tary rule. He appointed the younger William Sydenham governor of Weymouth and the Isle of Wight. Further fighting ensued, and in August 1644 a party of Royalist Dragoons killed Sydenham's mother. Francis killed the major held to be responsible for this act. Francis died in the Battle of Weymouth (1645), at which conflict Thomas was present. Ironically, so was the royalist Richard Wiseman (c. 1620–1676), who would later be considered the greatest surgeon of the age.

At the end of the first civil war (1646), Sydenham returned to Magdalen Hall. In May 1647, Parliament appointed visitors to purge Oxford of royalist opposition. On 30 September delegates were sent to colleges and halls to investigate the views of university members. Sydenham was appointed delegate to Wadham College, where he was made a fellow commoner. In 1648 he remained at the university, rooting out royalists. In April of that year, he was granted a BM, possibly as a reward for political services. He was elected to a fellowship of All Souls College, and in 1649 the visitors appointed him senior bursar. This position he held for a year, although he resided at the college until March 1651, when he again left for military service. On 21 April he accepted a commission as captain in a cavalry regiment. He served in the north of England and the Scottish borders and saw heavy fighting. It seems likely he was seriously injured. His troop was disbanded in October 1651. During the civil war, at least, Sydenham seems to have been committed to the Puritan cause of preparing for the Apocalypse. His career at this point is unclear, although it was not until 1655 that he resigned his fellowship at All Souls. He definitely returned to Oxford, and while there, he became a friend of Robert Boyle (1627–91). Sydenham was owed money for equipping his brother during the wars. On 16 March 1654, on Thomas Cromwell's endorsement, the council of state awarded him £600. He also was rewarded with employment as comptroller of the pipe. This office was within the exchequer and had responsibility for collecting and auditing receipts from the sheriffs. He apparently held this position from 1655 to 1660. In 1655 he married Mary Gee in his hometown of Wynford Eagle. They had three sons.

Sydenham recounted in his *Observationes medicae* (1676) that he decided to study medicine while at Oxford. He wrote that he accompanied Thomas Coxe (1615–85) to London around 1646 and had no plans, but influenced by Coxe, he turned his attention to physic. Self-taught in part (he read Latin fairly well), Sydenham is reputed to have traveled to Montpellier to study, but this is conjectural. Various Sydenhams are recorded as traveling to Italy and Leiden at this time to study medicine, but Thomas was probably not one of them. His foreign studies, if any, remain in doubt. At some point Sydenham moved to London, where he was definitely resident in late 1655 and probably practicing medicine. He lived in Westminster, a district in which he recorded seeing a case of dropsy in about 1656. He was living in Pall Mall in 1658. In this year he stood unsuccessfully for election to Richard Cromwell's parliament for Weymouth and Malcombe Regis. He was also calling himself 'Docktor' but had not yet been licensed by the RCP. It was not until April and May 1663 that Sydenham submitted himself to the college's three-part examination (the college was clamping down on unlicensed practitioners at this time). On June 25 he was voted licentiate. During the plague of 1665, he left London.

Medical Views

Sydenham's opinions on how medicine should be learned, practiced, and improved were distinctly colored by the views of Puritans and intellectual Parliamentarians. Coxe was associated with Samuel Hartlib and those of his circle who advocated promoting the progress of learning in the manner proposed by Francis Bacon (1561–1626), a writer much praised by Sydenham. Medical men who circulated among these thinkers, most prominently Sydenham himself, professed to eschew theory and invoked Hippocrates as the model medical practitioner. Hippocratic knowledge was praised as eminently practical, especially by radical popularizes such as Nicholas Culpeper (1616–54). Sydenham famously despised learning medicine from books rather than from the bedside (although, of course, Sydenham was widely read). Richard Blackmore (1654-1729) recalled that he had asked Sydenham what books a man should read to qualify him in physic, and Sydenham had replied, 'Read *Don Quixote*, it is a very good Book, I read it still.' In his 'Epistle to Dr Brady', Sydenham wrote that 'practice and that alone, will do good which elicits the indications of cure out of the phenomena of the disease itself. This made Hippocrates divine.' In an uncompleted fragment, 'De Arte Medica' (1668/69), Sydenham began to set out his vision of the role of clinical experience. It is a salutary reminder of Sydenham's place in his own time, however, that he upheld the claims for cure made by Valentine Greatrakes (1629–83), the Irish stroker.

It is notable that Parliamentarian healers, in respect of their praise of Hippocrates, differentiated themselves from Royalist physicians, especially the so-called Oxford physiologists around Thomas Willis (1621–75). These latter continued to summon up Aristotle and Galen or contemporary medical theorists such as René Descartes (1596–1650) and Marcello Malpighi (1628–94). Such authors were valued because they espoused dissection and the search for hidden causes; the works of Hippocrates were held in less esteem because they were concerned with outward signs only. But it was this latter approach that Sydenham and his like said that they valued. Man, wrote Sydenham, could only perceive the 'outer husk of things' (*Works*, I, p. 171). It should be noted, though, that many chemical physicians praised Hippocrates, and in spite of Sydenham's denunciation of theory, chemical views, especially those derived from Paracelsus (1493/4–1541)

through Joan Baptista van Helmont (1579–1644), permeate his writings. References to humoral theory also pervade his works, notably in a manuscript titled 'Of the four constitutions' (published for the first time in Dewhurst).

Sydenham became known in the eighteenth century as the 'English Hippocrates', and indeed, his published works contain reference to no other authority than the Greek physician. In the late 1660s Sydenham and John Locke (1632–1704) became friends. Like Sydenham, the mature Locke denounced the search for hidden causes, a view that was codified in his *Essay on Human Understanding* (1692). Sydenham and Locke held that not only was the search for causes useless to medicine, but furthermore, causes were unknowable for philosophical reasons. Boyle, who visited patients with Sydenham, was one of the most influential figures to take this empiricist view. Boyle's sister, and powerful intellectual patron, Lady Ranelagh, was Sydenham's neighbor and friend in Pall Mall.

Sydenham's Hippocrates was not, of course, the physician of antiquity, but one shaped for seventeenth-century use. The most important feature of Sydenham's Hippocrates (and the one so different from the ancient texts) is that he was a natural historian of the *species* of disease. Delineating diseases at the bedside, Sydenham never ceased to iterate, was the cornerstone of medical knowledge and the key to medicine being made a practical, useful art. One of Sydenham's most quoted aphorisms was 'It is necessary that all diseases be reduced to definite and certain species, and that, with the same care which we see exhibited by botanists in their phytologies' (*Works*, I, p. 13). The disease of a 'simpleton', he wrote, was no different from that of a 'Socrates'. It is here we begin to see clearly an intellectual formulation in Western medicine of how the diseases of populations were to be investigated and managed. This, in turn, can be seen to be derived from Puritan programs and methods that were advanced in the Commonwealth period, such as the extension of medical treatment to the poor and the statistical investigation of populations. The idea of specific diseases was also an important constituent of Paracelsianism.

In turning attention to the diseases of populations, Sydenham placed fevers at the center of the investigative enterprise. Thus it was that the Greek text *Epidemics* embodied Sydenham's ideal Hippocrates. It was Boyle, apparently, who encouraged Sydenham to study epidemic disease. Apart from his own practice, Sydenham visited patients at one of the London hospitals. The key concept he employed in his investigations was the 'epidemic constitution'. This latter was that conspiracy of factors: the environment, the individual's makeup (age, sex, inherited predisposition, etc.), and the cause of fever itself that gave rise to the clinical symptoms and signs that were characteristic of a certain epidemic. On the causes of fever, contrary to his denial of interest in theory, Sydenham flirted with chemistry and postulated a role for morbific particles (a concept probably borrowed from Boyle). Sydenham did not hold that particular fevers were always the same whenever and wherever they occurred. Rather, in similar conditions when a similar epidemic constitution prevailed, fevers took a similar shape. This was the basis of Sydenham's 'methodus medendi', or method of treatment, and his promotion of specific remedies. What was the best methodus medendi was widely discussed at the time. Sydenham claimed to draw his method directly from Hippocrates, and it delineated fevers, which it was hoped would lead to the discovery of specific cures. Thus, if a remedy (which might be as simple as bloodletting) had worked when a fever appeared under a distinct epidemic constitution, the same remedy, he reasoned, might work again when, under similar conditions, a similar fever appeared. The other pillar of Sydenham's method was the healing power of nature, again a theme recurrent in the Hippocratic texts. Observing fevers showed which route nature was using to rid the body of noxious matter in any particular epidemic, and so, encountering similar symptoms again showed that nature must be assisted in a similar way.

Besides general remedies such as bloodletting, which might be specific in certain circumstances, Sydenham also endorsed the view that drugs might be specific. Many orthodox physicians regarded specifics as a mark of quackery. In particular Sydenham pronounced the virtues of cinchona (Jesuits' or Peruvian bark) in intermittent fevers or agues. This agent began to be used in Europe in the 1640s. Sydenham advocated it increasingly throughout his career. He also believed his credit for promoting the drug had been stolen by a Cambridge apothecary, Richard Tabor or Talbor (c. 1642–1681), who had cured Charles II and earned a knighthood and a great deal of money.

Sydenham investigated fevers in London. Probably while he was away from the capital during the plague of 1665, he wrote *Methodus curandi febres, propriis observationibus superstructa* [Methods of curing fevers based on original observations], which appeared the following year. It was dedicated to Robert Boyle, and Sydenham was assisted with the Latin. He divided the work into four parts: continued fevers, special symptoms accompanying continued fevers, intermittent fevers, and smallpox (Sydenham thought the latter a mild disease that everyone naturally underwent). The second edition of the *Methodus* included remarks on the plague, and it was after reading this work that Locke sought out Sydenham. Sydenham was much praised in the eighteenth century for his treatment of smallpox. Seventeenth-century therapy for the disease was aggressive: patients were kept in dark, hot rooms, and bloodletting was employed. Sydenham, however, advised cooling therapy, fluids, the admission of light, and abandonment of bloodletting, all on the grounds that meddlesome physicians were the cause of smallpox's high mortality. He successfully treated smallpox in the family of the first Earl of Shaftesbury (Locke's patron) by this method. His opinion was also asked for in the case of Shaftesbury's own longstanding illness. The *Observationes medicae* (1676) was an extensive reworking and lengthening of *Methodus*. *Observationes* described the constitutions of 1661–64, 1665–66, 1667–69, 1669–72, and 1673–75. Consistent with his declared method, Sydenham gave detailed accounts of the epidemic fevers prevailing, correlating them with the seasons and atmospheric conditions.

Politics and Religion

Although Sydenham endeavored to use medicine for the Puritan project of improving the lives of the poor, he was never a radical iconoclast like Culpeper, who believed that through popularization everyone could be their own doctor (Culpeper translated learned works out of Latin. Sydenham wrote in English and had his manuscripts translated into Latin). Sydenham was an intimate of an elite reforming circle, not a revolutionary. He never joined the radical Society of Chemical Physicians, nor, on the other hand, was he elected to the Royal Society. Most of his patients were of the middling sort; a few had titles, but he also treated the poor *gratis*. Sydenham was a licentiate of the College of Physicians but no great friend of it. The period 1660–80 saw some sharp attacks on the college, especially by physicians with an enthusiasm for chemistry. Conservative practitioners accused Sydenham of subversion at this time when it was known that he was composing a manuscript attacking theory and anatomy. A contemporary mathematician, the Rev John Ward, recorded that Sydenham had said that medicine 'is not to bee learned by going to Universities, but hee is for taking apprentices; and says one had as good send a man to Oxford to learn shoemaking as practising physick' (Dewhurst, 1966, p. 17).

Sydenham never deserted his Puritan beliefs, and his medical ideas were deeply imbued with theological ones. He set down his views on God and nature in an undated manuscript titled 'Theologia rationalis' (printed in Dewhurst, 1966, pp. 145–159). In it Sydenham asked, 'How far the light of nature, if closely adverted to, may be extended towards the making us good men?'. Sydenham's answer was for the most part a meditation on the argument from design and on the existence of free will and a justification of the necessity 'to benefit mankind' and to improve 'human Society'. He could not comprehend the order of things and their subservience to each other without envisioning an 'admirable wisdom and power', which was 'the Contriver and Maker', the 'Supream nature'. He found man was 'a mixt Animal' in the 'scale of Beings'. But men, who have 'intellectual Natures', were put on earth to worship the deity and to 'exert Arts that flow from reason'. There is nothing in the manuscript about Christ, sin, or redemption, and it concluded with a quotation from Cicero (his favorite author). Clearly, however, Sydenham held that Providence was at work in the world.

Later Life

In 1676 Sydenham graduated MD from Pembroke College (a sign of his continuing links with the establishment). In 1680 he published two long letters in *Epistolae responsoriae duae*. In the letter to Robert Brady he described the epidemic constitution up to 1679 and gave instructions on the treatment of specific diseases and the use of the bark. In the letter to Henry Paman he discussed the treatment of venereal disease and recommended salivation. In 1682 he published in the *Dissertatio epistolaris* a letter to Dr William Cole on the treatment of smallpox and hysteria. His letters were written in English and translated for him. In 1677 Sydenham had an attack of gout that incapacitated him for nearly five months. He convalesced for five weeks at the Earl of Salisbury's Hatfield House. In 1683 he published *Tractatus de Podagra et Hydrope*. An English translation, *Treatise on gout and dropsy*, appeared the following year. Multiple editions of his collected works appeared. His descriptions of gout, scarlatina, and measles have become 'classics'.

Legacy

By the end of his life, and certainly within ten years of his death, Sydenham was recognized as a major figure. By this time the latitudinarian churchmen of Boyle's circle and the Whigs around the Earl of Shaftesbury and John Locke had come into power. Enthusiasm and doctrinal theory making were anathema. Cautious fact-gathering was applauded. Sydenham's installation as the first great, modern bedside practitioner was accomplished in this climate. The irony is that Sydenham's rhetorical eschewal of books and theory was forgotten as he was rapidly incorporated into the fold of orthodox medicine. To a great extent, this was the achievement of Herman Boerhaave (1668–1738) in Protestant, Newtonian, Anglophile, liberal Leiden. Here Sydenham's natural historical approach to disease was both applauded and built on to a massive infrastructure of medical theory. It returned to Britain with Boerhaave's pupils and flourished in the many firsthand descriptions of febrile diseases that graced the eighteenth century. The concept of species of disease was the foundation of nosology. The idea of the English Hippocrates was created by Sydenham himself and embellished in the Enlightenment, and it is venerated to this day.

Bibliography

Primary: 1696. *The Whole Works* (London); 1848. (Latham, R. G., ed.) *Works* 2 vols. (London).

Secondary: Cunningham, Andrew, 2002. 'The Transformation of Hippocrates in Seventeenth-Century Britain' in Cantor, David, ed., *Reinventing Hippocrates* (Aldershot) pp. 91–115; Martensen, Robert L., 2002. 'Hippocrates and the Politics of Medical Knowledge in Early Modern England' in Cantor, David, ed., *Reinventing Hippocrates* (Aldershot) pp. 116–135; Meynell, G. G., 1988. *Materials for a Biography of Dr Thomas Sydenham (1624–1689): A New Survey of Public and Private Archives* (Folkestone); Bates, D., 1977. 'Sydenham and the Medical Meaning of "Method".' *Bulletin of the History of Medicine* 51: 324–338; Keele, Kenneth D., 1974. 'The Sydenham-Boyle Theory of Morbific Particles.' *Medical History* 18: 240–248; Dewhurst, Kenneth, 1966. *Dr. Thomas Sydenham (1624–1689): His Life and Original Writings* (London); Wolfe, David E., 1961. 'Locke and Sydenham on the Limits of Anatomy.' *Bulletin of the History of Medicine* 35: 193–220; *DSB*; *Oxford DNB*.

Christopher Lawrence

SYLVIUS, FRANCISCUS DELE BOË (aka DU BOIS, FRANÇOIS)
(b. Hanau, Germany, 15 March 1614; d. Leiden, the Netherlands, 15 November 1672), *chemistry, natural philosophy, clinical medicine.*

Sylvius (the Latinized version of dele Boë) was the second son of Isaac dele Boë and Anne de la Vignette. For religious reasons, his grandfather had emigrated from Cambrai in French Flanders to Frankfurt-am-Main. Because the family were convinced members of the Walloon Church, Sylvius received his primary education at the Calvinist academy of Sedan. From 1633 to 1635, he studied medicine in Leiden, where his professors included Adolphus Vorstius and Otto Heurnius. His interest in chemistry made him decide to go to Wittenberg and Jena, where Paracelsianism—as mediated by Daniel Sennert—was taught. After taking his doctorate in Basel on 16 March 1637, he set up medical practice in Hanau. In 1638 he was back in Leiden again, trying to profile himself by teaching anatomy privately and by giving demonstrations on the circulation of the blood. Sylvius was among the first on the European Continent to defend William Harvey's theory. Descartes might have been present at one of these demonstrations. More importantly, however, Sylvius succeeded in converting Johannes Walaeus, who had just been appointed professor of medicine, from a critic into an advocate. Walaeus not only had one of his students, Roger Drake, defend Harvey's theory, but he wrote two letters to his friend Thomas Bartholin, who included them in his textbook *Institutiones anatomicae* (1641).

Sylvius thus contributed to the acceptance of the blood circulation, but the envisioned academic career in Leiden did not materialize. In 1641 he moved to Amsterdam, where he was very successful. He was appointed physician of the Walloon poor relief, he set up a private practice that was very lucrative, and he became a member (later inspector) of the Collegium Medicum. He also became one of the leading experimental philosophers of Amsterdam, surrounding himself with renowned scholars including Nicolaas Tulp, Johannes van Horne, Willem Piso, Paulus Barbette, Johann Rudolph Glauber, and Otto Sperling. In 1649 Sylvius married Anne de Ligne; she died eight years later. In 1666 he married Magdalena Schletzer. A daughter was born in 1669, but mother and daughter died the same year from an epidemic.

Sylvius greatly enjoyed the intellectual climate in Amsterdam, where he continued to engage in post mortem examinations and chemical experiments. The curators of Leiden University, keen on appointing him professor of practical medicine, had to use all their persuasive force—including twice the usual yearly salary—to make him leave Amsterdam. On 17 September 1658 Sylvius gave his inaugural address, *De hominis cognitione*, in which he positioned himself methodologically. Although he was to maintain some of Galen's physiological concepts all his life (such as innate heat and the animal spirit), he was opposed to all dogmatism. In the new epistemology that he was advocating, experimental observation guided by reason should be the leading principle of research in natural philosophy.

As an industrious anatomist and experimentalist himself, his physiological thinking was based on recent anatomical findings—such as those of the blood circulation, the lymphatic system, and the glandular ducts—and on the conviction that all life and disease processes are based on chemical reactions. Inspired by Paracelsus and Van Helmont, Sylvius considered the human body to be analogous to a chemical laboratory, thinking in terms of the opposition between acid and alkali and the effects of their effervescing fermentation. Together they drove all processes: digestive, emotional, and even rational. A balance between acids and alkalis implied a healthy condition, whereas imbalance or acrimony caused disease. Because he thought of his laboratory experiments as an imitation of nature, Sylvius considered it vitally important to be well-equipped. Thus, when he moved to Leiden, he bought a house and refurbished it according to his needs. Apart from a huge library and a tutorial room, it contained three laboratories and a distilling chamber. In 1666 he was also appointed professor of chemistry. Three years later a chemical laboratory was arranged at Sylvius's initiative; the laboratory was honored with a visit by Cosimo de' Medici the same year.

In 1636 Otto Heurnius had introduced clinical demonstrations into the academic curriculum. Sylvius picked up this tradition, and it was continued after him by Herman Boerhaave, that other chemist-clinician. Sylvius stepped up the frequency of bedside teaching using carefully chosen cases from twice a week to every day in an attempt to connect theory to practice and clinical findings to post mortem observation. In total, Sylvius is said to have performed some 300 dissections in fifteen years.

Sylvius was an excellent teacher who attracted and inspired many students. They included Reinier de Graaf, Jan Swammerdam, Florentius Schuyl, Cornelis Bontekoe, Niels Stensen, Frederik Ruysch, Lucas Schacht, and Burchardus de Volder. Still, for someone with the ambition to reform medicine, grounding a new pathology on anatomy, chemistry, and the clinic, it is remarkable that he did not publish much himself. It is perhaps characteristic for the era—a watershed between tradition and modernity—that Sylvius decided not to publish well-rounded monographs, but rather disputations defended by his students.

They were edited and several experimental observations were added. In 1663 *Disputationum medicarum decas* was published, bearing witness to the lively intellectual climate around Sylvius and the tentative character of the natural philosophical experiments, observations, and preliminary conclusions of the times.

Only in his late fifties did Sylvius decide to publish *Praxeos medicae idea nova* [New idea in medical practice], which may be called his programmatic *magnum opus*. In it he did not limit himself to clinical descriptions but elaborated on physiological processes in general. The first volume was published in 1671, the other volumes posthumously.

Bibliography

Primary: 1663. *Disputationum medicarum decas* (Amsterdam); 1671–74. *Praxeos medicae idea nova* (Leiden) [Translated in 1675 by Richard Gower as *A New Idea of the Practice of Physic* (London)].

Secondary: Beukers, Harm, 1999. 'Acid Spirits and Alkaline Salts: The Iatrochemistry of Franciscus dele Boë, Sylvius.' *Sartoniana* 12: 39–58; Smith, Pamela H., 1999. 'Science and Taste. Painting, Passions, and the New Philosophy in Seventeenth-Century Leiden.' *Isis* 90: 421–461; Gubser, Alfred, 1966. 'The *Positiones variae medicae* of Franciscus Sylvius.' *Bulletin of the History of Medicine* 40: 72–80; Baumann, E. D., 1949. *François dele Boe, Sylvius* (Leiden); *DSB*.

Frank Huisman

SYME, JAMES (b. Edinburgh, Scotland, 7 November 1799; d. Edinburgh, 26 June 1870), *surgery*.

Syme was the second son of John Syme, a lawyer, and Barbara Spottiswood. He was educated privately and at the High School in Edinburgh. He was fond of chemistry and was provided with a laboratory at home, in which he discovered a new solvent for Indian rubber (1818). He used this to waterproof a silk cloak and produce flexible tubing, and he published his results in the journal *Annals of Philosophy*. The method was later patented in Glasgow by Charles Mackintosh, who went on to develop his famous business in Manchester. Syme began studying at Edinburgh University (1815) and after initial studies in botany and philosophy, moved to medicine in 1817, when he took anatomy with John Barclay. In 1818 he became the assistant of his third cousin, Robert Liston (1794–1847), when Liston set up his own anatomy class. His first appointment came in 1820 as medical superintendent at the Edinburgh Fever Hospital, and in the following year he became house surgeon at the Edinburgh Royal Infirmary. He became a member of the Royal College of Surgeons in 1823 and the following year studied with M. Jacques Lilsfranc (1790–1847) and Guillaume Dupuytren (1777–1835) in Paris.

In the 1820s he developed a reputation as an inventive operator and effective teacher. He performed the first amputation of a leg at the hip joint in Scotland in 1824 and published on further innovative procedures with the excision of the elbow, leg bones, and jaw and on repair of blood vessels.

Having fallen out with Liston, in 1824 he set up a new medical school with Dr Mackintosh, which attracted large numbers of students. In 1829 he founded his own Clinical Surgical Hospital in order to gain greater clinical experience, given that an appointment at the Royal Infirmary was difficult as long as Liston held office. In 1833 he became professor of clinical surgery at the University of Edinburgh, having agreed to pay £300 per year pension to the retiring chair Mr Russell, and the following year, when Liston left for University College Hospital, London, Syme was at last appointed surgeon to the Royal Infirmary. This made Syme the most influential surgeon in Scotland—a popular teacher with a large surgical practice and a key hospital appointment. He maintained this position, apart from a short sojourn to University College Hospital (1849), until his retirement (1870). He was quick to adopt anesthesia and in the late 1860s championed the antiseptic methods of his son-in-law Joseph Lister (1827–1912).

Syme published regularly in the *Edinburgh Medical and Surgical Journal*, and his textbook *The Principles of Surgery* (1832) broadened his reputation and authority, going through four editions to 1856. He published a number of books on special operations and maintained a high professional profile nationally through his journal articles and the many disputes in which he became embroiled. He was a controversialist in almost every aspect of his professional work, from rivalries with fellow Edinburgh surgeons over access to patients and standards of practice through to conflicts over practical techniques. He brought the same abrasive qualities to medical politics, serving on the General Medical Council for ten years and holding positions in a number of Edinburgh societies. Given his standing, power, and style, it is perhaps unsurprising that he was once called 'the Napoleon of surgery'.

Bibliography

Primary: 1831. *Treatise on the Excision of Diseased Joints* (Edinburgh); 1831–32. *The Principles of Surgery* 2 vols. (Edinburgh) [2nd edn. 1837, 3rd edn. 1842, 4th edn. 1856, 5th edn. 1863]; 1848. *Contributions to the Pathology and Practice of Surgery* (Edinburgh); 1861. *Observations in Clinical Surgery* (Edinburgh).

Secondary: Paterson, R., 1974. *Memorials of the Life of James Syme* (Edinburgh); Shepherd, J. A., 1969. *Simpson and Syme of Edinburgh* (Edinburgh); 1870. 'Obituary—James Syme, FRSE, DCL, Etc.' *British Medical Journal* ii: 21–26; *Oxford DNB*.

Michael Worboys

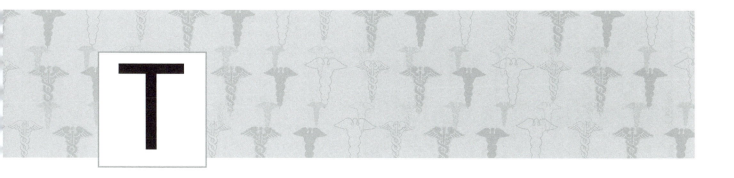

T

TADDEO ALDEROTTI (aka ALDEROTTO, DEGLI ALDEROTTI, TADDEO DA FIRENZE, THADDEUS FLORENTINUS) (b. Florence, Italy, 1206/1215; d. Bologna, Italy, 1295), *medicine, philosophy, medical education.*

Physician, philosopher, and scholar of the liberal arts, Taddeo was one of the three critical interpreters of Galenic translations from the Arabic and Greek in the late thirteenth century; the others were Arnald of Vilanova and John of Saint-Amand.

He was probably born into a Florentine family of modest resources, but with some medical affiliations. He married in 1274 into a more established family and to a woman notably younger than himself. With her, he had at least one daughter; through papal intervention, he also legitimized a natural son, Taddeolo. At his death, Taddeo was a wealthy man, with richly detailed preliminary and final wills and bequests.

We know he was a master at the University of Bologna in the mid-1260s, but his training to that point is enigmatic. His medical studies were in all likelihood taken at Florence and Bologna, perhaps with the Franciscans. He may, as a biographer asserted eighty-five years after his death, have been a slow learner, but his modern biographer finds both breadth and depth in his command of the liberal arts, philosophy, and, of course, medicine, suggesting dedicated instruction, particularly in medicine, at Bologna.

In his own turn, Taddeo's teaching was almost entirely in logic and in medicine, continuing until the early 1290s.

Although he may have taught on Aristotelian philosophy more broadly, there is little to support that conclusion. On the other hand, it is clear that Taddeo was one of the 'founders' of Bolognese medicine, at least at the University. His teaching enhanced his own reputation and led to both municipal privileges and a salary. Dante refers to him in the *Paradiso* (XII, 37–105) as a source of great medical learning, which can seduce others for its financial value. Unlike many of his colleagues who received similar benefits, Taddeo's role as a teacher was valued by the city even more than that as practitioner.

The success of his students attested both to Taddeo's importance as a teacher and to the pivotal times for medicine in which they lived. Numbered among this elite group were Bartholomew of Varignana, William of Brescia, Dino of Garbo, Turisanus, and Mondino De' Liuzzi, who between them helped revolutionize medicine, anatomy, and surgery, and whose authority reached into the papacy, numerous royal courts, and municipalities. A further didactic legacy may be the introduction of the *articella* into Bologna. The nature of his *consilia* corroborate that he had students with him when he visited some patients, although these texts do not attest to a consolidation of bedside instruction, as has been suggested. Taddeo does provide an early hint that anatomies may have been performed in Bologna in the third quarter of the thirteenth century, but he relates no concrete information.

complaints were his most common calls. He did offer advice for gynecologic conditions, including both sterility (masculine and feminine) and unwanted pregnancy. As a practitioner, Taddeo was probably well-known for his skill and, by the end of his career, for both greed and charity, as displayed in his wills. Other cities tried without success to attract him as practitioner and teacher.

His written output is noteworthy for its inclusion of both vulgar and Latin texts, including an Italian translation of the *Nicomachean Ethics*. His medical works number fourteen, extant in at least thirty-five manuscripts and several printed editions. He probably wrote these in the 1270s and 1280s. Among them, the works display a declining interest in Aristotelianism and a growing attention to Hippocrates and, especially, Galen. Taddeo was an attentive reader of translations, going so far as to compare three translations of one Galenic text and annotate his preferences. He wrote commentaries on Hippocrates' *Aphorisms*, *Regimen of Acute Diseases* (coauthored with, perhaps, his student Bartholomew of Varignana) and *Prognostics* (all unfinished); Galen's *Tegni*, *On Different Fevers*, and *On Crisis* (and a 'correction' of his *On the Interior Parts*); Johannitius's *Isagoge*; and Avicenna's (Ibn Sīnā) *Canon*, books one and four. Taddeo also wrote an *Introduction to Practice* and a *practica* on fevers, a table of remedies, a short poem on alchemy, a vernacular regimen for Corso Donati, and a well-known collection of 185 *consilia*.

In general, Taddeo's teaching favored the application of natural philosophy to the basis of medical science. His students continued the process into the fourteenth century. Interestingly, Taddeo's thought, as previously suggested, became increasingly practical throughout the course of his career, no doubt because of the influence of his medical practice. Nevertheless, he is well-known for philosophical emphasis within the *studium* in Bologna. In addition, he appears to have fostered in his students an interest in the Parisian philosophy of the time, which bolstered the Bolognese penchant for radical Aristotelianism into the fourteenth century. For example, Taddeo was a strong cardiocentrist, along the lines of Aristotle and Avicenna, although he softened his stance to accommodate the inflections of encephalocentrism, where it suited medical explanations. Taddeo was a less flexible Aristotelian than some of his students. Given his late entry into medical thought, it is little wonder that he favored more 'old-fashioned' interpretations, particularly of the internal faculties. And yet, he simultaneously expressed views of the mind that were radical and tended toward the Averroist. This Averroism, nevertheless, was very pragmatic and narrow, shying away from the more controversial notions of eternity and intellect.

In aggregate, Taddeo's life represents a remarkable degree of detail for a figure who was neither a religious nor political ruler, but it also embraces a 'triple threat' in thirteenth-century medicine—a figure who was influential in clinical practice, 'research', and education.

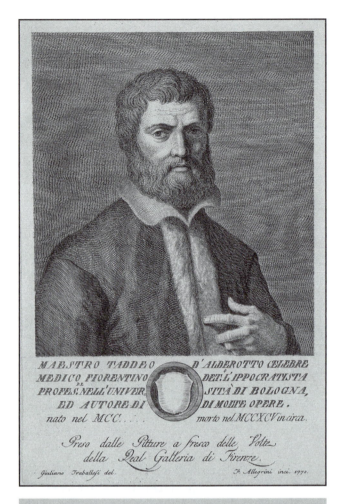

Taddeo Alderotti. Line engraving by F. Allegrini, 1770, after Giulio Traballesi. Iconographic Collection, Wellcome Library, London.

His practice was the source both of a large measure of his reputation and of his considerable wealth; it clearly affected his diminished capacity for writing and perhaps inspired his sleepwalking. Most prominent among his patients was the captive monarch, King Enzo (d. 1272, Bologna), but his other patients were geographically wide ranging, although almost wholly in Italy, favoring the north. He probably saw most of his patients in Bologna or prescribed by letter, but he also traveled to Ferrara and Venice on clinical business. His patients included the Venetian doge and, perhaps, Pope Honorius IV. Such was his reputation that the bishop-surgeon Theodoric of Lucca asked a *consilium* of Taddeo. From the meager details that survive, we gather that Taddeo saw patients at least from their teens into their sixties (excluding children) and of both sexes, socially ranging from a smith to the potentates just mentioned. The scope of his practice did not embrace wounds and fractures, which fell more clearly under the domain of the surgeon, but it was otherwise expansive. From his *consilia,* fevers and respiratory, urinary, and gastrointestinal

Bibliography

Primary: 1477. *Libellus de sanitate factus per Magistrum Thadeum de Florentia* (Bologna); 1522. *Thaddei Florentini medicorum sua tempestate principis in C. Gal. Micratechnen Commentarii* (Naples); 1527. *Thaddei Florentini Expositiones in arduum aphorismorum Ipocratis volumen* (Venice); Giorgi, Piero P., and Gian Franco Pasini, 1997. *Consilia di Taddeo Alderotti, XIII secolo* (Bologna).

Secondary: Garcia-Ballester, Luis, 1998. 'The New Galen: A Challenge to Latin Galenism in Thirteenth-century Montpellier' in Fischer, Klaus-Dietrich, Diethard Nickel, and Paul Potter, eds., *Text and Tradition: Studies in Ancient Medicine and Its Transmission: Presented to Jutta Kollesch* (Leiden) pp. 55–83; Siraisi, Nancy G., 1981. *Taddeo Alderotti and His Pupils: Two Generations of Italian Medical Learning* (Princeton); *DSB.*

Walton O. Schalick III

TAGLIACOZZI, GASPARE (b. Bologna, Italy, 27 February 1545; d. Bologna, 7 November 1599), *plastic surgery.*

Tagliacozzi was the son of Giovanni Tagliacozzi, a silk weaver, and Elisabetta Quaiarini. In 1565 he enrolled as student of medicine at the University of Bologna, where among his teachers were Ulisse Aldrovandi, Girolamo Cardano (1501–76), and especially Giulio Cesare Aranzio (*c.* 1530–89), who had been a pioneer in the field of reconstructive surgery and who had a profound influence upon him. On 12 September 1570, he was awarded a degree in medicine and was immediately asked to teach surgery. In 1576 he received a second degree in philosophy; after the death of Aranzio, he was made professor of anatomy in 1589–90 and, the following year, of theoretical medicine. In 1594 he was asked if he would be available to transfer to Padua to replace Girolamo Fabrici d'Acquapendente (*c.* 1533–1619), whose death seemed imminent. Two years later (1596), he was asked to go to Mantua to cure the Duke Vincenzo Gonzaga, with whom he established close relations and to whom he dedicated his magnificent book *De curtorum chirurgia per insitionem* (1597), devoted to reparative surgery to restore defects not only of the nose, but of the lips and ears as well. The work was illustrated with twenty-two plates, in which were shown the instruments; the deformities of the nose, the lips, and the ear; the seat and the various stages of the grafting; the preparation of the cutaneous flap; the positions to be maintained for the adhesion of the graft; the shaping of the flap; and, lastly, the various bandages and the vest or doublet employed to secure them.

Rhinoplasty had been empirically developed by members of the Branca family of Catania in the fifteenth century and the Vianeo (or Boiano) family of Tropea in the sixteenth century, in order to obviate the amputation of the nose caused by sharp-edged weapons. The method was improved and codified by Tagliacozzi and represents the so-called 'Italian method', which utilized skin from the arm in making

the graft, unlike the 'Indian method', which employed skin from the forehead. The skin flap for the reconstruction of the nose was obtained from the anterior surface of the arm using special instruments (forceps and knives in the form of a myrtle leaf). Using forceps, a fold of the skin was raised; the horizontal openings of the jaws guided the knife in order to obtain a regular cutaneous flap of the right size. This flap, cut off at its proximal extremity, was then applied to the scarified stump of the nose, the arm being kept in a raised position against the nasal region by a bandage attached to a doublet. The arm was immobilized in this position against the head until adhesion of the skin flap, i.e., usually in about twenty days. The flap was severed from the arm as soon as full union had occurred. Fourteen days after, the process of shaping the flap so that it resembled the nose began. A chapter was dedicated to the restoration of lips, and another dealt with the surgery of defects of the ear (in this case, the flap was taken from the hairless region just behind the ear).

Rhinoplasty, however, was almost completely abandoned for about two hundred years and only started to be performed again at the end of the eighteenth century, thanks also to the progress made in the study of animal regeneration.

Bibliography

Primary: 1587. *Epistola ad Hieronymum Mercurialem* [dated from Bologna on 22 February 1586] *de naribus multo ante abscissis reficiendis*, in Mercuriale, Girolamo, *De decoratione* 2nd edn. (Frankfurt) pp. 115–120; 1597. *De curtorum chirurgia per insitionem, libri duo* (Venice); 1598. *Chirurgia nova . . . de narium, aurium, labiorumque defectu, per insitionem cutis ex humero, arte hactenus omnibus ignota sarciendo* (Frankfurt).

Secondary: Belloni, Luigi, 1974. 'Empirismo e biologia sperimentale nella storia della chirurgia plastica.' *Simposi clinici* 11: xxv–xxxii; Teach Gnudi, Martha, and Jerome Pierce Webster, 1950. *The Life and Times of Gaspare Tagliacozzi, Surgeon of Bologna (1545–1599)* (Bologna and New York).

Giuseppe Ongaro

TAIT, (ROBERT) LAWSON (b. Edinburgh, Scotland, 1 May 1845; d. Llandudno, Wales, 13 June 1899), *surgery, gynecology.*

Tait, the son of Archibald Campbell Tait, a butler and vintner, and Isabella Stewart Lawson, was educated at George Heriot's School, at Edinburgh University from 1859, and at the Extramural School, being taught by James Young Simpson (1811–70), whose assistant Tait became. After graduating LRCPEdin and LRCSEdin (1866), Tait was appointed house surgeon to Clayton Hospital, Wakefield (1867), where he performed his first ovariotomy (29 July 1868) and was promoted to assistant surgeon. He purchased a practice in Birmingham (1870) and married Sybil Anne Stewart of Wakefield (28 January 1871). They had no children.

Tait launched himself into professional and public life with energy and achievement, writing for the medical and lay press, particularly the *Birmingham Morning News*. He was a founder and honorary surgeon of the Birmingham and Midland Hospital for Women (1871), instigating a nurses' training program. When it moved to larger premises (1878), he purchased the old building for his private clinic. An advocate of ovariotomy in the early stages of cystic disease, he demonstrated improved outcomes (139 sequential operations with no deaths, 1885) and modified the procedure by adopting silk intraperitoneal pedicle sutures instead of the external clamp devised by Thomas Spencer Wells (1818–97). He was among the first to perform the controversial 'normal ovariotomy' (1872). Tait received the BMA Hastings gold medal for 'the pathology and treatment of ovarian diseases' (1873) and performed his first hysterectomy for fibroids (1873). After initiating 'Tait's operation' (salpingo-oöphorectomy, 1877) for pelvic inflammatory conditions, he controversially advocated laparotomy in acute abdomen or when diagnosis was uncertain. He was also criticized for suggesting that large hospitals were responsible for high death rates (1877).

Tait came to dispute Joseph Lister's (1827–1912) antisepsis, believing that germs survived only in dead tissue such as pus. An ardent hygienist, he introduced a technique for cleansing the peritoneum and maintaining homeostasis. Contemporaries described his surgical technique as rapid, dexterous, and resourceful with the unexpected. He worked through small incisions with minimal disturbance to tissue and used few and simple instruments, many to his own design. A progressive abdominal surgeon, he performed some of the earliest appendectomies (1880), cholecystotomies (1879), and hepatotomies (1880). For his contribution to gall-bladder surgery, the Edinburgh College of Physicians awarded him the Cullen and Liston Prize (1890). He was the first to cut for ruptured tubal pregnancy (17 January 1883) and in five years had operated on thirty-nine women, with two deaths. Tait was variously president of the Birmingham Medical Institute (1889–93), the British Gynaecological Society, and the Medical Defence Union, which he helped establish. He and Sybil joined the Birmingham Natural History Society, and Tait found time to conduct botanical research, corresponding regularly with Charles Darwin.

Students flocked to Tait's clinic, and he toured Europe, the United States, and Canada (1884). Several American universities awarded him honorary degrees, and he was consulting surgeon to hospitals in West Bromwich, Nottingham, and Southampton. A persuasive public speaker, and occasionally pugnacious, Tait was early involved in Birmingham politics, being elected to the city council (1876) and chairing the health and asylums committees. He stood for Parliament as a Liberal (1884) but was defeated by the Unionist candidate. As professor of gynecology at Queen's College, Birmingham, he was instrumental in its transfer to Mason College, which became Birmingham University. At the height of his fame, he owned several country houses, a yacht, a houseboat, and many *objets d'art*. Of medium height and thickset, he enjoyed lavish meals, good company, and quantities of snuff, and he liked animals, being a vociferous antivivisectionist. He was kind to his patients, treating many poor women free of charge.

Among his colleagues, Tait's belligerence, dogmatism, and flouting of convention made him unpopular, and his last years were marred by dissension and decline. He began to suffer symptoms of chronic nephritis (1893) and relinquished nearly all his public appointments, although he saw patients and performed operations until a fortnight before his death.

Bibliography

Primary: 1874. 'The Hastings Prize Essay: pathology and treatment of ovarian diseases.' *British Medical Journal* i: 701–703, 733–736, 765–768, 798–800, 825–827; ii: 8–10, 27–29; 1877. *An Essay on Hospital Mortality: Based upon the Statistics of the Hospitals of Great Britain for Fifteen Years* (London); 1877. *Diseases of Women* (London); 1879. 'Removal of normal ovaries.' *British Medical Journal* i: 813–814; 1887. 'Presidential address on some pending questions in gynaecology.' *British Medical Journal* i: 145–148.

Secondary: Greenwood, Anna, 1998. 'Lawson Tait and Opposition to Germ Theory: Defining Science in Surgical Practice.' *Journal of the History of Medicine and Allied Sciences* 53: 99–131; Moscucci, Ornella, 1990. *The Science of Woman: Gynaecology and Gender in England, 1800–1929* (Cambridge and New York); Shepherd, John A., 1982. 'Lawson Tait: Disciple of Charles Darwin.' *British Medical Journal* 284: 1386–1387; Shepherd, John A., 1980. *Lawson Tait: The Rebellious Surgeon, 1845–1899* (Lawrence, KS); Flack, Harvey, 1949. *Lawson Tait, 1845–1899* (London); Martin, Christopher, 1931. *Lawson Tait: His Life and Work, with Personal Reminiscences* (Birmingham); McKay, W. J. Stewart, 1922. *Lawson Tait, His Life and Work: A Contribution to the History of Abdominal Surgery and Gynaecology* (London); [Anon.], 1899. 'Obituary, Lawson Tait, FRCS Eng & Edin.' *British Medical Journal* i: 1561–1564; *Oxford DNB*; *Plarr's Lives*.

Carole Reeves

TAKAKI, KANEHIRO (b. Mukasa, Hyūga domain [now Miyazaki Prefecture], Japan, 15 September 1849; d. Tokyo, Japan, 13 April 1920), *medicine, nutrition*.

In the 1880s Takaki Kanehiro demonstrated a causal connection between the high rates of beriberi in the Japanese Imperial Navy and the sailors' diet, which he argued was deficient in protein. Later, his protein-deficiency theory was disproved. Nevertheless, his research placed Takaki along with Christiaan Eijkman, Casimir Funk, Sir Frederick G. Hopkins, and Elmer V. McCollum in the genealogy of the discovery of vitamins.

In 1875 Takaki studied medicine at St Thomas's Hospital Medical School in London. Upon returning to Japan in 1880, he took the position of Chief Surgeon of the Naval Hospital in Tokyo, where he discovered an epidemic of beriberi in the navy. In 1880 alone the incidence rate was 36 percent.

Trained in British epidemiology, Takaki began searching for causes in the living conditions on ships and in barracks. Narrowing his focus to diet, he discovered a correlation between protein deficiency and rates of incidence. Beriberi was prevalent in the units where protein content was low, but, in units where the protein content was high, the incidence rate was low. Relying on the standards of nutrition found in Edmund Parkes's *A Manual of Practical Hygiene*, Takaki assumed that a healthy diet needed a 1:15.5 protein to carbohydrate ratio. In contrast, navy rations had an average ratio of 1:28. Takaki theorized that a dietary imbalance of too few proteins and too many carbohydrates was the cause of beriberi.

In October 1882 Takaki advocated Westernizing the rations by increasing the protein content of the navy diet with canned meat, powdered milk, bread, and barley. His reforms were implemented in January 1884. By 1886 Takaki claimed that he had eradicated beriberi from the navy. The incidence rate fell from 25 percent in 1883 to 12 percent in 1884 and then to 0.59 percent in 1885. By 1886 the incidence rate was 0.04 percent.

Japanese Imperial Army and Tokyo University doctors, however, did not recognize the effectiveness of Takaki's dietary reform. Trained in Germany, these doctors were interested in experimental medicine, and, believing beriberi to be an infectious disease like cholera, they sought its bacteriological origins. Because Takaki posited that beriberi was a dietary deficiency disease and backed up his assertions with medical statistics, not experimental data, many did not accept his work as scientifically valid. The army, however, could do nothing to mitigate the debilitating effects of beriberi. During the Sino-Japanese War (1894–95), the army suffered approximately 4,000 beriberi-related deaths. The navy did not incur even one case of the disease. Despite this record, it was not until the middle of the Russo-Japanese War (1904–05) that army doctors recognized the value of and need for dietary reform. By August 1904 between 12,000 and 18,000 soldiers with beriberi were triaged at the front. Because the disease was undermining the army's ability to wage war, the army high command ordered dietary reform as a preventative measure in August, and from September the incidence rate began to fall.

Takaki eliminated beriberi from the navy and set the standard for the dietary reform in the army. In 1890 he established the Tokyo Jikei Hospital and Medical School, which is famous for housing Japan's first college for nurses. It is still in operation. For these accomplishments, the Meiji Emperor awarded him the rank of baron in 1905. Takaki was also recognized for his contributions to the discovery of vitamins. In 1959 England named a series of promontories and glaciers in Antarctica after Takaki, Eijkman, Funk, Hopkins, and McCollum to commemorate this lineage.

Bibliography

Primary: 1993. *Takaki Kanehiro sensei gyōsekishu* [Works] (Tokyo); 1885. 'On the cause and prevention of Kak'ke.' *Trans. Sei.-I-Kwai* 4: 29–37 (reprinted in 1992, *Nutrition* 8(5): 376–381, 382–384).

Secondary: Carpenter, Kenneth J., 2000. *Beriberi, White Rice, and Vitamin B* (Berkeley); Matsuda, Makoto, 1990. *Kakke wo nakushita otoko: Takaki Kanehiro den* [The man who cured beriberi: life of Takaki Kanehiro] (Tokyo); Yamashita, Seizō, 1988. *Meijiki ni okeru kakke no rekishi* [History of beriberi in the Meiji era] (Tokyo); Itakura, Kiyonobu, 1988. *Mohō no jidai* [The age of imitation] (Tokyo).

Alexander R. Bay

TAO, HONGJING 陶弘景   (b. Nanjing, Jiangsu Province, China, 456; d. Mount Mao (now Zhongnanshan), Shaanxi Province, China, 536), *Daoism, alchemy, pharmaceutics.*

Tao Hongjing is celebrated in China as a patriarch of the Shangqing School of Daoism, as a historian, philologist, and bibliographer, and as one of the greatest herbalists and alchemists in Chinese history. He was born to a prominent aristocratic family. Because of his illustrious family background, he enjoyed an excellent worldly education as well as a Daoist discipleship that granted him access to esoteric scriptures and practices by initiation. Already at a young age, he became interested in pharmaceutical, alchemical, and spiritual studies related to the pursuit of immortality and transcendence of the mortal world. As an adult, he held the position Reader in Attendance, or tutor, to some of the Qi imperial princes, and then commander of the left detachment of the palace guards. After some years of successful government service, he resigned in 492 in order to withdraw as a recluse to Mount Mao, where he resided for most of the rest of his life.

At Mount Mao, he devoted himself to physical and spiritual self-cultivation and the study, collection, authentication, organization, and promotion of the sacred Daoist scriptures in his possession. Their distinguished literary style and calligraphy convinced him of their authenticity and divine origin and led him to compose several texts that represent Shangqing teaching, most notably the *Zhen gao* 真誥 [Declarations of the Perfected Ones, c. 492]. This collection includes poetry; instructions for physical and spiritual cultivation and attaining immortality, said to have been revealed to the medium Yang Xi 楊羲 in 364-70 by celestial visitors; and letters, records of dreams, Daoist genealogies, and historical information on the origin and transmission of the Shangqing scriptures. Taken together with Tao's other Daoist writings, all of which were most probably completed by 500, this collection was instrumental in establishing Shangqing Daoism as a highly influential school, with a body of literature, an organizational structure, and a comprehensive and codified system of religious practices aimed at attaining immortality by transcending the realm of ordinary existence. Moreover, they enable us to reconstruct the origin and development of the Shangqing School of Daoism in Southeast China over a century and a half.

In addition, and related to his textual studies of the Shangqing literary corpus, Tao Hongjing was also a renowned herbalist and alchemist. Perhaps his greatest work is the *Shennong bencao jing jizhu* 神農本草經輯注 [Collected Commentaries on Shen Nongs Classic of Materia Medica], in which he edited the Han period materia medica classic *Shennong bencao jing*, added his own commentary, and synthesized the current materia medica literature of his day. He thereby provided the basis for the preservation and transmission of China's earliest materia medica text. In layout, content, and organization, this text became the model for materia medica literature for the next 1,000 years.

Setting the pattern for later authors, he did not discard previous knowledge, but merely added information by lengthening the descriptions of individual drugs and by introducing new drugs, to a total of 730 medicinals. Using different-colored inks, he clearly differentiated between the original Han period classic, his own comments, and quotations from other texts. In an innovative scheme that was adopted by other authors for many centuries, he organized the drug monographs by their natural origins—stones and minerals, herbs, trees, fruits, vegetables and grains, insects, reptiles, birds, and beasts—which were then subdivided into the three grades of the original *Shennong bencao jing*.

In addition to his philological and alchemical studies, he established and supervised a monastic community of Daoist adepts on Mount Mao that continued to thrive long after his passing. He also provided guidance to political leaders of his time and formed a particularly close relationship with the Buddhist Emperor Wu of the Liang dynasty, who protected him and his community during the Daoist persecutions of 504 and 517.

Bibliography

Primary: c. 492. *Zhen gao* 真誥 [Declarations of the Perfected Ones]; before 500. *Dengzhen yinjue* 登真隱訣 [Hidden Instructions for the Ascent to Perfection]; c. 500. *Shennong bencao jing jizhu* 神農本草經輯注 [Collected Commentaries on Shen Nong's Classic of *Materia Medica*].

Secondary: Bokenkamp, Stephen R., 1996. '*Declarations of the Perfected;* Answering a Summons' in Lopez, Donald S., ed., *Religions of China in Practice* (Princeton) pp. 166–179, 188–201; Strickman, Michel, 1979. 'On the Alchemy of T'ao Hung-ching' in Welch, H., and A. Seidel, eds., *Facets of Taoism: Essays in Chinese Religion* (New Haven) pp. 123–192; Sivin, Nathan, 1968. *Chinese Alchemy: Preliminary Studies* (Cambridge, MA); *Nan shi* 南史 [History of the South] 76: 12810a–12812a; Jia Song 賈嵩, *Huayang Tao Yinju Nei Zhuan* 華陽陶隱居內傳 [Detailed Life of the Hermit Tao from Huayang], Tang period. TT 151.

Sabine Wilms

TARDIEU, AMBROISE-AUGUSTE (b. Paris, France, 10 March 1818; d. Paris, 12 January 1879), *medical jurisprudence, forensic pathology.*

Tardieu was the son of André-Ambroise Tardieu, a member of the renowned family of engravers, and of Charlotte Boulland. He attended Collège Charlemagne and then went on to study at the Paris École de Médecine. He became an interne of the Paris hospitals in 1840 and, three years later, received his medical degree, with a thesis on the subject of glanders, a topic that expanded the work of his professor, Pierre Rayer, with whom he was soon to quarrel. He was agrégé at the Paris Faculté de Médecine in 1844 and was made medical chief at Lariboissière hospital in 1851. During this period he published a manual of pathology, a study of cholera epidemics, and a dictionary of public hygiene.

In the mid-1850s Tardieu began to publish on medico-legal issues, beginning with abortion. He was elected to the Académie de Médecine in 1859. In 1862 he was named professor of hygiene in the Faculty of Medicine and in 1864 took over the position of dean, replacing Rayer, but he held that position for only two years. By 1867 he was president of the counsel of hygiene and president of the Académie de Médecine. As a physician at the Hôtel Dieu, he demonstrated how to recognize cases of infanticide, poisoning, suffocation, criminally caused wounds, and child abuse. He testified in more than 3,000 medico-legal cases, some of which were spectacular murder trials, most notably that of the journalist Victor Noir (Yvan Salmon) by Pierre Bonaparte in 1870. His testimony based on the autopsy exonerated Bonaparte, which led to an uproar among the students and the temporary closing of the medical school. For six years (1864–70) he was a member of the Municipal Council for the VIe arrondissement.

In recent years Tardieu has been quoted at some length. In 1972 Frederick N. Silverman, who was one of the first in recent years to describe the battered child syndrome, gave full credit to the earlier studies by Tardieu in 1860. Others have both praised and criticized Tardieu in the literature for his opinions on abortion, homosexuality, and child abuse. The best known of these is by Jeffrey M. Masson, who used Tardieu's reports on child sexual abuse to criticize Freud for abandoning his 'seduction' theory of neurosis.

Bibliography

Primary: 1856. *Étude médico-légale sur l'avortement* (Paris); 1859. *Étude médico-légale sur les attentats aux moeurs* (Paris); 1867. (with Roussin, Z.) *Étude médico-légale et clinique sur l'empoisonnement* (Paris); 1870. *Étude médico-légale sur la pendaison, la strangulation, les suffocations* (Paris).

Secondary: Cunningham, Jacqueline L., 1988. 'Contributions to the History of Psychology. French Historical Views on the Acceptability of Evidence Regarding Child Abuse.' *Psychological Reports* 63: 343–353; Masson, Jeffrey Moussaieff, 1984. *The Assault on Truth—Freud's Suppression of the Seduction Theory* (New York); Mosse, George L., 1982. 'Nationalism and Respectability: Normal and Abnormal Sexuality in the Nineteenth Century.' *Journal of Contemporary History* 17(2): 221–246; Silverman, F. N., 1972.

'Unrecognized Trauma in Infants, the Battered Child Syndrome, and the Syndrome of Ambroise Tardieu.' *Radiology* 104: 337–353; Hahn, Lucien, 1900. 'Tardieu, Ambroise-Auguste.' *La Grande Encyclopédie, inventaire raisonné des sciences, des lettres et des arts* (Berthelot et al., eds.) 30: 933.

Joy Harvey

TAUSSIG, HELEN BROOKE   (b. Cambridge, Massachusetts, USA, 24 May 1898; d. Kennett Square, Pennsylvania, USA, 20 May 1986), *pediatric cardiology.*

Taussig was the fourth child of Edith and Frank Taussig. Her mother died of tuberculosis when she was eleven. She was close with her father, a professor of economics at Harvard University, who appreciated her strength and helped her with her severe dyslexia and in her recovery from childhood tuberculosis. Taussig began college at Radcliffe College and graduated from the University of California at Berkeley (1921). She was an athlete and competed successfully in tennis and basketball. She considered Harvard; however, at the time, women were not admitted as degree candidates to the medical school. Therefore, she chose Boston University School of Medicine, where she worked in anatomy with Alexander Begg and began research in cardiac physiology. Encouraged by Begg, she transferred to Johns Hopkins School of Medicine. She graduated with an MD degree (1927), completed her postgraduate training, and joined the faculty (1930).

In 1930 Edwards A. Park, the newly appointed Chief of Pediatrics, wanted to develop outpatient specialty clinics at the Harriet Lane Home for children at the Johns Hopkins Hospital. He chose Taussig as the director of the cardiac clinic because of her interest and knowledge in heart disease. The Harriet Lane Home had acquired a fluoroscope, and Taussig began to use this tool to study children with congenital heart disease. She correlated clinical, electrocardiograph, and fluoroscopic findings with postmortem specimens and established a method to accurately diagnose congenital cardiac malformations. These observations were collected and reported as case studies in her textbook *Congenital Malformations of the Heart* (1947). Taussig's book added to previous autopsy studies by Maude Abbott and created for the clinician an exceptionally clear, concise clinical textbook with its anatomic drawings, schematic diagrams, radiographs, and detailed case reports.

Taussig observed that babies with Tetralogy of Fallot (blue baby syndrome) survived longer if they had a persistent ductus arteriosus, and she recognized that the major physiological alteration was the lack of blood flow to the lung. She reasoned that if a ductus could be created surgically, it would oxygenate the cyanotic child. She convinced Alfred Blalock, the new chief of surgery (1940), to study surgical intervention in a child with Tetralogy of Fallot. Blalock, with the assistance of his technician, Vivian Thomas, developed the 'Blalock-Taussig' shunt. The successful treatment was published in February 1945.

Taussig's principal contribution to medicine was the physicians she trained. During an academic career of thirty-five years at Hopkins, she trained generations of investigators and teachers who went on to become the leaders in this new field of pediatric cardiology. In 1962 she raised the alert concerning the association of phocomelia with thalidomide. Her efforts were instrumental in averting a disaster in the United States and in establishing Food and Drug Administration (FDA) requirements for drug testing.

Helen Brooke Taussig was a brilliant physician whose contributions advanced the status of women in medicine, her insightful observations influenced the development of cardiac surgery, and she developed a new subspecialty in pediatrics and wrote its first definitive textbook. In spite of many handicaps, particularly her hearing loss in her early thirties, she endured and excelled to become one of America's most famous and honored physicians. She lived a long life, one in which she was always intellectually active and productive.

Bibliography

Primary: 1945. (with Blalock, Alfred) 'The Surgical Treatment of Malformations of the Heart in Which There Is Pulmonary Stenosis or Pulmonary Atresia.' *Journal of the American Medical Association* 128: 189–202; 1981. 'Little Choice and a Stimulating Environment.' *JAMWA* 36(2): 43–44; 1992. (with Baldwin, Joyce) *To Heal the Heart of a Child* (New York).

Secondary: McNamara, Daniel, et al., 1987. 'Helen Brooke Taussig.' *Journal of the American College of Cardiology* 10: 662–671; Dietrich, Herbert J., Jr., 1986. 'Helen Brooke Taussig.' *Transactions and Studies of the College of Physicians of Philadelphia* 5(4): 265–271; Engle, Mary A., 1985. 'Helen Brooke Taussig, Living Legend in Cardiology.' *Clinical Cardiology* 8: 372–374; Taussig, Helen Brooke, 1973. 'Dr. Edwards A. Park, Physician, Teacher, Investigator, Friend.' *Johns Hopkins Med. J.* 132: 370–376.

Barry David Silverman

TENON, JACQUES   (b. Sépeaux [Yonne], France, 21 February 1724; d. Massy [Essone] France, 15 January 1816), *surgery, hospital architecture.*

'*Hospitals are a measure of a society's civilization.*' (Tenon, 1788, p. 1)

Tenon, a surgeon, is remembered mainly for his magisterial study of the Paris hospitals. His *Mémoires sur les hôpitaux de Paris* (1788) capped the work of a blue-ribbon committee of the Paris Academy of Sciences whose members included the philosopher Condorcet, the chemist Lavoisier, the mathematician Laplace, and the physicist Coulomb. In the 1780s these luminaries discussed the future of Paris hospitals, but it was Tenon who collected the information and wrote the reports. These remained a fundamental primer for hospital reform well into the following century.

Tenon's *Mémoires* embodied the French Enlightenment's response to a disastrous fire that destroyed a whole wing of the Paris Hôtel Dieu in 1772. Numerous architects submitted proposals for a new model hospital. The Academy of Sciences, backed by the Baron de Breteuil, one of the royal secretaries who had the king's ear, wanted to split up the huge and unmanageable central buildings. Tenon advocated an emergency and first-aid institution in the center of town, particularly to serve victims of accidents, together with specialized hospitals on the periphery of Paris.

These projects perished during the French Revolution, and a new Hôtel Dieu was not built until the 1860s, where it remains today just across the square from the site of the ancient hospital adjacent to Notre Dame Cathedral. Tenon's *Mémoires,* along with seventeen volumes of his manuscripts detailing his visits to hospitals throughout France and Europe, testify to their author's zeal for reform.

As the eldest of eleven children, five of whom died young, and as the descendant of modest provincial surgeons, Tenon made two obvious but weighty choices at an early age. In the early 1740s he left home for Paris to pursue a career in surgery, and he entered the Paris Hôtel Dieu. There he served three years in a surgical apprenticeship. He was shocked and angered by the unhygienic and thoughtless care that the indigent patients received. 'This horror became the initial and one of the chief motives of his life', remarked Georges Cuvier in his eulogy of Tenon at the Academy of Sciences.

Returning to Paris after a brief military campaign, he won the coveted position of chief surgical resident (*gagnant-maîtrise*) at the Salpêtrière Hospice. Completion of this six-year appointment entitled surgeons to the mastership degree without payment of the usual exorbitant fees. The Salpêtrière was then a teeming village of about 8,000 indigent and mostly old and invalid women, hundreds of whom were demented, insane, debauched, or imprisoned for some misdeed. A physician assigned to this hospice lived in town and came on weekly rounds, serving the administrative staff, the nurses, and the priests, while neglecting the poor. That left the hospital surgeon to treat the inmates' complaints, both medical and surgical. Tenon had to deal with the highly contagious scabies, ringworm, and venereal disease endemic in this hospice. He set up a center for the inoculation of smallpox. His medical experience also encompassed pregnant women, the unwanted children, the demented and the agitated insane, all hospitalized here, pell-mell. The *Mémoires* reveal that he observed details of hospital layout, management, and even practices such as the manner of preparing the infants' pap or the details of laundering the enormous number of sheets required for 8,000 persons.

In 1743 the government had added a master's degree in the liberal arts to the requirements for surgical certification, and Tenon therefore had to learn enough Latin to present a thesis. After fifteen months of study, asserts Cuvier, he 'spoke Latin fluently, understood Greek fairly well, and had distinguished himself in philosophy'. In 1757 he successfully defended a thesis on cataracts, a hotly debated ophthalmologic and surgical issue at that time. His name remains attached to a thin connective tissue capsule that forms the socket for the back of the eyeball. As a master surgeon, he became a member of the Paris College of Surgery, and the Academy of Surgery quickly elected him to membership.

Tenon served as professor of pathology at the College, and his course outline survives in manuscript. While teaching, he became increasingly aware of how useful a more varied clinical experience and opportunities for research would be for his colleagues. In 1764 he therefore wrote to the king's first surgeon, La Martinière, urging the creation of a hospice for the College of Surgery. The first surgeon convinced the king and contributed some of his own funds, with the result that such a research hospital, 'a unique and invaluable institution' (Tenon, 1888, p. 52), was established near the College and next to the magnificent new Academy of Surgery inaugurated in 1774. It eventually had twenty-two beds, twelve for men and ten for women, and accepted only the most complicated and interesting surgical patients, giving preference to gunshot and stab wounds, so that military surgery could profit from the investigations. The twelve attending surgeons took turns at presiding, first for six months, then for two years. Tenon took his turn in 1780, when he introduced practical innovations and urged the admission of a larger number of students, all of whom should be graduates of the practical dissection school across the street. This hospital thus represented a pioneering institution.

Tenon's busy life might have remained confined to the relatively narrow concerns of surgery had he not been elected to the Academy of Sciences, in 1759, on the strength of an elaborate paper on the exfoliation of bones, based on thirteen experiments on living dogs. His more than forty papers and two dozen reports presented to the Academy show that his research interests ranged broadly over comparative anatomy, osteology, odontology, stomatology, and, of course, surgery. Using conventional methods of descriptive and comparative anatomy, he presented significant details that ranged from the human skull and palate to the disease of hatters and the teeth of the horse, the elephant, and the crocodile. He emphasized 'natural anatomy', that is, research on living creatures, by injecting the blood vessels, lymphatic system, or excretory ducts, and by 'macerations and corrosions'. He believed that, once the 'natural anatomist' gained more knowledge, he could teach the physiologist, physician, surgeon, and even the painter and sculptor and thus contribute to the advancement of optics and acoustics.

During his fifty-seven years in the Academy, Tenon collaborated closely with some of the finest scientific minds. For example, he served on a commission with Pinel, Portal, Sabatier, and Cuvier, to report on Gall and Spurzheim's experiments on the anatomy of the brain, and with Percy, Portal, and others on the dangers to which dissection exposes anatomists. But nothing he undertook reached a national, international, or permanent importance comparable to his hospital book.

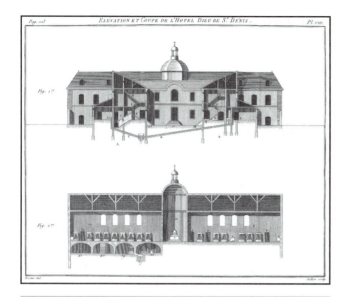

Architectural plan of the Hôtel Dieu de St Denis, showing staircases and drainage conduits (top) and wards (bottom). Engraving from *Mémoires sur les hôpitaux de Paris*, Paris, 1788. Rare Book, Wellcome Library, London.

When he was invited to join the hospital committee of the Academy of Sciences to respond to the king's request for the learned elite's recommendation regarding the future of the Hôtel Dieu, Tenon could display his unique experience. For at this very hospital, as an apprentice surgeon, he had observed the hundreds of details that abound in his *Mémoires:* the hierarchies and activities of nurses and servants; the hospital routines of feeding, cleaning, and laundering; the practice of accommodating over 3,000 patients in some 1,200 beds; the lack of adequate toilets; the poor quality of food, wine, and medicines. Tenon's book would document, for the first time, the staggering quantities of straw, sheets, wood, and candles, and the horrendous crowding, pollution, stench, and confusion. But he would also provide standards for the reformer, 'measuring stick in hand': the optimal size of a bed, so a patient could rest, sleep, and turn over; the minimum requirement of 'respirable air'; the width of staircases for a stretcher to pass; and the height of a stair that a convalescent could mount with ease. Tenon envisaged the transformation of the traditional hospital into an instrument for actively healing patients.

Patiently gathering information was no easy task, particularly because the Augustinian nursing sisters at the Hôtel Dieu refused him access to the hospital and would not open their account books. The most recent budget he used dated back to 1763. When no information came from England, the Academy agreed to finance a trip for Tenon and Coulomb. They were well received by Sir Joseph Banks, the president of the Royal Society. They were most curious about the Naval Hospital at Plymouth. They found an institution that had been functioning for twenty-four years and that embodied the pavilion plan, a model that the French committee had

laboriously perfected in the abstract. It was 'an experiment already completed', wrote chairman Bailly to Tenon. The admiration of the French Enlightenment for Great Britain was tellingly confirmed.

The most spectacular and direct result of Tenon's work was the transfer, during the penurious years of the Directory, of the whole lying-in service at the Hôtel Dieu—including the pregnant women, the babies, wet nurses, and midwives—to two salubrious institutions on the periphery of Paris, the former Port-Royal and Oratoire convents. Under the direction of Marie-Louise Lachapelle, the midwife-in-chief at the Hôtel Dieu, the municipal architects adapted the convent structures to the needs of a lying-in hospital. This included the transformation of the Oratoire chapel into a birthing room, soon to be followed by a small amphitheater for teaching deliveries. A midwifery school took shape here in 1802, with help from Jean-Antoine Chaptal, the physician–minister of internal affairs. Tenon's statistics and his compassion for the thousands of unwanted and doomed newborns and for the single girls, victims of 'a moment's weakness', had touched persons as different as the minister and the midwife.

The epithet 'venerable' recurs in comments about Tenon in his eighties. His tall, erect figure, old-fashioned dress, and white hair helped create the image that the only surviving likeness, the sketch by Jean-Noël Hallé, confirms. During the Revolution, Tenon was elected to the Legislative Assembly. He fought for moderation but failed to make himself heard. After the fall of the monarchy, he felt, like many Frenchmen, 'forced to seek safety in total solitude, in my home in the country'.

Honors did come his way. He figured among the charter members of the Institut de France in 1796 and among Napoleon's first awardees of the Legion of Honor in 1804. He won the approval of the pope and gold medals from Emperor Joseph II of Austria and King Victor Amadeus II of Sardinia. These distinctions came late in life, when the white-haired octogenarian bachelor journeyed to Paris, mainly to attend the weekly meetings of the Academy of Sciences, only to return to his books and papers at Massy. When, in 1815, soldiers of the Russian occupation forces sacked his home and destroyed his library, he fled to Paris, and, shortly thereafter, he died. He would have been deeply moved to know that, sixty-three years later, a major Paris hospital in the La Roquette district was named for him.

Bibliography

Primary: Tenon papers. Bibliothèque Nationale de France, NAF, 22742–22751, 11357–11368; 1785. *Observations sur les obstacles qui s'opposent aux progrès de l'anatomie* (Paris); 1788. *Mémoires sur les hôpitaux de Paris* (Paris); *Memoirs on Paris Hospitals* [ed., intro. notes, bib., and appendices Weiner, Dora B. (Canton, MA, 1996)]; 1791. *Réflexions en faveur des pauvres citoyens malades* (Paris).

Secondary: Gelfand, T., 1980. *Professionalizing Modern Medicine: Paris Surgeons and Medical Science and Institutions in the Eighteenth Century* (Westport, CT); Foucault, Michel, Blandine Barret

Kriegel, Anne Thalamy, François Beguin, and Bruno Fortier, 1976. *Les machines à guérir* (Paris); Greenbaum, Louis S., 1975. '"Measure of Civilization": The Hospital Thought of Jacques Tenon.' *Bulletin of the History of Medicine* 49: 43–56; Weiner, Dora B., 1972. 'The French Revolution, Napoleon, and the Nursing Profession.' *Bulletin of the History of Medicine* 46: 274–305.

Dora B. Weiner

TEZIAKOV, NIKOLAI IVANOVICH (b. Verkhnie Sergi, Russia, 29 November [10 December] 1859; d. Moscow, USSR, 2 January 1925), *community medicine, hygiene, epidemiology.*

Teziakov was born to a family of serfs who worked in the Urals mining industry. He studied at Kazan University (1879–84) and received a basic degree in clinical medicine. His teachers there included I. P. Skvortsov, one of the early Russian proponents of experimental hygiene science, and A. V. Petrov, a pathological anatomist. Under Petrov's influence, Teziakov became actively involved in the Kazan Society of Physicians [*Kazanskoe obshchestvo vrachei*], collecting epidemiological data and other statistics pertaining to local health conditions. This work inspired in Teziakov an interest in statistics and a recognition of the importance of training new generations of community physicians in the use of statistics to supplement the cultural, education-based tradition of community doctoring in rural Russia.

Following his graduation, Teziakov served as public health physician in the rural self-administration organizations (*zemstvos*) of the provinces of Perm (1884–89), Kherson (1889–96), Voronezh (1896–1903), and Saratov (1903–18). The presence of large agricultural enterprises in southern Russia had fostered increased migration of laborers, which in turn presented particular public health challenges. Teziakov was instrumental in creating new zemstvo-administered medical-nutrition points that provided migrants with basic medical care, food, and shelter, as well as performing epidemiological surveillance over this population. Teziakov also helped organize a network of nurseries to improve the health of infants and young children whose mothers were agricultural laborers. His volume on school hygiene for teachers in rural and church-administered schools filled a gap in good quality, comprehensible textbooks for this audience, and it was reprinted in eight editions until 1915.

Teziakov represented the segment of community physicians who embraced the available bacteriological solutions to infectious disease without turning their attention from the socioeconomic factors that contributed to infectious disease. After participating in smallpox vaccinations in Perm early in his career, Teziakov became one of the first community physicians in Russia to use antidiphtheria serum to fight an epidemic in the winter of 1894–95.

After the outbreak of the Russo-Japanese War in 1904, Teziakov was called up to serve in a field hospital for the Russian infantry in Manchuria. He returned to Saratov at the war's end, but the conflict and political crisis had seriously damaged his efforts to build a public welfare section in Saratov on the model of similar organizations he had observed in Voronezh and Kherson.

Teziakov's work with migrants highlighted the importance of controlling syphilis and tuberculosis, and, in the early twentieth century, Teziakov was active in the All-Russian Anti-Tuberculosis League. In 1918 he was invited to head the Section on Spas and Sanatoria of the People's Commissariat for Health. Teziakov was instrumental in developing and improving the existing network of health centers and in shaping programs to allow workers access to treatment for pulmonary infections and other conditions, which had been largely inaccessible to them before 1917.

Teziakov was an important leader among rural public health physicians, vocal on the national level, and contributed significant analysis and organizational efforts to the development of public health activities in Russia.

Bibliography

Primary: 1899. *Besedy po gigiene v primenenii ee k narodnoi shkole* [Lessons on hygiene and its implementation in the public school] (Voronezh); 1903. *Otkhozhie promysli i rynki naima sel'skokhoziaistvennykh rabochikh v Saratovskoi gubernii (k voprosu ob organizatsii vrachebno-sanitarnogo nadzora za peredvigaiushchimisia rabochimi massami)* [Migrancy and hiring markets for agricultural laborers in Saratov province (on the matter of organizing medical-sanitary surveillance over traveling workers)] (Saratov); 1965. 'Iz vospominanii' [Recollections] in Kal'iu, P. I., ed., *Ocherki istorii russkoi obshchestvennoi meditsiny* [Sketches from the history of Russian community medicine] (Moscow) pp. 239–262.

Secondary: Idel'chik, Khasiia Isaakovna, 1960. *N. I. Teziakov i ego rol' v razvitii zemskoi meditsiny i stroitel'stve sovetskogo zdravookhraneniia* [N. I. Teziakov and his role in the development of zemstvo medicine and the creation of Soviet public health] (Moscow); Idel'chik, Khasiia Isaakovna, 1960. 'N. I. Teziakov—stroitel' sovetskogo zdravookhraneniia' [N. I. Teziakov: builder of Soviet public health] *Sovetskoe zdravookhranenie* 19(1): 67–72.

Lisa K. Walker

THAYER, WILLIAM SYDNEY (b. Milton, Massachusetts, USA, 23 June 1864; d. Washington, D.C., USA, 10 December 1932), *medicine, pathology.*

Thayer's parents were James Bradley Thayer, professor at Harvard Law School, and Sophia Bradford Ripley. Thayer manifested his privileged New England background throughout his life, most offensively by his patronizing and sometimes derogatory comments about Jews, blacks, and other ethnic groups.

Following a happy and uneventful childhood, he entered Harvard College at age sixteen. He graduated in 1885—a year late, because of a college prank. Chastised and matured, he then studied medicine at Harvard and completed his MD in 1889. He was a member of the first generation of American doctors able to study laboratory science at home and a beneficiary of the most advanced medical education then available in the United States. He particularly appreciated studying pathology with Reginald Fitz.

After an internship at Massachusetts General Hospital, Thayer visited Europe for several months; his experience in Paul Ehrlich's laboratory made him an ardent advocate of clinical pathology. He returned to Boston, but when given the opportunity to serve as resident physician under Osler at the recently opened Johns Hopkins Hospital, he soon moved to that Baltimore institution. He became an attending physician in 1898 and was named associate professor of medicine in 1896 and professor of clinical medicine in 1905. He had hoped to succeed Osler, who left in 1903, and was disappointed when Lewellys Barker was chosen instead. Nonetheless, he decided not to accept a call to Harvard, and in 1919 he finally acceded to Osler's former positions as physician-in-chief and chair of medicine at Hopkins.

In 1901 he married Susan Read, a nurse of aristocratic southern background. They had one child, who died in infancy.

Thayer's initial research interest was blood disease. He published innovative works on leukemia in 1891 and malaria in 1893. In 1896 he organized a course in clinical microscopy that set the standard for such courses throughout the United States. His research later turned to the heart. After his appointment to the clinical professorship, he concentrated on teaching, consulting, and writing. Attuned to scientific medicine and not hesitant to use whatever treatment was indicated in any given case, he nonetheless would forego drugs if he thought physical therapy or psychological counseling would do the job.

In 1917 Thayer joined a Red Cross relief mission in Russia. His wife, who had been sick, died while he was away, and he was in Moscow at the time of the Bolshevik Revolution. The United States entered World War I almost as soon as he had returned from Russia, and he quickly joined the army medical corps in France, with the understanding that the chair of medicine at Hopkins awaited his return. In 1921, displeased with his own administrative performance, he took partial retirement from Hopkins. He left the hospital in 1925, while continuing to teach at the medical school and consult in the Baltimore-Washington area. He had been suffering symptoms for some time, and he knew he was quite sick, but his death from a heart attack was regarded as sudden.

Thayer was a highly literate man who published a volume of poetry and could readily converse in several languages. Regarded by some as a fop or aesthete, he clearly considered himself a gentleman physician in the mold of Osler. He was a superb diagnostician who sought to balance what he regarded as the scientific and humane sides of medical practice. Beyond his scientific contributions, his lasting importance lies primarily in those whom he mentored and trained.

Bibliography

Primary: 1897. *Lectures on the Malarial Fevers* (New York); 1908. 'On the Early Diastolic Heart Sound, the So-Called Third Heart Sound.' *Boston Medical and Surgical Journal* 158: 713–726; 1931. *Osler and Other Papers* (Baltimore).

Secondary: Reid, Edith Gittings, 1936. *The Life and Convictions of William Sydney Thayer, Physician* (New York); 1934. 'The Thayer Memorial Exercises.' *Johns Hopkins Hospital Bulletin* 55: 201–219; *DSB*; *DAMB*.

Edward T. Morman

THOMPSON, JOHN ASHBURTON   (b. Kensington, England, 31 July 1846; d. South Kensington, England, 16 September 1915), *public health, epidemiology*.

Thompson was the son of Emma Hitchcock and John Thompson, a lawyer, so a professional career was expected of him. Educated at St Paul's School and University College London, he studied medicine at Guy's and Middlesex Hospitals, London, gaining his LRCP MRCS LM LSA in 1868. Postgraduate study in Brussels led to the award of an MD degree (1876). Back in London, he combined private practice with work for the Great Northern Railway Company. Suffering poor health, he visited New Zealand and Australia to recuperate. On his return to England, he completed the Diploma in Public Health at Cambridge (1882).

As a result of his earlier visit, Thompson decided to migrate to Australia in 1884, working first at the Hospital for Pacific Islanders in Mackay, Queensland, where there was an outbreak of dengue fever. He was appalled by the conditions there, so he moved to Sydney, arriving in the middle of a smallpox epidemic. He accepted a position as temporary medical officer with the Board of Health but, before long, was appointed chief medical inspector in recognition of his unique qualifications as an epidemiologist, the only one in New South Wales.

He demonstrated his ability with a meticulous investigation of a typhoid epidemic in 1886. In a manner reminiscent of John Snow in London, he traced the disease to a polluted dairy, by careful mapping of all reported cases. As a result of his report, stronger legislative controls were introduced. He repeated this process with other infectious disease outbreaks in Sydney, in each case producing reports that established him as the authority on public health issues in the colony. In 1891 he was the official delegate to the International Congress of Hygiene and Demography in London.

In 1896 Thompson was appointed as the first full-time president of the New South Wales Board of Health. He proved to be a capable manager, who must be credited with the establishment of an efficient public health regime. This was achieved despite his difficult relationships with other board members, politicians, and professional colleagues. Based on the work of his predecessors, Thompson drafted a consolidated Public Health Act (1896) that provided improved regulation of environmental pollution, as well as measures for ensuring pure food and for the control of unhealthy buildings. Although he was an avid centralist, he was forced to accept that these public health responsibilities should be shared with local government.

Thompson stopped practicing clinical medicine upon taking up these administrative appointments, which suited him better. He always had been more interested in disease than people. He came to international notice with a prize-winning study of leprosy in Australia (1897). When bubonic plague struck Sydney in 1900, Thompson was the right man to be in charge. He reasoned that the disease bacillus was transmitted in some way by rats, so he organized an effective campaign to eradicate the city of these pests. His theories were vindicated by research carried out by his colleague, the microbiologist Frank Tidswell, who proved that the fleas carried by rats were the disease vector.

His work in suppressing the plague further enhanced Thompson's international standing, leading to invitations to address learned bodies in Boston, Berlin, and London. Unfortunately, he omitted any reference to the research of Tidswell, giving the impression that it was entirely his own work. When he retired from the Board of Health in 1913, he immediately returned to London, dying of a stroke two years afterward.

Bibliography

Primary: 1897. *A Contribution to the History of Leprosy in Australia* (London); Board of Health, 1898–1913. *Minutes of Proceedings* (Sydney).

Secondary: Cummins, C. J., 1979. *A History of Medical Administration in New South Wales 1788–1973* (Sydney); Armstrong, W. G., 1925. 'An Eminent Epidemiologist.' *Health* (Canberra) 3: 97–100; *AuDB*.

Peter J. Tyler

THOMSON, ARTHUR SAUNDERS (b. Arbroath, Scotland, 29 December 1816; d. Tientsin, China, 4 November 1860), *military medicine.*

Thomson, the son of Margaret Saunders and James Thomson (occupation unknown), graduated MD from the University of Edinburgh in 1837, receiving a gold medal for his thesis on the influence of climate on health. He joined the British Army and served in India, contributing several papers to the local medical journals, including one entitled 'Could the Nations of a Temperate Climate Colonise and Increase in a Tropical Country, and Vice-versa?' In January 1848 he joined the 58th Regiment in Auckland, New Zealand, during a period of peace between white settlers and Maori. Later that year he wrote an open letter to Maori, urging them to be vaccinated against smallpox. He soon learned to speak fluent Maori and traveled widely round the country, staying in Maori villages and conversing at length with their inhabitants.

Thomson remained in New Zealand for almost eleven years and contributed to various British medical journals; these papers, the first to be published from New Zealand, described conditions and diseases in the colony. In writing on epidemics of scarlet fever and of influenza, he took a statistical approach, which was unusual in those days. The figures were small and probably not statistically significant, but the statistician in him had to record the numbers. He sent the Statistical Society of London an excellent detailed description of Auckland as it was in 1848; this was read to the Society on his behalf. Another paper examined the effects of the New Zealand climate on the health of British immigrants. More important were papers on the anthropology of the Maori, their health, stature, customs, and tattooing. He measured the height and weight of young Maori men compared with British soldiers, finding correctly that Maori limb bones were significantly shorter and their trunks rather longer, so that, overall, the Maori was only slightly shorter on average than the European. Thomson saw six cases of 'Maori leprosy', more than any other doctor. He had seen leprosy in India, and, although the cases in New Zealand were rather different, he was convinced that they were a variety of the same condition. The disease has now died out and there are various opinions on its cause, but no one has the authority of Thomson.

In limestone caves in the central North Island, he discovered bones of a giant extinct bird called the moa (dinornis). He wrote the 700-page account *The Story of New Zealand* (1859), which traces, in fine fashion, the Maori and the European history of the colony, its geography, its flora, and its fauna. The book is authoritative yet easy to read. In particular, it contains an extensive bibliography of more than 400 items relating to New Zealand, dating from 1642 to 1859. It must have been a prodigious effort to collect all that material.

Late in 1858 Thomson reluctantly went back to England with his regiment. He had bought land in New Zealand and was determined to return, to spend the years of his retirement, and ultimately to die in the country that he had come to love so much. But it was not to be. In 1860 he volunteered to serve with the army in the small war then being fought in China, and he died there in his prime, aged forty-three, from a ruptured liver abscess. Thomson was a good scientist, a statistician, an anthropologist, and a climatologist in relation to medicine and health. His scientific endeavors tended to overshadow his work as a medical practitioner, but that was quietly carried on in the background of his published work.

Bibliography

Secondary: Wright-St Clair, R. E., 2002. 'Dr A S Thomson: Ethnographer and Historian.' *Journal of Medical Biography* 10: 155–159; Salesa, T. D., 2001. 'The Power of the Physician: Doctors and the "Dying Maori" in Early Colonial New Zealand.' *Health and History: Maori Health Special Issue* 3(1): 13–40.

Rex Wright-St Clair

THOMSON, SAMUEL

THOMSON, SAMUEL (b. Alstead, New Hampshire, USA, 9 February 1769; d. Boston, Massachusetts, USA, 4 October 1843), *botanical healing.*

Thomson was the second of six children of John Thomson and Hannah Cobb. In early childhood he became interested in the healing properties of plants, learning about medicinal roots and herbs both from a local botanical practitioner and through his own investigations in the fields and woods of the family farm. In 1790 Thomson married Susan Allen; they went on to have eight children. By that time, personal and family medical experiences had led him to distrust the skills of orthodox physicians and to develop his own set of therapies derived from his empirical knowledge of plants.

Initially, Thomson confined his medical activities to the treatment of family members and neighbors while making his living from farming. But in 1805 he decided that demand for his services was sufficient to occupy him full-time, and he dedicated the rest of his life to the promotion of a practice that became known as Thomsonism (or Thomsonianism), the first system of 'alternative medicine' developed in America. Having determined through clinical experience that patients benefited from botanicals that produced vomiting and purging or that had a heating effect, Thomson reasoned that all disease must be due to loss of heat from the body. Remedies therefore worked either by restoring heat to the system (accomplished by cayenne pepper, for example) or by removing internal obstructions to the production and distribution of heat (the effect of his favorite drug, the emetic lobelia). Other evacuative and heating plants were also employed, as well as tonic herbs to restore strength to the system after the debilitating first stage of treatment. In all, Thomsonian therapy utilized some seventy botanicals, supplemented with steam baths and enemas.

To protect his system from misuse by imitators, Thomson obtained a patent from the U.S. government in 1813. Backed by patent protection, he hired agents to sell so-called Family Right Certificates throughout the country. Priced at twenty dollars, the Certificates granted heads of families the privilege of treating all members of their household with Thomsonian remedies, as well as the right to purchase drugs from Thomsonian pharmacies and to form local Friendly Botanic Societies to share experiences with other Certificate holders. By 1839 Thomson could claim to have sold more than 100,000 Family Right Certificates. That estimate was perhaps inflated, but even mainstream physicians acknowledged that in some rural areas, as much as a third of the population adhered to Thomsonian practice.

The attraction of Thomsonism was as much political as medical. In the self-consciously democratic cultural climate following the 1828 election of Andrew Jackson (1767–1845, seventh president of the United States), the public was warmly receptive to Thomson's attacks on the pretensions of the educated medical elite and ready to answer his call to assume responsibility for their own health; 'every man his own physician' was the Thomsonian battle-cry. People were drawn as well by the presentation of botanicals as 'natural' remedies that supported the body's innate recuperative power instead of assaulting it with the harsh mineral drugs and bleeding trusted by orthodox physicians.

The Thomsonian movement was nevertheless turbulent with internal dissension, much of it occasioned by the acerbic personality of its founder, and it began to fragment even before Thomson's death in 1843. After that date, Thomsonism degenerated into competing splinter groups and steadily faded away over the second half of the century.

Bibliography

Primary: 1822. *A narrative of the life and medical discoveries of Samuel Thomson* (Bristol); 1822. *New guide to health; or, Botanic Family Physician* (Boston).

Secondary: Haller, John S., Jr., 2000. *The People's Doctors. Samuel Thomson and the American Botanical Movement, 1790–1860* (Carbondale, IL); Berman, Alex, 1951. 'The Thomsonian Movement and Its Relation to American Pharmacy and Medicine.' *Bulletin of the History of Medicine* 25: 405–428, 519–538; Halstead, Frank, 1941. 'A First-hand Account of a Treatment by Thomsonian Medicine in the 1830s.' *Bulletin of the History of Medicine* 10: 680–687; *DAMB.*

James Whorton

THOMSON, WILLIAM

THOMSON, WILLIAM (b. Paisley, Scotland, 1819; d. South Yarra, Australia, 22 May 1883), *medicine, epidemiology, medical controversy.*

Thomson, the son of Thomas, gentleman, and his wife, Agnes Robertson, studied at the Andersonian School of Medicine and Glasgow University, taking prizes in medicine and anatomy. He became MRCS Edinburgh in 1843 and FRCS Edinburgh in 1872.

As ship's doctor Thomson made six voyages to Australia. In 1852 he sailed from Liverpool for Melbourne on the *Wanata,* carrying about 800 ill-provisioned Scots and Irish with many children. Typhoid erupted before the vessel cleared the Mersey. Thomson worked devotedly, but deaths, especially among the children, continued throughout the passage. At Port Phillip, the ship was quarantined for pertussis, with ninety-six cases. Overall there were forty-six deaths at sea, thirty-five of them children. Thomson had observed that the fever cases were not concentrated, but spaced throughout the voyage, suggesting that the causes were not miasmatic, but issued from sequential infections. Thereafter, he always pressed the careful tracing of cases and contacts, stringent disinfection, and isolation.

The *Wanata* calamity enabled gasbag Herbert Spencer to wrongly blame Thomson. Possibly Thomson's acerbity in subsequent medical and literary rows stemmed from this episode. Spencer's branding probably led to Thomson's settlement in Melbourne in 1854. He was admitted to the Victorian medical register in 1855 and launched on a stormy, brilliant, thankless colonial career. Between 1856 and 1864, he was sometime committee member and librarian of the Medical Society of Victoria, from which he resigned (or was expelled) and secretary and editor (dismissed) of the *Australian Medical Journal*. He raised the motion in 1861 to expedite the founding of the University Medical School. A freethinker, in 1863 Thomson defended Wallace and Huxley against the antievolutionist foundation medical professor George Halford. Thomson's applications for posts in the School in 1865 and 1867 were rejected.

From about 1863 Thomson attacked local practitioners' boosting of Melbourne's climate to British consumptives. He used the relatively good Victorian statistics to show that incoming phthisics rarely lasted long and that pulmonary tuberculosis was spreading among the Australian-born.

Statistics and epidemiological investigations also underpinned his arguments that Melbourne's high typhoid and diphtheria rates were caused by 'pathogenic micrococci'. He wanted regulated notification and infection controls. Thomson won no medical or official friends by intruding on other doctors' patients to take case histories and inspect premises, notably in the hushed-up typhoid outbreak at the Kew Asylum in 1875–76. His effects on colleagues notwithstanding, Thomson seems to have been respected and trusted by ordinary people. He also sought bans on suspect imports in the mid-1870s to protect Victoria from foot and mouth, pleuropneumonia, and the phylloxera insect, but he lost to politicians and traders.

Bereft of clinical laboratory support, in 1876 Thomson reasoned the principle of modern chemotherapy: chemical substances could be used to kill 'germs in living tissue without at the same time destroying its integrity'. His fundamental insight passed unnoticed. In 1876 he stated that tuberculosis was caused by a specific germ although it might manifest variously. He surmised, from studying cases among domestic servants, that the organism could lurk for months in the dried phlegm among the fluff in consumptives' bedrooms. In 1882, after Koch announced his discovery of the bacillus, Thomson published *The Germ Theory of Tubercle Illustrated From . . . Victoria*, claiming priority.

He was a learned Baconian, small, sharp-eyed, with a neat beard, tirelessly warring with Shakespearians. He was wrong in some beliefs: he thought that pleuropneumonia and human measles were identical, and he overemphasized contagion, while not recognizing asymptomatic diphtheria and typhoid carriers. His death issued from a liver abscess related to a kick by a demented patient nine months earlier; until the final week he refused medical attendance.

Bibliography

Secondary: Smith, F. B., 2002. 'Disputes about Typhoid Fever in Victoria in the 1870s.' *Health and History* 4(2): 1–18; Ford, E., 1954. *A Bibliography of William Thomson* (Sydney); *AuDB*.

F. B. Smith

IBN AT-TILMĪDH, AMĪN AD-DAULA HIBAT ALLĀH IBN SAʿĪD
(b. Baghdad, Iraq, *c.* 1074; d. Baghdad, 12 February 1165), *medicine, pharmacy, medico-pharmacological glossography.*

Ibn at-Tilmīdh was born into a Christian Arab family of the Nestorian persuasion. Both his father and maternal grandfather were distinguished physicians, who fostered his interest in medicine. He began his apprenticeship with Saʿid ibn Hibat Allāh (d. 1102), physician to the Abbasid palace, who had the greatest impact on Ibn at-Tilmīdh's professional development. Apart from receiving a thorough medical training, the young Ibn at-Tilmīdh was also instructed in other branches of learning, such as Christian and Muslim theology, logic, poetry, music, and calligraphy. He thus deepened his knowledge of the Syriac language and also acquired a profound understanding of the Arabic language.

Ibn at-Tilmīdh then embarked on long journeys to Iran, where he seems to have practiced medicine in the Khorasan province. After many years abroad, he eventually returned to Iraq, now proficient in Persian.

In Baghdad, he set up a medical practice, and his clientele included members of the impoverished classes as well as wealthy dignitaries. He also started to give lectures on medicine, and before long he had fifty regular students. As his reputation as a physician and teacher spread, he was appointed head physician of the famous ʿAḍūdi hospital. In addition, he played an important role in the church of his community as a presbyter.

Ibn at-Tilmīdh had by now firmly established himself in Baghdad, as a physician, church representative, and an associate of the ruling classes and member of various literary and scientific circles. He was a man of wide interests; he liked to surround himself with musicians, poets, and men of letters, but also with philosophers, astrologers, and architects. He was, in fact, a keen poet himself, and over many years conducted a lively artistic correspondence with high-ranking government officials. Despite all this success, he remained a modest and down-to-earth person, kept treating the poor free of charge, and allegedly went so far as to take an oath not to accept any gifts except from the caliph himself. It was only a matter of time before the palace entrusted him with the supervision of medicine in Baghdad, which basically meant the promotion of some kind of licensing authority. The culmination of his career, though, was being appointed court physician, in which capacity he served the caliphs al-Muqtafī (r. 1136–60) and al-Mustanjid (r. 1160–70) until his own death.

Ibn at-Tilmīdh died aged ninety-one and was buried in a churchyard in the Christian quarter of Baghdad. He left to his son and only heir a considerable fortune and a huge library of inestimable worth.

In the Arabic tradition, Ibn at-Tilmīdh is famous for his prose writing. After his death, his letters were collected in a large volume now regrettably lost. His poetry, too, was deemed worthy of transmission. Otherwise, Ibn at-Tilmīdh was neither a prolific nor a particularly original writer. Of his independent works, his *Aqrabādhin*, or 'Dispensatory', is a notable exception, for it represents the apogee of scientific pharmacy among the Arabs, followed by his *Mujarrabāt*, or 'Empirical Drugs', a *Kunnash*, or 'Medical Handbook', and a few other medico-pharmacological writings. He also authored various commentaries and notes on Greek and Arabic medical texts. None of his major works have yet been published.

Bibliography

Primary: Kahl, Oliver, (forthcoming). *The Dispensatory of Ibn at-Tilmīdh*; Iskandar, Albert, 1977. 'An Autograph of Ibn al-Tilmīdh's Marginal Commentary on Ibn Sīnā's Canon of Medicine.' *Le Muséon* 90: 177–236.

Secondary: Ullmann, Manfred, 1970. *Islamic Medicine* trans. Watt, Jean (Edinburgh); Ibn Abi Usaibi'a (d. 1270), 1882–84. `*Uyūn al-anbā' fī ṭabaqāt al-aṭibba'* Müller, August, ed. (Cairo and Königsberg) 1: 259–276; *DSB*.

Oliver Kahl

TISSOT, SAMUEL AUGUSTE ANDRE DAVID (b. Grancy, Pays de Vaud, Switzerland, 20 March 1728; d. Lausanne, Pays de Vaud, Switzerland, 13 June 1797), *medicine, medical education, public health.*

Born to a family of professionals, son of Pierre, a land surveyor, and nephew of David, a Calvinist minister, Tissot grew up in the countryside above Lake Geneva. In 1741 he went to Geneva, where his mother, Jeanne Charlotte Grenus, had family ties, to enroll in the College and then the Academy. After his Master of Arts degree (1745), Tissot entered the Medical Faculty at Montpellier. He boarded with Boissier de Sauvages (1706–67), the school's most famous professor and proponent of vitalism. In his correspondence with Zimmermann (1728–97), Tissot credited what he learned of useful medicine to walking the Montpellier hospital wards with a Leiden graduate and training as a garçon-chirurgien. Upon receiving his MD (1749), he went back to his native village and then moved to Lausanne, where he was appointed physician to the poor in 1752.

Tissot contracted smallpox as a boy and helped fight smallpox epidemics in Montpellier and Vaud. Both experiences epitomized his medical praxis and philosophy. Observing his reactions to the treatment he was prescribed, Tissot rejected the traditional hot regimen for smallpox, instead unknowingly adopting the cool course of soothing drinks and fresh air advocated by Sydenham (1624–89). Confronting epidemics, Tissot learned to debunk charlatanism and superstition and to promote vitalism and education. Having heard from Tronchin (1703–81) of inoculation (variolation), Tissot published *L'inoculation justifiée* (1754), which led to fame and fights. Fame came as crowned heads entrusted him with their heir's inoculation or offered him positions as court physician. Tissot inoculated successfully;

however, he systematically refused the offers to leave Lausanne. Fights surged as other physicians, de Haen (1704–76) in particular, denounced inoculation's validity, later intertwining in their arguments the concept of irritability, developed by Haller (1708–77) and promoted by Tissot, to accuse both of atheism. Tissot devoted several open letters dedicated to colleagues to refute his opponents.

Steeped in ancient Greek medicine, Tissot advocated prevention of disease through regimens adapted to different groups of society. His first effort, often misunderstood as sexual repression, was *Onanisme* (1760), in which he presented a horrific tableau of the results of carnal excesses of any kind. Tissot condemned masturbation as a manifestation of homosexuality spreading from the nobility to the bourgeoisie. He denounced laziness, idleness, even strong ambitions, which led to unnatural behavior. He pursued the medicalization of morality and lifestyle in *De la santé des gens de lettres* (1768), *Essai sur les maladies des gens du monde* (1770), and *Traité des nerfs et de leurs maladies* (1778–80). With *Avis au peuple sur sa santé* (1761), an overwhelming success leading to numerous French and foreign editions, Tissot aimed to educate the public in the proper use of the emerging neo-Hippocratic medicine. To sustain the enlightened medicine he was promoting to the population, Tissot engaged in reforming public health, hospital structure, and medical studies.

In 1780 Tissot accepted a professorship at Pavia, where he taught clinical medicine until 1783; he then returned to Lausanne. Drawing from his teaching experience, Tissot wrote *Essai sur les moyens de perfectionner les études de médecine* (1785), which influenced Pinel (1745–1826) in organizing the Paris clinical program. Tissot, who admired Rousseau (1712–78) and had sojourned in Paris in 1779–80, first saw the French Revolution as an enlightened way to correct poor health bred by poverty or injustice; yet, recoiling from violence, he relied for his pursuit of societal health on a stable government listening to the advice of physicians. His notes from the Lausanne Health Council's meetings, over which he presided, testify to his efforts to improve medicine. In the whirls of wealthy patients and literary successes, Tissot never forgot that he was, foremost, the physician of the poor.

Bibliography

Primary: 1790. *Oeuvres de Monsieur Tissot* 15 vols. (Lausanne); 1797. *Vie de Zimmermann* (Lausanne) [not included in any edition of Tissot's works].

Secondary: Emch-Dériaz, Antoinette, 2005. *La correspondance entre Tissot et Zimmermann, 1754–1797* (Geneva); Barras, Vincent, et al., eds., 2001. *La médecine des Lumières: tout autour de Tissot* (Geneva); Emch-Dériaz, Antoinette, 1992. *Tissot: physician of the Enlightenment* (New York); Emch-Dériaz, Antoinette, 1992. 'The Non-naturals Made Easy' in Porter, Roy, ed., *The Popularization of Medicine 1650–1850* (London) pp.134–159.

Antoinette Emch-Dériaz

TOGBA, JOSEPH NAGBE (b. Sasstown, Liberia, 18 December 1915; d. Silver Spring, Maryland, USA, 13 June 2002), *medicine, medical politics.*

Togba was born of Kru parents in Sasstown (Sinoe County), Liberia. From his early childhood, Togba expected to become a physician: his uncle, a prominent indigenous healer, allegedly prophesied at Togba's birth that this baby would also become a doctor like himself.

Togba received his primary education from American Methodist and Lutheran missionaries at the St Paul Industrial School. He studied next at the College of West Africa (CWA) at Monrovia. At the age of seventeen (1932), he was introduced to the clinical practice of medicine and pharmacology at the Nana Kru Methodist Mission by Everett Veatch, an American physician from Texas. Togba graduated valedictorian from CWA aged twenty-one (1936). Since he was a 'tribal or country boy', as the Americo-Liberians called people from the interior, the Liberian government would not give him a scholarship to study in the United States. Togba received help from an American missionary, Susan Mitchell. Gathering together their resources, Mitchell agreed to assist Togba financially for study and Veatch agreed to help Togba find a scholarship. Eventually, in 1937, Togba boarded a ship for the United States with a scholarship from the Quaker Friends College at Wichita, Kansas.

When Togba arrived at Wichita, he was the first African student to attend Friends College with the aim of becoming a doctor. He subsequently studied premedical subjects, concentrating on biology and chemistry. An exceptional student from the outset, Togba appeared in the *Who's Who Among Students in American Universities and Colleges* (1939) and graduated (BA) in 1940. Since blacks were not permitted to treat white patients, Togba enrolled in the 'Negro' Meharry Medical College, Nashville, Tennessee, where he was able to gain broad clinical experience. Upon graduating with his MD from Meharry (1944), he began nine months of internship at Homer G. Phillips Hospital for Negroes in St Louis, Missouri.

In 1946 Togba returned to Liberia with an invitation to work for the government. Monrovia was just as he had left it: no port, rowboat taxis from the ships, unpaved streets, no electricity or piped water. On arrival, Togba found himself to be the only Liberian doctor among twelve others. His first assignment was at the Liberian Hospital at Snapper Hill, which was in a desperately rudimentary state. Together with his American wife, Jessye Helen Trent (an obstetric nurse), he assisted in the establishment of the Nursing School, the Liberian Nurses Association, and the Liberian Board of Nurse Examiners, with later membership in the International Council of Nurses and the West African College of Nurses. With further assistance from the United States Public Health Service, Togba went on to establish the National Public Health system in the late 1940s, which remained in service until the Liberian Civil War (1989), and to become the director of public health.

Togba was also important internationally. He headed the Liberian delegation to the United Nations International Health Conference in New York City: the conference that ratified the founding of the World Health Organization (WHO). As well as being a founding member, Togba had the honor, in 1954, of being the first African to serve as president of a WHO Assembly.

In 1949 Togba received his MPH from Harvard University. Afterward, he served as Minister (Secretary) of Health of Liberia (1953–60), executive director of the John F. Kennedy Medical Center of Monrovia (1968–72), and professor and chairman of public health and preventive medicine at the Doglotti Medical School, the University of Liberia (1972–86). Togba left Liberia (1990–91) because of the Civil War. His personal papers (and the Liberian National Archives) were destroyed during the war.

Bibliography

Secondary: Patton, Adell Jr., 2005. 'Liberia and Containment against Colonial Take-Over: Public Health and Sanitation Reform, 1912–1953' *Liberian Studies Journal* 30(2): 1–52; Patton, Adell Jr., 1982. 'Howard University and Meharry Medical Schools in the Training of African Physicians, 1868–1978' in Harris, Joseph E., ed., *Global Dimensions of the African Diaspora* (Washington, DC) pp. 142–162; Shick, Tom W., 1980. *Behold the Promised Land: An Afro-American Settler Society in Nineteenth-Century Liberia* (Baltimore).

Adell Patton Jr.

TORRELLA, GASPAR (b. Valencia, Spain, *c.* 1452; d. Rome, Italy, *c.* 1520), *medicine.*

Born in the bosom of a family in which at least his father and two brothers were university doctors, Torrella studied medicine—along with his brother Jeroni—in the Universities of Siena and Pisa during the 1470s. He obtained his degree of Magister in 1483, by virtue of his request to Pope Sixte IV.

Torrella's professional life took place almost entirely in Rome, where he enjoyed a comfortable social position as a member of Cardinal Rodrigo de Borja's court. When the latter became Pope Alexander VI (1492–1503), Torrella continued in his service as a personal doctor to his son Caesar. From 1504 onward Torrella was one of the archiaters of the new pope, Julius II (1503–13). Affiliated to the clerical state at least from the 1470s, he gathered many ecclesiastical privileges during his life, among them the domestic prelature close to both popes and the life bishopric of Santa Giusta, Sardinia (from 1494). Between 1498 and 1500, he was the librarian of the Vatican Library. From 1506 he seems to have been quite inactive as a medical practitioner.

Torrella's notable influence from the Neoplatonist tradition, as well as his permeability to the values of Latin humanism, may be related to his university medical training in Tuscany and to his residence at the papal court. Yet he kept himself intellectually identified to Avicennian Galenism, which was usual among most Italian physicians of his generation. His relations with powerful patrons of the sciences and arts and his residence in one of the centers of the earliest presses gave him the chance of publishing, repeatedly in two instances, all of his writings that are known to us, namely five medical works and an astrological prognosis, in the space of eleven years (1497–1507).

Of Torrella's medical works, the two about the French disease [morbus gallicus]—both of them dedicated to his master Caesar Borgia, a well-known early sufferer from this ailment—are among the earliest and most original medical writings on that 'new' condition, which he named pudendagra. The one work that Torrella published in 1497 has two different parts of similar length: the first contains his medical interpretation and treatment of the French disease, and the second collects five clinical accounts, chosen among the seventeen cases of sufferers from it that he had allegedly treated with success in only two months. This work was reedited under a new title (c. 1498) with a letter to the Bishop of Avranches (Normandy), Louis de Bourbon, who might have been urged to seek Torrella's medical advice for similar reasons as Caesar. Torrella's second work on the French disease (1500) gathers two independent studies on its pains and ulcers, for he claimed that these two major accidents could even lead the patient to die.

Torrella's other medical works were a *consilium*, doubly printed in 1505, about a 'new' pestilence popularly known as 'modorrilla', which broke out in the Castilian fleet at Flanders and spread over the Iberian kingdoms; a *consilium de peste* (after 1505), written on the occasion of a plague that ravaged Rome in 1504; and a *regimen sanitatis* (1506), a preventive regime presented as a dialogue addressed to his master Julius II—an early sufferer from the French disease. Finally, his *Judicium universale . . .* (1507), originally an epistle addressed to Caesar Borgia, was published only at the request of Giovanni Gozadini, an apostolic datary, who was intrigued by the astrological effects of a comet that appeared that year.

Bibliography

Primary: 1497. *Tractatus cum consiliis contra pudendagram seu morbum gallicum* (Rome) [2nd edn. *c.* 1498, *De morbo gallico cum aliis* (Rome)]; 1500. *Dialogus de dolore cum tractatu de ulceribus in pudendagra evenire solitis* (Rome); 1505. *Consilium de egritudine pestifera et contagiosa ovina cognominata nuper cognita quam hispani modorrillam vocant* (Rome and Salamanca); 1507. *Judicium universale de portentis presagiis et ostentis rerumque admirabilium ac solis et lune defectibus et cometis* (Rome).

Secondary: Arrizabalaga, Jon, John Henderson, and Roger French, 1997. *The Great Pox. The French Disease in Renaissance Europe* (New Haven) pp. 113–144, 311–317; Arrizabalaga, Jon, 1986. 'El "Consilium de modorrilla" (Roma y Salamanca, 1505): una aportación nosográfica de Gaspar Torrella.' *Dynamis* 5–6: 59–94.

Jon Arrizabalaga

TRALL, RUSSELL THACHER (b. Vernon, Connecticut, USA, 5 August 1812; d. Florence, New Jersey, USA, 23 September 1877), *hydropathy*.

A farm worker in his youth, Trall attended Albany Medical College, graduating in the mid-1830s, and then practiced conventional medicine for several years. In the early 1840s, however, he converted to hydropathy, an 'irregular' curative system developed in Austria in the mid-1820s by Vincent Priessnitz (1790–1851). Also commonly referred to in America as the water-cure, hydropathy relied on a variety of baths and other applications of cold water to stimulate the body to expel morbid matter, as well as to open the pores to facilitate such elimination. In 1844 Trall opened only the second water-cure institution in the United States, in New York City. He subsequently operated several water-cures in New York and New Jersey. He served as editor of *The Water-Cure Journal* (1849–61) and *The Herald of Health* (1863–66) and authored numerous books on all aspects of water-cure and health maintenance. He also directed several schools of hydropathy, most notably the Hygeio-Therapeutic College in Florence Heights, New Jersey (1867–77).

Trall was most influential for broadening the scope of hydropathy as it was practiced in America, into a system he called hygeiotherapy. Derived from the Greek word for health, 'hygeio' implied living in accord with nature's rules relating to diet, exercise, and other physical activities, so as to preserve health. Hygeiotherapy thus embodied the ideas that prevention was preferable to cure and that proper living habits constituted an essential component of therapy for those who had fallen ill: cold water treatments had to be complemented with good hygiene. To this end, Trall embraced the principles of Grahamism, the popular health-reform movement of the 1830s led by Sylvester Graham (1794–1851). Patients at his institutions were expected to adopt vegetarian diet, to abstain from alcohol, tobacco, and other stimulants, and to engage in vigorous exercise daily. In addition, women were urged to abandon fashionable dress (heavy skirts and tight-laced corsets) in favor of loose, light clothing; the Bloomer costume adopted by mid-century feminists was inspired by this 'wet dress' developed at water-cure institutions.

An important element of the hygeiotherapeutic philosophy was sexual hygiene, an area in which Trall was a radical reformer. Unlike the Grahamites, he considered sex an activity that should be engaged in for pleasure, not just procreation, and that should produce as much pleasure for women as men. Recognizing that fear of pregnancy could inhibit sexual pleasure and that repeated pregnancies could undermine health, he promoted contraception at a time when few physicians were so bold. The rhythm method he recommended, however, was based on erroneous assumptions about women's monthly cycle and advised intercourse be restricted to the time midway between menstrual periods. Fortunately, hygeiotherapy also included water treatments to facilitate natural childbirth for the women who followed his contraceptive advice.

For Trall, the laws of health were divine commandments that required as strict obedience as the moral commandments of scripture, and their observance could be expected to lead the human race to a millennial state of moral and social perfection. Hygeiotherapy's utopianism naturally attracted the politically liberal and was particularly appealing to, and supportive of, the early feminist movement. But although the system flourished in the reform-minded decades preceding the Civil War (1861–65), it faded as the horror of that war disabused Americans of notions of human perfectibility. Trall's Hygeian Home in New Jersey, where he practiced until his death from pneumonia, was one of the few water-cures to survive to the end of the 1870s.

Bibliography

Primary: 1852. *The Hydropathic Encyclopedia* 2 vols. (New York); 1860. *Water-Cure for the Million* (New York); 1866. *Sexual Physiology and Hygiene* (New York).

Secondary: Whorton, James, 2002. *Nature Cures: The History of Alternative Medicine in America* (New York) pp. 77–101; Cayleff, Susan, 1987. *Wash and Be Healed: The Water-Cure Movement and Women's Health* (Philadelphia); Donegan, Jane, 1986. '*Hydropathic Highway to Health': Women and Water-Cure in Ante-Bellum America* (New York); *DAMB*.

James Whorton

TRAUBE, LUDWIG (LOUIS) (b. Ratibor, Upper Silesia [now Poland], 12 January 1818; d. Berlin, Prussia, Germany, 11 April 1876), *medicine*.

Traube, the son of a Jewish wine merchant, began his medical studies in Breslau (Wroclaw) in 1835. Arriving in Berlin in 1837, he came under the influence of Johannes Müller. Soon he was studying the new French physiology in a private reading circle that included Rudolf Virchow, Arnold Mendelssohn, Hugo Rühle, Benno Reinhardt, and other young men oriented toward a scientific approach to medicine. After graduating with his MD, Traube spent several months in Vienna learning auscultation techniques with Joseph Skoda. Upon his return to Berlin, Traube began working in private practice, as academic careers were closed to Jews at this time. He nevertheless began to teach private courses in auscultation, using the patients who received poor relief assistance in Berlin as subjects, until the board of directors put a stop to this practice. Next Traube turned to experiments involving vivisection that he initially performed in his own home. Later Traube and his friends were able to use the facilities of the veterinarian school, where he conducted his famous experimental study on the 'pulmonary effects of dissecting the Vagus nerve'.

The turbulent months of the 1848 revolution brought Traube the academic opportunities that he had been denied for so long. Having received his Habilitation, Traube was able to enter the medical faculty of the Friedrich-Wilhelms-Universität in Berlin and to take up an appointment at the Charité Hospital in the same city, where he worked as Schönlein's assistant and as head of the ward for chest diseases. This made Traube the first civilian intern at the Charité, because this central Prussian hospital had formerly been exclusively reserved for the education of military surgeons.

At the Charité, Traube developed fruitful clinical research in auscultation, which resulted in the eponymous Traube's bruit, Traube's double tone, and Traube's space. He introduced the thermometer into clinical research and implemented a policy for the scientific measurement of hospital patients. Fever was previously regarded as characterized by rapid pulse and inner heat or shivering. Traube redefined it as high body temperature by outlining a new pathophysiological explanation. He also dealt with the issue of the treatment of fevers, testing cold water as well as digitalis or salicylic acid. He differentiated nephropathy from amyloidosis, as well as explaining high blood pressure in kidney diseases. Traube consistently argued for a close relation between experimental physiology and clinical medicine. Thus, following his programmatic principles concerning laboratory research in pathology, he typically tried to recreate his clinical observations in animal experiments. Combining clinical observation and the new physiology established by Emil Du Bois-Reymond, Ernst Brücke, and Hermann Helmholtz, Traube could be considered as one of the founders of German experimental pathology. Many researchers were also trained in Traube's laboratory, including such famous individuals as Julius Cohnheim, Ernst Leyden, Hermann Senator, and Theodor Billroth.

After Traube was appointed associate professor at the Medical Faculty in 1857, it appeared to be only a matter of time before the first-ever appointment of a Jew as full professor in Prussia. In 1857 Traube's ward was given the title of a teaching clinic. He rejected offers of professorships from Heidelberg and Breslau, preferring to stay in Berlin, even after Schönlein's retirement in 1859 deprived him of a valued colleague. Having succeeded to the chair of medicine, Frerichs began to challenge Traube's dominant position in Berlin medicine, but, after a hard fight, Traube was able to reinforce the position of his own clinic. In 1864 he was named professor at the Academy of Military Surgeons, and in 1865 he received the title of Medical Privy Councilor. He was also Director of the Department of Internal Medicine at the Jewish Hospital in Berlin. Finally, in 1872, Traube was promoted to a position equivalent to that of Frerichs, when he was appointed as both an ordinary professor at the faculty and a clinician at the Charité.

Bibliography

Primary: 1871–78. *Gesammelte Beiträge zur Pathologie und Physiologie* 3 vols. (Berlin).

Secondary: Hess, Volker, 2000. *Der Wohltemperierte Mensch* (Frankfurt am Main); Schmiedebach, Heinz-Peter, 1993. 'Pathologie bei Virchow und Traube. Experimentalstrategien in unterschiedlichem Kontext' in *Die Experimentalisierung des Lebens. Experimentalsysteme in den biologischen Wissenschaften 1850/1950* (Berlin) pp. 116–134; Berndt, H., 1981. *Zum Gedenken an Ludwig Traube (1818–1876)* (Baltimore).

Volker Hess

TREDGOLD, ALFRED FRANK (b. Derby, England, 5 November 1870; d. Guildford, Surrey, England, 17 September 1952), *mental deficiency, psychiatry.*

Tredgold, the son of a builder's foreman, Joseph Tredgold, and his wife, Bessey, studied medicine at Durham University and the London Hospital, winning prizes in anatomy, biology, physiology, pathology, and medicine. He qualified in 1899 and was immediately offered a research scholarship in insanity and neuropathology funded by the London County Council. Working at the Claybury Pathological Laboratory under the prominent psychiatrist Frederick Walker Mott (1853–1926), Tredgold began to focus particularly on the pathology of mental illness and deficiency. Although he entered general practice, he continued to work and publish in the field of mental deficiency, serving as consulting physician both to the National Association for Promoting the Welfare of the Feeble-Minded, founded in 1896, and to the Littleton Home for Defective Children.

In 1905 Tredgold was appointed as a medical investigator for the Royal Commission on the Care and Control of the Feeble-Minded, which provided the blueprint for the Mental Deficiency Act of 1913. In 1908 Tredgold published his influential textbook *Mental Deficiency (Amentia)*, in which he furnished a detailed account of the etiology, pathology, diagnosis, and treatment of all grades of deficiency. This book, which was based on his extensive clinical experience and which was illustrated with numerous tables, family histories, and photographs, established Tredgold's reputation as an expert in the field and was published in eight editions before his death. The later editions were prepared with the help of his son, Roger Francis Tredgold (1911–75), who continued to edit the book after Tredgold's death.

Tredgold regarded mental deficiency primarily as an inherited condition, linked to other forms of constitutional disease and social inadequacy such as alcoholism, syphilis, tuberculosis, epilepsy, and criminality. Mobilizing photographs of the anatomical anomalies (such as abnormalities of the skull and facial features) that were supposedly more common in defectives, Tredgold insisted that mental defectives were separated by an 'impassable gulf' from the normal population. Accordingly, he suggested that diagnosis should be based on careful physical examination by experienced clinicians, and he advocated treatment in special educational facilities, such as those established by Mary Dendy (1855–1933) in Manchester. His views were particularly influential in providing support for segregatory policies designed both to remove the 'social residuum' from the streets and to prevent defectives from producing more children.

Tredgold was also an important figure in the Eugenics Education Society, founded in 1907, presenting the Galton lecture to the Society in 1927. He published numerous articles in the *Eugenics Review* and in contemporary medical journals, in which he publicized the social dangers posed by the feeble-minded. In addition, he was a key figure in the National Association for Mental Health and subsequently expanded his views on mental diseases in his *Manual of Psychological Medicine*, first published in 1943.

Having fought in Gallipoli and Egypt during World War I, Tredgold returned home in 1916, suffering from dysentery. Over the following decades, while working primarily as a physician in psychological medicine at the London Hospital, he became increasingly influential in political and public debates about mental deficiency, serving on committees of the British Medical Association and the Board of Education during the 1920s. In the early 1930s he was a member of the government committee that, in its final report published in 1934, recommended the voluntary sterilization of mental defectives. In 1929 Tredgold was elected FRCP.

Bibliography

Primary: 1908. *Mental Deficiency (Amentia)* (London); 1909–10. 'The feeble-minded—a social danger.' *Eugenics Review* 1: 97–104; 1910. 'The feeble-minded.' *The Contemporary Review* 98: 717–727; 1911–12. 'Eugenics and the future progress of man.' *Eugenics Review* 3: 94–117; 1917. 'Moral imbecility.' *The Practitioner* 99: 43–56.

Secondary: Jackson, Mark, 2000. *The Borderland of Imbecility: Medicine, Society and the Fabrication of the Feeble Mind in Late Victorian and Edwardian England* (Manchester); Thomson, Mathew, 1998. *The Problem of Mental Deficiency: Eugenics, Democracy, and Social Policy in Britain, c. 1870–1959* (Oxford); *Munk's Roll*; *Oxford DNB*.

Mark Jackson

TREVES, FREDERICK (b. Dorchester, Dorset, England, 15 February 1853; d. Lausanne, Switzerland, 7 December 1923), *surgery.*

The son of a Dorset furniture maker, Treves received his early education from the 'Dorset poet' and polymath Rev William Barnes, before briefly attending Dorchester Grammar School and then, in May 1864, the Merchant Taylors' School, London. In 1871 he began medical studies at University College London, but attended for only a few months before beginning his training at the London Hospital. He obtained his diploma from the Society of Apothecaries (1874) and a year later gained his MRCS. The following year, he became the resident medical officer at the Royal National Hospital for Scrofula, Margate, where his elder brother William (1843–1908), FRCS, was honorary surgeon. After returning to Dorchester to take a bride, Treves bought a share in a practice in Derbyshire (1877), but in 1879, after obtaining his FRCS, he returned to the London Hospital to fill the post of surgical registrar. He was promoted to assistant surgeon there in the same year, to surgeon in 1884, and, finally, to consulting surgeon (1898) when, at the age of forty-five, he retired from the hospital in order to manage his extensive and hugely lucrative private practice based at 6 Wimpole Street. A decade later, he retired, devoting himself to performing public work, traveling, and writing books.

Treves was relentlessly ambitious and, like others of his generation who made their way into the medical elite, something of an ideologue of the work ethic. He rose every morning at 5:00 A.M. to spend two hours writing before commencing professional duties. His *Surgical Applied Anatomy* (1883), which reached the standard of a medical classic and, revised, remained in print until 1947, was the first of his publications to give full play to his not-inconsiderable literary talents. Several other more literary productions followed, including *The Tale of a Field Hospital* (1900), based on his experience in the Boer War; *The Other Side of the Lantern: An Account of a Commonplace Tour Round the World* (1905); *Highways and Byeways of Dorset* (1906); and, shortly before his death, *The Elephant Man and Other Reminiscences* (1923), which remains in print and was made into a film by David Lynch in 1980.

Treves achieved international fame (and a baronetcy) in 1902 when, two days before the coronation of Edward VII, the future king was diagnosed as suffering from an abscess on his appendicitis, which Treves successfully drained. Since the 1880s, when 'appendicitis surgery' had become more technically feasible and increasingly socially fashionable, Treves had carved himself a sizeable niche the field. It was almost wholly around this that his private practice revolved, while his leadership in general surgery rapidly fell into decline. Ironically, he was unable to save his youngest daughter from dying from appendicitis in 1900.

Although a conservative surgeon, Treves was radical in his advocacy of the need for operating on the appendix. Something of a showman, and dogmatic as a lecturer, he relished controversy over his opinions, just as he thrived on acrimonious institutional politics. In faith, too, he was 'muscular' and was proud to be appointed president of the evangelical Royal National Mission to Deep Sea Fishermen, to which his protégé, Wilfred Grenfell (1865–1940) was appointed surgeon. A keen sailor himself (he passed the Trinity House exams to become a Master Marine in 1892), Treves was a great supporter of open-air Christianity. It was within this militaristic frame in 1892 that he published a text on physical education. He also had more than a passing interest in the history of medicine, becoming in 1913 the vice president of the new Section of History of Medicine presided over by William Osler (1849–1919).

Bibliography

Primary: 1886. (ed.) *A Manual of Surgery* (London); 1892. *The Student's Handbook of Surgical Operations* (London); 1895. *A System of Surgery* 2 vols. (London).

Secondary: Gibbs, D. D., 1992. 'Sir Frederick Treves, Surgeon, Author and Medical Historian.' *Journal of the Royal Society of Medicine* 85: 565–569; Trombley, Stephen. 1989. *Sir Frederick Treves: The Extra-Ordinary Edwardian* (London); *Plarr's Lives*; *Oxford DNB*.

Roger Cooter

TRONCHIN, THÉODORE (b. Republic of Geneva [now Switzerland], 24 May 1709; d. Paris, France, 30 November 1781), *medicine, smallpox inoculation.*

Tronchin was the son of a banker, Jean-Robert Tronchin, and Angélique Calandrini, the daughter of a prestigious Italian family established in Geneva for several generations. Following his mother's early death, his father's second wife, Marthe-Marie Caussade, brought up Théodore in the countryside around Geneva. At the age of seven, he was sent to the school set up by Calvin, Geneva College, and, at the age of fourteen, as was customary, he moved on to the Academy of Geneva, where he followed classes in theology. In 1723 his father's difficult financial situation encouraged him to move to England, where he could count on the patronage of Lord Bolingbroke. The following year, he studied at Cambridge, without being officially registered, and there he decided to study medicine. The decision, prompted by his reading a book written by the famous Dutch physician Herman Boerhaave (1668–1738), induced him to consider studying in Holland. In 1727 he spent some months in London, walking the wards of the main hospitals. He then moved to Holland (where a branch of his family was established) and registered as a medical student in Leiden on 13 September 1728, becoming one of Boerhaave's students. On 22 August 1730, aged twenty-one, he graduated with a thesis about the clitoris, *De nympha*, and was awarded his MD.

After having been made a citizen of Amsterdam (26 October 1730) and admitted into the College of Physicians (31 October 1730) of that town, Tronchin established a private practice there. He profited from Boerhaave's protection, and he was soon to be recognized as his disciple, although he was not seriously considered as a potential successor after the latter's death in 1738. Tronchin remained in Amsterdam for twenty-four years. The war resulting from the troubled succession of Austria's throne, the consequent change in government in Holland, and a negative perception of the luxury in which the Dutch lived and their perspectives for the future all encouraged him to leave the country. After having declined the position of first physician to the Stathouder, he resigned from the College of Physicians on 8 December 1754 and returned to Geneva.

The arrival in Geneva of Tronchin, an international figure with invitations to establish himself in foreign courts, was met with great enthusiasm by most of the inhabitants but provoked jealousy in others. The city council, prompted by the Academy's senate, decided to establish a professorship in medicine for Tronchin without officially consulting the medical guild; in consequence, the guild persistently refused to admit him as a member. Tronchin therefore remained for ten years in the ambiguous situation of being the only professor of medicine in town, the most prestigious and sought after physician in the local medical marketplace, but the only medical doctor not to be officially licensed to practice medicine!

Tronchin published sparsely, and no important medical discovery can be associated with his name. He was, above all, a clinician and a great believer in the healing capacities of nature, and he regularly condemned excessive phlebotomy. In short, he was an advocate of noninterventionist therapies, an attitude that helped place him above the medical debates of the day. In certain circumstances, Tronchin, the careful physician, was also capable of taking risks when he thought the well-being of the patient was at stake, e.g., in his attitude to inoculation. As a father, in Amsterdam, he was among the first to inoculate his children in 1748 and thereafter one of the most ardent advocates of that procedure in Holland and then, from 1754, in Geneva.

Tronchin's prudence enjoined him to practice inoculation only in the most favorable circumstances. He carefully controlled the patient's diet and lifestyle in order to give the best chances of good health. In 1756 he played a symbolic role in promoting inoculation in France, where the practice had almost died out after the accidental death of a fourteen-year-old the previous year. Called upon by the Duke of Orléans to inoculate his children, the young Duke of Chartres and his sister Mlle de Montpensier, he secretly traveled to Paris and proceeded to inoculate both children. The operation was a success and contributed to putting inoculation back into fashion. On returning to Geneva, Tronchin helped associate the name of the town with inoculation, and many patients flocked to Geneva in order to consult him or to be inoculated by him. He also played an important role in promoting inoculation in Italy by inoculating the son of the Duke of Parma in 1764.

Tronchin was a member of many foreign academies and societies, but he was also a friend to his patients. Throughout his career, he was both a fashionable and a sociable doctor. He befriended many of the eminent families of his time and philosophers such as the Duke of Jaucourt, with whom he had studied, Voltaire, Rousseau, Diderot, and Grimm.

In 1766, possibly encouraged by the growing political tensions in Geneva, Tronchin accepted the position of first physician to the Duke of Orléans and moved to Paris. His medical practice there was often controversial because, through his responsibilities as physician to prominent members of the Royal Household, colleagues regularly attacked him. The death in March 1767 of Maire-Josèphe, the Dauphine, who had been treated by Tronchin, unleashed a great deal of hostility.

Bibliography

Secondary: Lindeboom, G. A., 1958. 'Tronchin and Boerhaave.' *Gesnerus* 15: 141–150; Tronchin, Henry, 1906. *Un médecin au XVIIIe siècle. Théodore Tronchin, 1709–1781 d'après des documents inédits* (Paris).

Philip Rieder

TROTA OF SALERNO (AND THE *TROTULA*)   (fl. Salerno, Italy, twelfth century), *medicine, women's health.*

It is a peculiar effect of medieval history that this entry should grant equal 'biographical' status to a medical author and practitioner, Trota of Salerno, and to a text named after her, the *Trotula*. Only one part of what became known as the *Trotula*—a compendium of materials on women's diseases, cosmetics, and even some andrology and pediatrics—can be linked directly to a twelfth-century Salernitan healer named Trota (or, as her name would have been spelled locally, Trocta), but it was the *Trotula* that was to have the most widespread historical impact, circulating all over medieval Western Europe and being translated at least twenty-one different times prior to 1500. Already by the early thirteenth century, people began to believe that 'Trotula' was not the title of the composite work, but the name of its author. This medieval misperception, in turn, led later philologists to question whether a woman could have authored such a work (which, in the parts we now know were not authored by Trota, there is a relatively high level of engagement with Galenic humoral theory). Debates about 'Trotula's' existence persisted until, in the 1980s and 1990s, new philological studies were able to untangle the textual history of the *Trotula* and identify the core elements of the text that can legitimately be connected with the historic Trota. Important as that work has been, it is still of historical interest why 'Trotula' and the larger question of women's capacities as medical authors have been such a persistent point of debate in medical history.

What we know of the historic Trota is almost entirely drawn from works attributed to her. In this respect, she is not unlike her twelfth-century male Salernitan peers, for whom, in most cases, we likewise have no biographical information other than what we can reconstruct from their writings. Salerno developed a reputation for the excellence of its empirical medical practices as early as the tenth century, and by the twelfth century, its most active period, it was distinguished for its theoretical medicine as well. Modern popular accounts often state that 'Trotula' was an eleventh-century figure; this supposed chronology rests solely on claims by a nineteenth-century historian that 'Trotula' was uninfluenced by the works of Constantine the African, a native North African who had come to southern Italy in the 1070s and translated several major Arabic medical works into Latin. In fact, one of the three *Trotula* texts (called *Conditions of Women*) is directly drawn from a Constantinian translation, the *Viaticum* of Ibn al-Ğazzār, and most likely dates from the first half of the twelfth century. Another text, *Women's Cosmetics*, opens with a direct quotation from Constantine's translation of the Hippocratic *Prognostics*. Trota herself likely flourished in the early or middle decades of the twelfth century, although there is currently no documentary evidence to pin her chronology down more precisely.

Trota's *oeuvre* is documented by three texts, none of which, apparently, present her work in the form she originally composed it, but all of which taken together show that she was an empirical practitioner of considerable clinical breadth. Her *Practical Medicine According to Trota* (in Latin, *Practica secundum Trotam*) is now extant in only two copies and is only a small portion of what once must have been a larger compendium. The *Practical Medicine* is a largely disordered assembly of cures for a variety of conditions from menstrual disorders to snakebites, from hair lice to burns, cancer, frenzy, eye problems, sprained foot, excessive sweat, toothache, scrofula, spleen problems, depilatories, hemorrhoids, and fevers. The text has no preface, nor are there any indications within the work to suggest what inspired Trota to record her practices. There are no references to fellow Salernitan practitioners, case histories, or other information that would help us date or localize the text.

The reason for believing that Trota's *Practical Medicine* had once been an even more sizable compendium comes from a different work, an anonymous compilation made in the late twelfth century called *On Treatment for Diseases* [*De egritudinum curatione*]. Found uniquely in a now-lost codex from Wroclaw, Poland, *Treatment for Diseases* is a very careful synthesis of excerpts from seven of the leading twelfth-century Salernitan medical masters: Johannes Platearius, Copho, Petrus Musandinus, Bartholomeus, Johannes Afflacius, Johannes Ferrarius, and Trota, whose name alone is never preceded by the honorific 'M.' for 'master' (magister). Here, the excerpts explicitly attributed to Trota range from treatments for epilepsy to eye diseases; conditions of the ears, gums, and teeth; and conditions of the respiratory and, most extensively, the digestive systems. Some of these excerpts are new; some of them overlap with material in her *Practical Medicine* (and often they are more extensive in *Treatment for Diseases*, thus suggesting the considerable size of Trota's original text). Some of them, moreover, overlap with a third text attributed to Trota, *Treatments for Women* [*De curis mulierum*].

Treatments for Women is the 'core' text of the *Trotula* ensemble, and it explains why, when *Conditions of Women* and *Women's Cosmetics* were later attached to it, the entire ensemble was called the *Trotula* (literally, 'the little Trota' or perhaps 'the abbreviated Trota'). Unlike *Conditions of Women*, which, as noted previously, was composed (probably by a male author) by adapting bits and pieces of the *Viaticum*, Trota's *Treatments for Women* relies not at all on previous gynecological texts, but is an entirely independent piece of work. Moreover, it reflects clear 'hands-on' practices, suggesting that its author had unmediated access to her female patients' genitalia, something that would not have been true of a male practitioner in this period. *Treatments for Women* may have been compiled, not directly by Trota herself, but out of her oral expositions about her practice, to which an anonymous redactor added various embellishments (including a case history in which Trota, referred to here in the third person, cures a young woman of 'wind in the womb' by carefully distinguishing a uterine disorder

from a supposed intestinal one). Also added were several references to the theories or practices of some male Salernitan practitioners, including Copho and Johannes Ferrarius. If they were in fact Trota's contemporaries, this would confirm her period of activity as the second quarter of the twelfth century.

In neither Copho's nor Ferrarius's works, nor in any other known Salernitan work, do we find further mention of Trota. The name Trota (or Trocta) became rather popular among southern Italian women after the 1080s, so we have no way of knowing at this point if any of the many dozens of 'Troctas' we find in Salernitan documents from the period are identical to this particular practitioner. Nevertheless, we do know that Trota was not unique as a female healer in Salerno, for Copho and several other male writers speak of the practices of the *mulieres Salernitane* ('the Salernitan women'). The *mulieres* are attributed with a variety of practices involving 'simple' medicines (i.e., uncompounded vegetable, mineral, or animal ingredients). Thus, for example, the *mulieres* are said to use oppoponax to treat epilepsy in children, calamint for drying out uterine superfluities, and aloe mixed with rose water to treat superficial swellings. There are, moreover, several interesting correspondences between practices we find in Trota's work and those attributed to the *mulieres*. For example, Johannes Platearius notes that the *mulieres* use cabbage leaves for pustules of the penis (one of several examples where it is clear that women practiced certain elements of andrology as well as care of themselves and their children). In Trota's *Treatments for Women*, we find a virtually identical treatment. What the *mulieres* and Trota also have in common is that they rarely seem to employ compound medicines and their range of materia medica seems overall to be less expansive than what is known to be have been employed by their male contemporaries. For example, neither the *mulieres* nor Trota ever seem to use sugar as an ingredient, which had come into regular use by male practitioners in the early twelfth century. In fact, the only thing that seems to broadly distinguish Trota from the other *mulieres* is that, for reasons we cannot yet explain, she crossed the boundary into the literate aspects of medicine, whereas the other *mulieres* never did.

Even if fellow Salernitan medical writers never mentioned her, Trota clearly developed a reputation outside of Italy for her medical practices. An early or mid-thirteenth century cosmetic writer repeatedly claims to have drawn some of his practices from 'Dame Trote', and the satiric French poet, Rutebeuf, crafted a savage caricature of her in his mid-thirteenth century parody of itinerant charlatans. As noted previously, Trota's work was not limited to women's medicine, and Rutebeuf gives no indication that he thinks she was the only expert in that field. Nevertheless, it was not Trota as the empiric of wide competence, but 'Trotula' as the expert on 'women's nature' that was to have the most widespread medieval fame. Although Trota's *Practical Medicine* seems to have been quickly forgotten (it was not to

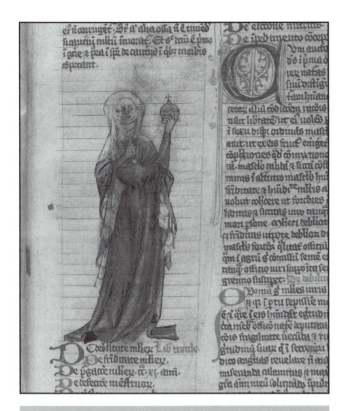

Trotula holding a urine flask. Pen and wash drawing from *Miscellanea Medica XVIII*, early fourteenth century. Archives and Manuscripts, Wellcome Library, London.

be rediscovered until 1985), the *Trotula* is now extant in over 130 copies, plus a variety of medieval translations. It was 'Trotula' the expert on women who was to be noted in a variety of contexts, including, most famously, in Chaucer's *Wife of Bath's Prologue* in the *Canterbury Tales*.

Male physicians relied heavily on the *Trotula* for their knowledge of women's medicine well into the fourteenth century. Thereafter, new gynecological texts (in addition to the substantial sections on women's diseases to be found in many medical encyclopedias) gradually eclipsed the *Trotula*. It was 'rediscovered' in 1544 when a German humanist physician, Georg Kraut, found a copy and decided to 'clean it up', rearranging the (unbeknownst to him) three different component texts into one more smoothly ordered tract on women's diseases. Moreover, Kraut attempted to weed the text of what he assumed were medieval corruptions; apparently, he believed the text to be of ancient origin, and his presentation of it as such was accepted for several decades. This assumption in turn led to another creative act of emendation: a philologist hypothesized that the author was not 'Trotula' but 'Eros', presumed to have been the freedman of the Roman empress Julia. Thus, by 1566, 'Trotula' had been eliminated as author of the text, and the debate about the text's authenticity was born.

A few believers in 'Trotula's' existence as a female author could still be found after the sixteenth century. In 1681 the Salernitan medical historian Antonio Mazza made the most important contribution to her postmedieval fame when he alleged that she, as well as several other women, had actually held professorial chairs at the University of Salerno. This assertion (counterintuitive though it may be, since Salerno had no university prior to the thirteenth century) was found to be attractive, both to later Salernitan historians and, at the beginning of the twentieth century, to first-wave feminist historians when they began to craft histories of women's place in medicine. The recent philological researches that have now separated the hitherto conjoined twins, Trota and 'Trotula', together with the modern theoretical perspectives of women's and gender history, raise new and ultimately more interesting questions about the range of women's medical practices in pre-modern Europe and the circumstances that foster or hinder their development as medical authorities.

Bibliography

Primary: Hiersemann, Conrad, 1921. *Abschnitte aus der Practica des Trottus in der Salernitanischen Sammelschrift De Aegritudinum Curatione. Breslau Codex Salern. 1160–1170* Inaugural dissertation, University of Leipzig; 1967. (De Renzi, Salvatore, ed.) *Collectio Salernitana ossia documenti inediti, e trattati di medicina appartenenti alla scuola medica salernitana* 5 vols. (Bologna); 2001. (Green, Monica H., ed. and trans.) *The 'Trotula': A Medieval Compendium of Women's Medicine* (Philadelphia).

Secondary: Green, Monica H. (forthcoming). *The Masculine Birth of Gynecology*; Green, Monica H., 2000. *Women's Healthcare in the Medieval West: Texts and Contexts*, Variorum Collected Studies Series, CS680 (Aldershot); Green, Monica H., 2000. 'From "Diseases of Women" to "Secrets of Women": The Transformation of Gynecological Literature in the Later Middle Ages.' *Journal of Medieval and Early Modern Studies* 30: 5–39; Green, Monica H., 1999. 'In Search of an "Authentic" Women's Medicine: The Strange Fates of Trota of Salerno and Hildegard of Bingen.' *Dynamis: Acta Hispanica ad Medicinae Scientiarumque Historiam Illustrandam* 19: 25–54; Green, Monica H., 1996. 'The Development of the *Trotula*.' *Revue d'Histoire des Textes* 26: 119–203 (repr. in Green, 2000, *Women's Healthcare*, as Essay V); Benton, John F., 1985. 'Trotula, Women's Problems, and the Professionalization of Medicine in the Middle Ages.' *Bulletin of the History of Medicine* 59: 30–53.

Monica H. Green

TROTTER, THOMAS (baptized Melrose, Roxburghshire, Scotland, 3 August 1760; d. Newcastle upon Tyne, England, 5 September 1832), *naval medicine*.

Trotter was the second son and the third of five children of John Trotter, baker, and his wife, Alison. He was educated at Melrose and Kelso academy until 1777, when he studied medicine in Edinburgh. In 1779 he became a surgeon's mate in the Royal Navy, serving on the *Berwick* in the Channel Fleet, which sailed for the West Indies in 1780. For his treatment of the wounded at the battle of Dogger Bank (1781), he was promoted to surgeon.

In 1783, after the American wars ended, Trotter took ship as a surgeon on a Liverpool slaver, the *Brookes*, for a fourteen-month voyage to the West Indies. Trotter was appalled by the conditions aboard and became a lifelong abolitionist. Clinically, he observed 300 cases of scurvy among the 650 slaves. His first publication, in 1786, was devoted to this subject. On returning to England (1784), Trotter practiced as a surgeon-apothecary at Wooler in Northumberland. He attended William Cullen's (1710–90) lectures in Edinburgh and graduated MD with a thesis on inebriation. This formed the basis of a publication on drunkenness (1804). In this and his *View of the Nervous Temperament* (1807), Trotter launched an attack on the ills of the age, notably commercialization and urbanization. The result of modern civilization, he said, was a swathe of nervous ailments and a consequent addiction to sedatives, drugs in general, and alcohol. Later writers have seen in Trotter's work the first delineation of a new disease entity: alcoholism.

After graduating, Trotter rejoined the navy. In 1790 he was surgeon to *Royal William*, the flagship of Vice-Admiral Robert Roddam. In 1793 he was surgeon to the *Vengeance* on a voyage to the West Indies. In December of that year, Trotter was appointed second physician to the Royal Naval Hospital at Haslar. His work there formed the basis of *Remarks on the Establishment of Naval Hospitals with Hints for Their Improvement* (1795). In 1794 he was appointed physician to the Channel Fleet. He served in this capacity through 1794–95, finally leaving the navy in 1802. Throughout his career, Trotter pressed for reform of the medical department of the navy. He insisted, as James Lind (1716–94) had before him, that health aboard ships was determined by a variety of moral and physical factors: discipline, fresh air, cleanliness, and a good diet. Trotter, ever since his work on scurvy, had insisted on the importance of the latter. He esteemed Lind and increasingly stressed the role of citrus fruits, especially lemons, as part of the regimen necessary to prevent this disease. All these proposals were the other side of the campaign to promote the role and status of medical men in the navy. Trotter agitated for a rise in the pay of naval surgeons, and in part owing to his efforts, 200 surgeons were added to the half-pay list after the 'glorious first of June' of 1794.

After Trotter retired from sea, he practiced in Newcastle upon Tyne. He married Elizabeth Everitt in 1802. She died in 1804, eleven days after the birth of a son. In 1810 he married Isabella Dixon. They had two sons. In these years Trotter published poetry and a play. He agitated for reform of the working conditions of coal miners and wrote a treatise against impressment.

Bibliography

Primary: 1786. *Observations on the Scurvy* (Edinburgh); 1797–1803. *Medicine Nautica: An Essay on Diseases of Seamen* 3 vols. (London); 1804. *An Essay, Medical, Philosophical, and Chemical, on Drunkenness, and Its Effects on the Human Body* (London) [reprint 1988, Porter, Roy, ed. (London)].

Secondary: Carmichael, J., 1993. 'Thomas Trotter, 1760–1832, Physician to the Fleet' in Gardner-Medwin, D., A. Hargreaves, and E. Lazenby, eds., *Medicine in Northumbria: Essays on the History of Medicine in the North East of England* (Newcastle upon Tyne) pp. 164–192; Lloyd, Christopher, and Jack L. S. Coulter, 1961. *Medicine and the Navy. Volume III—1714–1815* (Edinburgh and London); *Oxford DNB*.

Christopher Lawrence

TROUSSEAU, ARMAND (b. Tours, France, 14 October 1801; d, Paris, France, 23 June 1867), *medicine, therapy.*

The son of an impecunious school teacher, Trousseau was orphaned quite young and depended upon a scholarship to study at the lycée at Orléans and the lycée at Lyon. Upon graduating, he spent two years teaching first in Tours, then at the Collège de Châteauroux in 1820, where he taught rhetoric. He left to study medicine with Pierre Bretonneau at Tours, from whom he learned the technique of tracheotomy for diphtheria and with whom he remained in contact throughout his life. He completed his studies at the École de Médecine, Paris. He entered the Hospice of Charenton as an interne, where he continued studies in anatomy and comparative pathology and obtained his medical degree in 1825. He won a place as agrégé professor in 1827.

In 1828 Trousseau was sent by the government to study epidemics in the Midi and then took part in the commission to study yellow fever in Gibraltar along with the physicians, Pierre Louis and Nicholas Chervin. He fell ill with that disease and was decorated on his return. Trousseau wrote an important memoir on veterinary medicine and surgery in 1828. He became a hospital physician in 1831, assisting Joseph Récamier for three years at the Hôtel Dieu. In 1837 he shared the grand prize of the Académie de Médecine with Hippolyte Belloc for work on laryngeal tuberculosis, chronic laryngitis, and diseases of the voice, in which he advocated medical practices of both Récamier and Bretonneau. This book was warmly received and translated into German and English.

From the Hôtel Dieu, Trousseau went to Saint Antoine Hospital. After publishing a widely praised treatise on therapeutics in 1836, he competed successfully for the chair of therapeutics at the Paris Faculté de Médecine, where his teaching attracted a wide following. Trousseau played a political role in 1848 as a deputy from Eure-et-Loir in the Constituent Assembly, where he demonstrated a liberal and independent turn of mind. In 1850 he transferred to the clinical chair at the Hôtel Dieu, the leading Paris hospital appointment, where he became a remarkable clinician. During this period he published a number of books as well as numerous journal articles on tracheotomy, typhoid fever, and his clinical cases at the hospital. One of his best-known students, Guillaume Duchenne de Boulogne, first studied paralytic disease while in his service. In 1852, Trousseau took over A.-F. Chomel's chair in internal medicine when

Chomel, an Orléanist, refused to swear allegiance to the new regime of Napoleon III. In 1856 Trousseau was elected to the Académie de Médecine.

Ackerknecht considered Trousseau the last 'great man' of the clinical school and the best remembered. An eclectic physician, he was opposed to dogmatic theories and published a treatise on eclectic medicine in 1861. At the end of his life, Trousseau rejected both new diagnostic methods and laboratory medicine, possibly because of his unusual skill at physical diagnosis.

Bibliography

Primary: 1836–39. *Traité de thérapeutique et de matière médicale* 2 vols. (Paris); 1851. *Nouvelles recherches sur la trachéotomie pratiquée sur la période extrême du croup* (Paris); 1861. *Clinique médicale de l'Hôtel-Dieu de Paris* 2 vols. (Paris) [English edn., 1867–72, 5 vols. (London)].

Secondary: Peumery, Jean-Jacques, 2003. 'Armand Trousseau (1801–1867), 'médecin français par excellence.' *Histoire des sciences médicales* 37(2): 151–156; Ackerknecht, Erwin H., 1967. *Medicine at the Paris Hospital 1794–1848* (Baltimore) pp. 112–113: Hahn, Lucien, 1902. *La Grande Encyclopédie, inventaire raisonné des sciences, des lettres et des arts* (Berthelot et al., eds.) 31: 434 (Paris); Triaire, Paul, 1892. *Bretonneau et ses correspondants; ouvrage comprenant la correspondance de Trousseau et de Velpeau avec Bretonneau.* (Paris).

Joy Harvey

TROWELL, HUBERT CAREY   (b. Bexley, Kent, England, 8 August 1904; d. Salisbury, England, 23 July 1989), *medicine, nutrition, medical education.*

Trowell is most renowned for his nutritional work in East Africa. His father, William, was an active congregational minister, and his mother, Mabel, formerly worked as a Baptist missionary in China. Together they provided their three children with a strong Christian upbringing. Trowell's interest in a medical career was said to stem from his early experiences coping with tuberculosis, unfortunate circumstances that kept him out of Reigate Grammar School (1913–23) and in constant contact with doctors for three years. His desire to serve in the Colonial Medical Service was shaped by both the postwar idealism prevalent during Trowell's years at St Thomas's Hospital Medical School (1924–29) and his involvement in the Christian Student Movement.

Trowell was an accomplished student whose education was financed through awards and scholarships. Although his chief at St Thomas's, Dr Birley, cautioned Trowell not to join the Colonial Medical Service, Trowell was not so easily discouraged. Soon after taking his medical degree (1929) and gaining some experience as a houseman at St Thomas's under Sir Maurice Cassidy, Trowell secured a colonial appointment and set out for Kenya. Immediately upon taking up his first post, Trowell began pressing for improvements in the provision of medical supplies and services. His concern for African health and his willingness to criticize colonial medical practices was not well received and led to his transfer on more than one occasion. In 1933 Trowell took charge of the African Medical Training Depot in Nairobi and earned his Membership in the Royal College of Physicians, and he later became the first doctor in East Africa to be elected FRCP (1945). Unfortunately for Trowell, the white-settler politics then predominant in Kenya made one of his primary interests, the training of African medical personnel, an unpopular assignment. Uganda, on the other hand, provided a much more fertile environment for these educational ambitions; the Ugandan Makerere Medical School was already a blossoming focal point for the medical training of Africans in sub-Saharan Africa. For this reason, Trowell was only too delighted to transfer and join the colonial medical staff in Uganda when given the opportunity in 1937.

Trowell spent the next twenty years instructing students, treating patients, and conducting research in Uganda. His enduring commitment to medical training is evident in the two instructional manuals that he promptly published (1937 and 1939) and in his efforts to involve students in research. Trowell focused his research on finding the cause of an unrecognized and highly morbid illness he encountered among his pediatric patients, first in Kenya and then in Uganda. After more than a decade, and in spite of resistance from superiors and colleagues, Trowell and Jack Davies finally determined that the illness was due to a diet deficient in protein. These discoveries were part of a major breakthrough in nutritional science in which the disease, kwashiorkor, became progressively elucidated and understood.

In 1959 Trowell retired from the Colonial Medical Service in order to complete a study of the contrasting disease patterns in African and economically developed populations (1960). This work led to his most notable contribution to nutritional science, the identification (with Denis Burkitt) of dietary fiber as an essential nutrient lacking in processed food. After returning to England, Trowell sought ordination at Wells Theological College (1960), and, although he remained engaged in his medical and nutritional work up until his death, he was increasingly occupied with religion and ethics in the later years of his life.

Bibliography

Primary: 1937. *A Handbook for Dressers and Nurses in the Tropics* (London); 1939. *Diagnosis and Treatment of Diseases in the Tropics* (London); 1954. *Kwashiorkor* (London); 1960. *Non-Infective Disease in Africa* (London); 'Dr. Hugh Trowell OBE, MD, FRCP.' MSS.Afr.s. 1872 (144A), Rhodes House Library, Oxford.

Secondary: Iliffe, John, 1998. *East African Doctors: A History of the Modern Profession* (Cambridge); Bray, Elizabeth, c.1988. 'Hugh Trowell: Pioneer Nutritionist' (unpublished manuscript, Wellcome Library for the History and Understanding of Medicine, London); *Munk's Roll.*

Jennifer Tappan

TRUDEAU, EDWARD LIVINGSTON (b. New York, New York, USA, 5 October 1848; d. Saranac Lake, New York, USA, 15 November 1915), *tuberculosis, medicine.*

The third child born to a physician father and a mother whose father was a French physician, Trudeau was educated in Paris from 1851 to 1865. About to enter a U.S. Naval college, he elected to care for his brother, who had rapidly progressing tuberculosis. After his brother's death and various jobs, on impulse he entered the College of Physicians and Surgeons (later Columbia University), New York, graduating in 1871 after appointment as house physician to the Strangers Hospital.

During his training Trudeau developed a cold abscess, not then recognized as a feature of tuberculosis, and just after graduation, there were obviously tuberculous glands in his neck. After practicing on Long Island and in New York City, in 1875 he was found to have extensive tuberculosis of his left lung. Advised to go south, he chose the then-remote Adirondacks, staying at St Regis, New York. The results were so good that he decided to over-winter there, and next year, he moved to Saranac Lake, where he remained until his death. Trudeau had not expected to survive and so, financially comfortable, initially spent his time hunting and shooting. Nevertheless, in 1880 he started practicing medicine again, and two years later, after reading about Bremer's sanitarium in Silesia for tuberculosis, he decided to build a similar institution at Saranac. The beginnings were humble—a small cottage, costing $400, known as 'The Little Red'—but gradually more wards were built, with places for the poor added through public subscriptions together with a nurses' home, chapel, occupational therapy department, and offices. Subsequently, other physicians joined the team.

Once Robert Koch had discovered the causative organism, Trudeau built a laboratory, becoming expert in mycobacterial staining and exhorting other physicians to use the technique. He was advised by two eminent physician-friends, William Osler (who mentioned the Sanitarium in his *Principles and Practice of Medicine*) and William Welch (who had worked with Koch in Germany). He also participated in the unsuccessful therapeutic use of tuberculin and became a recognized world expert on all aspects of tuberculosis. Such was its fame that the sanitarium movement began to spread throughout the United States: by 1909, no fewer than 352 private and State institutions had been built. One of the famous who came to Saranac Lake was the author Robert Louis Stevenson, who was then, in 1887, not very ill and who subsequently became a lifelong friend of Trudeau. Tragically, however, Trudeau's daughter developed tuberculosis; he never recovered from her death and that of his eldest son from a stroke, and these were associated with a relapse of his own illness.

Initially, Trudeau decided to admit only favorable cases to Saranac Lake, holding that the regimen was best suited for arresting early tuberculosis. After receiving criticism, he amended this policy, building a Reception Hospital for patients with advanced disease. Like most of the developments, which included new wards and a nurses' training school, this relied on donations from philanthropists, public appeals, and Trudeau's personal funds. At his death, the sanitarium could hold 150 patients and had expanded from its original sixteen acres to sixty, accommodating thirty-six buildings.

Though any benefits of the sanitarium regimen were never subjected to formal trials, Trudeau was a major influence on the development of ideas about tuberculosis. He had been taught that the disease was noncontagious but generally incurable, being inherited and due to constitutional peculiarities. By the time of his death, his example and proselytizing had persuaded physicians and the general public not only of the need to segregate patients with open disease and of the benefits of a regulated regimen, but also that screening by staining for acid-fast bacilli was vital in early diagnosis. Until streptomycin was introduced, his example was the bedrock of the medical management of the so-called white plague.

Bibliography

Primary: 1899. 'The Adirondack Cottage Sanitarium for the Treatment of Incipient Pulmonary Tuberculosis' *Practitioner* 62[n.s. vol 9]: 131–146; 1916. *An Autobiography* (Philadelphia).

Secondary: Ellison, David L., 1994. *Healing Tuberculosis in the Woods: Medicine and Science at the End of the Nineteenth Century* (Westport, CT); *DAMB.*

Stephen Lock

TRUETA I RASPALL, JOSEP (b. Barcelona, Spain, 28 October 1897; d. Barcelona, 19 January 1977), *orthopedic surgery.*

Trueta was a member of a dynasty of physicians: his father was a doctor and his great-grandfather a surgeon in the Navy. After primary education at the religious *Escuelas Pías*, he followed the secondary school at the *Instituto General y Técnico*. He studied medicine at Barcelona Medical School (1916–21). A year later he obtained the doctorate, becoming resident at the *Santa Creu i Sant Pau* Hospital (Barcelona) under Manuel Corachán, professor of surgery. In 1933 he became assistant of the Chair of Surgery at the University of Barcelona and was appointed surgeon-in-chief at the Hospital.

During the decade 1929 to 1939, he was head of the surgical service of the *Caja de Previsión y Socorro,* an insurance company assisting about 40,000 accidents a year. At the beginning of the Spanish Civil War, Trueta was in a strategic position: head of surgery at the largest hospital of Catalonia and also at the largest insurance company. He was a liberal-conservative and did not assume any political responsibility during the Second Spanish Republic. When the advance of Franco's troops anticipated the outcome of the war, he was uncertain about remaining in Barcelona, but, being convinced that Catalonia would be devastated by the winner, he went into exile. In 1939 he had a solid scientific background and was a member of the Sociedad de Cirugía de Barcelona (1928), the Société Internationale de Chirurgie (1932), the Association Française de Chirurgie (1933), the Sociedad Española de Cirugía Ortopédica y Traumatología (1935), the Acadèmia i Laboratori de Ciències Mèdiques, the Societat de Cirurgia de Catalunya, and the Società Italiana di Anestesia e di Analgesia.

Arrival in England

On 3 February 1939 Trueta crossed the border to France, as did thousands of Spanish refugees, and got in touch with two British surgeons who invited him to England to discuss the best strategy for the civil defense of London. Without money or documentation, Trueta traveled to London, where he discussed the most suitable sanitary organization in the light of foreseeable German aerial attacks. The international conflict represented a threat for the care of the population, and a controversy was triggered in the British medical press. In addition, the accepted practice for the treatment of war wounds contradicted Trueta's experience during the Spanish Civil War, and his presence in London woke up the interest of surgeons to discuss the method he applied. He summarized his technique in *Lancet* and was invited to give a lecture to a selected group of British surgeons in the Royal Society of Medicine 14 July 1939. Shortly after, he received an invitation from G. R. Girdlestone to visit the orthopedic clinic in Oxford. Girdlestone obtained a fund of fifty pounds a month for Trueta and his family to remain in England for six months when the war started. As a provisional solution, he received a document from the Health Minister, as adviser to the Wingfield Hospital (Oxford), which allowed him to develop surgical operations without formal British medical accreditation.

The Treatment of War Wounds

As soon as the Spanish Civil War had begun, a great many wounded patients arrived on the surgical services. The dimension of the problem was unforeseeable, and Trueta thought it necessary to establish a protocol of action. The critical period for war wounds was about eight to ten hours after the provocation, and the final result could be anticipated at the end of the first week. Trying to avoid septic inflammation, some surgeons performed a succession of operations instead of a single initial one. But the use of the scalpel did not seem to prevent suppuration. The bacteria found excellent means of reproduction in the damaged soft tissue fragments. Trueta thought that the extirpation of all of the muscular tissue damaged by the wound was the best form of antisepsis. The better the cleansing, the more positive were the results. Four principles allowed him to obtain excellent results in the shortest period of time with the minimum of suffering for the patient: (a) immobilizing and pro-

tecting the wound; (b) avoiding the retention of fluids by means of drainage; (c) eliminating the dirt and bacteria by washing the wound and its surroundings with soap and water; and (d) applying treatment before bacteria reached the underlying healthy tissues. He thought that the best method to immobilize and protect a wound was surrounding the region with plaster and elevating the member. His results were spectacular. In 1938 a monograph was published in Catalan and immediately translated into English and Spanish. But Trueta's method was considered dangerous, and no other works gave support to his technique.

The greater difficulty derived from the reluctance of surgeons to plaster a wound and make resections of living tissues. But the numbers were undeniable: he had treated 1,073 patients by the end of the Spanish Civil War and only six of them were dead. Obviously, the aid of a good system of blood transfusions was necessary. According to Trueta, immobilization had a favorable effect because resting helped the natural defenses. Other immediate benefits were pain control, the fast disappearance of the shock, the recovery of sleeping and appetite, and a better consolidation of the fractured bone.

Orthopedic Surgery and Experimental Research at Oxford

When Trueta entered the Wingfield Morris Orthopaedic Hospital, G. R. Girdlestone had a reduced team of collaborators. The hospital had been created during World War I and was the only one in Oxford devoted to orthopedics. After some months working at the hospital, Trueta became a member of the Royal Society of Medicine, and a new Service for Accidents was inaugurated at the Radcliffe Infirmary (Oxford). Initially, the Canadian Jim Scott became head of that service, but, in 1942 he was required in the air force and Trueta assumed the post. The service initially had thirty beds and grew considerably during the next years.

Trueta gave more than eighty lectures between 1939 and 1944. Probably the most remarkable were the two given at the Royal Society of Medicine. During that period, the lack of official permission to work as a surgeon allowed him to carry out experimental investigations of wound treatment. With the aid of Girdlestone, he was accepted in the laboratory of Howard Florey in the William Dunn School of Pathology, where he started a fruitful collaboration with his team: Gardner, Chain, Scheontal, Abraham, Duthie, and Orr-Ewing. This laboratory pioneered the antibiotic era, introducing penicillin.

Scheontal called Trueta's attention to a recent publication devoted to biological antagonism between *B. pyocyaneus* and pyogenic microbes. This feature agreed with Trueta's observation in Barcelona of around seventy cases in which the presence of the *B. pyocyaneus* cleaned the wound of germs. The concept of 'biological antagonism' had been formulated in Trueta's book on the treatment of the war wounds and Scheontal suggested that he investigate its

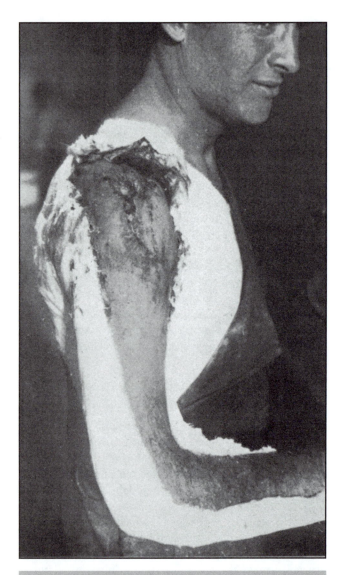

Severe gunshot wound of the shoulder with fracture of the humerus and soft tissue destruction treated by debridement and plaster. Photograph taken on removal of second plaster seventy days after injury. Halftone reproduction from *Treatment of War Wounds and Fractures . . . 1939*. Wellcome Library, London.

fundamental aspects of microcirculation in the kidneys. Another field of interest was the sequelae of poliomyelitis, which caused not only problems in development, but also dramatic respiratory paralyses in children during the final stage of the disease.

In 1949 Trueta was appointed to the chair of orthopedic surgery at the University of Oxford. In 1960 the clinical section of the Oxford Medical School included four Nuffield Chairs, one of them occupied by Trueta. With the foundation of the National Health Service, a change in the organization of the health care took place. Trueta considered that, whatever the effects of the new sanitary model, medical assistance was going to change during the following years. The chair offered him a unique opportunity to create a research center equipped with hospital facilities and a new laboratory, a room for x-rays, and a building for animal research. The institution designed by Trueta became a reference center where specialists met and young graduates became surgeons. Research in orthopedics was already impossible without hospital means, clinical x-ray apparatus, and other technical resources, external patients, and clinical files. The new center was inaugurated 27 October 1958 in the presence of the Queen Elizabeth and Lord Nuffield. It was the day of Trueta's sixty-first birthday.

Social Engagements

Although Trueta remained out of the Spanish Republican movements in his exile, he maintained close links with Spanish refugees. In 1946 he published a booklet entitled *The Spirit of Catalonia*, dedicated to his friend Pablo Casals, the 'great Catalan and big artist'. He showed a humanist dimension and a strong engagement with Catalan culture. After his retirement, he returned to Catalonia and published his memoirs (1978–80). He received an extensive list of distinctions. He was a member or honorary member of numerous societies around the world. Some days before Trueta's death, King Juan Carlos I bestowed on him the Great Cross of Charles III.

Bibliography

Primary: 1938. *Tractament de les fractures de guerra* (Barcelona) [English version, 1939, *Treatment of War Wounds and Fractures with Special Reference to the Closed Method as Used in the War in Spain* (London)]; 1943. *The Principles and Practice of War Surgery* (London); 1946. *The Spirit of Catalonia* (London); 1947. *Studies of the Renal Circulation* (Oxford); 1949. *An Atlas on Traumatic Surgery. Illustrated Histories of Wounds of the Extremities* (Oxford); 1956. (with Wilson, A. B. K., and M. Agerholm) *Handbook on Poliomyelitis* (Oxford); 1959. *Orthopaedics at Oxford. Past, Present & Future. Reflections after Ten Years in the Oxford Chair of Orthopaedic Surgery* (Oxford); 1971. *Girdlestone Orthopaedic Society* (London); 1978. *Fragments d'una vida* (Barcelona). [English version, 1980, *Trueta, Surgeon in War and Peace* (London)].

biological mechanisms. Trueta also investigated the influence of movement and immobilization of the limbs on lymphatic circulation and the effect on tissue absorption.

After a series of experimental works carried out in 1940 and 1941, Barnes and Trueta began to investigate traumatic shock after the German air raids. Trueta thought that a vascular and nervous factor could cause a spasm of the kidney's arteries, blocking blood circulation and the production of urine. The results were published in the *British Journal of Surgery* and demonstrated that a similar vascular spasm of the abdominal arterioles takes place when urine production is stopped.

In 1945 Trueta returned to experimental investigations of the physiological mechanisms of renal circulation, describing

Secondary: Barona, Josep Lluís, 2004. 'Josep Trueta I Raspall (1897–1977). La biografía científica de su exilio en Oxford.' *Laberintos* 3: 5–28; Prim, Josep M., 1997. *L'esperit de Josep Trueta.* (Barcelona); Rodrigo, Antonina. 1997. *Biografía del Dr. Trueta. Héroe anónimo de dos guerras* (Madrid); 1996. *Homenatge a Josep Trueta (1897–1977)* (Barcelona); *Oxford DNB.*

Josep Lluís Barona

TUỆ TĨNH 慧靖 (aka NGUYỄN, BÁ TĨNH, HỒNG NGHĨA) (b. Nghĩa Phú village, Vietnam, 1330; d. Nanjing, China *c.* 1389 or later), *Vietnamese traditional medicine, pharmacology, veterinary medicine.*

The Buddhist religious name Tuệ Tĩnh 慧靖 has been used by at least two men in Vietnam who were traditional healers as well as being Buddhist monks. Although to some extent the exploits of these two men have become merged in the popular imagination in Vietnam, the most important of the two is the earlier Tuệ Tĩnh 慧靖, who lived during the Trần Dynasty (1225–1400) and who is generally credited with having codified Vietnamese medicine, after he was sent as a living gift to the court of the Ming Dynasty (1368–1644) in China.

Early Life and Education

Tuệ Tĩnh 慧靖 was given the name Nguyễn Bá Tĩnh at birth. He was born in Nghĩa Phú village in present day Hải Dương province. After he became an orphan at the age of six, he was raised and educated by the Buddhist monks of two well-known pagodas in northern Vietnam. He studied not only the Buddhist classics but also Confucian texts in preparation for the imperial exams. He passed the exams at the age of twenty-two, but, instead of accepting the job as an official of the Trần Dynasty that his success had earned for him, he decided to become a monk, and he took the name Tuệ Tĩnh, meaning 'Tranquil Wisdom'.

Work as a Monk in Vietnam

At that time in Vietnam, it was common for Buddhist institutions to be involved in public health care, and, during the years when he lived in several different Buddhist monasteries, Tuệ Tĩnh 慧靖 became a highly respected doctor and pharmacist. He worked extensively with plants, growing or gathering many from the wild. He also prepared his own plants for use and made various powders, decoctions, and extracts from them. During this period of his life, Tuệ Tĩnh is credited with having founded medical gardens at several pagodas and with doing research into the medicinal properties of plants from many regions and microclimates in Vietnam. It was during this time that he acquired the nickname 'Master Hồng Nghĩa', referring to the fact that his home village was Nghĩa Phú in Thượng Hồng District.

It was also during this time that he compiled the first of his two classic works on Vietnamese medicine, *Hồng Nghĩa*

giác tư y thư [Medical Books by Hong Nghia]. His medical philosophy, as expressed in this and in his later work, consisted of several points. First, it is best to maintain good health through an appropriate diet relying on seasonal local fruits and vegetables and a lifestyle of adequate physical exercise and moderation in hedonistic activities. As a counterpoint, he discouraged the use and consumption of imported foodstuffs and medicaments. He also felt that the plant life of Vietnam, if properly investigated and used, was superior for the Vietnamese people to imported Chinese medicines, which often contained parts of one or more animal species. To this day, the defining difference between Chinese medicine, as practiced in Vietnam, and what the Vietnamese refer to as 'Southern' medicine, meaning Vietnamese medicine, is that Vietnamese medicaments are derived almost exclusively from plants.

Tuệ Tĩnh's medical philosophy is often summed up in the phrase 'Vietnamese medicine for Vietnamese people'. In its most profound sense, this philosophy assumes a physical and spiritual relationship between human beings and the land where they live and asserts that the earth, air, and water of a given place produce foodstuffs and medicines that are uniquely suited to the constitutions of people born and raised there.

The *Medical Books by Hong Nghia* presented this medical philosophy in poetic format that made it easy to remember for ordinary people, many of whom were illiterate. This text addressed the common everyday afflictions of ordinary people and of their livestock. Since most of the ingredients for his prescriptions, whether for maintaining health or treating disorders, could be found in or around most village gardens or in the surrounding forests, this work became the standard practical medical reference, centuries before it was first printed in 1717, for both Vietnamese families and Vietnamese traditional healers. It is still regularly used and consulted today.

China

At the time Tuệ Tĩnh lived, Vietnam, although independent, was required to regularly send tribute to China. Such tribute often included people with special talents or skills. When he was fifty-five, Tuệ Tĩnh was arrested and sent to China with the tribute mission of 1385, as a gift to the Ming royal family. Tuệ Tĩnh had a very successful career in China at the court of the Ming Dynasty. He is reported to have saved the life of a Chinese Empress who suffered severe postnatal complications. Tuệ Tĩnh's second major medical treatise, the *Nam Dược Thần Hiệu* 南藥神效 [Miraculous Drugs of the South], was written while he lived at the Ming court. This work was designed to systematize the use of Vietnamese medicaments within the parameters of Chinese drug theory and to present and explain Vietnamese medicine to Chinese physicians at the Ming court: Tuệ Tĩnh thus wrote in Chinese rather than in Vietnamese, which dominates his other work. The text takes up eleven volumes, with the first volume devoted purely to pharmaceutical ingredients and the rest covering 184 different medical situations, from epidemic disease, to chronic complaints, such as arthritis, to conditions such as pregnancy. Tuệ Tĩnh sent copies of the *Nam Dược Thần Hiệu* back to Vietnam via a Vietnamese diplomatic mission.

It was a sore point with the people of Tuệ Tĩnh's home village that he was never allowed to return home and that his remains were never returned after he died in China. Tuệ Tĩnh's tomb, in Nanjing, was a favorite pilgrimage site for Vietnamese visiting the area. Sadly, Tuệ Tĩnh had specified that his epitaph contain a request for anyone from Vietnam who came to his tomb to please carry his remains home. In 1676 a scholar from Tuệ Tĩnh's home village of Nghĩa Phú recorded the text on the commemorative stele at the gravesite and had it carved on another one that was erected in their home village. It can still be seen there today.

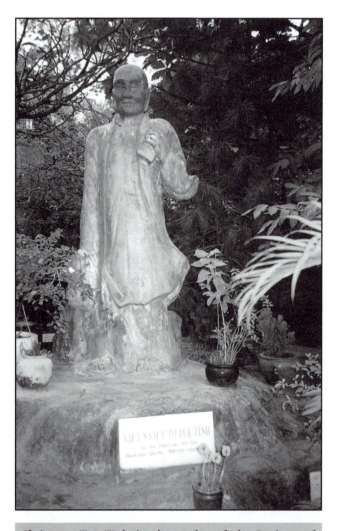

Shrine to Tuệ Tĩnh in the garden of the Institute of Traditional Medicine and Pharmacy, Hồ Chí Minh City, Vietnam. Photograph by Annick Guénel.

The two surviving works by Tuệ Tĩnh are essential reference tools for Vietnamese traditional healers today, and they are also still found on the bookshelves of many ordinary families. His practical, easily utilized medical formulas and advice have stood the test of time in helping everyday Vietnamese people treat the afflictions that abound in their tropical climate. The Vietnamese people have dedicated shrines to him, named streets and medical gardens after him, and honor him as the founder of Vietnamese traditional medicine: they remember him very fondly.

Bibliography

Primary: 1353–1885. *Hồng Nghĩa Giác Tư Y Thư* 洪義覺斯醫書 [Medical Books of Hong Nghia]; (n. d., but after 1385) *Nam Dược Thần Hiệu* 南藥神效 [Miraculous Drugs of the South].

Secondary: Nguyen Kiet Chi, 1986. 'Traditional Drugs of Vietnam in the Works of Tue Tinh.' *Vietnamese Studies* n.s. 12: 47–104; Hoang Bao Chau, 1993. 'Overview of Vietnamese Traditional Medicine' in Chau, Hoang Bao, and Huu Ngoc, eds., *Vietnamese Traditional Medicine* (Hồ Chí Minh City) pp. 5–29; Vũ Ngọc Khánh, 2004. 'Tuệ Tĩnh (1330–?)' in Thế Giới Publishers, *Renowned Vietnamese Intellectuals prior to the 20th Century* (Hồ Chí Minh City) pp. 38–42.

C. Michele Thompson

TUKE, DANIEL HACK (b. York, England, 19 April 1827; d. London, England, 5 March 1895), *psychiatry*.

Tuke was the youngest of thirteen children of Samuel Tuke (1784–1857), the Quaker philanthropist and lunacy reformer, and Priscilla Hack. Tuke's twin brother died at birth, and he himself was dogged by ill health for much of his life.

Tuke's great-grandfather, William (1732–1822), had been the prime mover in the founding of the York Retreat (1792). His father Samuel Tuke had authored a book on the new institution, *A Description of the Retreat* (1813), thereby drawing major attention to the therapeutic regime developed at that Quaker asylum. Indirectly and somewhat inadvertently, the book helped to launch a national campaign to reform existing madhouses and to copy the Retreat's emphasis on what was called moral treatment. Daniel grew up in the shadow of the asylum, but first sought a legal career, being articled to a solicitor in Bradford (1845). Unhappy with the work, he abandoned his training (1847) and took up the post of secretary and house steward at the Retreat, where he remained for three years. Now persuaded to build a career as an alienist, Tuke left his post in 1850 to undertake medical studies at St Bartholomew's Hospital in London, where he qualified MRCS (1852), before obtaining an MD from Heidelberg the following year. It was 1875 before he was elected FRCP.

For the first four decades of its existence, the Retreat had been essentially a lay-run institution. A series of visiting physicians had made no discernible impact on the state of its patients, and moral treatment, emphasizing kindness, work, and minimal restraint, had been developed in contradistinction to medical treatment. Tuke's great-grandfather had exhibited considerable skepticism about the value of contemporary medicine, and it was not until 1838 that John Thurnham (1810–73) was appointed as its first medical superintendent. Tuke's decision to qualify as a doctor thus marked a break with family tradition, and he now returned to the Retreat as its assistant medical officer. At the nearby York medical school, he introduced a course on psychological medicine, providing clinical instruction for those who enrolled in it at the Retreat.

In 1854 Tuke's essay on the moral management of the insane won a prize from the Society for Improving the Condition of the Insane. There was an irony here, for the Society, founded by Sir Alexander Morison (1779–1866) in 1842, was the center of resistance to many of the new-fangled ideas adopted by the lunacy reformers. Shortly thereafter, Tuke began the collaboration with John Charles Bucknill (1817–97), superintendent of the Devon County Asylum, that led to the publication of *A Manual of Psychological Medicine* (1858), a concise summary of the contemporary consensus on the care of the insane, which continued to be influential for a quarter of a century and which went through four editions. Tuke's contribution was the first half of the book, surveying the history of the treatment of the mentally ill and culminating in the abolition of mechanical restraint and the establishment of modern medico-moral treatment.

Contracting tuberculosis in 1853, Tuke soon moved to Falmouth for the sake of his health. A decade and a half later, somewhat improved, he moved to London and established himself as a consultant in psychological medicine. To most modern eyes, the Victorian asylums had by now degenerated into a caricature of their supposed inspiration, the York Retreat, but Tuke remained an unembarrassed apologist for what they had become (unlike his coauthor Bucknill). His *Chapters in the History of the Insane in the British Isles* (1882) contained a good deal of archival work and presented a story of progress echoed by many later historians. Late in life, he edited and made major contributions to a two-volume *Dictionary of Psychological Medicine* (1892) that summarized late Victorian thinking on the subject for a professional audience. Joint-editor of the *Journal of Mental Science* from 1880 (a journal founded by Bucknill), he was elected president of the Medico-Psychological Association the following year.

Bibliography

Primary: 1859 (with Bucknill, J. C.) *A Manual of Psychological Medicine* (London); 1882. *Chapters in the History of the Insane in the British Isles* (London); 1892. *Dictionary of Psychological Medicine* 2 vols. (London).

Secondary: Bynum, W. F., 1991. 'Tuke's *Dictionary* and Psychiatry at the Turn of the Century' in Berrios, German E., and Hugh Freeman, eds., *150 Years of British Psychiatry, 1841–1991* (London); Digby, Anne, 1985. *Madness, Morality and Medicine: A Study of the York Retreat* (Cambridge); *Oxford DNB*.

Andrew Scull

TÙNG, TÔN THẤT (b. Thanh Hóa, Vietnam, 10 May 1912; d. Hanoi, Vietnam, 7 May 1982), *surgery.*

Tôn Thất Tùng was the youngest child in a family belonging to a branch of the Vietnamese imperial family. He was born during the period of colonial domination, which had begun with the French conquest of the southern region (or Cochinchina) at the end of the 1850s. Tùng was a native of the central region (Annam), which, along with the northern region (Tongking), became a French protectorate in 1883 and was integrated into the Indo-Chinese Union (Vietnam, Laos, Cambodia) in 1887.

His father died shortly after Tùng's birth. The family then moved to Huê, the city where the Vietnamese Imperial Court had been located since the beginning of the Nguyên dynasty (1802). Tùng always expressed a strong antipathy toward the mandarins of the Court. Like some young Vietnamese of his generation, he opted for a Western course of training, and in 1931 he left Huê for Hanoi, where the French colonial government had established the Indochina University. Tùng obtained the baccalaureat degree at the Lycée du Protectorat before enrolling in the Faculty of Medicine in 1934.

The Medical School of Hanoi, created in 1902, was the oldest branch of the Indochina University. After a period of restrictions regarding educational standards and the number of students, the French administration made some improvements, including the conversion of the Medical School of Hanoi into a Faculty of Medicine in 1933. With a curriculum and degrees equivalent to those of the metropolitan faculties, this meant that Indo-Chinese students were not required to go to France to defend their theses and acquire the degree of Doctor of Medicine.

Medical Training and First Work in Liver Surgery

Tùng thus belonged to the first generation of Vietnamese doctors who followed a full course of study in Hanoi. Since the establishment of the medical school, Indo-Chinese students had received a practical training at the 'hôpital du protectorat' (or Yersin hospital). In 1935 Tùng was named to the post of extern at the Yersin hospital, which at that time specialized in surgery. There he began to be interested in liver disease, which occupied an important place among the local pathologies.

Tùng was the student and laboratory assistant of the French surgeon Pierre Huard, and he envisaged studying the anatomy of the liver during an autopsy on a liver where the biliary tree was infected with ascaris. Because he was able to trace the path of the ascaris with a curette, he thought dissection alone enabled him to understand the anatomy of the liver. The other investigation methods of this time were radiologic exploration and corrosion, both of which gave imprecise results. Tùng became an intern in 1938, the first Vietnamese granted this position, and was able to pursue his investigations on the vascularization of the liver at the Hanoi Institute of Anatomy, as well as to continue his work at the hospital. Between 1935 and 1939, he is said to have done more than 200 dissections. In 1939 he defended his medical thesis, *La vascularisation veineuse du foie et ses applications aux résections et lobectomies hépatiques*, which was awarded a Silver Medal by the Paris Faculty of Medicine.

Thanks to this work, he successfully performed during the same year—together with his professor, the surgeon Jacques Meyer-May—the resection of a tumor in the left lobe of the liver. The technique consisted in the progressive exposing and ligaturing of the vessels as they entered the hepatic parenchyma. However, for several years, Tùng had to give up his work on this surgical technique.

First, the report sent in 1939 to the Academy of Surgery in Paris was not well received, and, in addition, a patient affected with a massive hepatoma died during the operation. During the last years before the declaration of Vietnamese Independence in August 1945, he did more work on the particular forms of ascaridiosis he had observed among the Vietnamese and published *Chirurgie des pancréatites aiguës* [Surgery of Acute Pancreatitis] shortly after the Revolution. The second event, which interrupted his research on liver surgery for an even longer time, was the war.

War Surgery and Final Work in Hepatectomy

He had enthusiastically joined the Independence movement and served the new government in August 1945. Therefore, at the end of 1946, when Hồ Chí Minh decided to organize the resistance against the French outside Hanoi, he left the Yersin hospital. Between 1946 and 1954, he set up mobile surgical units, for which he had often to rely on rudimentary and ingenious means (such as bicycle headlights for lighting underground operating rooms). On Hồ Chí Minh's order, he participated, as a surgeon, in the decisive Battle of Dien Bien Phu. He also trained new surgeons in the North Vietnamese jungle.

In 1948 he was named vice-minister of health. From 1954 and until 1962, when he left the Ministry, he also was director of the Yersin Hospital, which became the Viet-Duc Hospital (Vietnam-GDR Friendship Hospital) in 1956. In the early 1960s, after the hospital was reorganized, partly thanks to foreign assistance, Tùng was able to return to his research on liver surgery. Meanwhile, the hepatic 'planned' resection was reintroduced by Westerners, in particular the French surgeon Jean-Louis Lortat-Jacob, whose technique involved the dissection and crushing of the vessels outside the liver, at the level of the hilum. This technique was difficult and required a long period of training. In 1961 Tùng attempted for the first time the removal of the right lobe of the liver on a patient put in hypothermy after he had opened the parenchyma with fingers and clamped the vessels inside the hepatic tissue. During that year about fifty patients successfully underwent the same operation, which lasted less than ten minutes.

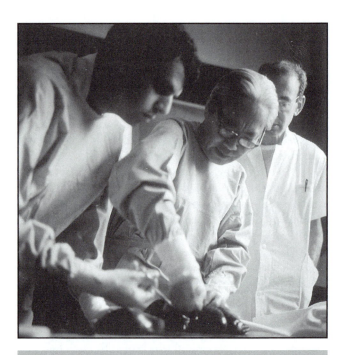

Tôn Thất Tùng (center) dissecting a liver, Eaubonne Hospital, Paris, early 1980s. Photograph by J. M. Krivine.

First published in an East Germany review before being published in *Lancet*, Tùng's technique gained international attention. In 1964 Tùng could finally demonstrate the efficiency of his method in French hospitals. Tùng's *Chirurgie d'exérèse du foie* was first published in French, in Hanoi in 1962, and later translated into several languages. In 1965 Tùng was elected to the USSR Academy of Medicine. His work was also acknowledged in Western countries, where he was invited to participate in surgical colloquia. In 1970 he was named a member of the Paris Academy of Surgery, where his work had been severely criticized thirty years earlier.

Tropical Pathologies and Dioxin

As he worked on refining his technique, he looked for pathologies other than tumors to which it could be applied. One such pathology was liver abscesses, some cases of which were caused by ascaris; another one was intrahepatic lithiasis. He also described a rather prevalent infectious disease in Vietnam, which involves hemorrhage of the biliary ducts, naming it 'tropical hemobilia' to distinguish it from hemobilia of traumatic origin. He discovered the cause of 'capsular hematoma of the liver', reporting a much higher number of cases than other investigators.

His findings were published mainly in French journals, but also in some American journals. The surgical treatments of these liver pathologies and others were described in a book published in 1979, *Les résections majeures et mineures du foie*, which remains a standard reference work in liver surgery. At this point, his own experience was based on more than 700 hepatectomies. In 1979 his work was awarded the

International Surgical Medal, a prize only given once every five years since it was established in 1911. Tung's technique, known as 'digitoclasie' ('finger-fracture'), or the crushing of the hepatic parenchyma and the locating of the vascular pedicles with the fingers, is still used in many cases of hepatectomy in Vietnamese hospitals. However, it was not widely adopted in foreign countries. In France, for example, surgeons have remained faithful to the 'planned hepatectomy', which consists of the clamping of the vessels before cutting the liver parenchyma (today with the use of ultrasound).

In 1970, during the American War, Tùng also had to supervise studies concerning the toxic effects of defoliants in addition to his surgical work. He set up a laboratory in his hospital where people who were victims of the chemicals spread on South Vietnam were examined. Although the scientific value of initial results, obtained in cooperation with a Chinese team, showing chromosomal alterations, was contested, they strengthened the arguments for a resolution against the American government. However, because of the lack of experts and funds and because of distance, the genetic studies on the effects of dioxin conducted under Tùng's direction did not go further. He could only note the marked increase in the number of liver cancers after 1962, which was certainly connected to the use of defoliants.

Throughout his career, he took an interest in the specific conditions in Vietnam that made some pathologies more prevalent there than in Western countries. He was also interested in the factors that gave them their local peculiarities. Nevertheless, he always stressed the importance of collaboration with foreign scientists, from the West as well as from the East. He always encouraged his students to go abroad for further training, especially in France, from the 1980s on. He died in May 1982, without having known the new policy of Doi Moi, established in 1986, which certainly has greatly facilitated scientific exchanges.

Bibliography

Primary: 1939. *La vascularisation veineuse du foie et ses applications aux résections et lobectomies hépatiques*, Thèse de Médecine (Hanoi); 1945. *Chirurgie des pancréatites aiguës* (Hanoi); 1962. *Chirurgie d'exérèse du foie* (Hanoi); 1979. *Les résections majeures et mineures du foie* (Paris); 1980. *Reminiscence of a Vietnamese Surgeon* (Hanoi).

Secondary: Krivine, Jean Michel, 2005. *Carnet d'un médecin au Viêt Nam, 1967–1983* (Paris); Vũ Quần Phương, 1998. 'Tôn Thất Tùng. Người đồng hành vĩnh cửu' [Tôn Thất Tùng, the Eternal Traveler], in Nguyễn Quang Ân, ed., *Lịch Sử và Văn Hóa Việt Nam. Những Gương Mặt Trí Thức* (Hanoi) pp. 667–673; M. Vigy, 1976. 'L'hépatectomie par digitoclasie' (Un entretien avec J.-M. Krivine), *Concours Médical* 98(7): 939–945.

Annick Guénel

TURNER, DANIEL (b. London, England, 1667; d. London, 13 March 1734), *surgery, venereology, medicine*.

Turner was the third son of John Turner, citizen and tallow-chandler of London, and his wife, Rebecca. He was apprenticed to the London surgeon Charles Bateman, but after two years was turned over to Thomas Lichfield, under whom he completed the remainder of his seven-year term. He became free of the surgeons' side of the Company of Barber-Surgeons in 1691, entering practice in the capital. He soon showed intellectual ambition. Reports of dissections in which he had taken part appeared in the *Philosophical Transactions* of the Royal Society in 1693–94, and in 1695 he published the first of thirty-four books. *Apologia Chyrurgica* attacked the quacks that he claimed infested the metropolitan medical world and called for the Barber-Surgeons to establish a much more rigorous system of examination of practitioners, backed by statutory powers. Both themes recurred throughout much of his other medical writings, and Turner, a pious Anglican Tory, frequently drew parallels between the disordered state of medicine and the rise of sectarianism.

Turner practiced surgery for two decades, treating patients from throughout the metropolis. However, in 1711 he left the Barber-Surgeons and was admitted as a licentiate of the College of Physicians. This doubtless reflected the success of his career. He commented that his new style of practice left him more time than the 'toilsome' nature of a surgeon's work, and in 1712 he married Elizabeth Altham. Nevertheless he continued to publish on surgery, most notably his major two-volume work, *The Art of Surgery*, published in 1722 and setting out the treatment of tumors, wounds, ulcers, fractures, and the diseases of women with numerous case histories.

In 1714 he published the first English work specifically dedicated to skin diseases—*De Morbis Cutaneis*. Whereas previous accounts of such conditions were organized according to the part of the body that was affected, Turner argued that such afflictions should better be divided into two sorts—those where the condition afflicted the inside of the body, but presented symptoms on the skin, and those that were of an outward origin. Turner further argued that this categorization was too simple because anatomical investigation had shown that matter could enter the body through the pores of the skin. As a result, he maintained, surgeons, who were traditionally supposed only to treat diseases of the surface of the body, should also be permitted to prescribe and administer internal medicines because their 'external' medicines were already entering the body—a reconceptualized model of the body thus encouraged a redrawing of the boundaries of medicine.

One chapter of Turner's book discussed marks on the skin produced by the mother's imagination during pregnancy. This was an unexceptional theory at the time, but it drew Turner into controversy. In 1727 James Blondel (1665/66–1734), writing in the aftermath of the Mary Toft case, when Toft claimed to have given birth to rabbits, dismissed this idea. A heated but inconclusive pamphlet war ensued between 1729 and 1730 in which Turner set out explanations of how the mother's passions could alter the body of the infant in her womb and rejected the iatromechanical ideas which underpinned Blondel's arguments. Although Whiggish histories of embryology have celebrated Blondel and dismissed Turner, it is important to note that at the time neither party could claim a clear victory. A similarly combative mode of writing can be seen in Turner's pamphlets on syphilis. In these works, Turner attacked what he saw as the excessive employment of mercurial treatments, but lambasted the purveyors of various proprietary remedies, such as Joshua Ward (1684/85–1761).

Bibliography

Secondary: Wilson, Philip K., 1999. *Surgery, Skin and Syphilis: Daniel Turner's London (1667–1741)* (Amsterdam); Wilson, P. K., 1992. '"Out of Sight, Out of Mind?" The Daniel Turner–James Blondel Dispute over the Power of the Maternal Imagination.' *Annals of Science* 49: 63–85; *Oxford DNB*.

Mark Jenner

TURNER, JOHN ANDREW (b. Portsmouth, England, 1858; d. London, England, 22 August 1922), *public health, sanitation.*

Turner completed his MB from Aberdeen and his MD from Edinburgh, earned a diploma in public health (DPH) from Cambridge, and trained in London, Paris, and Bonn. After serving as health officer in Leicestershire and Hertfordshire, he was posted to Bombay (1901–19). During these two decades, Turner made a distinctive contribution to tackling the health problems of the city. At his initiative, the Bombay Sanitary Association was established (1903) with the support of Indian doctors, philanthropists, and civic leaders. The objectives of the Association were to promote sanitary consciousness; disseminate knowledge of the 'laws' of health through public lectures, in English and Indian vernacular languages; appoint paid health visitors, who would visit a locality and report to the health department on unsanitary conditions or on overcrowding; and educate the residents in matters of personal hygiene. To spread this message, health exhibitions were organized (1905 and 1909), where sanitary appliances and apparatus were displayed and films were shown (1912) illustrating the sanitary and conservancy work being done. Leaflets and brochures on common diseases afflicting the population were prepared and also translated into the vernaculars. Sanitary classes were opened to train men and women who would teach elementary hygiene in primary schools and engineering and medical graduates who would be sanitary surveyors. This body led to the founding of similar associations in other cities of western India.

In his annual health reports, Turner made detailed observations on the condition of markets, slaughterhouses, and stables and advocated the seizure and destruction of unwholesome

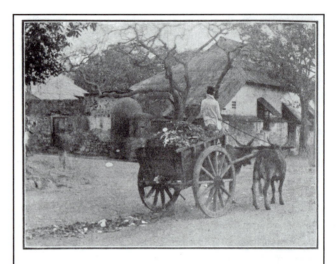

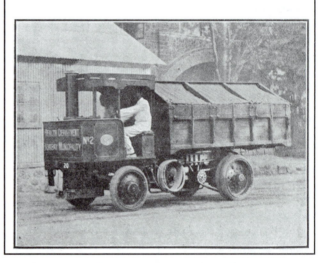

The removal of refuse in Bombay by 'old style' and 'new style'. Halftone reproduction from *Sanitation in India*, 1914. Wellcome Library, London.

food, a better system of registration of births and deaths, the notification of infectious diseases, and the medical inspection of school children. He also collated data for the Indian Factory Labour Commission (1908) comparing the health of Bombay mill workers with other laborers of the city. He found that the mortality rate was less among the former, though there were more deaths from phthisis. The Bombay Anti-Tuberculosis League (1912) was set up to promote awareness of the growing incidence of tuberculosis. It ran an information bureau, a dispensary, and later a sanatorium.

At Turner's initiative, a meeting of doctors was called to discuss the rising incidence of venereal diseases, which led to the foundation of the League for Combating Venereal Diseases (1916). This body aimed to disseminate information and provide treatment. Turner was also concerned with the high rates of infant mortality. Under his direction, the municipality appointed nurses to visit the homes of the poor, opened free maternity homes, and collaborated with the Lady Willingdon Scheme (1914) to provide treatment and proper care to infants after birth.

Turner championed W. M. Haffkine's plague prophylactic as a less interventionist alternative to the methods of evacuation, isolation, and disinfection, which had been very unpopular with the Indians. He zealously advocated the closure of wells as an antimalarial measure. During the influenza epidemic (1918–19), Turner's appeal for urgent public assistance received an overwhelming response, and an epidemic relief committee coordinated the efforts of twenty-five caste and community organizations. This collaborative effort between the public and the municipal health authorities reduced the number of casualties in the city.

Turner's enthusiasm, however, was not always matched with government support: some of his proposals for sanitary improvement were not implemented, owing to financial constraints. He believed that obstacles to sanitary progress could be overcome by patient and constant working, teaching, educating, gradually adopting modern appliances, and steadily enforcing laws and regulations that could be made sufficiently adaptable to the circumstances of the situation. He was among the few British medical men in India who held that there was no line of demarcation between Western and Eastern medicine. Turner was awarded the Commander of the Indian Empire (CIE) (1916) in recognition of his services to the city of Bombay.

Bibliography

Primary: 1914. *Sanitation in India* (Bombay); 1901–19. *Reports of the Health Officer in Reports of the Municipal Commissioner for the City of Bombay* (Bombay).

Secondary: Ramanna, Mridula, 2004. 'Perceptions of Sanitation and Medicine in Bombay, 1900–1914' in Fischer-Tiné, Harald, and Michael Mann, eds., *Colonialism as Civilizing Mission* (London) pp. 205–225.

Mridula Ramanna

TURQUET, THEODORE, DE MAYERNE   (b. Geneva, Switzerland, 28 September 1573; d. London, England, 16 March 1655), *medicine, iatrochemistry.*

Son of the noted Huguenot historian and political writer, Louis Turquet, who had fled to Geneva from Lyons after the St Bartholomew's Day massacre in 1572, Theodore completed the arts curriculum at Heidelberg University and studied at Montpellier for the MD, which he completed in 1597. Because Turquet was already committed at this time to the chemical and metallic medicaments of the Paracelsians—which, although tolerated, were not taught at Montpellier—it seems likely that he was influenced by a friend of his family, Joseph Du Chesne, or Quercetanus (1546–1609), one of Henry IV's (1553–1610) royal physicians. Turquet then moved to Paris to work with Quercetanus. Turquet, also appointed as a royal physician, began to build a wealthy clientele in his practice. When Quercetanus and his Paracelsian methods were attacked in print by the inflexibly orthodox Paris Medical Faculty, Turquet published a response in which he insisted that chemical remedies did not contravene the principles of Hippocratic or Galenic medicine (1603). From 1609, when Turquet was recognized as 'noble', he called himself Theodore de Mayerne. After the assassination of Henry IV, he was invited to England as first physician to James I (1603–25), and again, he was able to build up a highly lucrative practice.

He was elected a fellow of the RCP in 1616 and joined the project to produce an official London pharmacopoeia. When the first pharmacopoeia was published in 1618, it bore a dedicatory epistle to James by Mayerne and included a special section on iatrochemical remedies. Mayerne was by no means the prime mover in these initiatives, but he took a greater role in ensuring that apothecaries knew how to prepare the new chemical remedies. Together with Henry Atkins (1555–1635), the College's president on a number of occasions, he helped pharmacists to separate from grocers and to establish the Worshipful Society of Apothecaries in 1620. He was knighted by James I in 1624.

After James's death, Mayerne continued as royal physician, but Charles I (1600–49) clearly preferred William Harvey (1578–1657). Queen Henrietta Maria (1609–69), however, remained devoted to Mayerne. Charles seems to have been suspicious of Mayerne, who had certainly worked as a confidential agent for James, but whose Protestant sympathies were perhaps too extreme for the new king. Accordingly, Charles banned Mayerne from all foreign travel. Mayerne now saw his life at court as one merely of servitude, and he particularly resented not being able to visit his estate in Aubonne in France, which he had bought in 1620. In 1642, therefore, when Charles was preparing for war in York, Mayerne refused the royal summons to join him. He preferred to stay with his private practice and received no more salary from the crown.

Mayerne took consolation during these years of servitude in following various practical pursuits arising from his interest in chemistry. He experimented with artists' pigments and different kinds of varnish, and he improved the art of enameling. He produced cosmetics and perfumes for the ladies of the court, compiled a cookery book, and invented a delicious cordial. He also developed some medicaments of his own, notably *lotio nigra*, or black wash, a skin treatment containing mercuric oxide; and he advocated the use of calomel (mercury chloride) as a purgative. In 1636 Charles granted him a patent for distilling.

His major strength as a physician was a careful and continuous observation of his patients and a surprisingly nondoctrinaire response to changes in their condition. He was as ready to draw upon Galen as Paracelsus. His posthumously published case notes proved useful to subsequent generations, being published in different editions, the latest of which appeared in 1700.

Bibliography

Primary: 1603. *Apologia in qua videre est . . . remedia chymice preparata tuto usurpari posse, ad cujusdam anonymi calumnias reponsio* (La Rochelle); 1700. (Browne, Joseph, ed.) *Opera medica, complectentia consilia, epistolas, et observationes, phamacopeam, variasque medicamentorum formulas* (London).

Secondary: Nance, Brian, 2001. *Turquet de Mayerne as Baroque Physician: The Art of Medical Portraiture* (Amsterdam); Trevor-Roper, Hugh, 2000. 'Harriot's Physician: Theodore de Mayerne' in Fox, Robert, ed., *Thomas Harriot: An Elizabethan Man of Science* (Aldershot) pp. 48–63; Cook, Harold, J., 1986. *The Decline of the Old Medical Regime in Stuart London* (Ithaca and London); *DSB*; *Oxford DNB*.

John Henry

TZANCK, ARNAULT (b. Vladicaucas, Russia, 18 April 1886; d. Paris, France, 8 February 1954), *dermatology, hematology, blood transfusion.*

Born in the Russian Caucasus region north of Georgia, Tzanck emigrated to Paris with his family when he was four. He attended lycée at the height of the Dreyfus affair, and, drawn to medicine, he studied dermatology and venereal disease, most notably with Jean Darier. His thesis on 'Traitement de la paralysie générale' was completed in 1914. During World War I, Tzanck was attached to the ambulance service of the surgeon Antonin Gosset, one of France's pioneers of blood transfusion. After the war, he first took positions in dermatology and venereal disease at Broca and Saint-Louis Hospitals, but Tzanck was increasingly drawn to hematology and, specifically, blood transfusion when he moved to Saint-Antoine Hospital.

In 1923 Tzanck, along with Gosset and obstetrician Edmond Levy-Solal, organized one of the first transfusion donor services in Paris at Saint-Antoine. Their success and increasing demands from other hospitals led to the establishment in 1928 of the Transfusion Sanguine d'Urgence, in collaboration with Salpêtrière and Tenon Hospitals and with funding from the Paris hospital administration (Assistance Publique). This service identified and screened blood donors, who were called for transfusions at Paris hospitals. By 1937 the growth of the organization required construction of a new building for the transfusion center at Saint-Antoine with support from the government and private funds. The building was inaugurated in conjunction with the Second International Congress of Blood Transfusion, presided over by Tzanck.

Tzanck's contributions in hematology included early work in blood preservation and blood products (experiments with bovine plasma and storage of red blood cells). For treatment of nephritis, he pioneered techniques of exsanguino-transfusion and 'lavage du sang', a precursor to blood filtration and hemodialysis. His contributions in dermatology included development of the general concept of 'intolerance' to explain a variety of skin reactions, a large step toward the understanding of hypersensitivity, which he described in a 1932 book, *Immunité-intolérance, biophylaxie.* In 1947 he developed a simple test using a microscopic analysis of scrapings from skin cancer lesions, different ganglia, and some dermatitis, especially pemphigus. The Tzanck smear is now widely used as a test for herpes, among other diseases.

At the beginning of the 1930s, Tzanck campaigned unsuccessfully for organization of blood transfusion in the French army, but, at the outbreak of World War II, he led efforts to develop the transfusion service for what was expected to be a long conflict. After the armistice in 1940, Tzanck, a Jew, was threatened by arrest and escaped the country, eventually finding refuge in Chile. He returned first to Algeria, and, following the liberation of Paris, Tzanck was re-established at Saint-Antoine, where he coordinated the armed forces blood collection. In the postwar years, Tzanck was at the center of the creation of the academic and administrative institutions in France for the study and provision of blood for transfusion. He created, and was the first editor of, the *Revue d'Hematologie.* He served as president of both the Société d'Hematologie and the Société de Dermatologie. Tzanck was the driving force and first director of the Centre National de Transfusion Sanguine, which was established in 1949. In the process he educated a whole generation of serologists and immunologists, including Jean Dausset, Marcel Bessis, and Jean-Pierre Soulier.

Tzanck had broad eclectic interests in painting, music, and philosophy, the most important result of which was his book *Conscience créatrice* (1943).

Bibliography

Primary: 1932. *Immunité, intolérance, biophylaxie, doctrine biologique et médecine expérimentale* (Paris); 1933. *Problèmes théoriques et pratiques de la transfusion* (Paris); 1943. *La Conscience créatrice: entretiens sur la vie et la pensée* (Santiago, Chile); 1954. (with Melki, G. R.) 'Cyto-diagnosis in Dermatology' in MacKenna, D. M. B., ed., *Modern Trends in Dermatology* 2nd ser. (New York) pp. 87–103.

Secondary: Soulier, J. P., et al., 1964. *Hommage au Dr. A. Tzanck, 1886–1954* (Champigny); Baruk, H., et al., 1955. 'La vie et l'oeuvre du Dr. Arnault Tzanck' special issue of *Revue d'histoire de la médecine hébraique* 8: 69–103; Moline, R., 1955. 'L'oeuvre dermatologique et biologique d'Arnault Tzanck' in Charpy, Jacques, ed., *Accidents therapeutiques en dermatologie* (Paris) pp. 11–19.

William H. Schneider

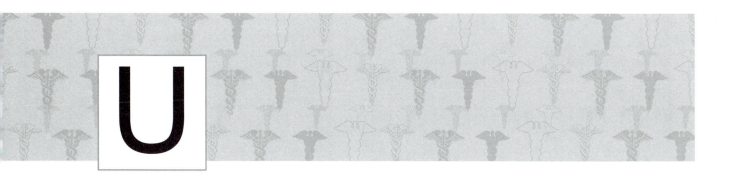

U

UGO, BENZI (b. Siena, Italy, 24 February 1376; d. Ferrara, Italy, 30 November 1439), *medicine, medical education.*

Ugo Benzi, son of Andrea, a magistrate from Siena, and of Minoccia Pagni, attended the Grammar School in Siena in his youth (1385–90). He studied philosophy at the Universities of Florence, Bologna, and finally Pavia, where he got his degree (1396) and where he became a lecturer of logic (1396–1402). Later he became a lecturer of philosophy at the University of Bologna (1402–5): his three philosophic commentaries to Aristotle's works date back to this period. There he started to study medicine at Marsilio of Saint Sofia's school. He then went back to Siena, where he started to teach medicine (1405). He was the personal physician of Cardinal Baldassarre Cossa from Pisa, later Pope John XXIII, moving then to Bologna after him and teaching medicine there until 1412. During those years, he came in personal contact and started academic disputes with the philosopher Biagio Pelacani from Parma and the physician Jacopo della Torre from Forlì.

Called to Parma by Nicolò III d'Este, Benzi taught medicine there (1412–15) and spent several years of particularly fervid work. He wrote three of his main medical commentaries: on Galen, on the Hippocratic *Aphorisms,* and on Avicenna (Ibn Sīnā). Such works, reflecting his academic teaching, were generated from the reading and commentaries of classical texts of Greek and Arabic medicine in the classroom, as was the habit among late medieval masters of

medicine. Benzi investigated matters relative to the scientific method and the cause and effect processes of medical science. He also wrote some *Quaestiones rerum naturalium* [Questions on Natural Things]. Later he moved again to the University of Siena (1416–21), leaving in 1423, probably because of the plague.

He was then hired by Filippo Maria Visconti as ordinary professor of medicine at the University of Pavia (1425–29). Benzi later left Pavia, after having completed the course on Hippocrates' *Aphorisms,* but leaving incomplete his commentary on Avicenna's *Canon,* Fen I, Book 4. Then he made a dissection at the University of Padua in 1430 for a didactic purpose.

Soon after having moved to Ferrara, he was called again by Nicolò III d'Este as court physician, without holding the chair at the university. His teaching in that period had to be carried out only privately or occasionally. Among his disciples was Angelo Decembrio, whose treatise about the plague echoed his tutor and defined Benzi as the most excellent prince of philosophers and doctors of the time.

Benzi's literary production in those years (1431–38) was quite outstanding, in particular concerning the writing of his *Consilia saluberrima ad omnes aegritudines* [Most Healthful Consultations for All Diseases], a wide collection of clinical cases containing the list of symptoms, prognostic judgments, and dietetic and pharmaceutical prescriptions selected to interest a wide sector of the medical community.

These *consilia* constitute one of the first examples of systematic collections of different diseases, displaying wide knowledge and hygienic-therapeutic experience.

Benzi was undoubtedly a man of broad culture, highly regarded in the most refined circles, who was able to join a humanist vocation and a brilliant medical career thanks to his competence in medical practice and his qualities as a scholar of theoretical medicine.

Bibliography

Primary: 1482. *Consilia medica* (Bologna); 1498. *Expositio super libros Tegni Galieni* (Venice); 1517. *Expositio Ugonis Senensis super Aphorismos Hippocratis et super commentum Galeni* (Venice); 1991. (Fioravanti, Gianfranco, and Antonella Idato, eds.) *Scriptum de somno et vigilia* (Florence).

Secondary: Lockwood, Dean Putnam, 1951. *Ugo Benzi Medieval Philosopher and Physician, 1376–1439* (Chicago); *DBI*.

Romana Martorelli Vico

UNANUE, JOSÉ HIPÓLITO (b. Arica, Peru, 13 August 1755; d. Lima, Peru, 15 July 1833), *climate, medical education.*

Unanue, son of the Spanish merchant navy officer Miguel Antonio Unanue and Manuela Pabón, attended the seminary of San Jerónimo de Arequipa and the Medical Faculty of San Marcos University, the main institution of higher learning of the Peruvian Viceroyalty.

Unanue's initial interests focused around experimental anatomy and medical education. In 1789 Unanue was appointed chair of anatomy at San Marcos University. Some years later, he helped organize the Royal Anatomic Amphitheater, encouraging experimentation among medical students. During the inauguration of the Amphitheater (1792), Unanue pronounced one of his most celebrated discourses, entitled 'Decadencia y Restauración del Perú'. This discourse stressed the relevance of Western medicine and medical education in the recovery of the demographic collapse produced by the Spanish conquest. Unanue also promoted the establishment of the San Fernando Royal College of Medicine and Surgery in 1811, aiming to abolish the division between medicine and surgery and to institute a practical medical instruction.

Unanue rose through the ranks of colonial bureaucracy and achieved important positions. His public career began in 1793, when he was named Official Cosmographer of the Peruvian viceroyalty and, as such, editor of the *Guía Política, Eclesiástica y Militar del Perú*, a publication that included information on geography, demography, natural history, climate, and diseases. In 1807 Unanue was appointed General Protomédico (a sort of medical inspector created by the Spanish Crown) and, seven years later, physician to the court of the king. Unanue was engaged in the improvement of urban environmental conditions and public hygiene. He encouraged the introduction of the smallpox vaccine, street cleaning, sanitary legislation, and the establishment in 1808 of the first cemetery outside the city walls of Lima, which replaced church burials. Unanue's goal was to diminish miasma emanation, considered the main reason for the spread of epidemics.

Unanue was also a founding member of the Sociedad de Amantes del País, a loose network of scholars and officers influenced by the Enlightenment, and editor of the *Mercurio Peruano*, a periodical publication that appeared between 1791 and 1795. Under the pseudonym of Aristio, he published articles on diverse issues such as natural history, botany, geography, economy, and medicine. His aim was to demonstrate that Buffon and other naturalists were wrong in considering American nature as derivative. Unanue's most influential work was on the medical implications of the climate of Lima (*Observaciones sobre el Clima de Lima*), a neo-Hippocratic medical treatise on the influence of climate on disease incidence and evolution. With this book, Unanue intended to respond to the eighteenth-century European philosophical perception of the New World as inherently degenerative and pathological. In the case of Lima, Unanue argued, mortality and morbidity rates could be easily reduced with a proper understanding of the uniqueness of local climates, diseases, and populations; with an increase in the number of university-educated physicians; and with more strict controls over charlatans, empiricists, and Andean healers. Unanue's *Observaciones* became a paradigm among the Peruvian medical community.

Unanue had an important political career. He was elected senator for the Province of Arequipa (1812) and, as such, was also a Peruvian delegate for the Cortes of Cadiz in Spain (1814). Despite his privileged position in the colonial administration during the tumultuous years of the Spanish-American Independence wars, Unanue embraced political liberal ideals and joined the revolutionary leaders. Between 1821 and 1826 he was deeply involved in politics and occupied high positions, such as minister of economy, president of the First Constituent Congress, and Interim Head of Government. By the end of 1826 he retired to a rural estate in Cañete, south of Lima, where he died.

Bibliography

Primary: 1806. *Observaciones sobre el Clima de Lima y su influencia sobre los seres organizados, en especial el hombre* (Lima).

Secondary: Woodham, John, 1970. 'The Influence of Hipólito Unanue on Peruvian Medical Science, 1789–1820: A Reappraisal.' *Hispanic American Historical Review* 50(4): 693–714; Lastres, Juan B., 1955. *Hipólito Unanue* (Lima).

Jorge Lossio

UNDERWOOD, MICHAEL (b. West Molesey, Surrey, England, 29 September 1736; d. Knightsbridge, London, England, 14 March 1820), *midwifery, pediatrics.*

A surgeon apothecary, Underwood studied at St George's Hospital, London. Subsequently he became a surgeon to the

British Lying-In Hospital, a member of the Corporation of Surgeons, and a Licentiate in Midwifery of the Royal College of Physicians (1784), a qualification now extinct. After several years he came to devote himself to midwifery and the diseases of women and children. His reputation grew. He was appointed as physician to the Princess of Wales. In this capacity he attended the princess at the birth of Princess Charlotte (1796). This boosted his practice and thus his wealth. However, he had a number of domestic anxieties, and he became severely depressed. He came to believe that he was unfit for professional duties, so in 1801 he gave up all professional work and lived in seclusion until his death.

By his publications on diseases of children, he opened the way to the great advances in this field in the nineteenth century. His most important book was *Treatise on Diseases of Children* (1784), which he revised for four editions. After his death further editions were edited in turn by Samuel Merriman (1771–1852), Marshall Hall (1790–1857), and Henry Davies (1782–1862). In addition there were American, French, and German editions (the last in 1848). This text remained current for sixty years. George Frederic Still (1931) stated that the book was manifestly superior to anything else yet written on the subject. Importantly, it gathered together all of the most recent research and discoveries in the diseases of children and thus initiated the modern study of disease in childhood, i.e., the field of pediatrics.

The first edition addressed itself to the laity, but, by the fourth edition (1797), he had changed the book to 'render the work appropriate to medical readers'. Perhaps most notably, the third edition considered the chemistry of milk. Underwood published a table showing the chemical analysis of human milk, as well as cow's, goat's, ass's, and mare's milk. For the first time, the subject of infant feeding was beginning to assume a scientific aspect.

Other firsts include his description of congenital heart disease. The morbid anatomist had first brought this topic to the attention of clinicians in an era when the stethoscope was still unknown. He described the morbid anatomy as the following example shows: 'The peculiarity is sometimes in the pulmonary artery, which is constricted or closed as it rises from the right ventricle; at other, in the septum cordis, which has an unnatural opening affording a free communication between the two ventricles: sometimes in the aorta, arising equally from the anteriour and posteriour ventricles: and sometimes in the imperfect closure of the foramen ovale or the canalis arteriosus' (Still, 1931, p. 485). He then endeavored to relate these findings to clinical features: 'Wheresoever any morbid structure may be, whenever it may prove of any consequence the constant symptoms attending it are discolouration of the face and the neck with a sloe-blue or leaden colour of the lips and sometimes unnatural coldness of the body' (Still, 1931, p. 485). He thus was describing cyanotic congenital heart disease, probably for the first time.

He is also credited with the first clinical description of poliomyelitis, or infantile paralysis, in the second edition of his *Treatise on the Diseases of Children* (1789) under a heading entitled 'Debility of the Lower Extremities'. This section was expanded in the fourth edition (1797), with a detailed account of diagnosis, treatment, and prognosis.

Underwood also wrote a treatise (1783) and surgical tract on ulceration of the legs (1784), which were combined in 1788.

Bibliography

Primary: 1784. *A Treatise on the Diseases of Children; with directions for the management of infants from the birth, especially such as are brought up by hand* (London) (2nd edn. 1789, 3rd edn. 1795, 4th edn. 1797).

Secondary: Maloney, W. J., 1950. 'Michael Underwood: A Surgeon Practising Midwifery from 1764 to 1784.' *Journal of the History of Medicine and Allied Sciences* 5: 289–314; Still, George Frederic, 1931. *The History of Paediatrics: The Progress of the Study of Diseases of Children up to the End of the XVIIIth Century* (London); *Munk's Roll*; *Oxford DNB*.

John Walker-Smith

URRUTIA GUEREZTA, LUIS (b. San Sebastián, Guipúzcoa, Spain, 3 March 1876; d. Madrid, Spain, 21 June 1930), *surgery, gastroenterology.*

Urrutia Guerezta, internal medicine specialist and surgeon, specialized in diseases of the digestive system and was one of the creators of digestive surgery. He studied at the schools of medicine of the Universities of Barcelona (1892) and Madrid (1893–99). On completing his studies, he devoted himself fully to gastroenterology on the recommendation of Juan de Madinaveitia (1861–1938), one of the founders of this specialty in Spain. From 1896 to 1897, he was physician-in-training at the department of surgery of San Carlos Hospital, Madrid, which influenced his later surgical approach to digestive diseases. During this period, he also maintained a good professional relationship with Luis Simarro (1851–1921), who taught him laboratory techniques. He further widened his studies with several trips to the best European departments of his specialty: Paris, Berlin, Vienna, London, and Halle. On his return to San Sebastian (1900), he devoted his time to developing gastroenterological surgery at different hospitals in the Basque capital, especially at San Ignacio, a hospital founded in 1906, where he was one of the directors. Until 1907, he was also a physician of the Beneficencia Provincial, the provincial Poor Law medical service. He received his doctorate in 1900, with a thesis on paraplegias by compression of the spinal medulla (1903).

In 1918 he created *Archivos Españoles de Enfermedades del Aparato Digestivo y de la Nutrición* in collaboration with Fidel Fernández Martínez (1890–1942) and Ramón Luis y Yagüe (1864–1939). This was the first Spanish journal of this specialty and continues in publication to this day. Urrutia

Guerezta presented the outcomes of his work as a digestive surgeon at numerous national and international conferences. At the National Congress of Medicine in Madrid (1919), he presented his wide resection approach to the treatment of gastric ulcers as an alternative to gastroenterostomy. One year later, he was invited to give a series of talks on his specialty at the clinic of the Mayo brothers in the United States. He also spoke in Cleveland, Chicago, and New York and participated in the Tenth Congress of the American College of Surgeons in Canada (1920).

In 1924 Urrutia Guerezta moved to Madrid at the invitation of Juan Madinaveitia, where he founded with other colleagues the Instituto Madinaveitia (1925), the first private institution in Spain exclusively devoted to digestive diseases, endocrinology, and nutritional diseases. It was generously endowed and had a clear orientation toward laboratory medicine. One year later, the Instituto published its *Anales*, which enjoyed great prestige among early practitioners of the specialty until its publication ceased with the Spanish Civil War (1936–39). Although his move to Madrid was professionally highly fruitful, he made enemies of most of his colleagues at the Instituto, including the family of Juan de Madinaveitia. He died of cardiac arrest in 1930.

Bibliography

Primary: 1920. *Enfermedades del estómago* (Madrid); 1921. *Enfermedades de los intestinos* (Madrid); 1923. *Enfermedades del hígado y del páncreas* (Madrid).

Secondary: Urquía Echave, José María, 1993. 'Urrutia Guerezta, Luis' in Granjel, Luis S., ed., *Diccionario Histórico de Médicos Vascos* (Bilbao) pp. 185–187; Gallart-Esquerdo, Antonio, 1955. *Historia de la Gastroenterología Española* (Barcelona) pp. 89–95; Luis y Yagüe, Ramón, 1930. 'El Doctor Luis Urrutia y Guerezta.' *Arch. Esp. Enf. Ap. Digest. Nutrición* 13: 641–647.

Guillermo Olagüe de Ros

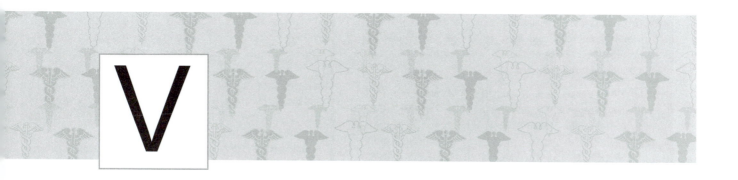

V

VAID, BHAI MOHAN SINGH   (b. Tarn Taran, Amritsar, India, 1881; d. Tarn Taran, 1936), *vaid, ayurvedic physician.*

Mohan was born into a devout Sikh family of hereditary medical practitioners and learned Sikh intellectuals, or Bhais (hence his name came to consist of Bhai, an intellectual or religious title; Singh, a Sikh title suffixed to his given name, Mohan, as commonly done in his time; and Vaid, referring to his role as an ayurvedic physician), in the Amritsar district of the British Punjab. Even in his youth in the 1890s, Mohan Singh began to attract widespread attention for his writings on ayurved, in vernacular Punjabi, and for his commitment to the cause of Sikh social reform, emerging as a response to Hindu revivalist movements.

Mohan Singh's career saw him establishing a well-known commercial pharmacy, the Khalsa Aushadalya, and his own printing press in his native town, near the city of Amritsar. He established links with local and provincial-level ayurvedic and unani corporate bodies and their campaigns for state patronage. By the1920s he was well known for his widely circulated tracts and pamphlets, written in Punjabi, on Sikh social reform and for his journal *Dukh Niwaran* (founded in 1906). He campaigned in all these publications for support for Sikh community reform and the popularization of ayurvedic medicine.

He also undertook prolific translations of classical ayurvedic texts into Punjabi and wrote numerous pamphlets on medical self-help and health, which continue to be popular and printed in local presses in the Punjab. Mohan Singh Vaid published much of this work in Punjabi in a series called the *Swadesh Bhasha Pracharak* series. His work and achievements to publicize ayurved in Punjabi assume particular significance because ayurved represented only a minor tradition of learning and practice in the nineteenth-century Punjab compared to Greco-Arabic, unani medical practice.

Mohan Singh Vaid chose to write and publicize in vernacular Punjabi when Sikh Punjabi writers were negotiating a new place and role for Punjabi writing as a vehicle of ethnic, political, and linguistic claims. His tracts and speeches in public gatherings reached out to ayurvedic and unani practitioners, as well as to the lay public, in his attempts to find support and patronage for local traditions of ayurvedic medical learning and practice in the vernacular. He resisted the setting up of ayurvedic curricula and degrees by corporate bodies such as the Ayurved Sammelan, as they imposed, from above, a 'uniform' Sanskrit-based learning and curricula. Mohan Singh Vaid argued that this would imply that both Hindu and Sikh practitioners with little access to the largely 'upper caste' Sanskrit tradition would find themselves relegated to a lesser 'status' among traditional practitioners. Mohan Singh Vaid's mission of ayurvedic 'prachar', or publicity, therefore sought to reconstruct histories of ayurvedic learning and employed arguments about the recovery of an indigenous, ayurvedic past that was not necessarily singular or 'Hindu' in its cultural bearings. In this way, he hoped to make a case for ayurveda as a unified indigenous or Indian sociocultural tradition that would also preserve its diverse ethnic composition. His tracts and journals are available in library holdings across Punjab, most notably in the university libraries of Amritsar and Patiala, and reprints of his tracts are currently available in many local bookshops in Amritsar.

Bibliography

Primary: 1912. *Arogta Prakash* [Light on Disease Prevention] (Tarn Taran); 1914. *Gauravta Ayurved* [Our Pride in Ayurveda] (Tarn Taran) [New edn., November 1995 (Tarn Taran)]; 1920. *Ayurvedic Shastar* [The Ayurvedic Treatises] (Tarn Taran); 1906–18 (old series). *Dukh Niwaran* (This was a health-cum-social-reform journal in vernacular Punjabi, published and edited by Mohan Singh Vaid from his home town. A new series of the journal was resumed by his sons after his death and is still published sporadically).

Secondary: Sivaramakrishnan, Kavita, 2006. *Old Potions New Bottles: Recasting Indigenous Medicine in Colonial Punjab* (Delhi); Amol, S. S., 1969. *Bhai Mohan Singh Vaid* (in Punjabi) (Patiala); Munsha Singh, 'Dukhi', 1939 (new edn., 1989). *Jeewan Bhai Sahib Bhai Mohan Singh Ji Vaid* [The Life of Bhai Mohan Singh Vaid] (Tarn Taran) (Contains a list of his publications).

Kavita Sivaramakrishnan

VAKIL, RUSTOM JAL (b. Bombay [now Mumbai], India, 11 July 1911; d. Bombay, 20 November 1974), *cardiology.*

Vakil, son of a general practitioner, Jal Vakil, and Jerbanoo, attended Elphinstone College and the Royal Institute of Science in Bombay. He then studied at St Thomas's Hospital Medical School, London, graduating in 1934. He passed his MRCP in 1935 and stood first in his MD examination at the University of London in 1937. Vakil returned to India in 1938 and set up a successful private practice as a physician, which he combined with teaching. He was assistant honorary physician at J. J. Hospital and Grant Medical College, which he gave up for a similar appointment at King Edward Memorial Hospital and G. S. Medical College, Bombay. Soon he developed a focus on the treatment of heart diseases and cardiology. Vakil married Jeroo Madan on 15 July 1968; they had no children.

Hypertension claimed many lives in India, and, of all available remedies, sedatives were proven to be the most effective. *Rauwolfia serpentina*, known to relieve symptoms of hypertension, was not new to India. The drug was first mentioned in Sir Ram Nath Chopra's 1933 survey of Indian remedies and had been studied extensively in the 1930s. However, it was B. B. Bhatia's account of the use of this drug in hypertension in the *Journal of the Indian Medical Association* in 1942 that inspired Vakil to conduct his own clinical trials on fifty patients in Bombay. The success of his trial, which he reported in *The British Heart Journal* in 1949, had a significant impact on the international medical community. Vakil's use of this indigenous remedy for the treatment of hypertension was given international recognition when he was awarded the Albert Lasker award in 1957, the first Asian to be so honored. Subsequent research into the toxic side effects of reserpine, however, reduced its use considerably.

Vakil was the first in India to carry out large-scale statistical analysis of various types of heart disease. Vakil maintained a strict confidentiality about most of his patients. In 1962 he published an epidemiological survey of cardiovascular disease in India, based on his study of 15,000 patients. In 1964 he reported in *The American Journal of Cardiology* on the 'pre-infarction syndrome' (a term he is credited with inventing), based on his studies of 360 cases. He introduced a new classification for abnormal heart rhythms and a number of new terms in clinical diagnosis: for example, 'hexalogy of the heart', 'transitory pulsation in coronary thrombosis', and 'subacute pulmonary oedema'. Vakil was also the first to establish normal electrocardiographic and blood pressure standards for young age groups in India. He was also among the few Western-trained doctors who took a serious interest in the clinical properties of medicinal plants mentioned in ancient Indian texts.

Vakil was awarded the Shanti Swarup Bhatnagar award (1966) and the B. C. Roy memorial award (1969) for his scientific research into medicine. He was elected FRCP (London) (1960) and was a member of the American College of Cardiology. Keen to establish cardiology as a specialist discipline in India, Vakil established the Dr Jal Vakil gold medal of the All India Heart Foundation and the Mrs Jal Vakil medal and lectureship in cardiology of the Association of Physicians of India. He founded the Vakil Institute of Cardiology and Research Centre at the King Edward Memorial Hospital, Bombay, in 1974.

Known as an efficient and competent clinician, a popular teacher, a popularizer of medicine, and an eloquent speaker, Vakil won the admiration of his students and the medical fraternity during his lifetime.

Bibliography

Primary: 1949. 'A Clinical Trial of *Rauwolfia Serpentina* in Essential Hypertension.' *British Heart Journal* 2: 350–355; 1964. 'Pre-infarction Syndrome: Management and Followup.' *American Journal of Cardiology* 14: 55–63.

Secondary: Gupta, S. P. K., 2002. 'Rustom Jal Vakil (1911–1974), Father of Modern Cardiology: A Profile.' *Journal of Indian Academy of Clinical Medicine* 3(1): 100–104; Golwala, Aspi F., 1979. 'Rustom Jal Vakil.' *Biographical Memoirs, Indian National Science Academy* 5: 102–108; *Munk's Roll*.

Indira Chowdhury

VALESCO OF TARENTA (b. Portugal, ?; d. France, after 1426), *medicine, surgery.*

Valesco was born in Portugal and began his liberal arts education in Lisbon before traveling to the University of

Paris, where he received his bachelor's degree. Around 1382 he moved to Montpellier, where he studied medicine under Jean de Tournemire, the university's chancellor, and Jean Jacme (Johannes Jacobi), a previous chancellor. He received his medical license in 1387 and soon thereafter was called to the court of Gaston III Fébus (r. 1343–91), count of Foix and *vicomte* of Béarn. He reports treating patients all over Spain and southern France, but his practice focused mostly in the region of Foix-Béarn, and he continued to treat people at the court of Foix under the three successive rulers following Gaston Fébus.

During his years of medical practice, Valesco wrote several shorter medical treatises, including the *Liber de regimine sanitatis* [Book of the regimen of health], now lost, and a plague treatise, *De epidemia et peste*, completed in 1401. His most influential work, the *Philonium*, completed in 1418, is a manual on medical practice that discusses the signs, causes, and cures of specific diseases from head to foot and includes a separate section on surgery. This scholarly text is unusual for having been written by a physician who never became a master and was not attached to a university school of medicine. On the contrary, Valesco emphasized that it was written 'after thirty-six years of practice'. Together, his medical writings reveal an emphasis on matters relating to *practica* (the medical genre that covered the problems of classifying and diagnosing different diseases and applying efficient cures in practice) over *theorica* (which covered the philosophy of medicine and the principles of physiology and pathology).

Valesco displayed a deep respect for the Greek and Arabic medical authorities in all of his writings. However, like many physicians in the late fourteenth and fifteenth centuries, he was increasingly concerned about inconsistencies in these authoritative texts and their presumed inability to satisfactorily explain, diagnose, and treat new diseases, such as the recurrent outbreaks of plague. Valesco responded to these challenges by drawing examples from his own practical experience to help settle questions regarding the causes of disease and the appropriate methods of diagnosis and treatment. For example, based on his own practice, he refined Avicenna's (Ibn Sīnā) definition and list of 'contagious' diseases, to better explain the transmission of plague and the observed differences in the symptoms and mortality of people suffering from pleurisy.

Valesco's surgical writings also reveal his reliance on both Greco-Arabic authorities and empirical knowledge. Like Guy de Chauliac, his predecessor at Montpellier, Valesco sought to elevate surgery as a learned discipline by putting it into a theoretical framework compatible with scholastic medical tradition. However, Valesco also valued the mechanical experience of craft surgeons and regularly incorporated knowledge gleaned from them alongside citations of ancient authorities in his surgical chapters in order to evaluate the merits of different operations.

Valesco's willingness to give an important position to empirical knowledge in his medical and surgical writings is representative of a shift toward practical medicine taking place in the post-plague years. Nonetheless, he still emphasized that a physician's theoretical and anatomical knowledge made him a superior healer compared to empirics and apprentice-trained surgeons, and he continued to hold the ancient authorities in high regard.

Bibliography

Primary: 1490. *Practica, quae alias Philonium dicitur* (Lyons).

Secondary: York, William H., 2003. 'Experience and Theory in Medical Practice During the Later Middle Ages: Valesco de Tarenta (fl. 1382–1426) at the Court of Foix.' PhD thesis, The Johns Hopkins University; McVaugh, Michael R., 1998. 'Treatment of Hernia in the Later Middle Ages: Surgical Correction and Social Construction' in French, Roger, Jon Arrizabalaga, Andrew Cunningham, and Luis García-Ballester, eds., *Medicine from the Black Death to the French Disease* (Aldershot) pp. 131–155; Wickersheimer, Ernest, 1936. *Dictionnaire biographique des médecins en France au Moyen Age* (Geneva) p. 772.

William H. York

VALLES, FRANCISCO (b. Covarrubias, Burgos, Spain, 1524; d. Burgos, 10 September 1592), *medicine, pharmacology, philosophy.*

It is said that Francisco Valles's father was a physician. The son studied medicine in the University of Alcalá de Henares (Madrid), in the Madre de Dios College, founded by Cardinal Cisneros for eighteen theology students and six medical students.

In Alcalá, he received the qualifications of Licentiate in Arts (1547), Bachelor (1550), Licentiate (1553), and Doctor in Medicine (1554). He was prima professor of the Faculty of Medicine from 1557 to 1572, when he was called to take on more important positions in the Kingdom.

He was the Royal Physician beginning 15 October 1572. His main patient was King Philip II, to whom, according to tradition, he owed the nickname of 'divine'. One day, when the king was tormented by gout pains and the remedies proposed by other Royal Physicians had failed, Valles decided to prepare a hot bath. When the king put his foot in the bath, he found immediate relief and gratefully exclaimed: 'Valles, thou art divine!'(an epithet added to his name).

For this or for other reasons, Philip II named him Protomédico (chief royal physician) of the Kingdoms of Castile, which in practice meant he had control over all aspects of Castilian medicine. In this post, Valles set regulations for pharmacological distillations, weights, and measures, editing a treatise called *Tratado de las aguas destiladas, pesos y medidas que los boticarios deben usar* (1592). In addition, on his advice, distillation laboratories were created in the Monastery of the Escurial, which were equivalent to advanced research centers.

He was said to be a good physician, erudite and expert in classical languages, for which he was named a member of the commission responsible for organizing the library of the Royal Monastery of the Escurial, together with such learned men as Benito Arias Montano and Ambrosio de Morales.

In 1592, after recommending one of the great Spanish Renaissance physicians, Luis de Mercado, as the new royal physician, he returned to his birthplace, where he died in the Augustinian convent in Burgos.

During his lectures in the Faculty in Alcalá, he introduced the novelty of trying to explain pathologies with the help of an anatomist, Pedro Jimeno, which set him on the road to the future pathological anatomy. It was not for this, however, that he received European recognition, but for a series of commentaries on the works of Galen and Hippocrates: *Claudii Galeni Pergameni de locis patientibus* (1559), *In Aphorismos* (1561), *In Prognosticum Hippocratis* (1567), *Galeni ars medicinalis* (1567), etc. and for *Controversiarum naturalium* (1563), a discussion of medical problems that includes personal experiences and had great repercussions in Europe. Also noteworthy are *Commentarii de urinis* (1565) and an attempt to link science and faith in *De iis, qua scripta sunt physice in libris sacris, sive de sacra philosophia* (1587). His *Methodus medendi* (1588) is valued as one of the best therapeutic treatises of the century.

Boerhaave said, of his study of epidemic illnesses, 'Whoever has the commentaries of this Spaniard needs no other, as all modern physicians write according to theories, and I only praise he who, with his own observations, explains that expounded by Hippocrates' (López Piñero, 1983, p. 393).

Bibliography

Primary: 1564. *Controversiarum medicarum & philosophicarum* (Alcalá); 1577. *In libros Hippocratis de morbis popularibus* (Madrid); 1588. *Methodus medendi* (Madrid).

Secondary: López Piñero, José M., 1983. 'Valles, Francisco' in López Piñero, José M., et al., eds., *Diccionario Histórico de la Ciencia Moderna en España*, vol. II (Barcelona) pp. 391–394; Granjel, Luis S., 1980. *La Medicina Española Renacentista* (Salamanca); Castellote Cubells, Salvador, 1963. 'Antropología filosófica en la obra de Francisco de Valles.' *Archivos Iberoamericanos de Historia de la Medicina* 15: 77–120.

Anastasio Rojo

VALLISNERI, ANTONIO (b. Trassilico, Garfagnana, Italy, 3 May 1661; d. Padua, Italy, 18 January 1730), *medicine, natural history.*

Son of Lorenzo, a judge, and Maria Lucrezia Davini, Vallisneri had a traditional education reserved for children of the best families. His studies progressed in accordance with the classical Jesuit model, going through courses of grammar, humanities, rhetoric, and philosophy. His education gave him a firm knowledge of the Latin language and litera-

ture, which accompanied him throughout his life, thus being the basis for his knowledge of the Italian Classics and his complete mastery of the Italian language.

In 1682 he moved to the University in Bologna, where he was a student of Marcello Malpighi (1628–94). He came into contact with the Cartesian and atomistic theses, but mainly with the Galileian experimentalism, integrated with the Baconian way of thinking by the most famous scholars of that environment, who aimed at neutralizing the dangerous metaphysical implications that led to the trial and condemnation of Galileo. The education of the young Vallisneri also benefited from the masterly skill of Giovanni Girolamo Sbaraglia, whose lessons he attended with attention, although unknown to Malpighi. From Sbaraglia's teaching, he learned about empiricism, which he removed from its traditionalistic context and inserted in a modern conceptual framework, making it comply with Malpighi's rational medicine, which he followed.

In 1685 Vallisneri graduated from the University of Reggio Emilia, and he practiced in Venice, Padua, and Parma, where he stayed until 1687, and where he was an apprentice of Jacopo Grandi and Lodovico Testi in Venice and of Giuseppe Pompeo Sacco in Parma.

He returned home, practiced medicine in different country districts under his care from 1687 to 1700, and devoted himself full-time to naturalistic observations, his main purpose being to confute the spontaneous generation thesis.

In 1700 he was appointed to the chair of practical medicine at the University in Padua, with the aim of affirming experimental philosophy. In 1709 he moved to the second chair of theoretical medicine, and in 1711 he was appointed to the first chair, where he stayed until he died.

In accordance with Francesco Redi (c. 1616–98) and Malpighi, Vallisneri emphasized the connection between naturalistic, anatomic, and medical studies in an open polemic with the Aristotelian and Galenic traditions, mainly using the empirical reductionism of Sbaraglia. In fact, the empirical approach could be fruitful only if included in a conscious theoretical context. To this end, Vallisneri envisaged an accomplishment in therapeutics, which, starting from Ippocrate's (Hippocrates) prescriptions and from anatomical and natural discoveries of modern authors, could test old and recent remedies continuously, thus building up a body of knowledge able to improve medicine's ability to intervene in ill health. The theoretical model had to match the empirical research, using the corpuscular and mechanistic paradigm that Vallisneri supported. He entrusted the general setting of phenomena to it, as well as the elaboration of theoretical interpretations and possible therapeutic hypothesis. The medicine obtained from there had to prove its effectiveness and, in the affirmative, take advantage of the various old and new proposals of the pharmacologic literature. Special attention was paid to specific remedies, such as mercury and cinchona, and, with extreme caution, to those obtained from chemical preparations and applied to medicine.

Finally, Vallisneri did not fail to consider the influence of psychological factors in therapy and, sometimes, the necessity to prescribe useless remedies, but he absolutely avoided using noxious ones just to tranquillize the 'opinion' that patients had of their disease.

Vallisneri's reputation as a practical doctor was great. Continuously called by the Venetian nobility and subject to an incessant request for consultations, he was asked by Clemente XI to be Giovanni Maria Lancisi's (1654–1720) successor, but without success, since Vallisneri did not want to renounce the safe chair at the University in Padua.

Bibliography

Primary: 1733. *Opere fisico-mediche* 3 vols. (Venice); 1991. (Generali, D., ed.) *Epistolario (1679–1710)* (Milan); 1998. (Generali, D., ed.) *Epistolario (1711–1713)* (Milan); 2006. (Generali, D., ed.) *Epistolario* (1714–1729) [1 CD] (Florence); 2004–. *Edizione Nazionale delle Opere di Antonio Vallisneri* (Florence).

Secondary: Generali, Dario, 2004. *Bibliografia* (Florence); Antonio Vallisneri—Edizione Nazionale delle Opere (www.vallisneri.it).

Dario Generali

VALSALVA, ANTONIO MARIA (b. Imola, Italy, 17 January 1666; d. Bologna, Italy, 2 February 1723), *anatomy.*

Valsalva, the third son of Pompeo Valsalva, goldsmith, and Caterina Tosi, began his education under the Jesuits in Imola. He subsequently moved to the University of Bologna, where one of his teachers was Marcello Malpighi (1628–94), and where he was awarded a degree in philosophy and medicine on 9 June 1687. While still a student, he attended the scientific reunions held at Eustachio Manfredi's house, which led to the foundation of the Accademia degli Inquieti, of which Valsalva was three times president. In 1697 he was nominated public anatomical dissector, and in 1705 he also became lecturer and demonstrator in anatomy. In 1718 he was appointed professor of surgery.

Valsalva devoted himself to teaching and scientific research, as well as to the practice of medicine and surgery. He attended the Bolognese hospitals, especially the S. Orsola Hospital, at that time called Ospedale degli Incurabili, of which he became head physician in 1697 and later surgeon.

In 1704 he published, with the active collaboration of Giovanni Battista Morgagni (1682–1771), the treatise *De aure humana*, the result of sixteen years of work, in which he made several important contributions, mostly concerning the anatomy of the ear. This work, containing ten plates that clearly illustrated the parts of the ear, was divided in two parts, the first anatomical and the second physiological; each part was composed of three chapters. Valsalva was the first to divide the ear into external, mid-

dle, and inner. He also described the small sebaceous glands of the skin of the auricle for the first time and provided a detailed and precise description of the auricular muscles and auricular ligaments (Valsalva's ligaments). He gave an exact description of the external auditory meatus, of which he prepared a wax cast to reproduce its course and diameters faithfully. In the middle ear, he clearly illustrated the auditory tube, which he called the Eustachian tube, examining the cartilaginous, membranous, and bony components, identifying the peristaphyline external muscle *(tensor veli palatini),* which dilates the tube. He also described the pharyngeal and uvular musculature in detail. He gave the name 'labyrinth' to the entire inner ear; working on fresh petrous pyramids, he discovered the endolabyrinthine liquid but did not identify the membranous labyrinth. Still adhering to the idea of the presence of air in the labyrinth, he simply attributed to it the function of moistening the *zonae sonorae* vibrating in the endolabyrinthine air, which he believed were the terminal expansions of the acoustic nerve. He recognized the bleeding area of nasal septum (also called the *locus Valsalvae)* before Kiesselbach. In the *De aure humana,* he also described his procedure, still known as Valsalva's test, which consists of a forced expiration with mouth and nose closed, later defined and developed by Morgagni (1761). He also described the dysphagia caused by a luxation of the hyoid bone (Valsalva's dysphagia) and established that, in hemiplegia, the lesion is in the contralateral cerebral hemisphere (Valsalva's rule).

Valsalva's other writings were studied and published posthumously by Morgagni (1740), who also wrote his teacher's biography and re-edited the *De aure humana.* Valsalva's name remains associated with the sinuses of semilunar valves and with the aortic sinus and aortic sinusal aneurysm. For aneurysms he employed the depletory treatment, consisting of a reduced diet and repeated bloodlettings, in order to diminish the volume of blood, and thus the force of the impact, against the arterial wall. As Morgagni reported, Valsalva was one of the first physicians to treat mentally ill patients in a more humane way.

Bibliography

Primary: 1704. *De aure humana tractatus* (Bologna) [1931, Italian trans. Mangano, Vincenzo (Rome)]; 1740. *Opera* 3 vols. in 2 (vol. 1: *Tractatus de aure humana . . . et Dissertationes anatomicae,* vols. 2–3: Joannis Baptistae Morgagni, *Epistolae anatomicae duodeviginti ad scripta pertinentes . . . Antonii Mariae Valsalvae)* (Venice).

Secondary: Barbieri, Luigi L., 1990. *Il dottor Antonio Maria Valsalva e la sua manovra* (Bologna); Belloni, Luigi, 1966. 'Suono e orecchio dal Galilei al Valsalva (Nel terzo centenario della nascita di A.M. Valsalva).' *Simposi clinici* 3: 33–42; Bilancioni, Guglielmo, 1911. *Valsalva. Le opere e l'uomo, secondo documenti inediti* (Rome); *DSB.*

Giuseppe Ongaro

VAN DYCK, CORNELIUS VAN ALLEN (b. Kinderhook, New York, USA, 13 August 1818; d. Beirut, Ottoman Empire [now Lebanon], 1895), *medicine, pathology.*

Van Dyck was born into a Presbyterian family. His father was an apothecary and medical practitioner. During his school years, he particularly excelled in Greek and Latin and helped his father in the pharmacy. He studied the local herbs and learned how to classify them according to the Linnaean system. A business partner betrayed his father, and the consequent loss of capital made it difficult for the children to go to university.

Van Dyck accomplished his secondary education partly as an autodidact and partly with the help of a local physician, who provided him with access to his private library. At the age of eighteen, Van Dyck started reading medicine at Jefferson College (Philadelphia), graduating with a diploma. In 1840 the American Board of Commissioners sent him to Beirut. Staying in quarantine for forty days, he learned his first 200 Arabic words, which laid the foundation for his subsequent excellent command of Arabic. Later, he polished his knowledge under the supervision of his Arab friends, the eminent *littérateurs* of the nineteenth century. In 1842 he was posted to the village of `Abeih, where he worked as a doctor and ran a school. Subsequently, he was employed as a doctor in various places in Syria and Lebanon. From 1867 until 1882, he held the chair in internal medicine and general pathology at the Syrian Protestant College (later the American University of Beirut). His colleague there was the American doctor John Wortabet (1838–1909), also an author of a well-known Arabic dictionary.

The medical and chemical laboratories were poorly equipped, with limited instruments and scientific literature. Van Dyck provided the students with textbooks and manuals, which he compiled and had printed at his own expense. The annual report of the Board of Managers for 1877 recorded that 'Besides giving instruction and lectures customary in such institutions the Professors have prepared in the Arabic language, edited and published . . . Pathology, Physical Diagnosis, Chemistry, Natural History, Physiology, Botany, Surgery, Materia Medica, Mental Philosophy'. Van Dyck also practiced in the Presbyterian Hospital (later American University of Beirut Medical Center), where he was an indisputable authority in medicine and the medical sciences.

In 1890 the local population celebrated the fiftieth anniversary of his residence and work in Lebanon. He received congratulations from the country's authorities and from the Islamic and Christian clergy. All of his biographers highlight his great ability for work and equally refer to his kind nature and deep understanding of the indigenous population. 'Of all foreigners, who came to work in Syria in the nineteenth century, he entered more intimately into the life of the people than any other', wrote George Antonius. Van Dyck ate local food, smoked the water-pipe [nargile], and even wore Lebanese costumes, which made him look like one of the locals and helped in his missionary work.

Van Dyck was a prolific writer, authoring twenty-nine books, eight of which were religious; all of the others discussed medicine and allied subjects. Among one of his greatest literary achievements was his translation of the Bible into Arabic from Hebrew, which he conducted in 1857–65 as a continuation of the unfinished translation by Eli Smith (1801–57). At that time, the Arabic Bible became the first major mass-printed volume in the Arabic language.

Bibliography

Primary: Zaidan, J., 1910–1911. *Tarājīm mashāhīr ash-Sharq* [Biographies of the Luminaries from the East] (Cairo). pt. 2, pp. 40–54.

Secondary: Glass, D., 1998. 'Der Missionar Cornelius van Dyck (1818–1895) als Lehrbuchautor und Förderer des arabischen Wissenschaftsjournalismus' in Preissler, Holger, and Heidi Stein, eds. *Annäherung an das Fremde, XXVI. Deutscher Orientalistentag vom 25. bis 29.9. 1995 in Leipzig* (Stuttgart) (*ZDMG* Suppl. 11) pp. 185–198 and bibliography.

Nikolaj Serikoff

VAN HOOSEN, BERTHA (b. Stony Creek, Michigan, USA, 26 March 1863; d. Romeo, Michigan, USA, 7 June 1952), *surgery, obstetrics, gynecology.*

Van Hoosen was born in Stony Creek, Michigan, the daughter of Sarah Taylor Van Hoosen, a teacher, and Joshua Van Hoosen, a farmer. She received her AB from the University of Michigan in 1884 and her MD from the University of Michigan Medical School in 1888. She was a resident at the Woman's Hospital of Detroit, worked at Kalamazoo State Hospital for the Insane, and interned at the New England Hospital for Women and Children in Boston. In 1892 Van Hoosen settled in Chicago, where she opened a private obstetrical practice and went on to fill various teaching, clinical, and surgical positions.

Van Hoosen served on the staff at several Chicago institutions, receiving her first positions at the Columbia dispensary, acting as a clinical assistant in gynecology and as an obstetrician in the outpatient department. Van Hoosen later worked in the clinic at the Charity Hospital as a surgical assistant before launching an independent surgical practice. She also served on the staff at the Wesley Hospital, the Women and Children's Hospital, the Cook County Hospital, and the Frances Willard Hospital. At the Cook County Hospital, she became chief of the gynecological staff, the first woman to receive this civil service appointment.

From the very start of her career, Van Hoosen combined teaching with her medical practice. First, she was a demonstrator of anatomy at Northwestern University Woman's Medical School, where she also became professor of embryology. She became a professor of clinical gynecology at the College of Physicians and Surgeons at the Illinois University

Medical School. She reached another great milestone in 1918, becoming professor and head of obstetrics at the Loyola University Medical School, where she was the first woman to head a medical division at a coeducational medical school.

Van Hoosen paved the way for other women physicians in surgery and gynecology. She trained several young women in surgery, calling her protégées her 'surgical daughters'. Frustrated by the marginal status of women in the profession, she was active in the founding of the American Medical Women's Association (AMWA) in 1915 and served as the organization's first president. In this role, Van Hoosen encouraged women physicians to organize and work cooperatively; she also fought, to no avail, for women physicians to serve in the military during World War I. Van Hoosen made her international mark by traveling the world, delivering speeches, demonstrating surgical techniques, and observing procedures.

Van Hoosen dedicated her career to improving the health of women. In addition to her clinical and surgical work, she taught sex education and hygiene through both private consultations and public lectures. Van Hoosen was also involved in the development of 'twilight sleep' (scopolamine-morphine anesthesia) to ease the burden of pain during childbirth. Despite opposition from colleagues, she employed twilight sleep in her own practice and had used it to deliver 2,000 babies by 1908. Serving the needs of mothers, she worked for the expansion of prenatal care and formed the first human breast milk bank in Chicago. Van Hoosen was also an active author, publishing numerous articles on obstetrics and gynecology, as well as her own autobiography *Petticoat Surgeon* (1947). Bertha Van Hoosen is remembered as an accomplished practitioner and surgeon, a vocal advocate for women physicians, and a strong activist committed to advancing the health care and livelihood of women and children.

Bibliography

Primary: 1915. 'The New Movement in Obstetrics.' *Woman's Medical Journal* 25: 121–123; 1947. *Petticoat Surgeon* (New York); 1950. 'Looking Backward,' *JAMWA* 5: 406–408.

Secondary: More, Ellen S., 1999. *Restoring the Balance: Women Physicians and the Profession of Medicine, 1850–1995* (Cambridge, MA); Fine, Eve, 1990. 'Separate But Integrated: Bertha Van Hoosen and the Founding of the AMWA.' *JAMWA* 45: 181–190; Morantz-Sanchez, Regina, 1980. 'Bertha Van Hoosen' in *Notable American Women* (Cambridge, MA) 4: 706–707; *DAMB*.

Carla Bittel

VARGAS REYES, ANTONIO   (b. Charalá, Colombia, 21 September 1816; d. Villeta, Colombia, 23 August 1873), *surgery, medical education.*

Vargas Reyes was born in the eastern province of Socorro, in a family of supporters of the Spanish colonial regime in its last years of existence in Colombia. After the battle of Boyacá in 1819—a battle that consolidated the local patriots' victory for independence over the Spanish—his family was scattered all over the country. In 1828 Antonio was brought back to Bogotá by one of his elder sisters.

He studied medicine at the Universidad Central and began his practice during the Civil War of 1839: one of the countless nineteenth-century Colombian civil wars. In 1842 he traveled to Paris and started again to study medicine from scratch, following theoretical and practical courses in anatomy, pathology, and surgery taught by Cloquet, Velpeau, Orfila, and other stars of French clinical instruction. He was also trained in the anatomoclinical method.

In 1846 he returned to Colombia and soon became the family doctor for Bogotá's elite. His practice and teaching took place amid the construction of an incipient nation-state. He joined the effort by promoting the constitution of a 'national pathology', by fostering a professional association for the few university-trained physicians, and struggling for improving medical education.

During this time, the country was ready to begin the 'Revolution of 1850', namely the prosperity brought by tobacco production and export. Supported by free trade policies, this 'Revolution' stimulated the diffusion of new ideas in all fields, particularly in science and industry. It was the ideal framework for consolidating (in Colombia) the scientific medicine that Vargas Reyes had observed and experienced in Europe.

Nonetheless, and in accord with the dominant liberalism at the time, a new law in 1850 allowed for the free teaching and exercise of all professions, with the exception of pharmacy. According to Vargas Reyes, this law deepened the chaos in medical studies and prompted empirics and quackery in the field. To counter these effects, Vargas Reyes, in coordination with other physicians, organized several lectures in different institutions, including Bogotá's public hospital. He also founded *La Lanceta* in 1852, the first Colombian medical journal devoted to scientific medicine and career regulation. Vargas's efforts were instrumental in creating a high standard and reinforcing the prestige of Colombia's medical elite.

After the 'Revolution', Vargas continued his medical work, provoking discussions and arousing the admiration of disciples and colleagues. The results of his studies appeared in two volumes (1859, 1862) entitled *Trabajos científicos*, which included a report on quinine, the well-known bark used for treating malaria fevers.

His contribution to Colombian surgery is also documented in his *Trabajos*: treatment of wounds caused by firearms, tumor extirpation, amputations, ligature of the arteries, hernia and fistula surgery, gynecological operations, etc. These were quite remarkable, as was his study on yellow fever and malarial fevers on the river Magdalena, which linked the southern region of the country with the middle-western region and the Atlantic Ocean and was thus essential for transportation and the import and export of goods.

In 1864 Vargas Reyes founded a new journal, the *Gaceta Médica de Colombia*. Based on his criticism of the public higher education system, the *Gaceta* proposed the creation of a private medical school with a sound curriculum. The proposal was the basis for the foundation of the Universidad Nacional de Colombia in 1867. Vargas Reyes was the first dean of the Medical Faculty of this University. Without doubt, Vargas Reyes was the most prominent figure in Western medicine and medical educational reform in Colombia during the nineteenth century.

Bibliography

Primary: 1859, 1862. *Trabajos científicos* 2 vols. (Bogotá).

Secondary: Miranda Canal, Néstor, 2002. *Librecambio y medicina en la Revolución Anticolonial de 1850* (Bogotá); Zubiría, Roberto de, 2002. *Antonio Vargas Reyes y la medicina del siglo XIX en Colombia.* (Bogotá).

Néstor Miranda Canal

VARIER, SANKUNNI PANNIYAMPILLY (VAIDYARATNAM)

(b. ?, 1869; d. ?, 30 January 1944), *vaidyan, ayurvedic medicine.*

Panniyampilly Sankunni (P. S.) Varier traced his professional lineage as a 'high caste' vaidyan or ayurvedic practitioner to one of the eight original Ashtavaidyan families of ayurvedic practitioners in the southern state of Kerala in India. Trained in a traditional school in the classical traditions of Hindu learning, Varier grew to be arguably the best-known leader of ayurvedic reform and a pioneer of the commercialized practice of ayurveda in South India in the first decades of the twentieth century.

Without overt contradictions, Varier combined in his career the traditional role of a vaidyan or practitioner of the 'varier', or 'ambalavasi', caste (dedicated to ritual service in temples) with the reformist vision of widening the base of ayurvedic education and practice. He founded a renowned pharmacy, the Arya Vaidya Sala, in the town of Kottakal in North Kerala in 1902, and fifteen years later he established the Ayurvedic Patasala, one of the first degree-based educational institutions for ayurvedic learning in South India. The Patasala introduced innovative methods of teaching orthodox ayurvedic therapies and attempted to combine scientific methods with a foundation in classical ayurvedic texts. At the Patasala, Varier deployed the knowledge of Western medicine that he had gained from Diwan Bahadur Dr V. Verghese in rationalizing traditional ayurvedic therapies and in restructuring his practice. Varier's practice was also notable for attracting patients from all castes and creeds, particularly significant in his times, when even temple entry in Hindu temples was forbidden to 'lower' castes and ritual purity by 'upper' castes was rigidly observed.

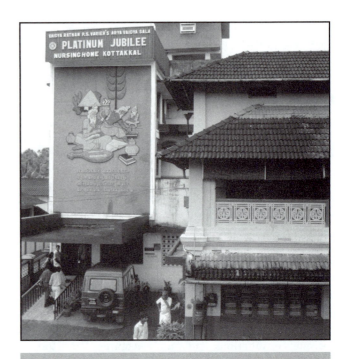

The main entrance of Arya Vaidya Sala Ayurvedic Hospital, Kottakal, Kerala Province. Photograph by Mark de Fraeye, Wellcome Photo Library, London.

Varier's interest in and patronage of local cultural traditions gave him a public profile beyond ayurvedic practice as he supported traditional drama troupes, performances, and the diffusion of vernacular Malayali literature. He authored many stage scripts, such as the Sanskrit classic *Abhinjanasakuntala* in vernacular Malayalam, for presentation by his dramatic troupe in public performances in South India. His commitment to social uplift, in particular his sympathy for the Mapila rebel uprising, triggered by landlord domination, made him a liberal figure in later years in the emerging nationalist politics.

Toward the end of his career, Varier gained widespread recognition for his contribution to ayurveda: titles were conferred on him by the British government (in 1933) and private bodies alike. He was also nominated to the Central Board of Indian Medicine and elected to head the All India Ayurved Mahasammelan, the apex national body of ayurvedic practitioners.

The Arya Vaidya Sala established by Varier endures as a family trust today, with expanded functions that include an extended range of commercialized ayurvedic products and syncretic healthcare therapies, attracting patients and visitors from across the world.

Bibliography

Primary: 1903–1926. *Dhanvantari.* (vols. I–XXII, total issues 552) (Kottakal) (The first medical journal in Malayalam, named after the divine god and source of ayurveda, who was also an incarnation of the Hindu god Vishnu, was published and edited by Varier from the year of its founding in 1903 until 1926.); 1907. *Chikitsasangraham* (Kottakkal) (in Malayalam); 1925. *Astangasariram* (Kottakkal) (in Sanskrit); 1942 (Part I)–1969 (Part II). *Brhaccariram* (Kottakkal) [These are treatises on ayurvedic theories, therapeutics, and drugs; the latter two have been reprinted in the Chowkamba Sanskrit Series (Varanasi) in 2005. All other works by Varier are available as manuscripts in the Arya Vaidya Sala Library].

Secondary: Krishnankutty, Geeta, 2001. *A Life of Healing: A Biography of Vaidyaratnam P. S. Varier* (Delhi).

Kavita Sivaramakrishnan

VELPEAU, ALFRED

VELPEAU, ALFRED (b. Brèches, France, 18 May 1795; d. Paris, France, 24 August 1867), *surgery, obstetrics, gynecology, oncology.*

Velpeau was born in a village in the Touraine region, the son of a blacksmith who, like many blacksmiths in the French countryside, practiced as a 'veterinary artist'. He did not attend school but received lessons from a priest, a schoolteacher, and, finally, on the recommendation of a local physician, the tutor of the children of a wealthy neighbor. He developed an early enthusiasm for medicine, which he studied in textbooks, and he began to treat patients in the vicinity. The physician first met Velpeau when he was summoned to help a girl whom the overconfident young man had treated for depression with a poisonous dose of hellebore. Impressed by his abilities, his patrons took him in 1816 to the hospital in Tours to train as a health officer, a lower-level medical practitioner intended to meet the needs of rural areas. He studied there with Pierre-Fidèle Bretonneau, the new chief of medicine, and qualified as a health officer in 1819. Like another protégé, Armand Trousseau, Velpeau remained Bretonneau's faithful disciple and worked to call attention to contributions that his mentor had left unpublished.

With Bretonneau's encouragement, Velpeau went to Paris to study for the doctorate, supporting himself by working as an anatomical assistant. When he received his degree in 1823, he was too old to apply for a prestigious hospital internship. Instead, he took the competitive examination for the newly introduced medical agrégation, intended for physicians interested in academic medicine. He succeeded and used the distinction to develop a distinguished and lucrative career in surgery. He was appointed surgeon at the Pitié Hospital in 1828 and then chief of surgery in 1833, the year in which he became professor of clinical surgery at the Paris Faculty of Medicine. He was elected to the Academy of Medicine in 1832 and served as its president in 1849; in 1843 he joined the Academy of Sciences.

Velpeau's many publications include books on surgical anatomy (1825), obstetrics (1830), physiology (1831), surgical operations (1832), embryology (1833), and diseases of the breast (1854). In this last work, he suggested that patients might have a constitutional predisposition to cancer; he distinguished benign from malignant tumors, which were incurable. Like Bretonneau, he embraced the contagion theory of disease and insisted on covering open wounds in his patients. Velpeau also took a strong interest in medical education and the organization of the profession; he advocated continuing to train health officers, arguing that the faculties could not produce enough doctors to meet the needs of the countryside.

Velpeau has sometimes been misleadingly depicted as excessively attached to the Paris clinical school of the early nineteenth century and opposed to innovation and the work of the enthusiasts of laboratory medicine, whom he dubbed the 'young Paris school'. Although he was unpersuaded by early experiments with anesthesia—in 1839 he famously dismissed the idea of painless surgery as a chimera—he accepted the use of ether in obstetrics and surgery. Similarly, his confidence that his clinical experience enabled him to make a more reliable diagnosis of cancer than the microscopists did not prevent him from sending them the tumors he removed.

Among the most prominent of French surgeons in the middle decades of the nineteenth century, Velpeau exemplified the Paris school's continuing commitment to hospital-based treatment and training at the highest level, combined with a sensitivity to the needs of the rural population in which he had his roots.

Bibliography

Primary: 1832. *Nouveaux éléments de médecine opératoire* 3 vols. (Paris); 1854. *Traité des maladies du sein et de la région mammaire* (Paris).

Secondary: La Berge, Ann, 1998. 'Dichotomy or Integration? Medical Microscopy and the Paris Clinical Tradition' in Hannaway, Caroline, and Ann La Berge, eds., *Constructing Paris Médicine* (Amsterdam) pp. 275–312; Aron, Émile, 1994. 'Alfred Velpeau (1795–1867): une carrière exceptionnelle.' *Histoire des sciences médicales* 28: 101–107.

Matthew Ramsey

VERSCHUER, OTMAR VON

VERSCHUER, OTMAR VON (b. Richelsdorf Hütte, Germany, 16 July 1896; d. Muenster, Germany, 8 August 1969), *Nazi eugenics.*

After serving as an infantry officer during World War I, Verschuer studied medicine in Marburg, Hamburg, Freiburg, and Munich. He was active in the nationalist Freikorps in 1920 in Thuringia. He received his medical degree in 1923 from Marburg, with a thesis on protein content in blood serum. The eugenicist Fritz Lenz found a position for Verschuer as an assistant physician to Wilhelm Weitz at the Tübingen Policlinic.

In 1927 Verschuer's Habilitation thesis was a study of twins. The anthropologist, Eugen Fischer, as director of the newly founded Kaiser Wilhelm Institute for Anthropology, Human Heredity and Eugenics (KWI for Anthropology), appointed Verschuer head of the Institute's Human Heredity section. In 1932 Verschuer supported the introduction of a sterilization law, and in 1935 he joined the hereditary health court of Charlottenburg to adjudicate on sterilization cases. Between 1932 and 1934, the Rockefeller Foundation provided some support for his research on identical twins. In 1933 Verschuer became a 'nicht beamteter' [unofficial] professor of human genetics and racial hygiene (eugenics) at the University of Berlin.

In 1934 the German Academy of Natural Scientists Leopoldina elected him a member. In 1935 Verschuer became professor at Frankfurt am Main and director of the Institute for Human Heredity. Josef Mengele was his assistant. Verschuer joined the NSDAP in 1940, yet, paradoxically, he was a member of the Protestant dissident German Confessing Church. In 1939 he addressed the International Congress of Genetics in Edinburgh and the Royal Society. In 1942 he returned to the KWI for Anthropology to succeed Eugen Fischer as its director. In 1943 the Prussian Scientific Academy named him a full member.

He published prolifically on the hereditary nature of human characteristics, including a medical textbook on *Erbpathologie* [Hereditary Pathology]. Between 1934 and 1944 he was also editor of *Der Erbarzt*. Verschuer achieved a reputation for research on the inheritance of susceptibility to infections. He published (with Karl Diehl) on the hereditary disposition to tuberculosis, comparing fraternal and identical twins. Verschuer was also involved with other doctors' medical studies on the hereditary nature of pathological conditions.

Verschuer was an energetic advocate of eugenics and racial hygiene, and he opposed socialized medicine on the basis that this undermined German national strength. He vehemently denounced foreign racial elements in Germany, distinguishing between two aspects of racial hygiene: maintaining the internal hereditary health of one's own race (*erbpflegerisch Seite*) and preventing the admixture of alien races (*rassenpflegerisch Seite*). Verschuer provided ideological and clinical support for Nazi racial policy in general and anti-Jewish policy in particular. He produced certificates of racial ancestry. From 1937 to 1941 he participated in conferences on the 'Jewish Problem' of the Reich Institute for History of the New Germany.

Verschuer maintained informal links with his former assistant from Frankfurt, Josef Mengele. The link became formalized, as Verschuer was a co-researcher on the project on specific proteins funded by the Deutsche Forschungsgemeinschaft, sending blood from Auschwitz. The link facilitated Mengele's supply of criminally obtained body parts to the KWI for Anthropology.

After the war Verschuer fled to his family estate at Sonthofen near Bebra. Efforts to establish himself as director of a revived KWI in Frankfurt were unsuccessful. He engaged in a bitter competition with his former colleague Hans Nachtsheim to re-establish a new research institute for human heredity. Briefly under a threat of arrest because of his Auschwitz links, he received only a nominal fine because his colleagues had argued tendentiously for his innocence. He was appointed professor and director of the Institute of Human Genetics at Muenster in 1951. He continued his twin research and commenced studies of the effects of radiation.

He died in 1969 from a car crash.

Bibliography

Primary: 1933–36. (with Diehl, Karl) *Zwillingstuberkulose. Zwillingsforschung und erbliche Tuberkulosedisposition* 2 vols. (Jena); 1934. *Erbpathologie: Ein Lehrbuch für Ärzte und Medizinstudierende* (Dresden and Leipzig); 1935. 'Zwillinge und Zwillingsforschung' in Dittler, R., et al., eds., *Handwörterbuch der Naturwissenschaften*, vol. 10 (Jena); 1941. *Leitfaden der Rassenhygiene* (Leipzig).

Secondary: Schmuhl, Hans-Walter, ed., 2003. *Rassenforschung an Kaiser-Wilhelm-Instituten vor und nach 1933* (Göttingen); Weindling, Paul, 1989. *Health, Race and German Politics between National Unification and Nazism, 1870–1945* (Cambridge).

Paul Weindling

VESALIUS, ANDREAS (b. Brussels, Belgium, 31 December 1514; d. Zakynthos, Greece, 15 October 1564), *anatomy, surgery.*

Andreas Wytinck van Wesel was born in Brussels on 31 December 1514 as the son of Andreas Vesalius, who was an apothecary of Emperor Charles V, and Isabel Crabbe. At the time, the Habsburg Netherlands were ruled by the authoritarian Margaret of Austria (1480–1506). The Ducal Court of Mechelen was the center of art and culture, from which humanistic ideas spread all over the Low Countries, fertilizing intellectual circles north and south. This also applied to the family Wytinck, originally from the duchy of Kleef, which had produced aristocratic and lettered notables for several generations, some of them reaching high rank medical positions in Burgundian Brabant.

Leuven and Paris

Vesalius grew up in Brussels, where he studied the *trivium*, consisting of grammar, dialectic, and rhetoric. On 25 February 1530 he matriculated at the University of Leuven in the Castle College, where he was taught natural philosophy. A year later he enrolled in the Collegium Trilingue, founded at the instigation of Erasmus of Rotterdam, where he especially studied Greek and Latin. Thanks to the intercession of Nicholas Flourens, court physician of the Emperor and a friend of the van Wesel family, Vesalius was allowed to study medicine in Paris in 1533. His teachers there included the Galenists Jacques Dubois (or Sylvius, 1478–1555), an authority in anatomy and medicine, and Johann Günther von Andernach (*c.* 1505–74), who had previously lectured on Greek in Leuven. In Paris, Vesalius was also influenced by such famous men as physician Jean Fernel (1497–1558) and surgeon Jean Tagault (?–1545).

On the basis of osteological findings on skeletons Vesalius had found at the Parisian cemetery of Montfaucon, Sylvius allowed Vesalius to carry out a dissection before his tutor and fellow students in 1535. This was rather unusual for an era in which anatomy was taught from the book by Mondino de' Luzzi (Mundinus). The dissection was a great success, if only because—contrary to his tutors—Vesalius used the knife himself. Being well versed in the classical languages, he was able to cooperate actively with Johann Günther, who was then working on an edition of the *Institutiones anatomicae*, a work by Galen. When it was published in Basel in 1536, Vesalius was not just celebrated for his anatomical dissections, but also for finding the origin of the testicular blood vessels.

Due to the war between France and the Holy Roman Empire, Vesalius had to leave Paris. He resumed his medical studies in Leuven in August 1536, where he became a friend of Reinier Gemma (1508–55), who originated from Friesland. At night, they went together, outside the ramparts of Leuven, to collect the bodily remains of hanged persons in order to be able to constitute a skeleton they would study more thoroughly afterward.

Vesalius stayed at Leuven University for only one semester, working very hard. Eighteen years after the last dissection in Leuven, he carried out a few dissections with the approval of burgomaster Adrian Blehenius and under the supervision of professor in medicine John Heems. He earned his bachelor's degree by commenting on the ninth book by Rhazes (al-Rāzī), *Ad regem Almansorem*. In this first work, edited in Leuven by Rutger Resck in February 1537, Vesalius gave an overview of all sorts of illnesses, together with their treatment. With his other professor, Jeremy de Drijvere (or Thriverius, 1504–54), Vesalius engaged in a dispute concerning the proper way to perform bloodletting for lung disease. Vesalius defended the Hippocratic method, by which venesection has to be carried out at the same side of the disease. This dispute must have been particularly lively; in his letter on venesection, Vesalius tried to substantiate his earlier viewpoint with anatomical evidence concerning the venous structure.

Padua and Bologna

Shortly after finishing his bachelor's thesis, Vesalius left for Italy, arriving in Padua in September 1537. The University of Padua had been under the supervision of the doge-state Venice since 1405, enjoying a great reputation. Alessandro Benedetti (*c*. 1450–1512) had founded a thriving school for anatomical research that attached great importance to the dissection of human cadavers. His colleague Giovanni Battista da Monte (or Montanus: *c*. 1489–1551) had introduced tuition at the sickbed. Under the supervision of this erudite scholar, Vesalius spent his clinical term at the San Vitale hospital in Venice. On 5 December 1537 the young Fleming passed his doctoral exam *cum ultima diminutione*. During previous months, he must have made such a favorable impression on the professors of the medical faculty that, already the day after his promotion, Vesalius was appointed lecturer in surgery and anatomy.

The need for Galenic textbooks most probably induced Vesalius to rework the version of Günther von Andernach's *Institutiones anatomicae* for the benefit of his students. More important than this edition, however, are the *Tabulae anatomicae sex* (1538). Until that day, almost no illustrations of human skeletons or organs had been available. The illustrations of the *Tabulae anatomicae* were jointly made by Vesalius and Jan Stevens (1499–1546/50), another Flemish citizen whose family originated from the German town of Kalkar. Vesalius had probably met him in Venice, where Stevens studied with Tiziano Vecellio (*c*. 1480–1576). It is assumed that Stevens was present at a dissection in December 1537, where he made drawings of the organ systems; Vesalius added explanatory texts for the sake of his students. His didactic enthusiasm was soon recognized by his academic superiors and the notables of Padua. It caused Marc Antonio Contarini, a criminal judge who had recently been appointed, to make the bodies of executed criminals available to Vesalius. These circumstances enabled Vesalius, together with his students, to carry out thorough research into the human body. His fame grew so quickly that in 1540 he was invited by students of Bologna University to give similar demonstrations on cadavers there.

The *Fabrica*

By this time, Vesalius had become convinced of the structural differences between human and animal skeletons. He realized the presence of 'mistakes' in the Galenic texts, which, in fact, contained descriptions of the human anatomy based on animal dissection, and devoted all of his energies to publishing a correct description of the human body. The concept for an ambitious project was made when Vesalius returned from Bologna to Padua.

His *De humani corporis fabrica libri septem* was finished in the summer of 1542 and published by John Herbst (or Oporinus) in Basel in July 1543. At the same time, he published an *Epitome*, being an abridged and much cheaper version of the *Fabrica*: a Latin version to be used by students, soon followed by a German one by Alban Torinus for German surgeons and other interested readers. Being a wealthy man, Vesalius could afford to hire the best artists, woodcutters, and printers. The folio-text, containing seventy-three true to nature illustrations, caused an innovation in anatomical textbooks. The seven books of the *Fabrica* dealt with bone structure, muscles, blood vessels, nerves, abdominal organs, organs of the chest, and, finally, the brain. The artistic quality and scientific value are particularly striking in the representation of the skeleton and in the 'muscle men'. Like the drawings, the text of the seven books of the *Fabrica* constituted no less than a revolution in descriptive anatomy. The traditional topographic tripartition of the human body by Plato was converted by Vesalius into a sevenfold organ- and tissue-related system that has been used in anatomy ever since. Vesalius adapted Galenic ideas, supporting his descriptions with visual assessments on human subjects. Twelve years later, a second edition was published, in which Vesalius included many corrections and additions to the first edition, especially with respect to abdominal and chest organs. In particular, Vesalius rejected the presence of pores, or openings, in the heart septum, discarded the Galenic concept of filamentous connections in the brain stem (the so-called rete mirabile), and pointed to the bilobular character of the liver.

Whereas Vesalius had dedicated his Opus Magnum to Emperor Charles V, the *Epitome* was dedicated to Prince Philip, the son of the Emperor. In early August 1543, Vesalius had traveled to the German town of Speyer, to personally offer a copy to the Emperor, who appointed him as his personal physician. During the summer of 1544, Vesalius joined the Imperial troops at the siege of Saint-Dizier. His anatomical knowledge greatly helped him as a surgeon; in turn, his experience at the battlefield led to several surgical innovations in diagnostics and treatment.

Response and Impact

Public response to the publication of the *Fabrica* varied widely, ranging from deep resentment to abundant praise. The fierce criticism of his former tutor and friend Jacques Dubois (Sylvius) must have hurt Vesalius deeply. In the spring of 1546, when he treated an emissary of the Emperor in Nijmegen, Sylvius's scathing judgment about the *Fabrica* reached Vesalius. The latter's *Epistola rationem modumque propinandi radicis chynae* was not just a treatise on a plant root, but also a defense of Vesalius against Sylvius's allusions.

A quite different response was published by Gabriele Falloppia (1523–62), who was the successor of Vesalius to the chair in Padua in 1551 (after Realdo Colombo and a few temporary instructors). Falloppia had an almost divine veneration for his predecessor. In 1561 he published his *Observationes anatomicae,* which contained numerous anatomical discoveries (among them being the oviducts that were to be named after him) and a few gentle suggestions for improvement of the *Fabrica.* Vesalius responded to Falloppia in his *Anatomicarum Gabrielis Falloppii observationum examen,* which was published posthumously in 1564. In this extensive letter, Vesalius commented on Falloppia's text with ample argumentation, accepting some criticisms and rejecting others.

Vesalius's renovating ideas, as well as the iconography of the *Fabrica,* conquered the entire medical world in just a few decades. Except for the Galenic school in Paris, his ideas were accepted by most of the university-trained medical doctors, as well as by most surgeons, representing a new and factual anatomical-descriptive representation of

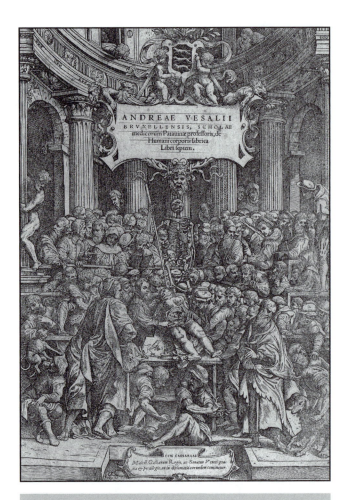

Vesalius dissecting a cadaver in front of a large audience. Woodcut, title page from *De Fabrica . . . 1543.* Rare Books, Wellcome Library, London.

the human body. The plagiarism of Vesalius's work was, although annoying to its author, the best expression of its acceptance. Whereas the German edition of the *Epitome* had probably been published with the consent of Vesalius, the same cannot be said about later works produced by anatomists and physicians who made public texts and illustrations, sometimes using the name of Vesalius, but more often publishing under their own names. Although Vesalius explicitly filed a complaint against this type of plagiarism in his publication concerning the China root, it shows the extent to which his method and his views had become commonplace in Europe.

For rather unclear reasons, Vesalius left Madrid early in 1564 to make a pilgrimage to the Holy Land. On return, his ship is said to have put the sick Vesalius ashore at the isle of Zante (now Zakynthos), where he died shortly afterward.

Like Paracelsus, Vesalius had no fear of getting rid of Galenic truths, pressing charges against this deity of all physicians, pointing out the inaccuracy of many of his claims. Considering the circumstances, this meant a real revolution, involving many risks. The innovation in the most basic science of medicine—anatomy—that had started with Leonardo da Vinci was consolidated by Vesalius. It induced people like William Harvey to integrate knowledge about the human structure with his theory of blood circulation and his ideas about procreation, thereby putting medical science on the inductive-experimental track of philosophers such as Francis Bacon or René Descartes.

Bibliography

Primary: 1537. *Paraphrasis in nonum librum Rhazae ad regem Almansorem* (Basel); 1539. *Epistola docens venam axillarem dextri cubiti in dolore laterali secundam* (Basel); 1543. *De humani corporis fabrica libri septem* (Basel). [2nd revised edn., 1555 (Basel)]; 1546. *Epistola rationem modumque propinandi radicis chynae decocti pertractans* (Basel); 1564. *Anatomicarum Gabrielis Falloppii observationum examen* (Venice).

Secondary: Nutton, Vivian, 2003. 'Introduction' to *On the Fabric of the Human Body.* Annotated translation of the 1543 and 1555 editions of Vesalius's *De humani corporis fabrica* by Garrison, Daniel, and Malcolm Hast (Evanston, IL). Also available at http://vesalius.northwestern.edu/books/FA.aa.html; Hee, R. van, 2000. 'Andreas Vesalius and His Pupils: The Breakthrough of Anatomy' in van Hee, R., ed., *Emperor Charles V and Medicine* (Ghent, 2000) pp. 37–62; O'Malley, C. D., 1964. *Andreas Vesalius of Brussels, 1514–1564* (Berkeley); Cushing, Harvey, 1962. *A Bio-Bibliography of Andreas Vesalius* (New York); *DSB.*

R. van Hee

VICQ D'AZYR, FÉLIX

(b. Valognes, France, 28 April 1748; d. Paris, France, 20 June 1794), *anatomy, epidemiology, public health, medical education.*

Vicq d'Azyr was the son of a successful physician in a town in the Cotentin Peninsula of lower Normandy that was favored as a provincial resort by the aristocracy and known as the 'Versailles of Normandy'. After completing his secondary schooling at Caen, he traveled to Paris in 1765, at the age of seventeen, to begin his medical studies. He learned anatomy from the surgeon Antoine Petit and the naturalist Louis Jean-Marie Daubenton, his grandfather by marriage. In 1772 he married Daubenton's niece. She died a year and a half later, and he never remarried. His studies were interrupted by a bout of ill health marked by coughing and bloody sputum, most likely the first manifestation of tuberculosis, and he returned home to recuperate. While in Normandy, he produced a series of studies of marine life, which he submitted to the Academy of Sciences. These papers helped win him election to the Academy as an affiliate in anatomy in 1774, shortly after he received his doctorate in medicine. He also won admission as a doctor regent of the Faculty of Medicine, which made him eligible to serve as a professor, and he was appointed as a physician to the Count of Artois, the king's brother.

Vicq d'Azyr rapidly carved out a career as a teacher, researcher, and administrator largely independent of, and often in opposition to, the Paris Faculty of Medicine. In 1775 he taught anatomy as a substitute for Petit at the Jardin du Roi, the royal natural history center. Petit hoped to see Vicq d'Azyr succeed him, but this plan did not have the approval of Buffon, the Jardin's director, and the appointment went instead to Antoine Portal in 1777. Vicq d'Azyr offered private courses on anatomy, physiology, and surgery and a public course on comparative anatomy at the Royal Veterinary School in Alfort, in the suburbs southeast of Paris, where he held a chair from 1780 to 1788. He was a charter subscriber of the Musée de Monsieur, a scientific educational center for the general public founded in 1781, and occasionally taught there. From 1778 he served as the permanent secretary of the new Royal Society of Medicine. In 1788 he was elected to the French Academy, taking the seat left vacant by the death of Buffon. After the death of Joseph Marie François de Lassone at the end of that year, Vicq d'Azyr succeeded him as first physician to Queen Marie-Antoinette, who fondly referred to him as 'mon philosophe'.

Vicq d'Azyr's most original work linked animal anatomy and veterinary medicine to their human counterparts. His broader contributions to human medicine were mainly those of a teacher and synthesizer. He edited the first six volumes (1787–92) of the thirteen-volume *Dictionnaire des sciences médicales*, part of the massive *Encyclopédie méthodique* launched by the printer and publisher Charles Joseph Pancoucke (1736–98). He summarized the contributions of eminent scientists and physicians in the more than fifty eulogies he delivered as secretary of the Royal Society of Medicine.

Anatomy and Veterinary Medicine

Anatomy, human and comparative, was the consistent focus of Vicq d'Azyr's teaching, research, and scientific publications. He contributed a 325-page article on pathological anatomy to the *Dictionnaire de médecine*. In 1792 he published the first volume of what became a five-volume set for the *Encyclopédie méthodique* entitled *Système anatomique*, on comparative anatomy and physiology. Hippolyte Cloquet (1787–1840) completed a second volume, which Vicq d'Azyr had left unfinished at his death, and produced the three additional volumes that appeared between 1819 and 1830. Vicq d'Azyr had a special interest in neuroanatomy: the one common eponymous medical term that bears his name, the thalamomamillary bundle of Vicq d'Azyr, designates a small structure in the brain. His work emphasized systematic comparisons of the same organs across species, but also of different organs within the same individual. He called for reforming anatomical nomenclature following the example of chemistry. His approach to anatomy had a strong physiological component; he practiced experiments on living animals as well as dissections.

Vicq d'Azyr's involvement in veterinary medicine began with a high-level government assignment in 1774. A major epizootic, most likely rinderpest, had broken out in south-western France in May of that year. The government's response was organized by the economist and administrator Anne-Robert-Jacques Turgot, newly appointed as Controller-General of Finance. Turgot was associated with the circle of Enlightenment thinkers known as 'Physiocrats', whose economic model emphasized agriculture on the grounds that only the soil produced a true surplus. At his instigation, the Academy of Science named a commission to deal with the emergency and appointed Vicq d'Azyr to chair it. For two years he oversaw a campaign to contain the disease, which involved establishing *cordons sanitaires*, destroying the affected animals, and disinfecting their quarters. Some of the animals that were sacrificed he used for physiological experiments. A convinced contagionist, he conducted other experiments in an effort to understand modes of transmission from animal to animal. He observed that infection conferred immunity and tried prophylactic inoculation on the model of variolation for smallpox, although he considered the method too dangerous for general use. He noted the parallels between epizootics and human epidemics, including plague. Vicq d'Azyr figured prominently among the advocates of veterinary medicine in the late eighteenth century who focused on the implications for human medicine rather than on agriculture, on the Physiocratic model.

The Royal Society of Medicine

The Royal Society of Medicine grew out of the work of the commission on epizootics. In April 1776, toward the end of Turgot's ministry, a decree of the Council of State established a new commission headed by Lassone, whose responsibilities were now extended to include human epidemics. By the summer of 1776, the commission was styling itself the Société et correspondance royale de médecine, with Vicq d'Azyr as its first correspondent; by September it had become the Société de correspondance royale de médecine, with Vicq d'Azyr as commissioner-general for epidemics. To the great consternation of the Paris Faculty of Medicine, which saw itself as the supreme authority in the kingdom on matters medical, the upstart society behaved increasingly like a royal academy, even organizing a prize competition, with awards announced in January 1778. Despite the faculty's continuing opposition, both court and government rallied behind the society, which received letters patent in August 1778, officially establishing it as the Royal Society of Medicine and appointing Vicq d'Azyr as permanent secretary, with Lassone as president. In contrast to the faculties and other academies, the Society was remarkably nonexclusive. Its regular members and associates (sixty of them foreign) included pharmacists, surgeons, and other nonphysicians, and it had an unfixed number of corresponding members, who sent reports on epidemics and other public health concerns. Under the influence of environmental medical theories, they were encouraged to submit meteorological data on standardized forms, and many wrote medical topographies of their regions. The Society was also charged with examining and approving mineral waters and proprietary remedies. Although it had no direct involvement in the oversight of medical and surgical practice—the jealously guarded prerogative of the medical faculties and colleges and the surgical communities—it regularly received complaints about quackery and malpractice in the provinces, and it modeled an approach that linked medicine, surgery, pharmacy, and veterinary medicine and emphasized the health of the population, not just the individual patient. An academy of medicine in all but name, the Society was regularly consulted by the government on medical questions and functioned in some respects like a ministry of health. It owed its success to the combined efforts of many 'enlightened physicians', as they liked to style themselves, but above all to Vicq d'Azyr, who handled the voluminous correspondence, edited the ten volumes of the Society's *Histoire et Mémoires*, and played the principal role in organizing the Society's many activities.

The French Revolution

Like many enlightened physicians, Vicq d'Azyr saw in the first phase of the French Revolution an opportunity to reform French medicine and public health along the lines advocated by the Royal Society of Medicine. With the help of colleagues from the Society, he drafted an ambitious proposal, a *Nouveau plan de constitution pour la médecine en France* [New Plan for the Organization of French Medicine], developed between August 1789 and November 1790. It called for a researched-oriented academy of medicine based on the Society, a new medical curriculum, and a national health care system. The old faculties, with their corporate privileges, would be replaced by a network of state-sponsored medical schools, each one associated with a teaching hospital. The curriculum would be grounded in the basic sciences; emphasize clinical training; and include such subjects as obstetrics, gynecology, pediatrics, hygiene, medical history, and forensic medicine. A second tier of practitioners would receive a practical training without charge in local hospitals and, upon graduation, would be placed around the district as salaried health officers, according to community needs. In November 1790 Vicq d'Azyr presented the plan to the National Assembly's Health Committee, a body formed the previous September that included the seventeen physicians, all from the provinces, who were members of the Assembly. The Committee agreed to take the *New Plan* as the working draft of its report. Over the course of its deliberations, it dropped most of the provisions on public health and health care, but, in the final bill that emerged in September 1791, the sections on education were close to those in the *New Plan*. The proposal died with the dissolution of the Assembly at the end of that month. Its influence was discernible, however, in the law on medical education presented after Vicq d'Azyr's death by his former protégé, Antoine de Fourcroy, and passed by the National Convention in December 1794.

As the Revolution turned increasingly radical following the fall of the monarchy in August 1792, Vicq d'Azyr anxiously watched the consequences for the world of medicine and science. The academies, including the Royal Society of Medicine, were closed in August 1793 and then the faculties in September. Friends such as the astronomer Jean Sylvain Bailly went to the guillotine; so did Vicq d'Azyr's royal patient and patron Marie-Antoinette on 16 October 1793. Vicq d'Azyr was reduced to working as a physician in the military hospitals and supervising saltpeter production for the national Gunpowder Commission. In December the National Convention established a Temporary Commission on the Arts to preserve objects of cultural and scientific value and appointed Vicq d'Azyr to the anatomy section. In May 1794 he joined the bibliographical section, charged with reviewing the library catalogues of émigrés and executed counterrevolutionaries to select volumes for the library of the Committee of Public Safety. On 8 June, a very warm day, he felt obliged to attend the elaborate Festival of the Supreme Being, arranged by Maximilien Robespierre to help promote deism as the religion of the Revolution. He developed what was described as congestion in the lungs and fever and died delirious twelve days later.

Vicq d'Azyr championed an Enlightenment vision of medical reform in which medical education and practice would draw upon the sciences, the clinic, and all the branches of the medical arts and in which the profession, in alliance with the state, would work to promote public health. His career also dramatically illustrated how a close connection with the royal court could raise a physician to rapid prominence under the Old Regime and then reverse that ascent with the monarchy's fall.

Bibliography

Primary: 1805. (Moreau de la Sarthe, J.-L., ed.) *Œuvres . . .* 6 vols. (Paris); 1776. *Exposé des moyens curatifs & préservatifs qui peuvent être employés contre les maladies pestilentielles des bêtes à cornes* (Paris); 1786–90. *Traité d'anatomie et de physiologie* (Paris).

Secondary: Weiner, Dora, 1993. *The Citizen-Patient in Revolutionary and Imperial Paris* (Baltimore); Wilkinson, Lise, 1992. *Animals and Disease: An Introduction to the History of Comparative Medicine* (Cambridge); Gillispie, Charles, 1980. *Science and Polity in France at the End of the Old Regime* (Princeton); Hannaway, Caroline C., 1972. 'The Société Royale de Médecine and Epidemics in the Ancien Régime.' *Bulletin of the History of Medicine* 46: 257–273; *DSB.*

Matthew Ramsey

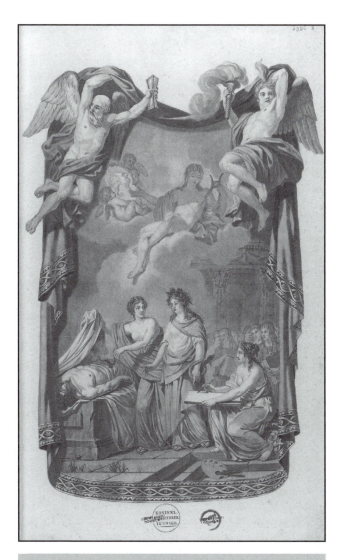

Preparation for anatomical dissection with seated female artist. Frontispiece to *Traité d'anatomie et de physiologie . . .* Paris, 1786–90. Rare Books, Wellcome Library, London.

VILLERMÉ, LOUIS-RENÉ   (b. Paris, France, 10 May 1782; d. Paris, 16 November 1863), *statistics, public health.*

Villermé grew up in Lardy, a small village in the department of the Seine-et-Oise, where his grandfather practiced medicine and his father had been an attorney at the law court in Paris (the Châtelet) before his retirement for health reasons. After attending the village school for several years, Villermé went to Paris to study. Upon completion of his education in 1804, he pursued medicine, and that same year he was admitted as a military surgeon. After spending ten years as a surgeon in the Napoleonic army, he left military service in 1814. He settled in Paris, where he cared for his widowed mother. That same year, he took his exams and received his MD from the Paris Faculty of Medicine with a thesis on false membranes.

At first Villermé embraced medical practice and pathological anatomy and, by 1818, was collaborating on the

Dictionnaire des sciences médicales. That same year, he married Mlle Morel-d'Arleux, with whom he had a son and a daughter. He was elected to the Société médicale d'émulation and was secretary general for several years. But his interest in the practice of medicine did not endure, and before 1820 he began to focus on public health and political economy, with a special interest in statistics.

By the late 1820s he had published two landmark studies on differential mortality and was the French authority on the influence of standard of living on health. He was a founding editor of and frequent contributor to the *Annales d'hygiène publique et de médecine légale*, founded in 1829 and the organ of the French public health movement. He was an associate member of the Conseil de salubrité de la ville de Paris et du département de la Seine [Paris Health Council] from 1831 to 1836 and was a member of the Royal Academy of Medicine (from 1823). Along with his friend and colleague, Alexandre Parent-Duchâtelet, Villermé was one of the leaders of the early nineteenth-century French public health movement.

The apogee of Villermé's career and the work for which he is best known today was his two-volume study of the material and moral condition of the French textile workers, the *Tableau de l'état physique et moral des ouvriers employés dans les manufactures de coton, de laine et de soie*, published in 1840.

Statistics: Studies of Differential Mortality

Villermé became interested in using quantification as a tool to study public health and social questions in the 1820s. The publication in 1821 and 1823 of the first two volumes of the *Recherches statistiques sur la ville de Paris et le département de la Seine* by the Prefecture of the Seine provided him with statistical data to investigate the causes of differing mortality rates in France and Paris. Villermé's most important statistical studies dealt with the causes of differing mortality rates in the rich and poor departments of France and in the twelve arrondissements of Paris.

Using numerical data, Villermé examined the relationship of misery, affluence, health, and mortality. In one study, he compared morbidity and mortality in the poor and rich departments of France and the poor and rich areas of Paris. The second investigation focused on Paris. Using statistical tables from the *Recherches statistiques*, as well as statistics gathered from prisons and other institutions, Villermé developed his 'thesis' on the relationship of poverty, disease, and mortality. He argued that social and economic factors—that is, the environment created by affluence or poverty—were the principal determinants of differing mortality rates among the French and Parisian populations.

Villermé's thesis differed from the point of view that prevailed in most medical topographies and hygiene manuals of the 1820s and earlier, which attributed differences in disease and death rates to climatic and topographical fac-

tors. Some hygienists, such as Villermé, had begun to shift their explanations of disease causation from climatic and topographical to social factors, namely wealth and poverty. But this social explanation was at first contested. Whereas most hygienists believed that misery deprived people of good health, others argued that wealth and luxury promoted excesses detrimental to health. Villermé's goal was to use statistical data to test these hypotheses scientifically.

Using property taxes to determine relative wealth or poverty, Villermé ranked the Parisian arrondissements from wealthiest to poorest. Correlating affluence or poverty with mortality rates, he found that, with one exception, the wealthiest neighborhoods had the lowest (at-home) mortality rates and vice versa. Comparing wealthy and poor departments in France, Villermé found similar correlations. In some poor departments, the mortality rate was more than twice a high as in the rich.

In the second study Villermé sought to identify specific causes of differing mortality rates. His final, revolutionary, conclusion was that the circumstances hygienists had claimed exerted a great influence on health—the location of dwellings, proximity to the Seine river, prevailing winds, agglomeration of dwellings, and population density—could not explain the differences in mortality. He argued that the effect of these causes was masked by the affluence or poverty of the population. His studies showed that affluence, wealth, and the material conditions they provided were the primary determinants of health. Villermé proved statistically what many French hygienists already believed, namely, that the poor were sicklier and died earlier than the comfortable and wealthy.

The Health of Textile Workers

By the 1830s Villermé had an international reputation as a statistician, social investigator, and public hygienist. Studies on differential mortality and other public health investigations had established Villermé's reputation as a sociohygienic investigator when his colleagues in the recently re-established (1830) Academy of Political and Moral Sciences asked him and former military surgeon and statistician, L. F. Benoiston de Châteauneuf to investigate the condition of the French working classes. Just that year, in a study on the health and longevity of British workers, Villermé found mortality rates higher in manufacturing than in agricultural areas. British statistical data supported his earlier research, allowing Villermé to contend that the low salaries of the workers—not industrialization—were at the root of the problem. The Academy asked the two investigators to determine if industrialization was harmful or beneficial to workers and if the physical and moral condition of French workers was as bad as the conservative and socialist critics claimed. Villermé was in charge of the departments with the highest concentration of textile workers.

After traveling from 1835 to 1837 to French textile centers and observing workers, Villermé reported that the overall condition of the working classes had improved, but that certain groups of workers, namely weavers and spinners, had not shared in these improvements. He described the filthy conditions in which the textile workers of Lille, Rouen, and Lyon lived, citing those of the cotton workers of Lille, one of the most industrialized of French cities, as the worst. He singled out the handloom weavers as being the unhealthiest of all workers, attributing their condition to long working hours, bad nutrition, and deleterious working conditions. One exception to this gloomy picture was the Lyonnais silk workers, whose situation had noticeably improved. Villermé found the silk-weavers living in better conditions than the cotton-weavers of Lille and the Haut-Rhin and noted their sobriety and intelligence.

Villermé believed that material conditions were related to moral conditions. Hence, he maintained that poor material conditions predispose people to bad moral behavior. For example, he observed that the more poverty-stricken the workers, the more alcohol they consumed. Workers were, to some extent, responsible for their behavior, but Villermé blamed factory owners even more. He accused factory owners of having little concern for workers' material and moral condition, contending that they regarded workers as 'simple production machines' (1840, vol. 2, p. 55).

Villermé's research on British manufacturing areas showed that industrialization was correlated with bad health, but in the *Tableau* he argued that, with a few exceptions, industrialization was beneficial to workers because it improved their standard of living. But there was a paradox: if industrialization was beneficial to workers, then what were the causes of workers' morbidity and premature mortality? Why were certain groups of workers exempt from the public health improvements of the era? Villermé shared the view of his colleagues that the real causes of workers' diseases were not industrial processes or working conditions, but too much work, too long working hours, insufficient sleep, lack of nutritious food and personal hygiene, and habits such as drunkenness and debauchery. At the root of all of these conditions were salaries inadequate to satisfy basic needs. Villermé's research on textile workers yielded results that supported his thesis on the relation of disease to poverty. Hence, he concluded that the main causes of workers' morbidity and premature mortality were poverty and concomitant bad living conditions—not industrialization or working conditions in factories. The solutions to workers' health problems were higher salaries, better living conditions, and shorter working hours.

Villermé's special concern was child labor, and he contended that the long working hours of children were not work, but torture. Hence, he argued for a national law to regulate child labor, with the goal of improving children's health and the public health. Partly as a result of Villermé's efforts, a child labor act was passed in 1841. Even though

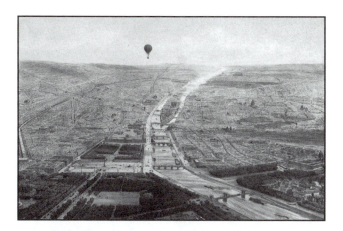

A hot-air balloon floats over the crowded quarters of Paris, 1846. Hand-colored lithograph by Jules Arnout. Iconographic Collection, Wellcome Library, London.

some historians have hailed the law as a landmark of social legislation, a concrete outcome of Villermé's study of textile workers, the law was unenforceable. It did not provide for salaried inspectors and applied only to large factories, thereby excluding most of French industry, which was still pre-industrial and conducted in small workshops.

Villermé's conclusions in the *Tableau* reinforced his thesis that poverty and bad living conditions were the main causes of disease and death. Hence, this work, like his other studies, exemplified the social theory of epidemiology favored by French public hygienists. Villermé and many of his colleagues found the origins of disease in social conditions, namely poverty, and advocated both socioeconomic and moral reform to improve public health. By moral reform, they meant *embourgeoisement,* or teaching the poor to adopt middle-class values and habits of organization, sobriety, and cleanliness. It is significant that the hygienists reached this consensus by what they considered scientific investigation, with an emphasis on gathering and analyzing statistical data. Quantification was a principal tool of hygienic investigation, one which hygienists believed gave public hygiene scientific status.

Villermé continued to work through the early 1860s. Pursuing his interest in the working classes, in the 1840s and 1850s he promoted the establishment of working-class housing projects, or *cités ouvrières*. Villermé believed that, if workers were given decent cottages to live in, they would become healthier and more moral. If poor material conditions predisposed workers to bad morals, then providing adequate residences would result in better morals and better health. Villermé's last studies dealt with statistical methods and army recruitment and the age of spouses in marriage. Villermé died in 1863 at the age of eighty-one.

Bibliiography

Primary: 1828. 'Mémoire sur la mortalité en France dans la classe aisée et dans la classe indigente.' *Mémoires de l'Académie royale de* *médecine* 1: 51–98; 1830. 'De la mortalité dans les divers quartiers de la ville de Paris.' *Annales d'hygiène publique et de médecine légale* 3: 294–341; 1834. 'Sur la population de la Grande-Bretagne considérée principalement et comparativement dans les districts agricoles, dans les districts manufacturiers et dans les grandes villes.' *Annales d'hygiène publique et de médecine légale* 12: 247–271; 1840. *Tableau de l'état physique et moral des ouvriers employés dans les manufactures de coton, de laine et de soie* 2 vols. (Paris).

Secondary: La Berge, Ann, 1992. *The Early Nineteenth-Century French Public Health Movement* (New York); Reddy, William, 1984. *The Rise of Market Culture: The Textile Trade and French Society, 1750–1900* (New York); Coleman, William, 1982. *Death Is a Social Disease: Public Health and Political Economy in Early Industrial France* (Madison, WI); Guérard, Alphonse, 1864. 'Notice sur M. Villermé.' *Annales d'hygiène publique et de médecine légale* 21: 162–177.

Ann F. La Berge

VINCENT, CLOVIS   (b. Ingré [Loiret], France, 26 September 1879, d. Paris, France, 14 November 1947), *neurosurgery.*

Vincent studied first at the lycée in Orleans and then medicine in Paris, where he also did his hospital internship. He was a student of Joseph Babinski, who was himself a disciple of famous French neurologist Jean-Martin Charcot. Just before World War I, Vincent became chief medical officer at the Pitié-Salpêtrière Hospital. At the time, French medicine was anchored in the anatamo-clinical method, which assumed that all behavioral disorders had an anatomical basis and that all anatomical lesions were manifested in symptoms analyzable by clinical examination. In neurology, Joseph Babinski brought anatamo-pathology to its apogee when, for example, he proposed a distinction between organic hemiplegia and hysterical hemiplegia, thus reducing hysteria to hypochondria that manifested itself in autosuggestive symptoms that could disappear through persuasion. After a meticulous clinical examination, Babinski could determine a medullar lesion within a millimeter of its location, thus opening the way, with his students Thierry De Martel and Clovis Vincent, to French neurosurgery.

When war broke out in 1914, Clovis Vincent followed his passion for active sports and engagement by becoming a combat stretcher bearer. One of his biographers related that in 1915, during the capture of a hill in Vauquois, 'he found the time while treating wounded French soldiers to kill some enemy soldiers'. This action won him the military Légion d'honneur. The war also gave him the chance to practice new methods of treating hysteria, and he developed a method for rehabilitation of combatants with shell shock. For the latter, he utilized the method of verbal suggestion inspired by his mentor Babinski, reinforced with electric shock treatment. The use of electric shock had the advantage of distinguishing malingerers from soldiers who were truly suffering, but, despite the praise of the General staff, Vincent's methods brought complaints from some

troops, which eventually resulted in his being transferred to a rear hospital in the city of Tours.

After the war Vincent moved from neurology to neurosurgery. He visited the United States to study with the acknowledged world leader in neurosurgery, Harvey Cushing, at the Peter Bent Brigham Hospital in Boston. Following a long French surgical tradition, Vincent developed 'careful manual technique and procedures', quickly becoming a specialist universally recognized for the extraction of pituitary and other meningeal tumors. His dexterity earned him the admiration of Cushing, who, during a visit to Paris, told the dean of the Medical school that he had 'seen the best neurosurgeon on the world operate'. This appreciation was shared by the Rockefeller Foundation, whose support in 1933 allowed Vincent to create the Neurosurgical Center of the Pitié-Salpêtrière, where he studied the physiology of frontal lobes of the skull and was named to the first chair of neurosurgery created at the Paris Medical School in 1939.

Bibliography

Primary: 1928. *Diagnostic des tumeurs comprimant le lobe frontal* (Paris); 1937. (with David, M., and H. Askenasy) *Sur une méthode de traitement des abcès subaigus et chroniques des hémisphères cérébraux* (Paris); 1939. *Leçon inaugurale de la Chaire de neuro-chirurgie.* Faculté de Médecine de Paris (Paris).

Secondary: 1949. *Hommage à Clovis Vincent composé par un groupe de ses élèves et de ses amis* (Paris).

Jean-François Picard

VIRCHOW, RUDOLF KARL   (b. Schivelbein, Pomerania, Germany, 13 October 1821; d. Berlin, Germany, 5 September 1902), *pathology, anthropology, social medicine, public health, politics.*

Virchow's life was relatively straightforward, and his career path was not dominated by outstanding events. Between 1839 and 1843, he studied medicine at the Pépinière, a medical school for military physicians in Berlin. In 1843 he got his MD and became assistant physician (Unterarzt) at the Charité, the Berlin Military Hospital. In 1844 he became the assistant of Robert Froriep (1804–61), who worked as prosector in the dead room of the Charité-Hospital. In 1846 Virchow became Froriep's successor. His teacher's license (Habilitation) followed in 1847. Although he was dismissed in 1849 because of his political activities in the course of the Revolution of 1848, he got the chair of pathological anatomy at the University of Würzburg in the very same year. Finally, in 1856, he obtained the chair of pathology at the University of Berlin and became again prosector of the Charité-Hospital. In 1893 he was director of Berlin University. Virchow died in Berlin in 1902.

Virchow is one of the most well-known German physicians of the nineteenth century. His work was a milestone in the history of pathology and scientific medicine, for two main reasons. First, he brought the project of the Viennese pathologist Carl von Rokitansky (1804–78) to a conclusion, namely the development of the field of morbid anatomy as a medical discipline. Second, Virchow went one step further when transforming pathology in general to the core discipline of the new scientific medicine. Virchow did this with his new conceptualization of pathology. First of all, he envisioned a new setting for pathology within the medical context when creating new methods and new aims for the field. Second, Virchow developed a new theory for pathology and for medicine. The basis for these achievements was his own research work, but also the mobilization and systematization of already existing contemporary research in medicine. Besides pathology, Virchow had two other subjects of interest, namely social policy and anthropology, which made him a broad-minded and versatile scientist.

The New Setting of Pathology

In 1839, when Virchow came to Berlin to study medicine, the Medical Faculty had discussed the best way to develop and practice its subject. Those favoring philosophy-oriented medicine stood against the representatives of a new medicine, favoring routine autopsy and the use of the laboratory to promote investigations into the nature of human diseases. This new medicine would no longer rely on individual experience and the intuition of the healer. In contrast, it aimed to question nature specifically, in both ward and laboratory, and to achieve precise knowledge on the pathology of man. This knowledge would be transferred to effective therapies. This approach mingled with a social reform movement within medicine, fostering democracy as a tool for the fight against social misery and, thus, against diseases. There were discussions on the health of people because of the effects of early industrialization in Germany. Physicians argued for better health care provisions for the poor, which led, inter alia, to the movement for medical reforms (Medizinalreformbewegung) in the course of the Revolution of 1848. The activities of the respective physicians were enveloped by efforts to create a sort of middle-class identity directed against the gentry, whose superior position they wished to undermine. One part of these efforts was symbolized by the foundation of laboratories, where accurate knowledge about the basic sciences could be acquired by experimental studies. In addition, these efforts were mingled with the philanthropic middle-class ideal that well-educated physicians might use their knowledge for the benefit of the poor.

Berlin stood for these new movements, and Virchow was involved in the respective discussions. He developed a new frame for pathology, based on the two most influential disciplines of nineteenth-century medicine: anatomy and physiology. In 1846, when he became Froriep's assistant as the prosector of the Charité-Hospital, Virchow viewed the dead room to be the 'vestibule of actual medicine' (Vir-

chow, 1847, p.10). He believed that this vestibule should not to be governed by hypothetical theories of natural philosophy. In contrast, detailed investigations on single problems should be carried out there without any prejudices. The examination of pathological changes of human morphology would provide the firm basis to elucidate laws of the causation and effect of diseases. These investigations should rely on the same principles as in the sciences of physics and chemistry. The disease process had to be examined with the help of experiment, including animal experimentation. The establishment of a 'pathological physiology' was the most important aim for Virchow. It was the 'fortress of scientific medicine', whereas morbid anatomy and clinical medicine were the 'outer wards', or the supporting fortification (1847, p. 19). Virchow's ideas on the setting and the aims of pathology were visible also in the title of a new journal, which he founded together with his colleague Benno Reinhardt (1819–52) in the very same year: *Archiv für pathologische Anatomie und Physiologie und für klinische Medizin* [Archive of Morbid Anatomy and Physiology and of Clinical Medicine].

Virchow was keen to set his ideas into practice. Morbid anatomy and the connections to the ward served to detect the causes of death of deceased patients. Furthermore, it served for teaching and research. Pathological anatomical specimens were collected for students as well as physicians at the Charité-Hospital. Virchow invaded the field of pathological physiology, e.g., with his first research work on the inflammation of veins (phlebitis), published between 1845 and 1847. He concentrated on the examination of the arteries of the lungs, which were obstructed due to clotted blood (a so-called thrombus). Virchow showed that these blood clots were not caused by phlebitis. On the contrary, the blood from the veins of the lower extremities to the arteries of the lung carried them, thereby causing what Virchow called 'embolism' (Embolie). Work in the dead room, as well as experiments on dogs, were combined with clinical experience. This way, Virchow refuted hypothetical theories on the character of phlebitis because he could elucidate the relationship between cause and effect of pathologically changed morphological conditions. Furthermore, Virchow opposed 'medical systems', which attempted to explain pathological processes with untested, easily understood general explanations. Therefore, Virchow criticized Rokitansky's hematopathology, which tried to explain nearly all diseases by changed conditions of the blood.

The New Principle of Pathology

Virchow had set up new coordinates for the performance of pathology within scientific medicine, but there was still no consensus in medicine about the general basic mechanisms of the origins of diseases. In the years to come, Virchow tried to solve exactly this problem. In 1847 he became successor of Froriep, but his involvement in the Revolution of 1848 made it difficult for him to work in Berlin any longer. In 1849 he accepted the call to Würzburg, as professor of pathology. After the political excitements of the previous years, he now devoted all of his time to the clarification of detailed problems of morbid anatomy. Above all, Virchow made extensive use of the microscope as a new tool within the daily routine of the physician. The result of his work was the foundation of a new 'principle' of pathology and medicine, the so-called 'cellular pathology'. This principle combined very effectively the already developed knowledge about the living cells of plants, animals, and human beings. In Virchow's view the cell was the smallest unit of life. Every cell generates from another cell (*omnis cellula e cellula*). On this basis the cell was the actual seat of disease. The origins and developments of diseases in cells were based on physiological, namely, chemical and physical, laws. Disease, for Virchow, was nothing else than life under changed conditions. The consequence was that diseases were not separate entities or living beings, as postulated by many contemporary physicians who were still devoted to philosophical theories of life. Virchow deepened organ and tissue pathology by introducing the field of cell pathology, and he strengthened the solidist attitude, which conceptualized the solid parts of the body as the seat of disease. Cellular pathology fostered, above all, histological examinations of specimens on a routine basis. Virchow thus examined the different types of cells of the body tissues, and he acquired knowledge on the specific character of cells. Remarkably, Virchow's 'cellular pathology' also had political implications. According to Virchow's liberal views, the body was a democratic cell state, governed by its parts, not by any seemingly most important organ.

In 1858, only two years after he returned to Berlin, Virchow presented his new brainchild from the Würzburg years to the public. In his Berlin Institute, he presented lectures to physicians, which were published in the same year as a book entitled *Die Cellularpathologie in ihrer Begründung auf die physiologische und pathologische Gewebelehre* [The Cellular Pathology in Its Foundation on Physiological and Pathological Tissue Theory]. Although Virchow did not want to give birth to a new general 'system', his new principle enabled contemporary scientific medicine to deal with human disease on a unified basis. Virchow's cellular pathology met the desire of his time to create a coherent synthesis of the knowledge acquired until then. The new principle promoted an effective communication within the medical scientific community. It became clear that the discipline of pathology not only applied to morbid anatomy, but also dealt with the theory of disease. Virchow's offer was soon well known. In contrast to all of the former systems, cellular pathology relied strictly on the experimental methods of the sciences, which also flourished in the nineteenth century. Because Virchow's work was related to the contemporary approaches of biological research, his cellular theory was a principle of life as such.

The Influence of Virchow's Pathology on Medicine

In his second period in Berlin, after he had developed a new organizational and theoretical frame for pathology, Virchow became well known. For many physicians and scientists, his institute became a place for basic education in pathology, advanced education, and research. Furthermore, it became the starting point for the foundation of pathology as a discipline in the medical faculties of the German-speaking countries, but also in foreign countries. In the second half of the nineteenth century, nearly all universities in Germany, Austria, and Switzerland founded institutes and chairs of pathology. Virchow's institute soon had an international reputation and became a model for other institutions of pathology, but also for the position of the field within medicine. Between 1896 and 1906, a new complex of buildings for pathology was erected in Berlin, on the grounds of the Charité-Hospital, due to the initiative of Virchow. Three large buildings covered the main house, the morgue, and, last but not least, the pathological museum. They were connected with each other and could be reached from the hospital as well as from the city. The new institute covered three departments. The anatomical department stood in the center; its purpose was the organization of the autopsies. Then there was a chemical-pathological department, which had to care for chemical examinations, showing the connection of Virchow's pathology with the sciences. The pathological museum was the third department. Pathological specimens were collected, prepared, and mounted there.

The institute expanded and developed its strength in morphological diagnostics and research. Although Virchow did not work in the morgue from about 1870, his pet child remained the pathological museum, and its growth promoted the foundation of pathological collections at the single institutes in Germany in the course of the second half of the century. Virchow's museum was opened in 1899, covering approximately 23,000 specimens on five levels. It served for teaching and research, but also for the education of the public. This stood in accordance with Virchow's middle-class mentality, making him feel obligated to inform the public about the results of research in morbid anatomy. In Virchow's view, physicians and lay people should meet in the museum. Pathology should influence scientific medicine, but also German society in general.

Although influential, the organization of Berlin pathology, as well as Virchow's new principle, was also controversial. Not only pathologists, but also anatomists, bacteriologists, and clinicians needed dead bodies. Furthermore, pathologists and clinicians discussed, in the dissection room, how to perform and utilize autopsies. In Germany, the professionalization of pathology had distanced the new field from clinical medicine. In 1897 the German Pathological Society was founded, and pathologists were divorced from the *Versammlung Deutscher Naturforscher und Ärzte* [Assembly of the German Natural Scientists and Physicians]. Virchow did not favor this decision because he viewed pathology as closely bound to the clinical disciplines, but the process of separation was already far developed by the end of the nineteenth century.

Furthermore, there was resistance to autopsy as a method. The relatives of deceased patients in the course of the nineteenth century increasingly refused autopsies. Although the administration of the Charité-Hospital basically supported Virchow's claims to maintain the effective performance of routine autopsies, it had, on the other hand, to acknowledge the interests of the public because the reputation of the hospital was at stake. Therefore, the administration supervised Virchow's management of the autopsy business in the Pathological Institute and reserved the right to interfere if necessary.

Virchow's principle, cellular pathology, was also controversial. Although it was supportive for invasive surgery in the last third of the century, problems occurred with its application to internal medicine: How should one carry out cellular therapy in case of the diverse infectious or feverish diseases? There was no clear answer. Also, some basic doubts remained: Were the cells really the most important entities of the human body or were other systems? This could be the blood (e.g., Rokitansky), but also the nerves. And how far was cellular pathology compatible with the newly acquired knowledge of bacteriology? If microbes caused diseases, was it then plausible to view the cells as the units being decisive for health and disease? Virchow discussed with bacteriologists the final cause of disease and remained skeptical toward the approach of Robert Koch (1843–1910).

Some physicians raised another point: Virchow's cellular approach seemed to be cold and mechanistic because it favored single parts of the human body, but not the body as well as soul of the whole individual. Indeed, if Virchow wrote about the organism of man as a whole, he had the tendency to come back very soon to the character and functions of the organs and body parts, using, e.g., the terms 'cell-organism' (Zellen-Organismus), and 'assembled organism' (zusammengesetzter Organismus). The critical attitudes in respect of such statements were fueled by the general unease of people at the end of the nineteenth century because rapid industrialization seemed to create a more and more mechanistic and materialistic world. Therefore, many physicians had doubts whether scientific medicine, as it stood, was really able to deal with people's health problems. They started to consider external and internal conditions of the causation and development of disease and the overall constitution and environment of the individual.

But keen defenders of a mechanistic worldview also attacked Virchow. Virchow had received his education in a time when philosophical approaches had a foothold in medicine, and this left traces. Virchow always kept vitalistic thoughts about life forces, which could not be explained at all. These explanations invaded his writings on the cells, especially at points where his knowledge came up against limiting factors.

Finally, Virchow was not able to establish pathological physiology as the 'fortress' of pathology and medicine. In contrast, the 'outer ward', namely, morbid anatomy, always remained at the core of Virchow's work. His strength was the description of static morphological conditions of the human body. One of his most important concerns was to sort out and collect pathological specimens. Animal experimentation as a decisive method of experimental pathology was neglected. Virchow had only visions about the development of pathological physiology. It was one of his students, the Leipzig pathologist Julius Cohnheim (1839–84), who especially cultivated the field in close contact with clinical medicine, and it was Cohnheim who thereby influenced the rise of 'clinical pathology' in twentieth-century England. Clinical pathology could break up the alienation between pathology and practical medicine in the long run. In Germany, the dead room remained the intellectual center of pathology in the first half of the twentieth century. The new strand of clinical pathology came back to Germany only after 1945.

However, cellular pathology was increasingly accepted as an effective principle in Western scientific medicine during the second half of the nineteenth century. When Virchow died in 1902, he was viewed as one of the most important representatives of scientific medicine. His work had brought a certain unification of medicine. The cellular view opened new pathways for the research of the ill human body. This was based on the introduction of the routine autopsy, with a firmly established dissection technique and macroscopic as well as histological examinations. The blank landscape of the human body was filled continuously in the course of the nineteenth century. Virchow's work decisively shaped the morphological age, when pathological conditions of cells, tissues, and organs were investigated.

Social Policy

As already indicated, Virchow's work was strongly correlated with political ideas and visions. An important event for the development of his political attitudes was the outbreak of a typhus epidemic in Upper Silesia in 1847–48. Virchow stayed there between 20 February and 10 March 1848. The result was a report to the Prussian government, indicating clearly that medical sanitary improvements were linked with the introduction of democracy, educational measures, and freedom, as well as prosperity. Virchow developed liberal attitudes; he called himself a 'republican'. In the course of the Revolution of 1848, Virchow was a member of democratic associations and fought on the street. His engagement was mainly devoted to the realization of the already-mentioned 'medical reform'. Together with the psychiatrist Rudolf Leu-buscher (1821–61), he founded a journal with a correspond-ing name, *Die medicinische Reform* [Medical Reform]. The journal called for radical changes of the health system, with new health laws improving the working conditions of the physicians, as well as the health care for the people. But the revolutionary efforts of Virchow and his co-combatants failed. The journal was suspended, his company flat was sub-ject to notice, and his salary was reduced. In 1849 he resigned his post in Berlin and became professor of pathology in Würzburg.

In Würzburg, politics receded in favor of keen work on pathology. But this did not mean he abandoned his liberal ideas and political activities in the long run. After his appointment as pathologist in Berlin, Virchow was elected member of the Ber-lin City Council (1859). Virchow's work for the City of Berlin, which he maintained until his death, included, among others, several fields of public health care, e.g., the organization of drainage and hygienic measures, the administration and setup of city hospitals, and the health care of school children. These efforts corresponded with Virchow's view that politics would be nothing else than medicine on a higher level (*Medicin im Gros-sen*, 1848). Therewith, Virchow continued, after 1856, what he had started in his first Berlin period, not, of course, as a revolu-tionary, but as a settled, middle-class elite scientist. This also meant that Virchow took up again anticonservative initiatives. In 1861 he belonged to the founding members of the German Liberal Party (Deutsche Fortschrittspartei), which promoted the unification of Germany under democratic headings. In the same year, he became a member of the Prussian Parliament, where he actively opposed Otto von Bismarck (1815–98), who, in 1871, would unify the German territorial states on the basis of the Franco-Prussian War. To influence state policy, Virchow used the only effective tool of the parliament at these times, namely, the approval of the budget. He spoke and worked against increased expenditures for the military and in favor of investing in social and health care. He proceeded with this pol-icy between 1880 and 1893, when he was member of the parlia-ment of the newly founded German Empire. There he was a fierce critic of German colonial politics, which he judged as an expensive, risky, and useless undertaking.

Virchow's regional and national support for the improvement of public health care was without doubt suc-cessful. This cannot be said about his engagement in gen-eral politics, where he was not so effective as he was in scientific medicine. But Virchow at least contributed to the upkeep of democratic thinking and tradition in German society, which surely was a backbone for all of the twentieth-century efforts to set up a democratic state in the country, namely after 1918 and after 1945.

Anthropology

Since the 1860s, simultaneously with his growing interest in continuous political activity, Virchow's research interests were focused very much on anthropology. It was then a very young discipline, and Virchow bolstered its development with his activities. His aim was to establish a comparative anatomy of human cultures. One important point was the question of the origins of the human beings, which was hotly debated then by scientists from divergent backgrounds. Virchow sym-pathized with the theories of Charles Darwin (1809–82) about the origins of species and saw some evidence for the idea that the development of animals and human being took place in steps. But, in contrast to his student Ernst Haeckel (1834–1919), who applied Darwin's theory to the develop-ment and relationship of human races (social Darwinism), Virchow was reluctant to accept it definitely. In his view, it remained a hypothesis that needed further clarification. In this sense, based on his own research on school children and in contrast to fashionable contemporary notions, Virchow refuted any identification of races with specific nations. Vir-chow's own investigations concentrated more or less on anthropometrics, the measurement of different parts of human skeletons and their pathological changes. There he focused mainly on research of the skull base, which, in his view, could show formative relations between face, brain, and cranium. His research therefore shows similarities with the *Völkerpathologie* [people's pathology], which was promoted by the Freiburg pathologist Ludwig Aschoff (1866–1942) in the 1920s. The aim was an unprejudiced investigation of the morphological manifestation of different pathological condi-tions of humankind. Virchow finally helped institutionalize anthropology. In 1869 he became a member of the German Anthropological Society (Deutsche Anthropologische Gesell-schaft), which he headed over many years. In the same year, he founded the Berlin Society for Anthropology, Ethnology, and Prehistory (Berliner Gesellschaft für Anthropologie, Eth-nologie und Urgeschichte).

Virchow did this work in close relation to archaeological research. His contacts with Heinrich Schliemann (1822–90), who in the late 1870s tried to find the site of the his-toric Troy, were famous. Virchow himself contributed to archaeological excavations and to the examination of the material. Besides the site of Troy, Virchow visited different sites in the German-speaking countries, and also in Egypt and the Caucasus.

When Virchow died in 1902, he was one of the most influential German physicians and scientists of his time, whose approaches and attitudes had ruled over all of medi-cal Berlin for decades. He was so well-known that thou-sands of people attended the mourning events. But at the time of his death, it was also clear that Virchow had remained a nineteenth-century man whose notions about contemporary issues had been shaped, above all, by his pre-revolutionary experiences of politics and medicine. At the end of the nineteenth century, it was often felt that his invocations lacked flexibility and did not correspond to current discussions about respective topics of modern culture. But his work influenced the development of

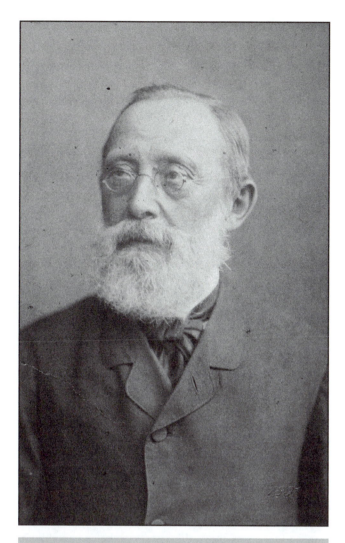

Rudolf Virchow. Photograph by J. C. Schaarwächter, 1891. Iconographic Collection, Wellcome Library, London.

twentieth-century scientific medicine most decisively as a guideline, as a starting point for further developments, and for discussions about the character of modern medicine with its chances, risks, and dangers.

Bibliography

Primary: 1992–. (Andreé, Christian, ed.) *Rudolf Virchow. Sämtliche Werke,* vols. 4(1), 21(1), 32(2), 59(4) (Bern); 1847. 'Über die Standpunkte in der wissenschaftlichen Medicin.' *Archiv für pathologische Anatomie und Physiologie und für klinische Medizin* 1: 3–19; 1849. 'Mittheilungen über die in Oberschlesien herrschende Typhus-Epidemie.' *Archiv für pathologische Anatomie und Physiologie und für klinische Medizin* 2: 143–322; 1858. *Die Cellularpathologie in ihrer Begründung auf die physiologische und pathologische Gewebelehre* (Berlin) (English trans., 1860); 1901. (Schwalbe, Julius, ed.) *Virchow-Bibliographie 1843–1901* (Berlin); 1906. (Rabl, Maria, ed.) *Rudolf Virchow, Briefe an seine Eltern 1839–1864* (Leipzig); 1958. (Rather, L. J., trans. and intro.) *Disease, Life, and Man: Selected Essays* (Stanford); 1985. (Rather, L. J., ed.) *Collected Essays of Public*

Health and Epidemiology 2 vols. (Canton, MA); 1990. (by Rather, Lelland J.) *A Commentary on the Medical Writings of Rudolf Virchow: Based on Schwalbe's Virchow Bibliographie, 1843–1901* (San Francisco).

Secondary: Prüll, Cay-Rüdiger, 2003. *Medizin am Toten oder am Lebenden?—Pathologie in Berlin und in London 1900 bis 1945* (Basel); McNeely, Ian F., 2002. *'Medicine on a Grand Scale': Rudolf Virchow, Liberalism and the Public Health* (London); Goschler, Constantin, 2002. *Rudolf Virchow. Mediziner-Anthropologe-Politiker* (Cologne, Weimar, and Vienna); Schipperges, Heinrich, 1994. *Rudolf Virchow* (Reinbek); Bauer, Axel, 1989. *Die Krankheitslehre auf dem Weg zur naturwissenschaftlichen Morphologie. Pathologie auf den Versammlungen Deutscher Naturforscher und Ärzte von 1822–1872* (Stuttgart); Mazzolini, Renato, 1988. *Politisch-biologische Analogien im Frühwerk Rudolf Virchows* (Marburg); Vasold, Manfred, 1988. *Rudolf Virchow: Der große Arzt und Politiker* (Stuttgart); Maulitz, Russell C., 1978. 'Rudolf Virchow, Julius Cohnheim and the Program of Pathology.' *Bulletin of the History of Medicine* 52: 162–182; Andreé, Christian, 1976, *Virchow als Prähistoriker* (Cologne and Vienna); Ackerknecht, Erwin, 1953, *Rudolf Virchow. Doctor-Statesman-Anthropologist* (Madison, WI); Pagel, Walter, 1931. *Rudolf Virchow und die Grundlagen der Medizin des XIX. Jahrhunderts* (Jena).

Cay-Ruediger Pruell

VOGT, CÉCILE AUGUSTINE MARIE (b. Annécy, Haute Savoie, France, 27 March 1875; d. Cambridge, England, 4 March 1962). **VOGT, OSKAR GEORG DIECKMANN** (b. Husum, Germany, 6 April 1870; d. Freiburg im Breisgau, Germany, 31 July 1959), *neurology, psychology, neuroanatomy.*

The daughter of the French brigade officer Pierre Louis Mugnier, Cécile Mugnier studied medicine in Paris (1893–99) and graduated MD with a neuroanatomical dissertation in 1901. In the same year she was given the doctor's certificate in France. Oskar, eldest son of the parish priest Hans Friedrich Vogt, who had died prematurely, and his wife Maria, studied medicine and biology at the Christian-Albrechts-University of Kiel and the Friedrich-Schiller-University of Jena (1888–94). Based on his neuroanatomical work, he obtained his MD from Jena University in 1894. During his medical studies, Walther Flemming, Ernst Haeckel, Max Fuerbringer, and Otto Binswanger counted among his teachers. On the occasion of Oskar's residency in the Paris laboratories, Cécile and Oskar had met in the French capital and got engaged in 1899. Together with her daughter Claire, who was born before their marriage, Cécile accompanied Oskar on his way back to Berlin.

Oskar Vogt had already served as assistant to Otto Binswanger in Jena and Robert Binswanger in Kreuzlingen (1883–84). In 1884 he visited August Forel in Zurich, learned the technique of hypnosis, and was made editor of Forel's *Zeitschrift für Hypnotismus, Psychotherapie sowie anderer psychophysiologischer und psychopathologischer Forschungen,* which he continued from 1902 onward as *Journal für Psychologie und Neurologie.* In 1894–95 he proceeded with his internship at the Leipzig Clinic for Psychiatry and Neurology of Paul Flechsig and earned his living in private practice with hypnotic therapy. On their return from Paris, Cécile and Oskar developed the so-called 'Neurologische Centralstation', formerly established as a neuroanatomical laboratory in Oskar's flat, into a major institute for brain research. Due to their common efforts, the 'Neurobiological Institute', as it was now called, was integrated into Friedrich-Wilhelms-University in 1902, and Oskar Vogt was appointed university professor. Their institute was the kernel of the Kaiser-Wilhelm-Institute for Brain Research, established in 1914, which later moved to Berlin-Buch during the Weimar Republic.

Together with Korbinian Brodmann, the Vogts laid the foundation for what they called a 'cytoarchitectonic and myeloarchitectonic classification of the cortex' and defined the areas of the brain in humans and other mammals. Their pathogenetic assumptions were molded after their concept of 'pathoclisis', i.e., the view that circumscribed architectonic defects of brain tissue were responsible for psychiatric disorders. Apart from these findings, Cécile decisively formed our understanding of the thalamus and the basal ganglia, and both Vogts were able to distinguish electrophysiologically between the motor and the sensory cortex. Together with the appreciation of Cécile's doctor's certificate, in 1920 she was made head of the neuroanatomical department. Between 1925 and 1930 Oskar moved frequently between Berlin and Moscow, as he was made scientific head of the creation of the State Institute for Brain Research in the Soviet Union. In the beginning, it was the aim of the Russian institute to investigate the neuromorphological properties of the revolutionary leader Vladimir Ilji Lenin. Oskar Vogt's research and organizational talent led to a steady increase in German-Soviet relations in science and education.

The Vogts continued to develop the Berlin Institute into a research foundation with extensive dimensions. By 1928 there existed eleven distinct research departments, each of which was led by a scientist; e.g., Nikolai Vladimirovi Timoféeff-Ressofsky was in charge of the department for neurogenetics, and Max Bielschowsky headed the neuropathological department. This fruitful scientific endeavor was abruptly disturbed by the Nazi regime. Due to their leftist political attitudes and the influence of personal intrigues, the Vogts had to leave Berlin, in 1937, and sought refuge in a private Institute for Brain Research and General Biology in Neustadt, Black Forest. After Oskar's death, in 1959, Cécile moved to Cambridge, England, where their daughter Marthe had emigrated in 1933.

Bibliography

Primary: 1907. 'Zur Kenntnis der elektrisch erregbaren Hirnrindengebiete bei den Säugetieren.' *Journal für Psychologie und Neurologie* 8 (suppl.): 277–456; 1937–38. 'Sitz und Wesen der Krankheiten im Lichte der topistischen Hirnforschung und des Variierens der Tiere, 1. u. 2. Teil.' *Journal für Psychologie und Neurologie* 47: 237–457, 48: 169–324; 1941–42. 'Thalamusstudien I–III.' *Journal für Psychologie und Neurologie* 50: 32–154.

Secondary: Hagner, Michael, 1999. 'Gehirnführung. Zur Anatomie der geistigen Funktionen, 1870–1930' in Hagner, Michael, ed., *Ecce Cortex. Beiträge zur Geschichte des modernen Gehirns* (Göttingen) pp. 177–205; Satzinger, Helga, 1998. *Die Geschichte der genetisch orientierten Hirnforschung von Cécile und Oskar Vogt in der Zeit von 1895 bis ca. 1927* (Stuttgart); Satzinger, Helga, 1996. 'Das Gehirn, die Frau und ein Unterschied in den Neurowissenschaften des 20. Jahrhunderts: Cécile Vogt (1875–1962)' in Meinel, Christoph, and Monika Renneberg, eds., *Geschlechterverhältnisse in Medizin, Naturwissenschaft und Technik* (Stuttgart) pp. 75–82.

Frank W. Stahnisch

VOUROS, IOANNIS (b. Chios, Ottoman Empire [now Greece], 1808; d. Athens, Greece, 23 January 1885), *pathology.*

Vouros undertook his general studies in Trieste and in 1825 began medical studies in Vienna, where he formed a lasting friendship with Baron Sinas. He received his doctoral degree in Heidelberg in 1832 and continued his studies in Berlin and Paris, where he became acquainted with Adamandios Korais, one of the most important personalities of the modern Hellenic Enlightenment, who supported his studies.

Upon his return to Athens in 1834, Vouros was appointed initially as a regional doctor in the islands of the Cyclades. The edict of 30 October 1833 stipulated that ten regional doctors were to be appointed, one in each national region, to police medical practice in the newly established Hellenic state and to survey the health system of the countryside. In 1835 he was appointed as a professor of nosology and clinical medicine at the Medical-Surgical School. Established in Athens for the training of 'empirical doctors', its students and staff became the target of 'scientific doctors', who attempted to dominate the medical field and to discredit 'empirical practice' during the nineteenth century.

In 1837, with the establishment of the Athens University Medical School, Vouros was appointed professor of pathology and therapy and gave lectures in the methodology of medicine. Later, he was appointed as a member, secretary, and eventually chairman of the Medical Board, a central political body established in 1834 to create and operate systematically the 'health police' and to work for the advancement of the scientific and rational medical knowledge within the independent Hellenic state. In 1839 he became the personal doctor of King Othon, the first King of the independent Hellenic state.

In March 1842, with the opening of the state hospital, Elpis (Hope), one of the first hospitals established in Athens, Vouros undertook management of the pathology clinic. During 1841–42 and again in 1845–46, he served as dean of the Medical School, and from 1836 onward he was chairman of the Medical Society of Athens, established 5 June 1835. On 1 August 1836 the Medical Society of Athens published its first medical magazine, *Asklipios*, with the mission of developing a professional body of scientific doctors.

Among his publications is 'On Hospitals: A Sketch' (Paris, 1831), an early article on the foundation and function of hospitals as places for the isolation and the treatment of illness in the newly independent Hellenic state. The lack of hospital-asylums during the pre-revolutionary period had fueled a pressing need to establish hospitals as therapeutic institutions. In the new hospitals, as Vouros noted, the doctors became the main figures. Formerly providing medical care only by traveling to the patient's home, the doctors now became responsible for the entire medical therapeutic procedure within the hospital, with the help of nurses and assistants. Under this new paradigm, geared to the production of medical knowledge, the doctors would make continuous contributions. On a daily basis, they would supervise the observation of an illness, note its symptoms and progression, and carry out treatment.

With X. Landerer and I. Sartori, Vouros wrote *Pharmacopoea Graeca* [Hellenic Pharmaceuticals] (1837), the first pharmaceutical text used as a guide for doctors and chemists of the Hellenic state during the nineteenth century. He also wrote *The Medical Situation of Cyclades during 1834*.

Bibliography

Secondary: Korasidou, Maria, 2002. *When Illness Threatens. Surveillance and Health Control of the Population in Greece in the 19th Century* (in Greek) (Athens).

Maria Korasidou

VULPIAN, (EDMÉ-FELIX) ALFRED   (b. Paris, France, 5 January 1826; d. Paris, 18 May 1887), *neurology, medical administration.*

Vulpian was the son of a lawyer who also wrote for the theater. He began his schooling at Prytané de Ménars outside Paris and then at Lycée Louis-le-Grand in Paris. Although his parents wished him to attend the École normale supérieure, his interest in physiology led him to enter the École de Médecine in 1848. An interne at La Pitié hospital at the same time as his friend Jean-Martin Charcot, Vulpian wrote his medical thesis on the origin of the cervical nerves and received his medical degree in 1853.

For three years Vulpian served as an assistant to Pierre Flourens at the Musée d'Histoire Naturelle in Paris, lecturing in comparative physiology. He incorporated these lectures in an important publication on the comparative physiology of the nervous system. His work in this area won him prizes from the Académie des Sciences. In 1860 he wrote on secondary pneumonias for his agrégé thesis. Between 1861 and 1869 he joined Charcot in a post at the Salpêtrière hospital, and together the two published a large number of significant papers on pathological anatomy of the nervous system. In 1867 he was named professor of anatomical pathology at the Faculté de Médecine and in 1872 was awarded the chair of comparative and experimental pathology. With Charles Édouard Brown-Séquard and Charcot, he founded the *Archives de physiologie normale et pathologique* in 1868. In that same year he married Inès Mantoux, a friend of Charcot's wife.

When Vulpian was made dean of the medical faculty in 1875, he reorganized and expanded the experimental laboratories of the medical school and the École pratique until his resignation in 1881. He had been a member of the Académie de Medécine since 1869, but in 1876 he was also inaugurated into the Académie des Sciences and became the perpetual secretary of that body ten years later. He published a lengthy study of diseases of the nervous system in two volumes between 1879 and 1886. During this period, he encouraged laboratory-based medical research, animal experimentation, and the use of the microscope.

Vulpian became an active supporter of the work of Louis Pasteur, first as a member of the commission on hydrophobia. He recommended that Pasteur proceed with his use of antirabies inoculations in human cases of rabies and continued to defend him before the Académie de Medécine and the Académie des Sciences in the mid 1880s. Among Vulpian's students were the neurologists Jules Déjerine and his wife Augusta Klumpke-Déjerine, who both wrote of their admiration for him. He died of pneumonia at the age of sixty-one.

Bibliography

Primary: 1866. *Leçons sur la physiologie générale et comparée du système nerveux* (Paris); 1874. *Leçons sur l'appareil vaso-moteur* 2 vols. (Paris); 1879–86. *Maladies du système nerveux. Leçons profesées à la Faculté de Médecine* 2 vols. (Paris).

Secondary: Goetz, Christopher G., Michel Bonduelle, and Toby Gelfand, 1995. *Charcot: Constructing Neurology* (New York, London); Ebner, Anton, 1967. *Edmé Felix-Alfred Vulpian, 1825–1887.* (*Zurcher Medizingeschichtliche Abhandlungen* NR 49) (Zurich); Laignel-Lavastine, M, 1927. 'Edmond-Felix-Alfred Vulpian [*sic*] (1826–1887).' *Bull. Soc. Franç. Hist. Med.* 21: 287–303.

Joy Harvey

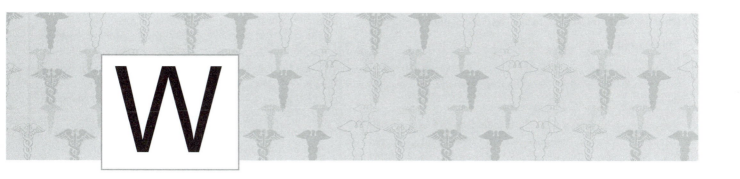

W

WAGNER, GERHARD (Neu-Heiduk, Upper Silesia [now Poland], 18 August 1888; d. Munich, Germany, 25 March 1939), *eugenics, Nazi medicine*.

Wagner, son of the surgeon Wilhelm Wagner, studied medicine in Munich until 1912. He was a volunteer during World War I and came back from the front a decorated soldier. After the war, he worked as a general practitioner and as an assistant at the gynecological hospital in Munich. Because Upper Silesia was to be separated from the Reich, he decided to join a nationalist fighting group (Freikorp) (1921–23) and headed the German nationalist League of Upper Silesia. After returning from Upper Silesia to Bavaria, he became a member of the NSDAP (Nazi Party) in 1929 and headed a local branch of the party. The National Socialist German Physician's League (NSDÄB) was founded in 1929; he served as its treasurer and from 1932 he was its third president. After Hitler came to power, Wagner was active in many National Socialist institutions and above all took a key role in the Gleichschaltung (enforcement of political conformity) of the medical profession.

As head of both of the medical associations in Germany, the German Physician's League and the Hartmannbund that was institutionalized in 1900 to defend the economic interests of the profession, Wagner began in 1933 the Nazification of German physicians and the removal of Jews from the medical profession. In April and June 1933 'non-Aryans' were excluded from medical insurance practice. As Reich Physician Leader (1934), he centralized the various medical organizations and unified medical periodicals, while placing them at the service of the Nazi Party. In spring 1936 a Reich Medical Chamber was established and all previous medical associations were dissolved.

From 1933 Wagner was a major influence in public health and racial hygiene. He was head of the party expert committee for public health, a member of the expert committee for population and racial policy at the Reich Ministry of Interior, and adviser to Rudolph Hess in medical affairs. Moreover, he was the middleman between NSDAP and the Red Cross and between NSDAP and the Labor ministry. In 1934 he joined the SA as a medical squad leader, headed a department for genealogical research, and reorganized the National Socialist Union of students. In 1935 he called for the formation of a working group on the Neue Deutsche Heilkunde [New German Alternative Medicine]. He wanted to increase the influence of alternative medicine, while tying it to orthodox medicine and placing it under his control. In 1936 he was decorated by the party. In 1937 he became supreme judge of the Labor organization 'Deutscher Arbeitsfront'.

Wagner always served National Socialist racial hygiene zealously. He pressed for radicalization of the sterilization law. In September 1934 he decreed that carrying out abortions where the parents were apparently degenerate was legal. With Gross and Bartels (both medical ideologues of the NSDAP), Wagner urged the passage of a strong law to eliminate Jews from German life. The result was the Nuremberg laws of 15 September 1935, to 'Protect German Blood and Honor'. Hitler is reported to have secretly informed Wagner of the intention to implement euthanasia in 1935. In 1936 Wagner encouraged discussion of euthanasia.

As a power struggle occurred between state and party for control of health care, Wagner wished to unify professional and public health administration under the auspices of the party Gauleiter. Wagner's power was limited by Gütt, the head of the Reich Ministry Department of Public Health, who used his position to strengthen a centralized state structure. In 1939 Wagner retired, and he died on 25 March in Munich. His successor was Leonardo Conti, who worked closely with Himmler on medical and racial policies.

Bibliography

Primary: 1933. 'Arzt und Volk im Dritten Reich.' *Deutsches Ärzteblatt* 63: 4–6; 1934. 'Rasse und Volksgesundheit.' *Deutsches Ärzteblatt* 64: 917–923.

Secondary: Weindling, Paul, 1989. *Health, Race and German Politics between National Unification and Nazism* (Cambridge); Zunke, Peter, 1972. *Der erste Reichsärzteführer Dr. med. Gerhard Wagner* (Kiel).

Anne Cottebrune

WAGNER-JAUREGG, JULIUS VON (b. Wels, Austria, 7 March 1857; d. Vienna, Austria, 27 September 1940), *psychiatry*.

Wagner-Jauregg (his father, Adolf Johann Wagner, had been bestowed the title, 'Ritter von Jauregg') was one of the leading psychiatrists in the early decades of the twentieth century and the first psychiatrist to win the Nobel Prize (1927). After attending the prestigious Catholic Schottengymnasium in Vienna, Wagner-Jauregg studied medicine at the University of Vienna (1874–80). Wagner-Jauregg's career reflects the expansion and professionalization of psychiatry as an academic discipline, as well as its scientific ambitions to understand and control insanity. In 1883 he started training in psychiatry at the state mental asylum of Lower Austria. After spending three years as an adjunct professor of psychiatry at the University of Graz (1889–92), Wagner-Jauregg returned to Vienna and accepted a professorship in psychiatry at the University of Vienna. At the time, Wagner-Jauregg had been studying the connection between endemic goiter and cretinism. By carrying out a number of experiments in the Austrian province of Styria, he proved that the routine ingestion of iodine prevented goiter.

Wagner-Jauregg's career made headway in Vienna. In 1902 he succeeded Richard von Krafft-Ebing (1840–1902) as full professor (Ordinarius) of psychiatry and director of the Psychiatric Clinic within the General Hospital. Three years later, in 1905, Wagner-Jauregg took over the influential position of director of the newly constructed Psychiatric Clinic Am Steinhof. During World War I, Wagner-Jauregg was in the van of Viennese psychiatry through his treatments of a large number of soldiers suffering from 'war neuroses'. Because he used electric currents (faradization) to make soldiers fit for duty again or to single out soldiers whom he believed were malingerers, Wagner-Jauregg was accused of being a militaristic doctor. After the war, when a commission investigated a large number of 'military breaches of duty', Sigmund Freud (1856–1939) was the scientific expert at Wagner-Jauregg's hearing. Freud took advantage of this opportunity to profess the superiority of psychoanalysis over biological psychiatry, but displayed solidarity with Wagner-Jauregg by rejecting most of the accusations against him.

Interestingly, World War I was also the time when Wagner-Jauregg laid the foundation for his greatest success. In 1927 Wagner-Jauregg was awarded the Nobel Prize for, to quote the committee's explanation, 'his discovery of the therapeutic value of malaria inoculation in the treatment of dementia paralytica'. Dementia paralytica, or general paresis, was a common, fatal mental disease caused by syphilis, and until then none of the several treatment efforts had turned out to be effective.

Though Wagner-Jauregg had already made plans to experiment with artificial fever in cases of general paresis as early as the late 1880s, it was the overcrowded situation at the clinic under war conditions that enabled him to carry out the risky experiments. In 1917 Wagner-Jauregg inoculated nine soldiers suffering from general paresis with malaria, a disease that could already be cured with quinine. After undergoing severe bouts of fever, six of the patients exhibited milder symptoms. After carrying out further experiments with good results, Wagner-Jauregg was able to convince the psychiatric community that he had found a powerful method of treatment against the manifestations of general paresis. In the 1920s his malaria therapy found acceptance in many European and American psychiatric hospitals and asylums, and continued to be used well into the early 1950s, when penicillin made this therapy obsolete.

After his retirement in 1928, Wagner-Jauregg remained active in his scientific writing, concentrating on the hereditary aspects of mental disease, forensic medicine, and racial hygiene. Deeply committed to the German nationalistic mentality, he even became a member of the Nazi party in 1940, the year of his death.

Bibliography

Primary: 1914. (with Bayer, Gustav) *Lehrbuch der Organotherapie* (Leipzig); 1936. *Fieber- und Infektionstherapie. Ausgewählte Beiträge 1887–1935* (Vienna); 1950. (Schönbauer, Leopold, and Marlene Jantsch, eds.) *Lebenserinnerungen* (Vienna).

Secondary: Hofer, Hans-Georg, 2004. *Nervenschwäche und Krieg. Modernitätskritik und Krisenbewältigung in der österreichischen Psy-*

chiatrie, 1880–1920 (Vienna); Brown, Edward M., 2000. 'Why Wagner-Jauregg Won the Nobel Prize for Discovering Malaria Therapy for General Paresis of the Insane.' *History of Psychiatry* 11: 371–382; Whitrow, Magda, 1993. *Julius Wagner-Jauregg (1857–1940)* (London).

Hans-Georg Hofer

WAKLEY, THOMAS (b. Membury, England, 11 July 1795; d. Madeira, 16 May 1862), *medical journalism, medical reform, legal medicine, politics.*

Wakley was the youngest son of Henry Wakley (1750–1842), a successful Dorsetshire farmer, and his wife Mary. Although he enjoyed a conventional education at various local grammar schools, the young Wakley expressed an earnest desire to go to sea. At the age of ten he was made midshipman on a merchant clipper captained by a friend of his father, and set off on a voyage to Calcutta. On the trip home the captain died, and on his return to England Wakley's father insisted he pursue a less dangerous career. Wakley's experiences on this voyage were reflected in his later campaigns against the flogging of sailors. He changed his allegiance to medicine and in 1810 was apprenticed to an apothecary in nearby Taunton. He spent some time working for a surgeon in Beaminster before finishing his apprenticeship with his eldest sister's husband, a surgeon in Henley-on-Thames.

In 1815 Wakley traveled to London, seeking to improve his practical knowledge of medicine by 'walking the wards' under one of the great surgeons of the day. After experiencing the neglect and confusion then prevalent in London hospital medical schools, he settled on the united hospitals of Guy's and St Thomas's, where Astley Cooper (1768–1841) was at the height of his didactic and technical powers. He began to question his apothecary training, settling instead on anatomy as 'the foundation of all medical knowledge: there can be no good surgeon who is deficient in anatomical knowledge' (Anon., 1862, p. 609). After only eighteen months of study, during which he attended the Grainger brothers' private anatomy school, Wakley passed the College of Surgeons examination with ease. He later characterized the exam as 'the veriest farce imaginable' (Anon., 1862, p. 609).

In 1817 Wakley took up private practice in the City. During this period he met and proposed to Elizabeth Goodchild, the daughter of wealthy lead merchant Joseph Goodchild. In 1819 Joseph gave Wakley a large loan, enabling him to buy a successful practice in the fashionable West End of London and a large house nearby. Wakley and Elizabeth were married in February 1820.

In August 1820, however, this comfortable life was rudely interrupted. After deceiving their way into his home, a gang of men stabbed and beat Wakley into unconsciousness before setting fire to the house. His assailants may have been friends of the Cato Street Conspirators, the last men in Britain to be sentenced to the traitor's death of hanging, drawing, and quartering, and whose (postmortem) beheading was wrongly supposed to have been performed by Wakley. Although he recovered and escaped, his house and possessions were destroyed. His insurance company would not pay, implying that Wakley had started the fire himself. He sued the company and received full compensation with costs, but in the meantime was forced to move his household and practice to the poorer, shabbier Strand area.

Wakley and *Lancet*

'The biography of Mr. Wakley may almost be said, since the time he established THE LANCET, to be the history of the Medical Profession' (Anon., 1862, p. 609). Although perhaps hyperbole, *Lancet*'s assessment of its own founding editor contains a kernel of truth. The rise of *Lancet* (and, starting from 1857, the *British Medical Journal*) took place at a time of great cultural change in British medical practice. Physicians, surgeons, and apothecaries began to contest their traditionally mediocre social and economic status, citing the new European 'laboratory medicine' as a fresh source of scientific authority for medical practice. They sought to reconstruct their manual trades as scientific professions: occupations suitable for intelligent, cultivated gentlemen. Wakley's style of journalism—bold, bombastic, and radical—was perfectly suited to this new mood.

In the early 1820s a number of factors prompted Wakley to reconsider his career in medicine. Elizabeth was dissatisfied with life in the Strand, and urged her husband to find a more satisfactory source of income. This coincided with Wakley's friendship with the radical journalist and politician William Cobbett (author, in 1830, of the influential *Rural Rides*) and his encounter with Walter Channing, a Boston physician and the founder of the *New England Journal of Medicine and Surgery*. Wakley left his practice in the spring of 1823. He spent the summer generating interest in his new periodical and preparing the first issue for publication. *Lancet* was named with care: it describes both an incising tool for puncturing abscesses, and also a tall window for letting sunlight into darkened rooms.

Three factors separated *Lancet* from its competitors and contributed to the journal's immediate success. It was the only weekly medical journal in Britain: other monthly periodicals could provide learned articles but not fresh news and comment. It was written not for the leaders of the profession but for the 'ordinary' surgeon or physician, thus ensuring a wide circulation. And it reflected Wakley's interest in reform (albeit expressed via anonymous editorials): whereas other journals were interested only in the parochial concerns of the medical profession, *Lancet* engaged with the major political issues of the day.

Wakley spent much of his first decade as editor in the courtroom. He sought to make *Lancet* an organ of education as well as reform, and his chosen method was to transcribe and publish, without permission, the lectures given by eminent London clinicians. Some (such as Cooper) did not object; others, seeing the knowledge and experience from which they made their livelihoods pirated in the pages of a popular and inexpensive journal, fought back. John Abernethy (1764–1831), a surgeon at St Bartholomew's Hospital, sued for damages (1824). After a series of trials lasting over a year, *Lancet* was given permission to print public lectures as a service to medical education. Some surgeons resorted to the law when they found themselves the subject of one of Wakley's articles on botched operations or misdiagnosed diseases. Cooper's nephew Bransby was one such litigant, but after successfully suing Wakley over his description of a failed bladder stone removal, the two men became firm friends.

Lancet's early campaigns generally targeted the medical elite. His experience as a student had convinced Wakley that the system as it stood was corrupt, incompetent, and hypocritical. He attacked the large metropolitan teaching hospitals for refusing to publish mortality statistics, and campaigned for democratic reform of the RCS. The College's Council resisted this assault through a series of ferocious public debates, and only in 1843 was the category of Fellow of the RCS established to involve less exalted practitioners in the running of their profession. Perhaps Wakley's most ambitious notion, proposed in the early 1830s, was the creation of a London College of Medicine to provide a universal standard of medical training and qualification. Although he pursued this radical concept well into the 1840s, Wakley received little support from his colleagues, and the idea was quietly dropped. As he matured, Wakley's style became less aggressive and more calculated. Many nineteenth-century reforming journalists—from Cobbett via Thackeray to Dickens—admired his ability first to capture the public's imagination with a campaign and then to achieve material results.

Wakley and Politics

In *Lancet* Wakley sought to synthesize the medical and the political, and he quickly expanded his interests beyond the strictly clinical. In the months before the passing of the Great Reform Act (1832), he edited *The Ballot*, a political newsletter. This experience whetted his appetite for hands-on politics and led him to the conclusion that his reforms might be better achieved from within Parliament. Using Cobbett's inside knowledge, he stood as an independent radical candidate for the seat of Finsbury in the first election after the Reform Act. Although defeated, he returned in the 1834 election and was finally successful in January 1835.

Wakley's agenda as an MP was, true to form, radical: his first speech defended the Tolpuddle Martyrs (a group of laborers sentenced to transportation because they had formed an illegal trade union), and in the first years of his

THE LANCET.

Vol. I.—No. 1.]   LONDON, SUNDAY, OCTOBER 5, 1823.   *Price* 6d.

PREFACE.

IT has long been a subject of surprise and regret, that in this extensive and intelligent community there has not hitherto existed a work which would convey to the Public, and to distant Practitioners as well as to Students in Medicine and Surgery, reports of the Metropolitan Hospital Lectures.

Having for a considerable time past observed the great and increasing inquiries for such information, in a department of science so pre-eminently useful, we have been induced to offer to public notice a work calculated, as we conceive, to supply, in the most ample manner, whatever is valuable in these important branches of knowledge;—and as the Lectures of Sir Astley Cooper, on the theory and practice of Surgery, are probably the best of the kind delivered in Europe, we have commenced our undertaking with the introductory Address of that distinguished professor, given in the theatre of St. Thomas's Hospital on Wednesday evening last. The Course will be rendered complete in subsequent Numbers.

In addition to Lectures, we purpose giving under the head, Medical and Surgical Intelligence, a correct description of all the important Cases that may occur, whether in England or on any part of the civilized Continent.

Although it is not intended to give graphic representations with each Number, yet we have made such arrangements with the most experienced anatomical draughtsmen, as will enable us occasionally to do so, and in a manner, we trust, calculated to give universal satisfaction.

The great advantages derivable from information of this description, will, we hope, be sufficiently obvious to every one in the least degree conversant with medical knowledge; any arguments, therefore, to prove these, are unnecessary, and we content ourselves by merely showing in

1

Preface to the first copy of *Lancet*, October 5, 1823. Wellcome Library, London.

Parliamentary career he edited yet another reformist periodical, *A Voice from the Commons*. Although laconic in debate, he quickly made a name as a passionate speaker on subjects ranging from electoral reform to religious tolerance and military punishment. Medicine, however, remained his major interest, and his contributions to a series of Medical Acts in the 1840s were (with *Lancet*) his most significant influence on British practice. The 1858 Medical Act, although passed six years after Wakley's retirement from the House of Commons, established many of the reforms for which he had spent his career campaigning: the formal demarcation of medical and surgical practice, the creation of a Medical Register in which all practitioners were listed, and the establishment of a General Medical Council to regulate the profession and to set clinical standards.

One piece of legislation in which Wakley took particular interest was the 1837 Medical Witnesses Act, which for the first time enabled coroners to be paid for their services. He had initially stood for election to the West Middlesex coronership in 1830, and when elected to Parliament added the coroner system to his list of reform interests. He was eventually elected coroner in 1839. Medieval coroners had been lawyers, but Wakley brought a new medical authority to this archaic post: he investigated every suspicious death in the district, calling multiple medical witnesses when he felt it necessary, and made a point of involving the police when he suspected foul play. This new rigor was time-consuming and expensive, but an 1840 Parliamentary committee defended Wakley's approach and recommended that it become the norm. Wakley again used his official status to push for reform, arguing that deaths in Poor Law infirmaries and industrial accidents should fall under the coroners' jurisdiction.

In his later years the strain of a turbulent public life began to take its toll on Wakley's previously robust constitution. In 1851 he passed out in the doorway of *Lancet*'s offices after a twenty-three-hour working day. This incident, and the advice of his family, persuaded Wakley to withdraw from the Commons and to allow his sons, both physicians, to gradually take over his editorial duties. Elizabeth died in 1857, and by 1860 he had developed pulmonary tuberculosis. He spent the winter of 1861–62 recuperating in Madeira, but died there in the spring of 1862 after a fall on the beach.

The key to Wakley's influence on the history of British medicine lies in his willingness to mix medicine with politics at a time when the conservative British medical establishment felt the two to be utterly separate. His expression of this synthesis in *Lancet* gave a radical impetus both to the theory and the practice of modern medical politics.

Bibliography

Primary: 1823. 'The Lancet: Sunday, October 5, 1823.' *Lancet* i: 10–12; 1824. 'Hospital Reports.' *Lancet* i: 188–190; 1829. *A Report of the Trial of Cooper v. Wakley, for an alleged libel, taken by shorthand writers employed expressly for the occasion; with an engraving of the instruments, and the position of the patient. Together with Mr. B. Cooper's "Prefatory remarks" on the evidence, and a copious explanatory appendix* (London); 1839. 'Election of Coroner for Middlesex.' *Lancet* i: 697–699.

Secondary: Hostettler, John, 1993. *Thomas Wakley: An Improbable Radical* (Chichester); Loudon, Irvine, and Jean Loudon, 1992. 'Medicine, Politics and the Medical Periodical, 1800–50' in Bynum, W. F., S. Lock, and Roy Porter, eds., *Medical Journals and Medical Knowledge: Historical Essays* (London) pp. 49–69; Bostetter, M., 1985. 'The Journalism of Thomas Wakley' in Weiner, J., ed., *Innovators and Preachers: The Role of the Editor in Victorian England* (Westport, CT) pp. 275–292; Sprigge, S. Squire, 1897. *The Life and Times of Thomas Wakley* (London) (reprinted 1974, Hungtingdon, NY); Anon., 1862. 'Memoir of Thomas Wakley, Esq.' *Lancet* i: 609–612; *Oxford DNB*.

Richard Barnett

WALDMEIER, THEOPHILUS (b. Basel, Switzerland, 1831; d. Beirut, Lebanon, 10 March 1915), *psychiatry.*

Waldmeier, a Swiss Quaker, attended the missionary college of St Crischona, near Basel, before serving as a missionary in Abyssinia (Ethiopia) from 1858. He left Ethiopia for Syria in 1868 after being imprisoned by the Ethiopian Emperor Theodore and rescued by General Sir Robert Napier. He was married twice, the second time to the Ethiopian Fareedy Josephy Saleem (m. 17 April 1896).

From 1874 he worked with the Brummana Lebanon Mission (supported by the Society of Friends in Britain), helping with the Brummana High School. From 1894, he turned his attention to helping the mentally ill in Mt Lebanon. In his letters Waldmeier noted that the only acknowledged form of insanity in the Middle East was 'demonomania', i.e., the possession of a devil. This disease was generally cured by exorcisms and compulsory seclusion. There was no medical treatment: patients often died after being chained to blocks in the cave of the monastery of Kuzheya, deep in the Lebanese mountains, or in a cave near Mt Carmel.

The suffering of the insane prompted Waldmeier to improve the welfare of the mentally ill. To do this he had to resign from his post at the Brummana mission, thus losing his institutional support. However, he was a gifted speaker and endowed with exceptional organizational and fund-raising skills. During a quarter of a century of work in Lebanon, he won the respect and friendship of prominent people within the country, including Henry H. Jessup of the American Syrian Mission. Jessup helped Waldmeier establish his mental hospital in Lebanon by facilitating his appointment as a general agent with a mandate to visit Europe and the United States, where most of the money for the construction of an asylum was raised.

In 1898 the asylum site at Asfouriyeh (three miles away from Beirut) was purchased. The first buildings consisted of separate male and female wards for thirty patients each and an administration building, which housed Waldmeier and his wife and the medical director's family. The first director was Dr Wolff from Switzerland, and the nursing staff initially consisted of two European male attendants, three European female attendants, and a number of locals in training. In 1912 the property became a wakf, i.e., dedicated as a religious foundation (under the code of law prevailing in Lebanon), to be held by the Chairman of the London General Committee (who became the 'Trustee' or mutawallī). This set down the responsibilities of the 'Trustee' and his agents (in this case the Beirut Executive Committee) for managing the property. It was made a condition that the Hospital should be international and interdenominational. In planning the hospital, Waldmeier followed the advice of Henry Yellowlees (1888–1971) of the Glasgow Asylum, and employed the cottage system. He subsequently developed his own opinions about the nature and treatment of mental illness.

For the next fifty years, the Lebanon Hospital for the Insane at Asfouriyeh was the only institution of its kind in Lebanon, and its name was changed in 1914 to the Lebanon Hospital for Mental Diseases and again in 1950 to the Lebanon Hospital for Mental and Nervous Disorders.

Waldmeier introduced the British way of treating the insane to Lebanon. The medical directors of the Asfouriyeh eventually included the Lebanese physicians affiliated with the hospital, who had obtained their training in Great Britain. Furthermore, close ties were established between the Asfouriyeh hospital and the American University of Beirut. Since the latter had not developed independent psychiatric facilities, the teaching of psychiatry became entrusted to the medical staff of the Lebanon Hospital, which further enhanced the British model of psychiatric theory and practice in Lebanon.

Bibliography

Primary: 1925. (Hobhouse, Stephen, ed.) *The Autobiography of Theophilus Waldmeier, Comprising Ten Years in Abyssinia and Forty-six Years in Syria.* (London).

Secondary: Katchadourian, H., 1980. 'The Historical Background of Psychiatry in Lebanon.' *Bulletin of the History of Medicine* 54: 544–553.

Nikolaj Serikoff

WANG, JI 王省之 (aka WANG, SHENGZHI 王省之; WANG, SHISHAN 王石山) (b. Pushu, Qimen county, Huizhou prefecture, Anhui Province, China, 1463; d. Pushu, China, 1539), *Chinese medicine, surgery.*

Wang Ji was a Confucian physician (ruyi), the son of the physician Wang Wei. According to contemporary biographies, Wang studied the classics in his youth and made repeated, but unsuccessful, attempts at the civil service examinations. He is said to have given up his studies and put all his efforts into reading the medical classics on being told by his father of the famous motto of the Song dynasty vice grand councillor Fan Zhongyan 範仲淹 (989–1052): 'If you cannot serve as a good minister, you should hope to serve as a good doctor.' With his father's help, he quickly became an accomplished physician. His reputation spread far and wide, and within a short time he is said to have successfully cured several thousand patients.

As well as being a practicing physician with many disciples, Wang was a prolific author. Eleven books on topics as diverse as acupuncture and moxibustion, poxes, materia medica, and surgery are attributed to him. These include entirely new texts, revised editions of classic texts, general readers, case histories, and annotated compilations of key specialist texts. Wang's most notable work is the *Shishan yi'an* 石山醫案 [Stone Mountain medical case histories], a compilation of over 100 case histories taken from Wang's clinical practice and published by one of his disciples, Chen Jue 陳桷, in 1531. This work is the earliest extant example of

a specialist case history medical text and marks the emergence of case histories as a distinct genre of medical writing in China.

Wang aligned himself with the medical lineage of Zhu Zhenheng 朱震亨 (1282–1358) and Li Gao 李杲 (1180–1251), adapting and extending the ancient medical theory, popularized by Zhu, that in the human body Yang is in excess and Yin insufficient. He believed that Yang, or *qi* too, could be depleted and need replenishing. The case histories show that Wang often found depletion disorders of Yin and Yang, blood and *qi*, for which he would routinely prescribe replenishing treatments incorporating ginseng and astragalus root. As such, the *Shishan yi'an* was more than just a medical 'how-to' manual, in that it demonstrated the practical application of a specific theoretical stance, with cases showing the use and efficacy of warming and replenishing treatments in clinical practice. Although Wang was not alone in advocating this warming and replenishing approach, he encountered resistance to his theories from patients and rival physicians. Both the theoretical premise and its application in practice were controversial, particularly with regard to the use of ginseng for disorders of Yin depletion.

Wang was an active participant in the flourishing medical culture of sixteenth-century China, where social and economic developments such as improved transportation networks and a boom in medical publishing stimulated intellectual debate and fostered links among physicians. Wang sought to bring his teachings to a wide audience that included the general public as well as other physicians, commenting that the achievements of his long career would be pointless if he could not communicate his knowledge to future generations. He appears to have achieved this aim with further editions of his medical texts being published both in China and abroad long after his death, including a Japanese edition of the *Shishan yi'an*, which appeared in 1696.

Bibliography

Primary: 1522–1633. *Wang Shishan yishu bazhong* 汪石山醫書八種 [Eight medical books of Stone Mountain Wang] (Pushu); 1531. *Shishan yi'an* [Stone Mountain medical case histories] (Pushu).

Secondary: Grant, Joanna, 2003. *A Chinese Physician: Wang Ji and the 'Stone Mountain medical case histories'* (London).

Joanna Grant

WANG, WEIYI 王惟一 (aka WANG, WEIDE 王惟德) (b. ?, *c.* 987, d. ?, *c.* 1067), *Chinese medicine.*

Wang Weiyi was the Chief Steward of the Palace Medical Service; he flourished during the 1020s and 1030s. The information we have on his life is scarce, but we know Wang revised and edited authoritative editions of classical canons, aiding the revival of classical Han-dynasty medicine during the early years of the Song dynasty (960–1276). His most important contribution was redefining and standardizing acu-moxa therapy (i.e., acupuncture and moxibustion). Only a few incomplete and inaccurate acu-moxa manuals survived to the Song dynasty before Wang's book, which was why the eighth-century physician Wang Tao 王燾 warned that 'acupuncture kills patients whereas moxibustion cures them.'

The fourth Song emperor, Renzong 仁宗 (1023–66), assigned Wang, among others, to revise and edit two of the most important classical medical canons: the *Yellow Emperor's Inner Canon* and the *Yellow Emperor's Canon of Eighty-One Problems*. This was the first revision and printing of these canons since Wang Bing's revision (Tang dynasty). While studying these canons, Wang realized that acu-moxa, the main therapy utilized in these texts, was problematic because of the imprecise anatomical location of the acu-points. Even the course of the tracts, which represent the path in which the *qi* flows, was uncertain during his era. Accordingly, Wang headed another project, under imperial sponsorship, to revise and standardize acu-moxa knowledge.

Reviewing all the available literature, Wang compiled a systematic work on acu-moxa therapy. He designed this book to serve as a standard manual for acu-moxa therapy focusing on the correct location of the acu-points. The project lasted almost four years, concluding with the publication (1026) of *Tongren shuxue zhenjiu tujing* 銅人腧穴針灸圖經 [Illustrated Canon of Acu-moxa Therapy [Depicting] the Acu-points of the Bronze Figure]. This book, the first government-sponsored acu-moxa text, differed from its predecessors in contents and organization. Besides discussing each acu-point, Wang considered the body's physiology, the circulation tracts, and their association with medical disorders. A year later, probably as Wang realized that textual knowledge alone was insufficient to locate the acu-points precisely, he supervised the casting of two identical life-size bronze models of the human body mapping the acu-points and the courses of the circulation tracts discussed in his book. Wang's book was so highly regarded that in 1029 the emperor issued an order to carve it on stone tablets in an attempt to immortalize its contents.

The bronze models served as the standard for the location of acu-points on the body and for the courses of the circulation tracts. By depicting both the acu-points and the tracts, Wang emphasized the connection between them. The model's exact measurements, aside from the statement 'life-size', are not specified in the records. A similar Ming dynasty version, though not as elaborate as the Song model, was recorded as approximately one meter, sixty centimeters (sixty-three inches) tall. According to surviving records, the Song model was made up of a few detachable pieces. Inside were representations of internal viscera. On the outer shell the channels were carved with all the corresponding acu-points. Small holes piercing the surface corresponded to the acu-points listed in the *Illustrated Canon of Acu-moxa*.

The bronze model was the basis for a new, hands-on method of examining medical students. During the exam, students were asked to assess cases of patients presented by the examiners and, accordingly, to perform the acupuncture on the wax-covered bronze model, needling the acu-points that should treat the disease condition they diagnosed. Standardization was achieved not only by these examinations, but also by having one of the two models sent to different places where officials and physicians studied and recorded the correct locations of the acu-points.

Bibliography

Primary: 1026. *Tongren yuxue zhenjiu tujing* 銅人腧穴針灸圖經 [Illustrated Canon of Acu-moxa Therapy [Depicting] the Acu-points of the Bronze Figure].

Secondary: Goldschmidt, Asaf, 2001. 'Changing Standards: Tracing Changes in Acu-moxa Therapy during the Transition from the Tang to the Song Dynasties.' *East Asian Science, Technology, and Medicine* 18: 75–111.

Asaf Goldschmidt

WARBURG, OTTO HEINRICH (b. Freiburg im Breisgau, Germany, 8 October 1883; d. Berlin, Germany, 1 August 1970), *cell physiology, organic chemistry, oncology.*

Warburg, son of the physicist Emil Gabriel Warburg, studied physics and chemistry at the Albert-Ludwigs-University of his hometown (1900–02). In 1903 he continued his studies under Emil Hermann Fischer at the Friedrich-Wilhelms-University of Berlin, where he received his PhD with a thesis *Über Derivate des Glycocolls, Alanins und Leucins. Über l-Brom-propionsäure und das l-Alanylglycin* (1906). He decided to continue with medical studies at the Ludwig-Maximilians University in Munich and the Ruprecht-Karls-University of Heidelberg (1907–11). In 1908, under the influence of Jacques Loeb, he turned toward the analysis of biological oxidation processes. Warburg not only pursued experimental studies similar to Loeb's on the physiology of developmental processes, but also quantitative analyses of biochemical reactions, as described in 'Beobachtungen über die Oxydationsprozesse im Seeigelei' (1908). Warburg graduated MD from Heidelberg University in 1911 with a thesis *Über die Oxydation in lebenden Zellen nach Versuchen am Seeigelei*. The eggs of the sea urchin remained Warburg's central experimental model until 1914, because he saw that the formative processes underlay rapid changes, ideal for the study of oxidative processes in embryonic tissue.

Warburg conducted most of his experimental investigations at the Zoological Station of Naples, where he used to stay for many months during his university studies. Additional residences in the laboratories of Joseph Barcroft in Cambridge and Paul Ehrlich in Frankfurt am Main followed. In 1912 Warburg received his 'venia legendi' for physiology from the University of Heidelberg and volunteered as a cavalry officer at the beginning of World War I. After two years he was recalled from the battlefields to take on the directorship of the division for physiology at the Kaiser-Wilhelm-Institute for Biology. In selecting his staff, Warburg laid strong emphasis on precision engineers who provided him with specific technology for his experimental system. As a consequence of his achievements, Warburg was made a permanent member of the Kaiser-Wilhelm-Institute in 1921. Hans Krebs, who was Warburg's most prominent pupil, and many other scientists held his laboratory in high esteem, because its novices were trained in a wide variety of methods, ranging from chemical physiology and tissue culture to analytical chemistry.

Warburg's work was significantly funded by the Rockefeller Foundation, which perceived his research on tumor metabolism as exceedingly forward-looking. In 1923 he received a fellowship of the Rockefeller Foundation as 'an exceptionally promising scientist'. According to his own recollection, it was through the invitation of Johns Hopkins University in Baltimore, where he delivered the Herder Lecture under the title *Das Enzym-Problem und die biologische Oxydation* (1929), that officials of the Rockefeller Foundation remained aware of his research. Only with external funding was he able to direct his laboratory through the economic crisis of the Weimar Republic. Eventually, in 1930, Warburg founded the new Kaiser-Wilhelm-Institute for cell physiology, which provided access to made-to-measure experimental equipment of the highest standards. His discovery of the nature of respiratory fermentation was awarded with the Nobel Prize for Physiology or Medicine (1931).

During the Nazi regime, Warburg had been expelled as institute director because the Ministry of Education was told about his Jewish family origins. However, in 1942 he was reinstated as director for cancer research in what was now called a defense institute ('Wehrinstitut'), directly related to the High Command of the German Army. After World War II, Warburg worked in the United States before returning to his home country, where he was engaged with the reshaping of the former institute. It was reunited with the Max-Planck-Society in 1953. Until his death, Warburg continued to publish on the biochemical paradigm of cellular metabolism and tumor growth.

Bibliography

Primary: 1908. 'Beobachtungen über die Oxydationsprozesse im Seeigelei.' *Hoppe-Seyler's Zeitschrift für physiologische Chemie* 57: 1–16; 1926. *Über den Stoffwechsel der Tumoren* (Berlin); 1928. *Katalytische Wirkungen der lebenden Substanz* (Berlin).

Secondary: Werner, Petra, 1991. *Ein Genie irrt seltener . . . Otto Heinrich Warburg. Ein Lebensbild in Dokumenten* (Berlin); Höxtermann, Ekkehard, 1984. *Otto Heinrich Warburg (1883–1970), ein "Architekt" der Naturwissenschaften* (Beiträge zur Geschichte der Humboldt Universität zu Berlin, 9) (Berlin); Krebs, Hans, and Roswitha Schmid, 1979. *Otto Warburg. Zellphysiologe—Biochemiker—Mediziner 1883–1970* (Stuttgart) (English edn., 1981); DSB.

Frank W. Stahnisch

WARREN, EDWARD (b. Tyrell County, North Carolina, USA, 22 January 1828; d. Paris, France, 16 September 1896), *surgery, medical education.*

The son of William Christian Warren, a physician, and Harriet (Alexander) Warren, he followed in his father's footsteps by attending the University of Virginia and later Jefferson Medical College in Philadelphia, from which he received medical degrees in 1850 and 1851, respectively. In 1857 he married Elizabeth Cotton Johnstone, with whom he had four children.

Warren's morphia injection procedure and his subsequent role as medical correspondent in Paris (1854–55) won him notoriety. In addition, Warren's award-winning essay, 'The Influence of Pregnancy on the Development of Tubercles' (1856), earned him recognition as a leader in obstetrics and gynecology, although from his position as editor of the *Medical Journal of North Carolina* he severely criticized an article describing the benefits of silver suture by a young J. Marion Sims, who would later distinguish himself partly on the basis of this innovation. By 1860, despite his colorful and opinionated stands, the irascible Warren had firmly established his reputation as a prominent physician.

In 1856 Warren gave a scathing indictment of medical education in North Carolina and in the United States generally, and championed a medical practice law in his home state that passed in 1859. Warren was initially opposed to secession while he was a newly appointed professor of medicine at the University of Maryland and editor of the *Baltimore Journal of Medicine*, but with the outbreak of hostilities in 1861 he returned south and volunteered his services for the Confederacy. Warren carried his outspoken advocacy of high standards for medical practitioners into the war by insisting upon testing the competency of surgeons in the medical corps, and his vote against the relaxation of the standards of the Confederate Medical Examining Board earned him criticism. During the conflict, Warren served with distinction as surgeon general of North Carolina and as a medical inspector. His *Epitome of Practical Surgery for Field and Hospital* (1863) was widely distributed and used throughout the Confederacy.

Following the war, Warren re-established Baltimore's Washington University School of Medicine in 1867, becoming a faculty member and director of the institution. He also became the founding editor of the official mouthpiece of the state medical society of Maryland, *Medical Bulletin*, in 1868. In 1872 he cofounded the College of Physicians and Surgeons of Baltimore and that same year invented a splint for clavicle fractures.

Despite Warren's prominence, trouble seemed to follow him. He was subjected to severe public criticism in a famous murder trial in which his expert testimony provided the basis for the acquittal of a Baltimore woman. His unsuccessful bid for a position as Baltimore's coroner and failure to secure a professorship at the University of the City of New

York caused him to search for a post abroad, which he eventually obtained from the Khedive of Egypt.

He returned to Paris briefly in 1873 on his way to serve as physician to Ismail Pasha, then embroiled in efforts to secure independence from Turkey. After successfully treating a hernia for a top Egyptian official, he was awarded the honorific title Bey, and thereafter was frequently called Dr Warren Bey. Warren remained in this position until 1875, whereupon he started a practice in Paris. He remained there the rest of life, becoming a physician to the rich and famous. Warren received numerous honors: the Order of Isabella (1877), French Legion of Honor (1879), and the Egyptian Order of the Osmanich (1882).

Bibliography

Primary: 1856. 'Address Delivered Before the Medical Society of North Carolina,' *Transactions of the Medical Society of North Carolina* 7: 19–36; 1885. *A Doctor's Experiences in Three Continents* (Baltimore).

Secondary: Rutkow, Ira, 1989. Biographical sketch in the reprint edition of *An Epitome of Practical Surgery* (San Francisco); Vandiver, Frank E., 1977. *Biographical Dictionary of the Confederacy* (Westport, CT); Long, Dorothy, 1972. *Medicine in North Carolina* 2 vols. (Raleigh, NC); *DAMB*.

Michael A. Flannery

WARREN, JOHN COLLINS   (b. Boston, Massachusetts, USA, 1 August 1778; d. Boston, 8 May 1856), *medical education, surgery.*

Warren's father, John (1753–1815), was himself a man of considerable medical reputation, generally credited with the founding of Harvard Medical School. Yet the closest the younger John Warren came to medicine while at Harvard was participating in occasional body-snatching expeditions.

After graduating from Harvard College (1797), Warren spent a desultory year studying French, idly hoping for an opportunity in the mercantile world. He then at last began medical studies—in his father's office. (Like father, like son; later he would tutor his own son, Jonathan Mason Warren, the third of a distinguished six-generation sextet of Warren physicians.) The turning point came when Warren went to London for further study, where he worked under the surgeon (later Sir) Astley Cooper. Warren attended lectures in both Edinburgh and Paris before returning to Boston, where he found his father recovering from paralysis. The younger man promptly took up the challenge of managing his father's large practice.

Warren married Susan Powell Mason in 1803. She died in 1841, and in 1843 he married Anne Winthrop (who died eight years later). By 1806 he had been made an adjunct professor of anatomy and surgery at Harvard, as his father's assistant. He inherited the surgical chair when his father died, in 1815. A year later he was made Harvard Medical School's first dean; he was dean again from 1821 to 1826.

In 1812 Warren was instrumental in founding a medical journal (ancestor of today's *New England Journal of Medicine*), and he was author of a paper in its first issue. He was appointed surgeon at the Massachusetts General Hospital (MGH) in 1817, four years prior to its actual opening, and was for years the guiding spirit of the institution that he, with his close friend James Jackson, Sr., had helped found. In 1824 Warren became a consulting physician to the city of Boston.

In 1837 Warren made a return visit to Europe. London's Athenaeum Club bestowed an honorary membership on him; in Paris, he met and worked with Pierre-Charles-Alexandre Louis, whose numerical methods he subsequently promoted in the United States.

The date most often associated with John Collins Warren is 16 October 1846, when he carried out the first public clinical demonstration of surgery on a patient under ether anesthesia. Warren made a remarkably understated comment in his personal journal: 'Did an interesting operation at the Hospital this morning, while the patient was under the influence of Dr Morton's preparation to prevent pain. The substance employed was sulphuric ether' (Warren, 1860, vol. 2, p. 39). Shortly after that first ether demonstration, in early 1847, Warren resigned from Harvard, having performed some 5,000 operations and given more than 4,000 medical school lectures. He gave Harvard his collection of anatomical specimens, which today forms the basis of the Warren Museum there. At the 1850 annual meeting of the American Medical Association, he stepped down from the presidency of that organization.

Warren wrote on an impressive range of surgical topics. His major work on tumors (1839) was favorably reviewed internationally and translated into German. He published numerous articles on anesthesia, and he wrote on nonscientific subjects as well. Prominent among nearly a dozen social and professional organizations in which Warren was active was the Temperance Society. He remained to the end—literally and figuratively—a sober opponent of using alcohol as a beverage, late in life giving $10,000 to promote temperance and another $2,000 to subsidize publications on the topic.

Bibliography

Primary: 1839. *Surgical Observations on Tumours, with Cases and Operations* (Boston); 1846. *Physical Education, and the Preservation of Health* (Boston); 1848. *Etherization; with Surgical Remarks* (Boston).

Secondary: Truax, Rhoda, 1968. *The Doctors Warren of Boston* (Boston); Warren, Edward, 1860. *The Life of John Collins Warren, M.D., Compiled Chiefly from His Autobiography and Journals* 2 vols. (Boston); Arnold, Howard Payson, 1852. *Memoir of John Collins Warren, M.D.* (Cambridge, MA); *DAMB*.

Constance Putnam

WARREN, MARJORY WINSOME

WARREN, MARJORY WINSOME (b. Hornsey, London, England, 28 October 1897; d. Metz, Germany, 5 September 1960), *geriatrics*.

Warren, eldest of five daughters of Walter Richard and Annie Warren, was tall, redheaded, and freckled, and is generally accepted as the 'Mother of British Geriatric Medicine'. She was educated at North London Collegiate School and Royal Free Hospital, London, qualifying LRCP, MRCS (1923). She held junior medical posts at Queen's Hospital for Children, Hackney, at Royal Free Hospital, and at the Elizabeth Garrett Anderson Hospital, London, before being appointed assistant medical officer at the West Middlesex Hospital, Isleworth (1926). Although this appointment to a previously all-male domain was not greeted with universal approval, she soon became deputy medical director (1931) and consultant physician (1948). She was appointed Commander of the Order of the British Empire (1959). She died following a traffic accident in France that occurred when she was on the way to give a lecture in Germany. She was unmarried.

When Warren was first appointed to the West Middlesex Hospital, her interests were initially mainly surgical. She performed over 4,000 operations and gave about 3,500 anesthetics. During this period she lectured to nurses, eventually becoming an examiner for the General Nursing Council. When the Hospital took over the control of the neighboring Public Assistance Institution in 1935, she was put in charge of the 874 inpatients. Thus began her life's work and interest in the physical and social care of elderly people, especially those who were sick. She arranged the transfer of 160 maternity and 'mental observation' patients to their appropriate departments, leaving 714 patients for further assessment. She found that the same ward could contain an ill-assorted mixture of young and old, healthy and sick, as well as restless, noisy, and incontinent patients. The untreated patients had lost all independence, self-respect, morale, and hope of recovery. Some were totally contracted into a fetal position. Into this depressing arena Warren brought a complete break with the existing custodial attitude to care. She classified the patients and introduced a vigorous multidisciplinary rehabilitation and social care approach to treatment. She remedied deficiencies in the ward environment by arranging extensive redecoration, improving ward lighting, and bringing in new equipment, beds, and bedding. The result was improved patient mobility, which enabled many to be discharged from hospital, relieving pressure on beds to such an extent that three wards were released for other use. Her successes in mobilizing bedridden patients, previously thought to be untreatable, caused her medical colleagues to admit that their patients did better in her care than theirs. She was the first British geriatrician to publish inpatient admission/discharge data. This dynamic approach to patient care fired her staff with enthusiasm, even though they rather feared her.

These achievements led to increasing national and international recognition of Warren's highly effective, modern approach to the treatment of the 'chronic sick'. Senior medical officers of the Ministry of Health became her trusted allies. Her unit became the mecca for all those wishing to learn about her methods. She was Secretary of the International Association of Gerontology and lectured in many countries.

Warren, together with a small group of like-minded geriatricians, founded the Medical Society for the Care of the Elderly, which later was renamed the British Geriatrics Society. She was a member of the important 1947 British Medical Association working group, which published guidance on the modern management of sick elderly people for the benefit of the newly created NHS regional health authorities.

Bibliography

Primary: 1943. 'Care of Chronic Sick.' *British Medical Journal* ii: 822–823; 1946. 'Care of the Chronic Aged Sick.' *Lancet* i: 841–843.

Secondary: Sheridan, Alice M. (interviewee), 1991. 'Oral History of Geriatrics as a Medical Specialty', British Library, National Sound Archive F3284; Matthews, D. A., 1984. 'Dr. Marjory Warren and the Origin of British Geriatrics.' *Journal of The American Geriatrics Society* 32: 253–258; Adams, G. F., 1961. 'Dr. Marjory W. Warren, C.B.E., 1897–1960.' *Gerontologia Clinica* 3: 1–4; *Oxford DNB*.

Michael Denham

WASSERMANN, AUGUST PAUL VON

WASSERMANN, AUGUST PAUL VON (b. Bamberg, Germany, 21 February 1866; d. Berlin, Germany, 16 March 1925), *clinical chemistry, serology*.

Wassermann was born in Bamberg and began to study medicine in the nearby university town of Erlangen, before heading to Munich, Vienna, and Strassburg. In 1888 Wassermann graduated MD at the German university of Strassburg and began to work as research assistant to Robert Koch in the Institute for Infectious Diseases of Friedrich-Wilhelms-University of Berlin. Here he was introduced to the methods of laboratory experimentation and to Koch's concept of the relevance of bacteriology for clinical medicine. At the Institute for Infectious Diseases, Wassermann worked on immunity phenomena related to cholera infection and tried to develop antitoxins against diphtheria. As a result of these experimental investigations, he received the 'venia legendi' for hygiene in 1901. Following Paul Ehrlich's advice, Wassermann began to study the binding of toxin and antitoxin in the blood. He then investigated the differing reactions of blood groups in response to various precipitating blood sera. In 1902 Wassermann was made 'Extraordinarius' at the institute and in 1906 received the directorship of the division of experimental therapy and biochemistry. He then began to work on the complement-binding reaction, together with Albert Neisser and his research assistant

Carl Bruck. Those researchers had given experimental proof of the transmission of syphilis from one organism to another. It is debated whether Wassermann had been asked by the director of the Prussian Ministry of Education, Friedrich Althoff, to collaborate with the Breslau group. At that time, the national consciousness was sensitive to the relative state of cutting-edge research, and Wassermann's investigations were of both medical and political significance, because the French serologists were still much ahead of the German scientists.

The collaboration between Wassermann, Neisser, and Bruck laid the ground for the development of a serodiagnostic method for syphilis infection. This method later bore Wassermann's name as one of the central eponyms in clinical chemistry. In his original publication, Wassermann described the reaction as follows: Inactive serum of infected monkeys is combined with complement factors of the guinea pig. When specific hemolytic serum is added and corresponding erythrocytes are included, hemolysis is blocked. Already in 1927 a general review showed that at least 1,500 articles in clinical medicine mentioned the Wassermann reaction. However, as Ludwik Fleck has shown, this was an indirect success, because the identification of syphilis was the initial aim of the research collective, but their work led instead to an experimental system for the identification of syphilis antibodies.

In 1911 Wassermann was promoted to honorary professor for hygiene, and in 1913 the Kaiser-Wilhelm-Institute for Experimental Therapy in Berlin-Dahlem was created especially for him. When World War I broke out, all his technical supplies and the laboratory staff were moved to the Eastern Front in Russia. During the latter half of the war, Wassermann was made chief executive of the section for hygiene and bacteriology in the Prussian War Ministry, and thus was not able to pursue his research. In 1921 a reorganization of his institute took place, along with a change of its name to Kaiser-Wilhelm-Institute for Experimental Therapy and Biochemistry. Although Wasserman later intensified his work on tumor physiology and therapy, as well as on the complement-binding reaction in tuberculosis, he was never as successful later as he had been with the research on syphilis before.

Together with Rudolf Kraus he founded the 'Freie Vereinigung für Mikrobiologie' in 1906. Additionally, Wassermann served as chairman for the 'Akademie für die Wissenschaften des Judentums', and in 1921 he was awarded the Hans-Aronson-Prize. After his death in 1925, Wassermann's institute was closed down and thereafter continued only as a department for immunochemistry within the Kaiser-Wilhelm-Institute for Biochemistry.

Bibliography

Primary: 1894. (with Ehrlich, Paul) 'Über die Gewinnung der Diphterie-Antotoxine aus Blutserum und Milch immunisierter Thiere.' *Zeitschrift für Hygiene und Infektionskrankheiten* 18: 239–250; 1906. (with Plaut, Felix) 'Ueber das Vorhandensein syphilitischer Antistoffe in der Cerebrospinalflüssigkeit von Paralytikern.' *Deut-sche medizinische Wochenschrift* 32: 1769–1772; 1906. 'Eine serodiagnostische Reaktion bei Syphilis.' *Deutsche medizinische Wochenschrift* 32: 745–746.

Secondary: Krause, Peter, 1998. *August von Wassermann (1866–1925): Leben und Werk unter besonderer Berücksichtigung der Wassermannschen Reaktion* (MD thesis, University of Mainz); Fleck, Ludwik, 1980. *Entstehung und Entwicklung einer wissenschaftlichen Tatsache. Einführung in die Lehre vom Denkstil und Denkkollektiv* 2nd edn. (Frankfurt am Main) (English edn., 1979); Friedberger, Ernst, 1925. 'August von Wassermann.' *Zeitschrift für Immunitätsforschung und experimentelle Therapie* 43: I–XII.

Frank W. Stahnisch

WATERHOUSE, BENJAMIN (b. Newport, Rhode Island, USA, 4 March 1754; d. Cambridge, Massachusetts, USA, 2 October 1846), *medicine, natural history, smallpox vaccination.*

Waterhouse, son of the Quakers Timothy Waterhouse, who was a chair-maker and later judge of the Court of Common Pleas and member of the Royal Council for the Colony of Rhode Island and Providence Plantations, and English-born Hannah Proud, who was a relative of the physician John Fothergill, apprenticed with the Scottish surgeon John Halliburton, who had served in the British Navy. He also studied with Judge Robert Lightfoot, an Oxford graduate, and read extensively in the renowned library of Abraham Redwood. In 1775 he sailed to London and stayed with Fothergill, who directed his medical education. Waterhouse attended lectures in medicine at Guy's and St Thomas's Hospitals. In 1775–76 he studied in Edinburgh for nine months. He then returned to London and met many leading scientists and physicians at Fothergill's house, with whom he remained in correspondence after his return to America. In 1778 Fothergill sent Waterhouse to Leiden University in order to get a MD degree, which he received in April 1780. Waterhouse angered university authorities by adding 'Liberae Reipublicae Americanae Foederatae Civis' (Citizen of the free, confederated American Republic) to his signature upon matriculation. (The Dutch Republic had not recognized the new United States.) While in Leiden, he lived with the American ambassador John Adams and his sons, Charles and John Quincy, with whom he remained friends throughout his life. Waterhouse traveled extensively in Europe and met many distinguished individuals, including Benjamin Franklin.

After returning to Newport in 1782, Waterhouse set up a practice there, but soon moved to Boston, Massachusetts, to take the professorship of the theory and practice of physic in the newly established medical department at Harvard University (1783). His appointment was not without opposition; some pointed to the fact that he was not from Massachusetts, nor had he graduated from Harvard. (The patriots John Hancock and Sam Adams supported the appointment of Adams's son, Sam Adams, Jr., a physician who had served in the Continental Army.) In the end, his extensive medical education in Europe and his numerous medical and scientific acquaintances outweighed his disadvantages. Waterhouse also encountered wider professional opposition, and was initially denied membership to the Massachusetts Medical Society and the American Academy of Arts and Sciences.

Waterhouse developed a set of lectures on clinical medicine and on natural history, the latter of which he first delivered at the College of Rhode Island (now Brown University) in 1786–87. He also established the first mineralogical collection at Harvard and contributed to the zoological collection. To augment his income, he wrote many pamphlets and books.

Waterhouse's fame rests on the role he played in introducing smallpox vaccination into the United States. The Quaker physician John Coakley Lettsom sent to Waterhouse a copy of Edward Jenner's *An Inquiry into the Causes and Effects of Variolae Vaccinae* (1798), which detailed the procedure of using cowpox to inoculate individuals against future cases of smallpox. The use of cowpox rather than smallpox made vaccination a far safer procedure. Waterhouse tried to secure cowpox from England and succeeded in July 1800, whereupon he vaccinated several family members. Following the success of these vaccinations, he became the leading advocate of and expert on smallpox vaccination in the United States. He wrote numerous articles and pamphlets and corresponded with many individuals, including President Thomas Jefferson, about the procedure.

Waterhouse also tried to maintain a monopoly on the supply of cowpox. The initial cowpox shipped to the United States had been handled so casually that it shortly came to lose its efficacy. Waterhouse sought to prevent this corruption of the cowpox vaccine by monopolizing its distribution. He profited from this arrangement, but exposed himself to charges of improper ethical behavior and accusations that his motives were mercenary rather than humanitarian, and his behavior further alienated him from the Boston medical community. By 1801 Waterhouse had abandoned the attempt to control vaccination.

Jefferson, in recognition of Waterhouse's efforts to promote smallpox vaccination, appointed him head physician to the U.S. Marine Hospital in Charlestown in 1807. Waterhouse tried to reorganize the hospital and strengthen clinical teaching, but once again he ran into political difficulties. In 1809 President James Madison removed Waterhouse from this position. In May 1812 Waterhouse lost his professorship at Harvard. In 1813 he was appointed the hospital surgeon to the First Military District, and between 1818 and 1821 he was the medical superintendent of the military posts in New England. After 1821 Waterhouse left active medical practice and devoted his time to writing.

His first marriage (1788) was to Elizabeth Oliver, granddaughter of the Tory exile Peter Oliver. They had six children and lived in Cambridge. Elizabeth died in 1815, and Waterhouse married Louisa Lee in 1819; they had no children.

Bibliography

Primary: 1786. *A Synopsis of a Course of Lectures on the Theory and Practice of Medicine* (Boston); 1800. *A Prospect of Exterminating Small Pox* (Cambridge, MA); 1805. *Heads of a Course of Lectures on Natural History* (Cambridge, MA).

Secondary: Cash, Philip, 1992. 'Setting the Stage: Dr. Benjamin Waterhouse's Reception in Boston, 1782–1788.' *Journal of the History of Medicine* 47: 5–28; Cohen, I. B., ed., 1980. *The Life and Scientific and Medical Career of Benjamin Waterhouse: With Some Account of the Introduction of Vaccination in America* 2 vols. (New York); Blake, John B., 1957. *Benjamin Waterhouse and the Introduction of Vaccination: A Reappraisal* (Philadelphia); *DAMB*.

Andrea Rusnock

WATERSTON, JANE ELIZABETH (b. Inverness, Scotland, 18 January 1843; d. Cape Town, South Africa, 7 November 1932), *missionary medicine, general practice.*

Jane Waterston was the daughter of Agnes Webster and the banker Charles Waterston, who were cousins, and was one of six children. Inspired by David Livingstone at an early age, she determined to become a medical missionary. However, medical training seemed unattainable for a woman, and she went to the Free Church of Scotland's premier mission school, Lovedale, in the Eastern Cape, as superintendent of women students (1867–74). Her Xhosa pupils called her 'Noqakata'—the mother of activity—a name that epitomizes her later career. Still ambitious to become a medical missionary, she returned to Britain and, despite parental opposition, was among the first students to enter the London School of Medicine for Women (1874–78). She completed her training at the Rotunda Lying-in Hospital, Dublin, at the Royal Free Hospital, and at the British Lying-in Hospital, finally obtaining the Licentiate of the Kings' and Queens' College of Physicians of Ireland (1878). She received the LRC (Edinburgh), the MD (Brussels, with Great Distinction), and a Certificate in Psychological Medicine from the Medico-Psychological Association of Great Britain (1888). In 1906 she became a MRCP in Ireland, and in 1925 was elected a Fellow of the College, the second woman to be so honored.

After four years as a mission doctor at Livingstonia, Malawi, and at Lovedale (1879–83), she opened a private practice in Cape Town (1883), where she quickly established herself and, unusually for that time, saw patients of both sexes and all races. Waterston's successful private practice provided for her daily needs and helped support her family in Scotland, but her calling was to work among the poor. She led the establishment of the Ladies Department of the Free Dispensary (1888), which was the first institution to train colored and white midwives in the city and provide domiciliary maternal care. A Xhosa-speaker, she ministered to migrant dockworkers from the Eastern Cape, providing them with amenities at her own expense, and, despite advancing years, she nursed the poor during the 1918 influenza epidemic.

Staunchly pro-imperial, Waterston during the Anglo–South African War (1899–1902) organized relief for the refugees and the soldiers who poured into the city; more controversially, she also served on the women's commission appointed by the British government to inquire into health conditions in the concentration camps and rebut allegations of military culpability for their excessive mortality (1901). She received the Royal Red Cross for her services.

Waterston was South Africa's first professionally qualified woman medical practitioner and was fully accepted by colleagues, as her public medical activities demonstrate. She was Official Visitor to the Old Somerset Hospital and the leper settlement on Robben Island; when the mentally ill were moved to the new Valkenberg Hospital (in the 1890s), she became its Official Visitor, penning forthright quarterly reports on every aspect of the patients' medical and social condition.

Keenly involved in medical politics, Waterston participated in the founding of the South African Medical Association at the Cape (1883) and attended its first congress (1893). She was elected President of the BMA's Cape of Good Hope (Western Province) branch (1905–06) and actively supported the introduction of full medical education at the Cape. As the first woman to receive University of Cape Town's honorary LLD (1929), she was described at the time as 'the doyenne of women scientists [in South Africa] and the [most] senior qualified woman on the British Medical Register' (*Dictionary of South African Biography*, vol. I, p. 868).

Honored and revered in her lifetime, Waterston was 'a woman of rare determination, courage and intelligence' (Bean and van Heyningen, 1983, p. 11). She pioneered the entry of women into the medical profession in South Africa.

Bibliography

Primary: Bean, Lucy, and Elizabeth van Heyningen, eds., 1983. *The Letters of Jane Elizabeth Waterston 1866–1905* (Cape Town).

Secondary: van Heyningen, Elizabeth, 1996. 'Jane Elizabeth Waterston—Southern Africa's First Woman Doctor.' *Journal of Medical Biography* 4: 208–213; Robertson, Isobel, 1988. *The Life and Times of Dr Jane Elizabeth Waterston, Missionary and Physician 1843–1932* (Women's Section of the Presbyterian Church of Southern Africa); 1968. 'Jane Elizabeth Waterston' in de Kock, W. J., ed., *Dictionary of South African Biography* vol. I (Cape Town) pp. 866–868.

Shula Marks

WELCH, WILLIAM HENRY

(b. Norfolk, Connecticut, USA, 8 April 1850; d. Baltimore, Maryland, USA, 30 April 1934), *pathology, medical education, medical philanthropy, public health.*

Welch's father, William Wickham Welch, was a physician, as were four of his uncles and his grandfather. His mother,

Emeline Collin Welch, died when he was six months old, and he was raised by his paternal grandmother. At first intent on not becoming another of the 'Doctors Welch of Norfolk', he earned a BA at Yale in 1870, with the thought of teaching Greek. After unhappily serving as an apprentice to his father in the summer and fall of 1871, he returned to the Sheffield Scientific School at Yale to study chemistry. He enrolled at the College of Physicians and Surgeons (P&S) in New York in 1872.

At P&S Welch was offered a relatively good medical education, considering what was available in the United States at the time: didactic lectures and no laboratories, with limited clinical opportunity. He did, however, develop his skills in dissection and his knowledge of anatomy by working as prosector for the professor of anatomy. After completing his MD in 1875, he began an internship at Bellevue Hospital. Here he worked with Francis Delafield, who took a special interest in pathology and encouraged Welch to become familiar with the work of Rudolf Virchow. Interestingly, Welch recalled never having had the chance to slice, stain, or examine tissue while working with Delafield. By the end of his internship, though, he was certain that, rather than practice, he wanted to pursue a career in medical science. After learning of the plans for the Johns Hopkins Hospital and School of Medicine—intended to be a medical institution unique in America for its support of basic science—he began to seriously consider how to maximize his chances of ultimately working there.

In April 1876 Welch left for Europe, where he was among the most serious of the thousands of young American medical graduates traveling to German-speaking countries for advanced training in investigative or clinical techniques. Welch sought out the laboratories of two students of Virchow—Friedrich von Recklinghausen in Strasbourg and Julius Cohnheim in Breslau—but spent most of his time in Leipzig working with Carl Ludwig. His first publication, on edema of the lungs, appeared in a German journal in 1878. At Ludwig's laboratory he first met John Shaw Billings, who, as adviser to the Board of Trustees of the Johns Hopkins Hospital, would have much to say about the staffing of the planned institution. Welch sailed back in February 1878, knowing that the institutional basis for the type of work he wished to do did not exist in New York, but hoping that the new hospital and medical school in Baltimore would provide what he needed.

In New York he assumed a junior faculty position at Bellevue and joined other young German-trained doctors in an informal network dedicated to bringing scientific medicine across the ocean. He convinced Bellevue to equip a facility where he could teach what is now acknowledged as the first laboratory course in an American medical school. However, because of the pressure of earning a living from teaching, writing, and clinical practice, Welch was unable to continue with the type of investigations he had done in Germany.

Meanwhile, in Baltimore, leaders at Hopkins were actively searching for the right men to serve in the planned medical school and hospital. They had already been considering Welch, and contacted Julius Cohnheim, who strongly endorsed him for the chair of pathology. When Welch accepted the appointment in March 1884, it caused a stir among some of his New York associates, who could not understand why he would abandon the possibility of a lucrative practice in the metropolis for a position at an as yet nonexistent medical school in a provincial city.

German medical science had advanced rapidly since Welch's first visit; most stunningly, in 1882 Robert Koch had identified the pathogen of tuberculosis, an accomplishment that tipped the scale of opinion in favor of the germ theory of disease. Accordingly, Welch planned another trip to Germany, this time to include a short bacteriology course with Koch himself. He spent the academic year 1884–85 in Europe and then returned to Baltimore to join the faculty of the Johns Hopkins University. The hospital would open only in 1889, and the medical school did not open until 1893.

With Welch in the chair of pathology and William Osler having agreed to leave the University of Pennsylvania for the Hopkins chair of medicine, it was now up to Osler to recommend Philadelphian Howard Kelly for the chair of obstetrics, and to Welch to bring with him from New York the surgeon William Halsted. To complement these 'Big Four', Welch recruited three other first-rate young German-trained men for positions in the basic sciences: Franklin P. Mall in anatomy, John Jacob Abel in pharmacology, and William H. Howell in physiology.

Welch resumed scientific investigations when he arrived in Baltimore and made some modest contributions in both pathology and bacteriology. However, in 1893, when he assumed the position of dean at the newly opened medical school, he deliberately gave up research and turned his efforts to first, teaching and encouraging young scientists; second, the reform of medical education; and third, the advancement of scientific medicine in the United States. His students (from both Bellevue and Hopkins) later filled important positions in government agencies and medical schools around the country, and over the course of decades he was consulted on almost every appointment in pathology in an American medical school.

In 1901 Welch was invited to be president of the Board of Scientific Advisors to the Rockefeller Institute, an event placing him at the center of the effort to institutionalize scientific medicine in the United States. This position was not always comfortable for Welch. Although Hopkins was the model for the reforms proposed in Abraham Flexner's 1910 report on medical education, one element of the Flexnerian prescription caused great contention within the Hopkins faculty: on the advice of Mall and Halsted, Flexner recommended full-time appointments for clinical faculty members. Although Osler protested vigorously from Oxford

(where he was by then regius professor of medicine), in 1913 Welch—as acting president of the Johns Hopkins University—implemented the full-time plan at the school of medicine. Both Howard Kelly and Osler's successor, Lewellys Barker, resigned from Hopkins rather than give up lucrative private practices.

In 1904 Welch lobbied Theodore Roosevelt to appoint his former Bellevue student William C. Gorgas to take charge of mosquito control on the Panama Canal project, which up to this point had been controlled entirely by engineers. Gorgas had been responsible for eradicating yellow fever in Cuba, and his work ultimately guaranteed the success of the canal's construction. Welch served as president of the American Association for the Advancement of Science in 1906 and president of the National Academy of Sciences (NAS) from 1913 to 1916. He was also chairman of the Executive Committee of the Carnegie Institution of Washington from 1909 to 1916. During World War I Welch was instrumental in establishing the National Research Council within the NAS. He also participated in the Rockefeller Commission on the Peking Union Medical College and helped lead the struggle against antivivisectionists in the United States. From 1922 to 1932 he was chair of the Council of the Milbank Fund, an early health policy think tank.

Welch was a figure of international importance, but he made a point of demonstrating to Marylanders that Hopkins was part of their community. As president of the state medical society in the 1890s, he helped establish Maryland's first board of medical examiners. He was prominent in the effort in Baltimore to filter tap water and pasteurize the milk supply, and he served as chairman of the Maryland Board of Health and the Baltimore City Charter Commission.

Like many contemporary American intellectuals, Welch was sympathetic to the idea of massive programs (whether state-supported or philanthropic) to assist the poor, while wary of the masses acting in their own interest. He therefore was particularly interested in public health, but felt the need to define and contain it. In the interest of Southern 'poor whites', Welch participated in the 'Country Life' movement that led to the Rockefeller-funded campaign to eradicate hookworm in the American South.

Regarding education in public health, Welch, Flexner, and their associates at the Rockefeller Foundation—as well as staff at Harvard, MIT, and elsewhere—were at the time considering new models for the training of public health professionals. Welch, of course, was well placed to see that funds made available by the Rockefeller Foundation would come to Hopkins, and in 1918 he was appointed as the first dean of the Johns Hopkins School of Hygiene and Public Health (now the Bloomberg School of Public Health). He insisted that that term 'hygiene' come first, because he associated 'hygiene' with bacteriology, and his vision of public health was that it be as scientific as medical practice. Over the years, the school of hygiene at Hopkins has consistently been among the more

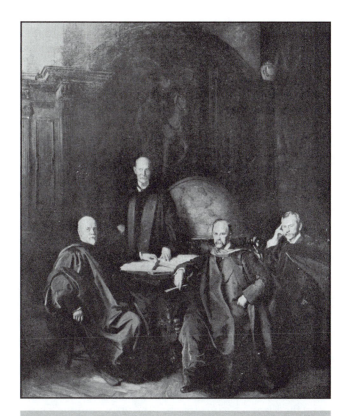

'The four doctors' (L–R): William Henry Welch, William Stewart Halsted,* William Osler,* Howard Atwood Kelly* (*see biographical entries). Oil painting by John Singer Sargent, Wellcome Library, London.

laboratory-oriented among the twenty or so public health schools that have since developed in the United States.

Welch, who never married, was close to seventy by the time the School of Hygiene was founded, and he never became very directly involved in its administration. In 1926 the Rockefeller Foundation funded a chair in medical history in Welch's name, and Welch was appointed to this position. Rockefeller also committed itself to the construction of a new building where the libraries of the Hopkins hospital, the school of medicine, and the school of hygiene would be merged—with space for a medical history department on the top floor. The Welch Medical Library and the Johns Hopkins Institute of the History of Medicine both opened in October 1929.

Welch, who was not pleased that a self-described dilettante like himself had been placed in the medical history chair, was willing to take the position only on the condition that he be allowed to visit Europe to purchase books and to search for a proper historian to succeed him as director of the Institute. During this trip he met Henry E. Sigerist, who had recently become director of the Leipzig medical history institute, and Welch—impressed by Sigerist's accomplishments as both a scholar and as an institution builder—subsequently succeeded in having Sigerist take over the Hopkins chair in history of medicine. Welch retired from Hopkins in 1931. He was hospitalized with

cancer in January 1933 and remained in the Johns Hopkins Hospital until his death. Although he claimed to have had a religious conversion as a child, he made clear to his friends that he had since become an agnostic, and he died a nonbeliever.

Welch was a promising scientist in his youth, but he parlayed his seriousness about research into advancing himself in an endeavor where he had greater genius, the transformation of medical science in the United States. He was a popular, if very private, figure, who equally enjoyed being photographed riding a donkey in China or in the company of movie stars in California, and being feted at testimonial dinners attended by leaders in science, medicine, and government. Although a supporter of Progressive-era reforms, he ultimately saw the advance and application of what was to become known as biomedicine as the most important good that he could contribute to humankind.

Bibliography

Primary: 1920. *Papers and Addresses in Three Volumes* (Baltimore); 1881. 'General Pathology of the Solid Parts of the Body and of the Blood' in Flint, Austin, *A Treatise on the Principles and Practice of Medicine for the Use of Practitioners and Students of Medicine* 5th edn.(Philadelphia); 1911–12. 'Urgent Needs in State and National Legislation.' *Bulletin of the Medical and Chirurgical Faculty of Maryland* 4: 135–137.

Secondary: Turner, Thomas B., 1974. *Heritage of Excellence: The Johns Hopkins Medical Institutions 1914–1947* (Baltimore); Fleming, Donald, 1954. *William H. Welch and the Rise of Modern Medicine* (Boston); Chesney, Alan M., 1943–63. *The Johns Hopkins Hospital and the Johns Hopkins School of Medicine: A Chronicle* 3 vols. (Baltimore); Flexner, Simon, and James Flexner, 1941. *William Henry Welch and the Heroic Age of American Medicine* (New York); *DSB*; *DAMB*.

Edward T. Morman

WELLS, THOMAS SPENCER (b. St Albans, Hertfordshire, England, 3 February 1818; d. Hotel du Cap d'Antibes, near Cannes, France, 31 January 1897), *surgery, ovariotomy.*

The eldest of five children of a builder in the market town of St Albans, Wells received his early education at St Albans Abbey School before undertaking a year's apprenticeship in 1835 with a surgeon in Barnsley, Yorkshire. Afterward he lived for a year with a parish surgeon in Leeds, where he also attended the lectures of several notable medical men. In 1837 he went to Trinity College Dublin for a two-year study under the physicians Robert Graves (1796–1853) and William Stokes (1804–78), the surgeon Philip Crampton (1777–1858), and the ophthalmologist Arthur Jacob (1790–1874). There Wells acquired an understanding of the clinical methods of the new Paris medicine, and subsequently moved to London to amass experience in hospital practice by walking the wards of St Thomas's.

In September 1841, shortly after obtaining his MRCS, he accepted a Royal Navy assistant surgeonship and was dispatched to Malta. There, besides treating a wide range of infectious diseases and injuries among sailors, he established a civilian practice, submitted articles to leading British medical journals, and, in 1844, was elected FRCS. He left Malta in 1846 and for the next decade embarked on a number of Royal Navy voyages, all of which afforded him opportunities to gather information for publications and thus further cultivate his professional profile. Promoted to surgeon in 1848, he was granted leave to go to Paris to study the treatment of gunshot wounds, a visit he extended in order to take in the clinics of Guillaume Dupuytren (1777–1835) and Joseph-François Malgaigne (1806–65) and the work of Claude Bernard (1813–78) and François Magendie (1783–1855).

Tiring of naval life but remaining on half pay, Wells returned to London in 1853, taking himself a wife (with whom he would have five children) and establishing a private practice in Grosvenor Square, where he first concentrated on ophthalmic surgery. In 1854 he gained an appointment as surgeon to the dispensary of the Samaritan Free Hospital for Women and Children, where, over the next two decades, he carved out his reputation as Britain's leading 'women's surgeon'. However, it was not until he returned from the Crimean War (after having volunteered for a civilian posting with the army) that he began his pioneering work in abdominal surgery and gynecology. Surgical interventions on battle casualties convinced him that abdominal surgery need not be tantamount to murder and that the techniques deployed there could be applied to women. Wells successfully did so, thereby contributing as enormously to his own pocketbook as to the development of gynecology, completing his thousandth ovariotomy in 1880.

It is hard to get the measure of Wells; he was clearly avaricious, greedily volunteering to serve in Crimea for £1,500 while still on half pay from the Royal Navy and, later, frequently demanding the contemporary maximum medical fee of 100 guineas for an ovariotomy. A social climber keen to make it into the London elite, he was as fastidious over his dress as he was over the selection of his instruments in the operating theater. He became an excellent horseman and judge of horseflesh, and maintained a lavish London residence in addition to owning a house and fine gardens at Golders Green, Hampstead. He used his editorship of the *Medical Times and Gazette* (1851–58) to puff up his own work and disparage that of others, was an ardent advocate of cremation (as well as a proponent of quarantine and vaccination at a time when they were not universally favored), and was a fierce defender of his own surgical techniques, especially against the claims of his bitter rival, Lawson Tait (1845–99). Yet he does not emerge from contemporary accounts as noticeably mean spirited and grasping; he did not blindly rush into the operation for which he became famous; he never omitted to mention his own failures or to include them in his statistical summaries of cases; and he frequently sided with those who denounced operations such as the removal of ovaries as depriving women of their 'true essence'. Of his religion nothing is ever said.

Bibliography

Primary: 1865. *Disease of the Ovaries* (London); 1872. *Surgery Past, Present and Future* (London); 1891. *Modern Abdominal Surgery: with an appendix on the castration of women* (London).

Secondary: Moscucci, O., 1990. *The Science of Woman: Gynaecology and Gender in England, 1800–1929* (Cambridge); Shepherd, J. A., 1965. *Spencer Wells: The Life and Work of a Victorian Surgeon* (Edinburgh and London); *Oxford DNB*; *Plarr's Lives*.

Roger Cooter

WENCKEBACH, KAREL FREDERIK (b. the Hague, the Netherlands, 24 March 1864; d. Vienna, Austria, 11 November 1940), *medicine, cardiology.*

Wenckebach was born into a wealthy family, whose members distinguished themselves with their technical, artistic, and scientific talents. Originally from Braunschweig, the Wenckebach family fled the turmoil of the Thirty Years War to settle as merchants in the Dutch Republic—first in Friesland, later in Amsterdam. Wenckebach's father, Eduard, played a crucial role in the construction of the Dutch telegraph service, thus greatly facilitating communication with the Dutch East Indies. As a student at Utrecht University, Wenckebach developed an interest in comparative anatomy and embryology and engaged in research at the Institutes for Zoology and Anatomy. In 1888 he earned his PhD (*cum laude*) with a thesis on *bursa fabricii* in thirty-two bird species. Part of his research had been carried out at the Institute for Biology in Naples. His publications from this period are evidence for his growing scientific interest.

After his marriage (to Catharina Henny) in 1892, Wenckebach set up practice in the town of Heerlen. In 1896 he returned to Utrecht to continue his physiological research with T. W. Engelmann. Five years later (in 1901), he was appointed professor of internal medicine at Groningen University. While there, Wenckebach made an early use of the new possibilities created by the discovery of the Roentgen rays. In 1911 he moved to the Imperial University at Strassburg and three years later (in 1914), to Vienna University. He was to stay in Vienna until his retirement in 1929, notwithstanding a tempting call from Amsterdam University.

Wenckebach's main research interest was in cardiac rhythm disorder. In 1903 he published his first book on the topic, which caught the attention of William Osler. Using cardiograms, sphygmographs, and esophagograms, he succeeded in describing the extra systole in man as well as the rhythm disorder that was to become known as AV-Block II type Wenckebach. After Willem Einthoven developed the electrocardiograph, Wenckebach made extensive use of this new technology, contributing considerably to its further improvement. His two-volume book on cardiac arrhythmias—coauthored with Heinrich Winterberg and published in 1927—contained a whole volume with illustrations. It remained the standard work on the subject for many decades.

Wenckebach did thorough research on quinine, publishing one of the first descriptions of the beneficial effects of the quinine alkaloids on arrhythmias. One of his patients, who had been given digitalis for atrial fibrillation, had pointed out to him that also taking an antipyretic containing quinine caused a regular pulse. Thus prompted, Wenckebach studied the therapeutic value of the combination of digitalis and quinine, which is still used today in cases of atrial fibrillation.

Other research focused on cardiac changes occurring in cases of beriberi. After he retired, Wenckebach traveled with W. C. Aalsmeer to Java, to do the research on this topic that resulted in his final book. With this work, he continued a Dutch tradition that had started with Jacobus de Bondt (1592–1631), who had published his *De paralyseos quadam specie, quam indigenae beriberi vocant* in the early seventeenth century.

Leading cardiologists of his time (including Thomas Lewis, James MacKenzie, and Arthur Keith) thought highly of Wenckebach, as did his students. Wenckebach's ability for self-criticism becomes clear from the phrase that he often used to start his lectures: '. . . our so-called facts of today may very well be the rubbish of tomorrow'.

Bibliography

Primary: 1903. *Die Arhythmie als Ausdruck bestimmter Funktionsstörungen des Herzens* (Leipzig) [English trans.1904, Snowball, T., *Arrythmia of the Heart* (Edinburgh)]; 1918. 'Über Chinin als Herzmittel.' *Berliner klinische Wochenschrift* 22: 521–525; 1927. (with Winterberg, Heinrich) *Die unregelmäßige Herztätigkeit und ihre klinische Bedeutung* (Leipzig); 1934. *Das Beriberi Herz. Morphologie, Klinik, Pathologie* (Berlin and Vienna).

Secondary: Scherf, David, 1968. 'A Cardiologist Remembers.' *Perspectives in Biology and Medicine* 11: 615–630; Pick, Ernst, 1955. 'Karl Friedrich Wenckebach und seine Bedeutung für die Wiener medizinische Schule.' *Wiener klinische Wochenschrift* 67: 636–637.

Armin Prinz

WEST, CHARLES (b. London, England, 8 August 1816; d. Paris, France, 19 March 1898), *pediatrics, midwifery.*

The son of a Baptist lay preacher, West was educated at his father's school at Chenies, Buckinghamshire. He became apprenticed to Mr Gray, a general practitioner in Amersham (1831). In 1833 he entered St Bartholomew's Hospital as a medical student. After two years he transferred his studies to Bonn, followed by Paris and then Berlin, where he graduated MD (1837). He had an unsuccessful attempt at general practice on his return to London. He then went to Dublin to study midwifery. On return to London he was appointed as a physician to the Dispensary for Women and Children, Waterloo Road (1842). He began to lecture on midwifery at the Middlesex Hospital (1845), and his lectures were published, first in the *Medical Gazette* (1847) and then as a book entitled *Diseases of Infancy and Childhood* (1848), which ran to a seventh edition and was translated into several foreign languages. It was this book that gave him the fame that led some to call him 'father of British pediatrics'.

In 1848 he became FRCP. In the same year he was appointed as joint lecturer on midwifery, with Edward Rigby, at St Bartholomew's Hospital. His lectures were said to be delivered in beautiful English, with a musical simplicity. He continued alone as lecturer after Rigby resigned in 1849. In 1861 he resigned because the hospital authorities did not give him recognition in the list of physicians, although he was in charge of the lying-in department and responsible for a ward of thirteen beds. He was, however, perceived at St Bartholomew's Hospital to be a difficult colleague who readily became involved in feuds. One of his notable publications from this time was a case report and literature review of the dangers of caesarian section in 1851.

However, his greatest achievement was to found the first children's hospital in the UK. West had tried to convert the Waterloo Road Dispensary into a children's hospital in the 1840s. He embarked on a fundraising campaign to establish a hospital specifically for children. He pointed out that neither in London 'nor throughout the whole British Empire is there any hospital exclusively devoted to the reception of children'. His campaign was ultimately successful. On 19 March 1851 he convened a public meeting, chaired by Lord Ashley, which founded the first children's hospital in Britain. Two weeks later the hospital was housed at 49 Great Ormond Street, formerly the home of Richard Mead (1673–1754), who had been physician to Queen Anne. It had ten beds. Charles West was the hospital's first physician. He continued in this post until 1875, when he resigned, although he continued as a member of the hospital's management committee. In 1877, following a disagreement with the committee, his formal connection with the hospital came to an end. In his own account, West believed that the heart of the disagreement was the opinion that his conversion to Roman Catholicism meant that he 'could not be trusted for the future'.

West also had an important role at the RCP, where he became Senior Censor. He later was to be a stern critic of the Censor's Board. He delivered the Croonian Lectures (1854), the Lumleian Lectures (1871), and the Harveian Oration (1874). This latter lecture was commended for its fine turn of phrase: 'We, with our narrow span of life, are naturally in a hurry for results. What comes not in our own time seems delayed indefinitely and we feel as little children do when they dig up the ground in their impatience to learn whether the seeds they have planted have yet begun to sprout.' This statement reveals his understanding and sympathy for children. He was known to have in the two bottom drawers of his consulting table 'a treasure house of marvellous toys'. Ever disputatious, he complained that the *British Medical Journal* had published the oration without his permission.

Throughout his career he fiercely opposed the admission of women to the medical profession. There were two notable occasions at the RCP when, in 1878 and 1895, he spoke strongly against the admission of women. He stated that if women were admitted, this would revolutionize society. In his view women did not generally wish for the admission of their own sex to medicine and most preferred to be treated by men.

After his retirement from Great Ormond Street Hospital, he continued in private practice in London, but London's fogs led him to winter in Nice between 1880 and 1885. In 1891 he had an attack of neuralgia, from which he never fully recovered, and in 1897 he returned to the French Riviera. In Nice he had an acute attack of herpes, and on his way back to London he was forced to break his journey in Paris, where he died. He had married twice and left behind a son and a daughter from his first marriage.

Bibliography

Primary: 1848. *Lectures on Diseases of Infancy and Childhood* (London) (2nd edn. 1852, 3rd edn. 1854, 4th edn. 1859, 5th edn. 1865, 6th edn. 1874, 7th edn. 1884); 1850. *The profession of medicine: its study, and practice; its duties, and rewards* (London); 1851. *Account of a Case in which Caesarean Section was Performed: with Remarks on the Peculiar Sources of Danger Attendant on the Operation* (London); 1854. *How to nurse sick children: intended especially as a help to the nurses at The Hospital for Sick Children* (London); 1856–58. *Lectures on the diseases of women* (London); 1874. 'Harveian Oration.' *British Medical Journal* ii: 1–8; 1885. *The mother's manual of children's diseases* (London).

Secondary: Moore, N., 1918. *The History of St. Bartholomew's Hospital* (London) pp. 727–729; 1898. Obituary. *Lancet* i: 968–970; 1898. Obituary. *British Medical Journal* i: 921–923; *Munk's Roll*; *Oxford DNB*.

John Walker-Smith

WHITE, PAUL DUDLEY (b. Roxbury, Massachusetts, USA, 6 June 1886; d. Boston, Massachusetts, USA, 31 October 1973), *cardiology.*

White was the son of a family practitioner who was also on the faculty at Tufts University. As a youngster, White often accompanied his father on house calls, and was undoubtedly influenced by him. They had much time to talk because they traveled in a horse-drawn buggy. His father

had tuberculosis, but died at the age of seventy-one of coronary disease. His mother died of pneumonia at the age of eighty-eight. She did much volunteer work with sick people.

His sister, Dorothy, died of rheumatic heart disease. His brother, Warren White, became an orthopedic surgeon and practiced in Hawaii. He had an older sister, Miriam, but little is known about her. His father and his sister Dorothy stimulated his interest in medicine, and his mother stimulated his humanitarian feeling, which persisted and grew as the years passed.

He was a superb grammarian and writer, which had much to do with his success in cardiology. He had studied science, mathematics, and history and, equally importantly, had mastered English, Greek, Latin, French, and German. As will be discussed later, this knowledge allowed him to read the original medical reports of the physicians of the past. It also permitted him to study the classical literature, which contributed to his general knowledge and understanding of the world and the people in it.

As a teenager, he was influenced by Theodore Roosevelt, and for a while considered becoming a forester, but decided to become a physician like his father, although his interest in preserving the natural environment never left him. He entered Harvard College at age eighteen and graduated cum laude in 1908. He took additional courses at the Massachusetts Institute of Technology, and entered Harvard Medical School and graduated in 1911.

He was not happy with the lectures given by the Harvard faculty. He, like others of his era, believed that bedside teaching was the superior method of teaching and that the content of lectures was often forgotten by those in attendance.

Little known today is the fact that White was interested in pediatrics. He became the first pediatric intern at the Massachusetts General Hospital in Boston. He served as a house officer on the medical service in 1912 and 1913. It was during this period that he created, along with Roger Lee, the Lee-White Method of measuring the coagulation time of the blood.

White intended to return to pediatrics, but was offered a Harvard Traveling Fellowship by David Edsall, who was chief of medicine at the Massachusetts General Hospital. He would have the opportunity to study electrocardiography and cardiac physiology with Thomas Lewis in London. With the agreement of the chief of pediatrics, Richard Smith, he began his work with Lewis in London in 1913.

The easygoing White initially found it difficult to work with Lewis. White was annoyed that Lewis ignored visitors who came great distances to see him. This influenced White, to have an open-door policy throughout his life; he would see and welcome anyone, at any time, who wanted to see him. In time, however, White was able to win Lewis's friendship and respect. They then worked intensely in what might be called the beginning of electrophysiology. They produced important research, and White's fame began to take shape.

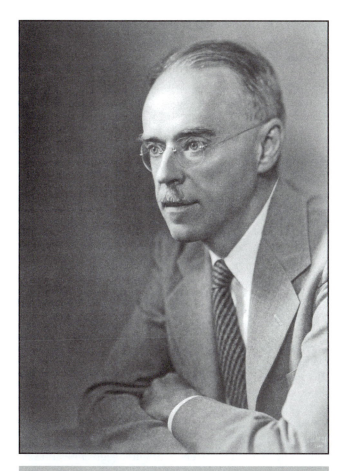

Paul Dudley White. Photoprint, courtesy of the National Library of Medicine.

While in London, White also became friends with James MacKenzie, John Parkinson, Frank Wilson, and others who became internationally known figures.

The likelihood of war was increasing, and so White returned to the Massachusetts General Hospital in 1914. He was given space in the basement of the 'skin ward' to develop a cardiac laboratory and was one of the first to use electrocardiography in the United States. His friends warned him that he could not be successful by being only a cardiologist, but he persevered despite their pessimistic advice. He created cardiology teaching clinics and taught students and other trainees, as well as practicing physicians. During this period, he became friends with Sam Levine at the Peter Bent Brigham Hospital.

His plans for the immediate future were interrupted by a call to service in the United States Army. He spent twenty-five months in the armed forces and returned to the Massachusetts General Hospital in 1919. He hated war, and this experience fueled his later view that doctors must encourage world leaders to promote world peace.

White continued to teach, write, and visit the leaders of cardiology in Europe. He always said that he took care of patients with heart disease. That was his definition of a car-

diologist. He married Ina Reid in 1924. She became his partner, helping him in every way. She became the gracious hostess to the world-famous physicians who visited them frequently. They later adopted two children, Penny and Sandy.

In 1920 White organized the training program in cardiology at the Massachusetts General Hospital. The trainees came from many countries, and many of them, due to White's influence, would return to their country to teach and engage in research. White not only developed the cardiac fellowship program, but also had programs for practicing physicians, in which they could learn more about the heart.

He, along with other physicians, insisted that the New England Association for the Prevention and Relief of Heart Disease join other organizations to form the American Heart Association. He became the first treasurer of the new organization. He fretted that the word 'prevention' was not retained in the name of the new heart association. He did not become its president until 1940. He traveled the world for the American Heart Association, urging numerous countries to create similar associations. He later supported the view that nondoctors should be able to join the American Heart Association. He saw in the move an opportunity to teach the lay public about heart disease and to gain financial support for cardiac research.

In the early twenties, he, along with M. M. Meyers, developed a method for classification of heart disease that included the recording of a statement of the etiology, altered anatomy, and functional status of the patient. Almost simultaneously, the New York Heart Association urged doctors to do the same thing. This was a giant step forward in ensuring the creation of a medical record for cardiac cases that could be analyzed at a later time. By the latter part of the decade, White had made clinical observations on 12,000 patients and was prepared to write his first book, *Heart Disease*. He was given another traveling fellowship in 1928, and he and Ina went to the Isle of Capri to write the book. Before settling in on the island, he visited the medical libraries in Italy and elsewhere in Europe, and talked to numerous friends. The book, now considered a classic, was published in 1931 and established cardiology as a specialty of medicine and White as its leader. The references show White's scholarship, and his reading of the original references, which were in several foreign languages, reflecting his rigorous early schooling.

White urged the development of the National Heart Institute. For eight years he spent about one-third of his time in Washington, D.C., as the institute's executive director. He saw in the institute a way to increase the funding for research in heart disease. He was not a scientist, but saw clearly the great need for more basic science and training in order to solve the problems caused by cardiovascular disease.

White and Louis Katz created the International Cardiology Foundation in 1957. The foundation's goal was to raise money and support for the International Society of Cardiology. White hoped that the latter organization could use its influential membership in efforts to eliminate violence and war.

White's personality also helped in his efforts to establish cardiology as a specialty. He was a kind and patient listener who took notes on what every doctor told him about patients and about their clinical problems. His reputation as a peacemaker was so respected that he could cool a heated argument by simply speaking a short sentence or by standing up.

White contributed to medical knowledge through his books, articles, and lectures. He pioneered electrocardiography and, along with Lewis Wolff and John Parkinson, identified the WPW syndrome. He contributed something about almost all of the types of heart disease recognized today. He was adept at untangling a patient's complex story of angina and anxiety. Already in the 1940s, White believed that cigarette smoking, high blood pressure, diabetes, lack of exercise, and a high-fat diet all contributed to the development of coronary atherosclerosis. He was also among the first to push the development of the risk factor concept. More than fifty years ago he believed that although coronary atherosclerosis was genetically predetermined, the risk factors could accelerate the development of disease. He believed that heart attack victims should return to the same work they did before the attack, and that a more optimistic attitude on the part of doctors would decrease the morbidity and mortality of heart disease. He predicted much of what we are seeing today.

He was forever optimistic and excited about medicine. He rode a bicycle and walked everywhere.

At the top of his profession, he saw many world leaders who had heart disease, including President Dwight D. Eisenhower. His friends arranged his nomination for the Nobel Prize and for his portrait to be on a U.S. postage stamp.

He died on 31 October 1973 at the age of eighty-seven. He had had angina pectoris, a small myocardial infarction, and a stroke from atrial fibrillation, subdural hematoma, pulmonary emboli, and finally another stroke.

Bibliography

Primary: 1921. (with Myers, M. M.) 'The Classification of Cardiac Diagnosis.' *Journal of the American Medical Association* 77: 1414–1415; 1971. *My Life and Medicine. An Autobiographical Memoir* (Boston).

Secondary: Hurst, J. Willis, 1991. 'Paul Dudley White: The Father of American Cardiology.' *Clinical Cardiology* 14: 622–626 [material from this article has been used here, with permission]; Paul, O., 1986. *Take Heart* (Boston); Hurst, J. W., 1985. 'Paul Dudley White: To Know Him Better.' *American Journal of Cardiology* 56: 169–177; Hurst, J. W., 1974. 'I'm Not Through Yet.' *Circulation* 49: 199–204; *DAMB.*

J. Willis Hurst

WHYTT, ROBERT (b. Edinburgh, Scotland, 10 September 1714; d. Edinburgh, 15 April 1766), *medicine, neurology, physiology.*

Whytt was the second son of a Scottish lawyer who died six months before he was born. His widowed mother moved from Edinburgh to Kirkcaldy, where Robert was educated at the public school. Whytt's mother died about 1720, and he was placed under the guardianship of his older brother, George, who died in 1728. Whytt inherited his estate. Although it is generally held that Whytt entered St Andrews, his name does not appear in the University records. However, a 'Robert Whyt' is recorded as having matriculated at Edinburgh University (1729). 'Robert White' is noted as having studied medicine at Edinburgh in 1731–32 and 1734, where he studied under Alexander Monro *primus* (1697–1767). In 1734 Whytt moved to London, with Monro's recommendation, to continue his studies under William Cheselden (1688–1752). After two years he completed his education on the Continent, attending lectures by Jacob Winsløw (1669–1760) in Paris and by Herman Boerhaave (1668–1738) and Bernhard Albinus (1668–1770) in Leiden. In 1736 Whytt took his MD at Rheims, and in 1737 was awarded an MD by the University of St Andrews and granted licentiate of the Royal College of Physicians of Edinburgh. In 1738 Whytt was elected a Fellow of that body and that same year commenced medical practice. In 1747 he was appointed professor of theoretical medicine in the University of Edinburgh, a position he held until his death. In 1752 Whytt was elected a FRS. In 1761 he was appointed First Physician to the King in Scotland, and in 1763 was elected President of the Royal College of Physicians of Edinburgh.

Whytt's modification of an existing preparation for bladder calculi, published in *Edinburgh Medical Essays* (1743), made his reputation, and he was able to build a secure practice. Whytt's abiding interest, however, lay in physiology (the *animal œconomy,* as it was then called). His first work on this subject, an inquiry into the 'sentient principle' that he believed governed voluntary and involuntary motions, was read before the Philosophical Society of Edinburgh ('An Enquiry into the Causes which Promote the Circulation of Fluids in the Small Vessels of Animals', 1745/46). Whytt sought to explain nervous activity on the basis of a fluid substance ('animal spirit'). To this he added the notion of an immaterial soul that acted on the body. This soul (also called by him the 'active power', 'nervous influence', or 'superior principle') was located in the brain and spinal cord. It was this power, acting through the animal spirit, that was thought to be responsible for nervous action. Whytt believed that muscle contraction was dependent on the nervous system, and therefore attempted to undermine the iatromechanical hypothesis of Albrecht von Haller (1708–77) and his school, who maintained that muscle and nerve fibers possessed an innate contractility or irritability. Whytt also denied the doctrine of a nervous fluid, a notion maintained by animists such as Georg Ernst Stahl (1659–1734). Although it could be argued that Whytt's 'animal spirit' made him an animist by other means, the animist hypothesis denied the primacy of the brain and nerves, which Whytt vigorously championed.

Whytt is an important figure of the Scottish Enlightenment. He was the first to describe 'hydrocephalus internus' (tuberculous meningitis of children). He elucidated the pupillary light reflex ('Whytt's reflex'), and experimentally determined that part of the spinal cord is required for reflex action, although Whytt did not use the term 'reflex', describing such action as due to 'sympathy'. Whytt sought to bring order to the several competing theories of nervous action. If his search for synthesis was not entirely successful, his studies paved the way for later investigators, and Whytt can with good reason be called a founder of neurophysiology.

Bibliography

Primary: 1768. *The Works of Robert Whytt, M.D.* (Edinburgh).

Secondary: Rocca, Julius, 2000. 'Robert Whytt (1714–1766): The Sceptical Neuroscientist' in Rose, F. Clifford, ed., *A Short History of Neurology. The British Contribution, 1660–1910* (London) pp. 93–107; French, Roger, 1969. *Robert Whytt, the Soul, and Medicine* (London); *DSB*; *Oxford DNB*.

Julius Rocca

WICKRAMARACHCHI, GABRIEL PERERA (b. Gampaha, Ceylon [now Sri Lanka], 20 September 1889; d. Gampaha, Sri Lanka, 1975), *ayurvedic medicine.*

Wickramarachchi, the son of a notable indigenous, ayurvedic medical practitioner, had his early schooling in a village school and his higher education at the Vidyodaya Pirivena in Colombo, under the internationally famous monk, the Venerable Hikkaduwe Sri Sumangala Maha Nayake Thero.

The Vidyodaya Pirivena was famous in South Asia for studies in the arts and the humanities, attracting scholars from South and Southeast Asia. Wickramarachchi graduated in Sinhala, Pali, Sanskrit, and ayurveda, and the British governor of Ceylon, Sir Robert Chalmers, conferred the title 'Pandit' on him in 1913.

In 1917, described as 'an outstanding person interested in Traditional Medicine' (Sessional Paper, 1927), he commenced postgraduate studies under the eminent Indian physician and scholar Kaviraj Jamini Bhusana Roy at the Astanga Ayurveda Vidyalaya (College) in Calcutta, India, and was awarded the final degree of Licentiate of Ayurvedic Medicine and Surgery—*Bhisagratna*; his 'subsequent contributions to the profession were outstanding'. While in India, he familiarized himself with Indian culture, Indian life, and the practice of ayurveda. He returned to Ceylon (1921) and then engaged in the practice of indigenous medicine, becoming the most distinguished ayurvedic physician of the day.

In Ceylon he edited the *Sinhala Bauddhaya,* a publication of the Mahabodhi Society of Ceylon that featured in the revival of Buddhism and Buddhist culture in Ceylon during the nineteenth and twentieth centuries. This was a period during which ayurveda in Ceylon had lost its prestige and the patronage of the British colonial government. Wickramarachchi did much toward the revival of ayurveda, traditional culture, and especially Buddhism, which he brought to bear on his teaching of ayurveda. It is noteworthy that a strong link was present then, as now, between traditional medicine in Ceylon, which includes the Indian component ayurveda, and Buddhism. In 1929 he founded the Ceylon (now Sri Lanka) Siddhayurveda Vidyalaya (College) at Gampaha, his native village, and maintained it at his personal expense, as the British colonial government gave no financial support for the teaching of traditional medicine.

After they graduated, Wickramarachchi's students received financial support and traditional medicinal preparations for their practice from the Pandit. By 1968, over six hundred students had graduated from his institution. His contributions to ayurveda resulted in his reputation as the 'Father of Revived Ayurveda' during this period, known as the 'Wickramarachchi period' of ayurveda in Ceylon. As a prominent citizen, he was appointed Notary Public.

His writings were on ayurveda and appeared in poetic and literary articles in journals, magazines, and newspapers. In addition, he organized cultural and dramatic events in his college, some of his own composition.

After the promulgation of the new constitution that gave Ceylon dominion status, Wickramarachchi was appointed a member of the Senate (the Upper House) in 1947. The honorary degree of Ayurveda Chakravarti was conferred on him in 1960 by the Vidyodaya University, Ceylon, (the former Pirivena, which had attained the status of a modern university by this time) and he was later appointed as a professor and as dean of the Faculty of Ayurveda there. He was also a member of the Das Gupta Commission on Indigenous Medicine and Traditional Medicine and Ayurveda in Ceylon (1947), coeditor of the *Charaka Samhita*, president of the Ayurvedic Medical Council, and a member of the Ayurvedic Research Board and the Ayurvedic Pharmacopoeia Committee.

His role models were Mahatma Gandhi, Pandit Nehru, Sardar Patel, and Rabindranath Tagore of India, and he shared their ideals, always wearing the national dress of Ceylon, and encouraging self-sufficiency in food through home-grown vegetables and a simple lifestyle.

Bibliography

Primary: Balasingham, K. (Chairman), 1927. *Sessional Paper I. Report of the Committee on the Indigenous Systems of Medicine* (Colombo); Das Gupta, K. M. L. (Chairman), 1947. *Sessional Paper XXIV. Report of the Commission on Indigenous Medicine* (Colombo).

Secondary: Karunaratna, W. S., Ram Raksa Pathak, D. M. Jayasingha, M. B. Ratnayaka, and J. Jayasingha, eds., 1968. *Wickramarachchi Felicitation Volume* (Kelaniya).

S. N. Arseculeratne

WIDAL, FERNAND (b. Dellys, Algeria, 9 March 1862; d. Paris, France, 1 January 1929), *medicine, internal pathology, serology.*

Widal originated from an Alsatian Jewish medical family. His father was a military doctor, and Widal was born in an Algerian village. He was sent to school in the metropolis, and his entire medical career took place in Paris. After his internship, he became an agrégé in 1894, a department chief in 1902, and obtained one of the four chairs of clinical medicine in 1918. He was a member of the academies of sciences and medicine.

Widal devoted his whole life to clinical teaching and research, at a time when the discovery of germs was having a profound impact on all aspects of the medical profession. He divided his time between the patients' bedside and the laboratory adjoining the ward. Although Widal greatly admired Claude Bernard and Louis Pasteur, and was a personal friend of Emile Roux, he did not join their laboratories, preferring to remain at the Cochin Hospital and to adapt it to the new standards of medical care. In addition to animal experimentation and microscopic observation, he emphasized the heuristic importance of 'spontaneous experiences', i.e., the investigation of individual cases.

The discovery to which his name is most closely attached illustrates his conception and practice of medicine. Gruber and Williams wrote in 1896 that the sera of people who had contracted typhoid fever agglutinated the bacteria described by Eberth in 1880. The same year, Widal showed that this reaction, which appeared at an early stage of infection, could serve as a laboratory test for the diagnosis for typhoid, which until then had been based only on observation of symptoms. However, it had no predictive value: the Widal (or Gruber-Widal) reaction indicated infection, but not protective immunity. Nevertheless, serodiagnosis, a term coined by Widal, was applied to many diseases in the following years, and eventually turned out to be a fruitful application of basic immunological research.

Widal explored organic fluids in various pathological conditions. He popularized the spinal tap, using the procedure to classify meningitis. He explored hemolytic anemias, those linked to congenital anomalies of red blood cells, as well as those occurring under the influence of cold or infections.

Despite its early promise, bacteriology did not lead to a complete reclassification of diseases in terms of specific germs. Nor did germ theory address the whole range of pathological phenomena. Thus Widal redefined nephritis, for example, around three cardinal signs: blood pressure, and the levels in blood of sodium chlorates and of urea.

Looking for clues to therapy, Widal conducted experiments on living patients with a recklessness that was not uncommon at the time. He repeatedly alleviated and induced cases of clinical edema by alternating a no-salt diet and one with a salt overload, thus demonstrating both the risk of cardiac failure and the therapeutic impact of dietary regimens on renal disorders.

The last part of Widal's life was dedicated to anaphylaxis. Charles Richet had shown that the injection of tiny amounts of a substance that was otherwise harmless could trigger cardiac and respiratory shock. Widal aggregated under the umbrella of anaphylaxis a number of poorly understood disorders, such as asthma, urticaria, and migraine, and did not flinch in making people inhale, eat, or be injected with a suspected agent. For him, the notion of individual susceptibility or 'idiosyncrasy', previously labeled as 'terrain', usefully completed the picture of pathogenesis. The influence of such endogenous factors shed light on pathological phenomena that could not be completely explained by the sole action of bacteria external to the body.

Widal attracted hundreds of students, who later moved to key university positions. His lessons at the bedside, unfortunately not preserved, reflected how Pastorian science revitalized the Paris School of clinical medicine.

Bibliography

Primary: 1896. 'Recherches de la réaction agglutinante dans le sang et le serum desséchés des typhiques.' *Bulletin des membres de la Société des médecins des hôpitaux de Paris* 13: 681–682.

Secondary: Contrepois, Alain, 2000. *L'invention des maladies infectieuses* (Paris); Lemierre, André, 1955. *Un grand médecin français, Widal* (Paris).

Anne Marie Moulin

WIER, JOHAN (aka **WEYER, JOHANNES**) (b. Grave, the Netherlands, 1515; d. Tecklenburg, Germany, 24 February 1588), *medicine, demonology.*

Wier was the eldest child of Agnes and Theodorus Wier. His father was a hop merchant in Grave, a Dutch town near Nijmegen. Around 1528, Johan became a pupil of the learned but rather unorthodox Cornelius Agrippa of Nettesheim, who was then living in Antwerp. He moved to Bonn in 1532 with his mentor. In 1533 or 1534 he went to Paris to study medicine, but without concluding his education with a medical doctorate. It has often been asserted—incorrectly—that he had received a degree in Orleans. In Paris he became acquainted with (among other people) Michel Servetus, the anti-Trinitarian and future discoverer of the pulmonary blood circulation, who was studying there under the pseudonym of Michael Villanovanus. Wier is also likely to have become acquainted with Jean Bauhin during that period. Bauhin later moved to Basel, where he became the personal physician of the Dutch spiritualist David Jorisz and a close friend of Sebastian Castellio, the famous advocate of religious tolerance. Toward 1540 Wier set up medical practice in his hometown Grave. In 1545 the town of Arnhem appointed him town physician; five years later, he became personal physician to the Duke of Cleves and Jülich.

In the 1550s Wier showed great interest in individualized, free religious beliefs. He asked Oporinus, his future publisher, who had been a servant of Paracelsus, for an assessment of the character of that physician, and he corresponded with David Jorisz, who in the 1540s had fled to Basel for his religious convictions. He consulted his brother Matthias, who was himself a spiritualist, about the ideas of the founder of the 'Family of Love', Hendrik Niclaes. Spiritualists like Niclaes, Joris, and Matthias Wier believed that man should strive for personal unification with God through mystic introspection. They felt that religious ceremonies were useless and that prosecutions of dissenters were un-Christian.

In 1563 Wier published his *De praestigiis daemonum*, the book that earned him fame as a major opponent of the prosecution of witches. The book contains quotations from the fierce words that the spiritualist Castellio had published in 1553 to protest against the execution of Michel Servetus earlier that year in Geneva. Wier argued that witches were innocent and that what seemed to be the result of their actions was really the doing of demons. Women who confessed to have engaged in witchcraft were actually suffering from melancholy caused by an excess of black bile, and they were tricked by demons into believing that they had concluded a pact with the devil and were guilty of witchcraft. On these grounds Wier argued that the supposed witches were in fact not *compos mentis* and should therefore not be liable to prosecution. His plea for tolerance caused an international scandal, although it was not the medical dimension of his argument that was disputed, but rather the legal one.

Wier was a confirmed humoral pathologist, as can be seen in the collection of observations of new diseases he published in 1567. Two of these case studies were published again in the following century. In 1624 Daniel Sennert inserted Wier's observation of the character and treatment of scurvy in his own book about this illness. In 1684 the Amsterdam physician Steven Blankaart incorporated Wier's treatise about the pox in a book about venereal disease.

Bibliography

Primary: 1660. *Opera omnia* (Amsterdam); 1563. *De praestigiis daemonum et incantationibus ac veneficiis, libri V* (Basel) [Eng. trans. 1991 (Binghamton, NY)]; 1567. *Medicarum observationum rararum liber I* (Basel).

Secondary: Waardt, Hans de, 2002. 'Johan Wier's *De praestigiis*. Mythes en motivatie' in Cobben, Jan Jacob, ed., *Duivelse bezetenheid beschreven door dokter Johannes Wier 1515–1588* (Rotterdam) pp. 17–74; Valente, Michaela, 2002. *Johann Wier* (Florence); Cobben, J. J., 1976. *Jan Wier. Devils, Witches and Magic* (Philadelphia).

Hans de Waardt

WILDE, WILLIAM ROBERT WILLS (b. Kilkeevin, near Castlerea, County Roscommon, Ireland, 1815; d. 19 April 1876, Dublin, Ireland), *ophthalmology, otology, anatomy.*

The youngest child of a prominent Roscommon practitioner, Thomas Wills Wilde, Wilde was apprenticed in 1832 at Dr Steevens' Hospital, Dublin, to Abraham Colles. He also studied anatomy, medicine, and surgery at the Park Street school and midwifery at the Rotunda Hospital, where he wrote a prize essay on spina bifida shortly before becoming a Licentiate of the Royal College of Surgeons in Ireland in 1837. He toured the Levant later that year, encountering widespread ophthalmic trachoma in Egypt, and thereby acquired an interest in diseases of the eye. The 1840 book of his travels gave him savant status in elite circles in Ireland and Britain, and its sales enabled him to study eye surgery at Moorfields in London under John Dalrymple (1803–52), Frederick Tyrell (1793–1843), and George Guthrie (1765–1856), and in Vienna with Anton Rosas (1791–1855) and Friedrich Jaeger (1784–1871). In Vienna he also encountered Joseph Skoda (1805–81) and studied pathological anatomy with Carl Rokitansky (1804–78). Wilde also worked at Johann Dieffenbach's (1794–1847) plastic surgery clinic in Berlin.

Wilde established a specialist practice in eye and ear surgery in Dublin, and in 1844 he established St Mark's, which was the first hospital in the British Isles to teach aural surgery and the first Irish hospital to treat the ear alongside the eye. He was an active member of the Dublin Pathological Society, and his 1853 textbook was the first to classify ear diseases by pathology as opposed to symptomatology and to foreground the importance of the tympanic membrane and the middle ear in aural infections. Wilde introduced Gruber's ear speculum into Irish practice and designed an aural snare, the first forceps for dressing the ear, and a new incision for mastoiditis. In the field of eye surgery, he and Thomas Wharton Jones (1808–91) established asymmetry of the cornea as the primary cause of astigmatism.

Wilde was closely involved with the Irish Census between 1841 and 1871, and he used the statistics on the Great Famine that he compiled for the 1851 Census in *On the physical, moral and social condition of the deaf and dumb* (1854). Between 1846 and 1849 he edited the *Dublin Quarterly Journal of Medical Science*, contributing a series of lives of eighteenth and early-nineteenth century Irish medical men to it, and also to the *Medical Times and Gazette* and the *Dublin University Magazine*. He was medical referee for the Victoria Assurance Company.

A polymath who stood out in a generational cohort of polymaths, Wilde was also one of the most distinguished antiquarians and field archaeologists of his day. He published a book on Jonathan Swift and a series of best-selling works on Irish topography and folklore (medical and otherwise), was prominent in the British Association for the Advancement of Science as an ethnologist, and was a leading light of the Statistical and Social Inquiry Society of Ireland and the Royal Irish Academy. He compiled a definitive three-volume catalogue of antiquities for the latter. He was appointed Queen Victoria's Oculist in Ireland and in 1864 was knighted for his statistical work for the Irish Census.

Bibliography

Primary: 1847. 'Report on the progress of ophthalmic surgery, for 1846. With original cases and illustrations.' *Dublin Quarterly Journal of Medical Science* 3: 209–216; 1853. *Observations on Aural Surgery and the Nature and Treatment of Diseases of the Ear* (Dublin); 1862. *On the Malformations and Congenital Diseases of the Organs of Sight* (London).

Secondary: McGeachie, James, 1999. '"Normal" Developments in an "Abnormal" Place: Sir William Wilde and the Irish School of Medicine' in Malcolm, Elizabeth, and Greta Jones, eds., *Medicine, Disease and the State in Ireland* (Cork and Portland, OR) pp. 85–101; Somerville-Large, L. B., 1960. 'The Development of Ophthalmology in Ireland.' *Irish Journal of Medical Science* 6th ser. 411: 97–129; Guthrie, Douglas, 1937. 'The Renaissance of Otology: Joseph Toynbee and His Contemporaries.' *Journal of Laryngology and Otology* 52: 163–176; *Oxford DNB*.

James McGeachie

WILLAN, ROBERT (b. Marthwaite, Yorkshire, England, 12 November 1757; d. Funchal, Madeira, 7 April 1812), *dermatology.*

Willan was the youngest of six children born to Robert Willan and Ann Weatherald, who each came from prominent Quaker families in the Sedbergh region of Yorkshire. His father was a medical practitioner, possibly an apothecary by training, and was well respected in the community. Willan attended the nearby Sedbergh School, obtaining a strong background in classics before studying medicine at the University of Edinburgh (1777–80), one of the few educational options open to Nonconformists. His MD thesis was titled *On Inflammation of the Liver.*

Armed with his MD degree, he went to London for further training under the guidance of the prominent London physician John Fothergill (1712–80), a family friend and fellow follower of the Society of Friends. Willan had intended to at a later time assume the country practice of a relative, Dr Trotter, in Darlington, County Durham. However, within the next several months, Fothergill died, followed shortly thereafter by Dr Trotter. Consequently, Willan moved much sooner than expected to the Northeast to begin practice. He found the atmosphere there oppressive, with two other medical men opposing him and a stultifying small-town life; however, he was able to accomplish a small project, comparing the sulfurous mineral waters at nearby Croft with those at Harrogate.

In 1782 Willan returned to London. Without an English medical degree, he could not readily obtain a hospital appointment, but, through Fothergill's sister, he received a position the next year at the newly opened Public Dispensary

on Carey Street (which years later moved to Drury Lane), and subsequently one at the Dispensary in Finsbury. In 1785 he successfully took the membership examination for the Royal College of Physicians. The questions and responses were given in Latin, but Willan, upon completion of the ordeal, responded in Greek, much to the amazement of the examining board.

The ensuing years proved to be most fruitful. Willan embarked upon a series of lectures directed toward the 'principles and practice of medicine'. Few students bothered with the Carey Street Dispensary sessions, until he changed his approach by pioneering bedside teaching in London. Willan's ability, both to make keen observations and to record them accurately and concisely, made 'his clinical school' highly successful. He taught a wide range of subjects, including public health, climatology, and industrial medicine. Willan called attention to lead colic and to the problems of infant mortality. He was also instrumental in the opening of a fever hospital in London (1802), much after similar facilities had been started in Chester, Manchester, and elsewhere.

Most important was his work on cutaneous disease. Although Daniel Turner's (1667–1741) book on skin disease had appeared earlier in the century, the only practical classification of skin diseases had been submitted by Josef von Plenck of Vienna (1776). Beginning in 1784 or 1785, Willan began to formulate a nomenclature for describing skin disease based on morphology, utilizing eight classical terms: papulae, squamae, exanthemata, bullae, pustulae, vesiculae, tubercula, and maculae. In 1798 he published the first of four installments of what would be called *On Cutaneous Diseases* (1808), containing thirty-three hand-painted illustrations and describing 119 skin diseases. A German edition may have preceded the London compilations, and in 1809 the first of several American editions appeared. Ashby Smith, his stepson-in-law, and Thomas Bateman (1778–1821), the most loyal of his pupils, also edited various posthumous editions of his works. Willan's reputation spread rapidly, and about forty students are known to have come from England and abroad to study at the Carey Street Dispensary. The French physician Laurent Biett (1781–1840), who was in London in 1816, returned to Paris to successfully lead the Willanist movement against the French school started by Jean Louis Alibert (1768–1837) at l'Hôpital St Louis.

Willan's reputation escalated, and in 1790 he received the coveted Fothergillian Medal for his essay *Cuticulam curare paratus*, becoming the second of six physicians to ever win this distinguished prize (including Edward Jenner, who received it in 1803). In 1809 he was elected a FRS, although the only medical group to which he is known to have belonged was the Society for Promoting Medical Knowledge. He was also a distinguished member of the Society of Antiquaries.

By 1811 Willan's health had gradually deteriorated to such a low ebb (possibly due to pulmonary tuberculosis) that he set out for the salubrious climate of

Madeira. Following a strenuous fifty-three day voyage, his condition worsened to congestive heart failure, and he died soon after arrival and was buried on the island. His widow, whom he had married in 1801, survived him, along with their son and his stepson-in-law, Ashby Smith, who was married to Mrs Willan's daughter by her first marriage.

Bibliography

Primary: 1782. *Observations on the Sulphur-Water, at Croft* (London); 1808. *On Cutaneous Diseases. Vol. I. Containing Ord. I. Papulae. Ord. Ii. Squamae. Ord. Iii. Exanthemata. Ord. Iv. Bullae* (London).

Secondary: Tilles, G., and D. Wallach, 1999. 'Robert Willan and the French Willanists.' *Br. J. Dermatol.* 140(6): 1122–1126; Booth, C., 1981. 'Robert Willan and his kinsmen.' *Medical History* 25(2): 181–196; Crissey, J. T., and L. C. Parish, 1981. *The Dermatology and Syphilology of the Nineteenth Century* (New York); Lane, J. E., 1926. 'Robert Willan.' *Arch. Dermatol. Syphilol.* 13(6): 737–760. [Bateman, Thomas], 1812. 'Biographical Memoir of the Late Dr Willan.' *Edinburgh Medical and Surgical Journal* 8: 501–512; *Oxford DNB.*

Lawrence Charles Parish

WILLEBRAND, ERIK ADOLF VON   (b. Vasa, Finland, 1 February 1870; d. Helsingfors, Finland, 12 September 1949), *medicine.*

Von Willebrand, son of Fredrik Magnus von Willebrand, an engineer, and Signe Estlander, went to the College Vasa svenska lyceum, from which he graduated in 1888. After that he attended the Faculty of Medicine at the Imperial Alexander University of Finland (1889–99), graduating MD.

His scientific work was initially devoted to laboratory research on blood diseases, starting with his thesis 'Zur Kenntnis der Blutveränderungen nach Aderlässen' (1899). He specialized in internal medicine.

In 1900 he married Walborg Maria Antell, with whom he had two children. He started his career as an assistant physician at the hospital of the Helsinki Deaconess Institute (1897–1900), and held a docentship of physical therapy (1903–08) and one of internal medicine (1908–30) at the University of Helsinki. In the summertime he also served as an assistant physician and as a head physician at the spa in Mariehamn (1894–95) and at the spa in Heinola (1899–1906).

However, he did his main work as a chief physician for the medical branch at the Helsinki Deaconess Institute and later as the head physician for the whole hospital at the Institute, 1922–31. He also served as a temporary professor of internal medicine at the University of Helsinki for some short periods (1910–22).

The discovery that made von Willebrand famous was of a previously unknown hereditary hemorrhagic disease. In 1924 he examined a small girl from Föglö, Xland, who suffered from a hemorrhagic disposition. What was extraordi-nary was that in her family there were several members, males as well as females, children and their parents, suffering from the same disease. At that time no hemorrhagic diseases were known other than hemophilia in young boys. Because von Willebrand was an able hematologist, he was able to explain the diagnosis precisely. In his investigations he proved that bleeding was prolonged in the patient as well as in her relatives, and that in most of them the number of thrombocytes (platelets) was normal. The disease was clearly different from classical hemophilia. In 1926 he published his findings in an article in Swedish with a German summary, 'Hereditäre Pseudohämophili', in *Finska Läkaresällskapets Handlingar* [Proceedings of the Medical Society of Finland].

Later von Willebrand returned to Föglö and further investigated the same families. The published reports were partly written together with the German hematologist Rudolf Jürgens, who had found a patient of the same type in his own country. In their common publication from the 1930s they called the disease 'constitutional thrombopathy', to which others attached the eponym von Willebrand-Jürgens, although in the German literature this disease is named after its real first describer, von Willebrand. Patients suffering from this disease have since been found elsewhere in the world.

It was only shown after von Willebrand's death that when he clarified the diagnosis of the small girl, he had discovered a disease that is the most common cause, worldwide, of prolonged bleeding. In 1971, forty-five years after he published the first paper on the disorder, the so-called von Willebrand factor (VWF) was found. It is a blood protein that is necessary for proper blood coagulation or clotting. When there is not enough VWF in the blood, or when it does not work the way it should, the blood takes longer to clot. The disease had not been understood until the discovery of this mechanism.

Bibliography

Primary: 1926. 'Hereditär Pseudohämophili.' *Finska Läkaresällskapets Handlingar* 67.

Secondary: Ignatius, J., 1992. 'von Willebrand ja hänen tautinsa.' *Duodecim* 108.

Hindrik Strandberg

WILLIAM OF BRESCIA (aka GUGLIELMO DE' CORVI) (b. ?, *c.* 1250; d. Paris, France, 1326), *medicine, medical education.*

William was born to an Italian merchant, Giacomo de Corvi, who subsequently moved to Brescia in the middle of the thirteenth century. His early training is unclear, but William was teaching logic and philosophy at Padua in 1274 under salary of the city. There he attracted a student, Engelbert, later abbot of Admont. Engelbert tells that William left Padua around 1279 to study with Taddeo Alderotti in Bologna and became a master in medicine by 1286. Although William's later teaching career is also murky, we know of at least one more student of his, Pancius of Lucca, who became personal physician to the bishop-surgeon Theodoric.

By 1298 William had become personal physician to Pope Boniface VIII, and he was later both physician and chaplain to Benoit XI, Clement V, and John XXII. In compensation, he held prebends of Brescia, Lincoln, Paris, and Constance and archdeaconries of Bautois (Constance) and Bologna. The latter was crucial because the role included the at least nominal supervision of the *studium* at Bologna. Within the hierarchy of the Church, William was a member of the minor orders, becoming a subdeacon in 1314. His duties kept him near the popes, including a sojourn in Avignon with Clement, but toward the end of his life, he settled in Paris, where he died. While at Avignon he may have had contact with the prominent papal physician, Arnald of Vilanova.

His influence on medical education was both potent and material. William was one of the three experts (along with Arnald of Vilanova and John of Alès) called to Montpellier on 8 September 1309 by Pope Clement V to help create the regulations for bestowal of medical degrees. William supposedly emphasized a conservative approach to the curriculum, offering up the 200-year-old texts of Rhazes (Al-Rāzī), Constantine the African, and Isaac Israeli as alternatives to Avicenna (Ibn Sīnā).

In his Paris will of 1326, following the Parisian model, he founded a college for poor scholars, perhaps the first of its kind at the University of Bologna. The will indicates that he had amassed a great deal of wealth by the time of his death, represented by holdings in Brescia, Bologna, and beyond. The bequest entitled fifty scholars to be housed in a college built for the stated purpose. His bequest began with the subvention of eight scholars, two each in canon law and medicine and four in liberal arts and philosophy. In addition, he willed his books to the college.

He was clearly occupied with clinical medicine and professional education, but because of his role at court and at the University of Montpellier, William also evinced significant attention to arts and philosophy, perhaps under the influence of his Parisian stay. William was likely a significant conduit of ideas between the three major medical schools of the day—Bologna, Montpellier, and Paris, by way of the papal court. He is credited in some manuscript sources with inspiring Henry of Mondeville. As witnessed by Henry's comments, William was a proponent of the Italian model of surgery and of the literacy of its practitioners. At least one translation from Hebrew into Latin was also inspired by William, the translation by John of Capua of Maimonides' *On diets*.

William's own medical writings include *Practica*, an encyclopedia of diseases from head to toe that included citations from Aristotle's *Libri naturales* and in which he also invoked both Avicennan and Averroistic philosophical precepts. While typical in many respects, the text also offers a description of the medieval pulmonary sign of orthopnea, which has attracted modern notice. He also wrote a brief *practica* on surgery.

William's scholastic orientation is reflected in *questiones* on Hippocrates' *Aphorisms* one through seven and on a portion of Avicenna's *Canon*, as well as on theriac, the panacea. He also left medical *consilia*, including those for the bishop of Brescia's brother and a Brescian lord, as well as a popular consideration of breast cancer. It is less clear whether he authored certain treatises on memory, on plague, and on fevers.

His work on theriac is significant for a reference to a royal autopsy (likely that of either Philip IV or Philip V of France); the text also reveals the influence of Arnald of Vilanova's thought at this time, as well as William's associations with Montpellier and Bologna. William's consideration of poisons and their remedies led to the first Montpellieran description of the Averroistic connection between magnets and theriac.

William represents to historians an uncommon example of the medieval physician. Because of the demands of his clinical and ecclesiastical commitments, he in all likelihood did not produce a large number of texts or students. Nevertheless, he had a notable influence on the state of medieval medicine—as an incipient regulator, as an advocate in educational policy, as a purveyor of ideas from Italy to France, as a mediator between medicine and surgery, as a sponsor and intellectual inspiration for translations and text production, and doubtless as a practitioner in his care of the popes.

Bibliography

Primary: 1508. *Excellentissimi medici Guielmi brixiensis dictorum illustrium medicorum ad unamquamque egritudinem a capite ad pedes practica* (Venice); Schmidt, Erich Walter Georg, 1922. *Die Bedeutung Wilhelms von Brescia als Verfasser von Konsilien* (Leipzig); McVaugh, Michael, 1972. 'Theriac at Montpellier, 1285–1325 (with an edition of the 'Questiones de tyriaca' of William of Brescia).' *Sudhoffs Archiv* 56: 113–144.

Secondary: Demaitre, Luke E., 2002. 'Straws in the Wind: Latin Writings on Asthma between Galen and Cardano.' *Allergy and Asthma Proceedings* 23: 61–93; Keil, Gundolf, and Thomas Holste, 1997–98. 'Randnotizen zu Wilhelm von Brescia.' *Jahrbuch der Schlesischen Friedrich-Wilhelms-Universität zu Breslau* 38–39: 181–184; Sirais, Nancy G., 1981. *Taddeo Alderotti and His Pupils: Two Generations of Italian Medical Learning* (Princeton).

Walton O. Schalick III

WILLIAM OF SALICETO (aka GUGLIELMO DA SALICETO, GUGLIELMUS PLACENTINUS, SALICETTI) (b. Saliceto, Lombardy [now Italy], *c.* 1210; d. ?, 1276/80), *medicine, surgery*.

William was born in the village of Saliceto, in Piacenza, a province of Lombardy, in the first third of the thirteenth century (*c.* 1210). There is no information concerning his family or early education other than that he learned Latin before coming to Bologna around 1230, where he studied under Buono di Garbo. Lanfranc de Milan, whom William taught in Bologna, was William's most famous student. Though most of his time was spent in Piacenza and Verona, William also practiced medicine and surgery in Milan, Cremona, Pavia, and Bologna. The date of William's death, like that of his birth, is uncertain, and estimates range from 1276 to 1285. The general consensus is that William died before the end of 1280. In 1552 the Collegio Medico Piacentiono placed a marker above his remains in the basilica of St Giovanni in Canale.

William's major works are his *Summa of Treatments* and a *Surgery*, each divided into five books; Pifteau also credits William with a work on practical medicine. William saw surgery and medicine as parts of a continuum of knowledge, and both surgical and medical topics are included in his two works. The *Surgery* focuses on the manual procedures of surgery, including medicinal treatments. The *Summa*, dedicated to his son Leodardino, is a general treatise on medicine. For these two texts William drew on the recently translated works of Galen (the 'new Galen') and Aristotle. There are two versions of the *Surgery*, which relates diagnoses and treatments of conditions, dated 1268 (finished in Bologna) and 1275 (finished in Verona). Agrimi and Crisciani have identified twenty-six extant manuscripts of the *Surgery*. Between the two versions of the *Surgery*, William composed his *Summa*. The *Summa* focuses primarily on medical theory and medicines. It makes rudimentary use of the scholastic question for analysis. There has not been a systematic examination of its sources or methods.

William wrote and organized the *Surgery* and the *Summa* in order to facilitate their use by students and practitioners. The *Surgery* achieved greater popularity in the Middle Ages than did the *Summa*. Included in the *Surgery* are William's personal anecdotes and experiences. The preamble to Book I includes instructions on the proper behavior of surgeons, their assistants, and patients.

According to his *Summa* and *Surgery*, William treated people from a variety of social backgrounds and of all ages. William saw surgery as 'a body of knowledge', which enabled one to perform manual operations. These treatments included medications, later the purview of scholastic physicians. The surgeon was the 'minister of nature'. William was the first medical writer to emphasize the importance of anatomy in surgery; Book IV of the *Surgery* contains basic anatomical information aimed at informing the surgeon so that he is able to incise, cauterize, and otherwise operate successfully. Book V introduces the West to the cautery of Albucasis (Al-Zahrāwī).

Bibliography

Primary: 1489. *Cyrurgia & Summa conservationis et curationis* (Venice) (held at the New York Academy of Medicine); 1898. (trans. and with commentary by Pifteau, Paul) *Chirurgie de Guillaume de Salicet, achevée en 1275* (Toulouse); 1965. (Tabanelli, Mario, ed.) *La Chirurgia Italiano nell'Alto Medioevo* Vol. II: *Guglielmo-Lanfranco* (Florence) pp. 499–800.

Secondary: Agrimi, Jole, and Chiara Crisciani, 1994. 'The Science and Practice of Medicine in the Thirteenth Century According to Guglielmo da Saliceto, Italian Surgeon' in García-Ballester, Luis, et al., eds., *Practical Medicine from Salerno to the Black Death* (Cambridge) pp. 60–87; Siraisi, Nancy, 1994. 'How to Write a Latin Book on Surgery: Organizing Principles and Authorial Devices in Guglielmo da Saliceto and Dino del Garbo' in García-Ballester, Luis, et al., eds., *Practical Medicine from Salerno to the Black Death* (Cambridge) pp. 88–109; Martini, R., 1955. 'Guglielmo da Saliceto' in *Piacenza Sanitaria IX* (Piacenza) pp. 3–59.

Michelle Garceau

WILLIAMS, CECILY DELPHINE (b. Darliston, Westmoreland, Jamaica, 2 December 1893; d. Oxford, England, 13 July 1992), *nutrition, pediatrics, tropical medicine.*

Williams was born in Jamaica to a well-off land-owning family. After attending Bath High School for Girls, she took her BA at Oxford (1917–20) and studied medicine at King's College Hospital, London (BM, BCh 1923). After graduation, Williams began to specialize in pediatrics, taking up her first hospital post at the South London Hospital for Women and Children (1923–29). She desired to work abroad and, after sitting on the waiting list for a colonial medical appointment for two years, was finally offered an appointment as a Medical Officer in the Gold Coast (now Ghana). In preparation, she took the Diploma in Tropical Medicine and Hygiene shortly before she departed for West Africa in 1929. This was the beginning of more than twenty-five years' work abroad.

Once in West Africa, Williams devoted her attention to setting up child welfare clinics and the further study of maternal and pediatric health. Her most important contribution was her diagnosis of the common childhood disease kwashiorkor (a disease that previously had often been misdiagnosed as another vitamin deficiency disease, pellagra). This work was based on the close observation of sick African children with characteristic swollen bellies and on the results of regular postmortems conducted on disease victims. She noted that many of the children that she examined had a tendency toward a fatty liver, a discovery that encouraged her to further explore the relationship between these symptoms and child nutrition. She wrote many articles on maternal and child care in the developing world, and her recommendations concentrated on education about the nutritional needs of weaned children.

After returning for a brief sojourn in England, during which time she was elected MRCP (1935) and was awarded her MD from Oxford (1936), she was transferred within the Colonial Service to Malaya, where she also undertook regular lecturing work at the University of Singapore. It was during this period (1936–48) that she began her vocal campaign against milk-producing firms that offered sweetened condensed milk for children instead of breast milk. Speaking on 'Milk and Murder' to the Singapore Rotary Club in 1939, Williams accused the producers of callous neglect of infant life in the pursuit of profit.

Her world was torn apart in 1941, when she was interred in Changi jail in Singapore by the Japanese. For four years Williams was moved between camps, sometimes tortured, and starved almost to the point of death. She was eventually released in 1945. Undeterred, however, Williams returned to Malaya after a brief recuperative stay in Britain and continued her work for a further three years (1945–48). It was during this period that she became the first woman to be put in charge of all maternity and child welfare services of the country.

Subsequently Williams held a variety of prestigious posts. She was elected FRCP (1949) and appointed Advisor in Maternal and Child Health for the World Health Organization, Geneva (1948–51) and Southeast Asia (1951–53). She was also Senior Lecturer at the London School of Hygiene and Tropical Medicine (1953–55), and held various consultancies and teaching appointments in Jamaica, Beirut, the United States, and London (1955–78). She retired to Oxford in 1978, although she continued to be a tireless speaker on child nutrition into her nineties, giving talks in countries such as Nepal, Pakistan, and Israel.

Bibliography

Primary: 1994. (compiled by Hunter, Isobel) *Dr. Cicely Delphine Williams (1893–1992), Nutritionist and Paediatrician: List of Papers in the Contemporary Medical Archives Centre at the Wellcome Institute for the History of Medicine* (London); 1985. (with Baumslag, Naomi, and Derrick Jelliffe) *Mother and Child Health: Delivering the Services* (London); 1978. 'Cultural and Other Barriers in the Implementation of Health Programs.' *American Journal of Clinical Nutrition* 31: 2037–2039.

Secondary: Baumslag, Naomi, ed., 1986. *Primary Health Care Pioneer: The Selected Works of Dr. Cicely Williams* (Geneva); Craddock, Sally, 1983. *Retired Except on Demand: The Life of Dr. Cicely Williams* (Oxford); Dally, Ann, 1968. *Cicely: The Story of a Doctor* (London); *Munk's Roll; Oxford DNB.*

Anna Crozier

WILLIAMS, DANIEL HALE (b. Hollidaysburg, Pennsylvania, USA, 18 January 1856; d. Idlewild, Michigan, USA, 4 August 1931), *surgery, medical education, hospital administration.*

Born to Daniel Williams, Jr. and Sarah Price Williams, the boy who would become known as 'Doctor Dan' apprenticed to a shoemaker, worked as a barber, and played guitar and sang for Anderson's string band before attending Chicago Medical College, from which he graduated in 1883. Though he was described as 'looking white', Williams's career took place in a world where race mattered and at a time when any African American heritage formed a barrier to professional acceptance and success. Yet succeed he did.

Williams is best known for successfully suturing the pericardium of a twenty-five-year-old stabbing victim, James Cornish, in 1893 at the interracial Provident Hospital that he had founded just two years before in Chicago. Although Henry C. Dalton of St Louis had performed a similar emergency operation two years before, Williams's superior clinical account of the procedure rightfully deserves credit for freeing cardiac surgery from the scorn of the medical profession. In 1902 Williams again displayed his surgical skill when he successfully sutured a spleen in a twenty-seven-year-old man.

By 1895 black physicians had a collective professional voice in the form of the National Medical Association with Williams as its vice president, although Doctor Dan had little time for national politicking. In the year of his famous pericardial suturing, Williams received a government appointment as surgeon-in-chief of the Freedman's Hospital in Washington. He found the Freedman's Hospital in a deplorable condition. He completely reorganized the surgical department, dramatically lowered the hospital's shameful mortality rate, and established a nursing school. However, he became caught up in political difficulties between the Freedman's Hospital and Howard University, and in 1896 a new Republican administration ended his tenure at the hospital.

Late in life Williams moved to Idlewild, Michigan, where built a successful hotel named Oakmere and retired to his home of the same name. Diabetes and a debilitating stroke made his final years ones of quiet difficulty. But he had made his mark. By the time of his death, Williams had received honorary degrees from Howard University and Wilberforce University, and was the only African American to be named a charter member of the American College of Surgeons. Williams went back to Chicago after marrying Alice Johnson on 2 April 1898. A year later he was invited by George W. Hubbard, president of Meharry Medical College, to teach as a visiting professor, and for many years thereafter the annual Williams surgical clinics were the Meharry College event of the year. Williams also served as professor of theory and practice of medicine at Knoxville Medical College. From 1900 to 1906 Williams was an assistant attending surgeon at Cook County Hospital in Chicago, and from 1912 to his death he was an attending surgeon at Chicago's St Luke's Hospital.

Williams is remembered in medical history for the synergy of his achievements, and Ulysses Grant Dailey, who had trained under Williams and knew him well, referred to his mentor as 'a veritable Moses to the Negro profession'. It may be said that Williams led the way in training a whole generation of black physicians in professional excellence.

Bibliography

Primary: 1897. 'Stab Wound of the Heart and Pericardium— Suture of the Pericardium—Recovery—Patient Alive Three Years

Afterward.' *New York Medical Record* 51(March 27): 437–439; 1904. 'Penetrating Wounds of the Chest, Perforating the Diaphragm, and Involving the Abdominal Viscera; Case of Successful Spleen Suture for Traumatic Haemorrhage.' *Annals of Surgery* 40: 682–683.

Secondary: Reed, Theresa Greene, and C. Carnot Evans, 1996. 'Essayists, Essays, and Hosts: Daniel Hale Williams' Medical Reading Club.' *Journal of the National Medical Association* 88(10): 663–664; Beatty, William K., 1971. 'Daniel Hale Williams: Innovative Surgeon, Educator, and Hospital Administrator.' *Chest* 60 (August): 175–182; Buckler, Helen, 1954. *Doctor Dan: Pioneer in American Surgery* (Boston); *DAMB*.

Michael A. Flannery

WILLIS, THOMAS (b. Great Bedwen, Wiltshire, England, 27 January 1621; d. London, England, 11 November 1675), *medicine, anatomy, physiology, chemistry.*

Although Willis rose to prominence as the Sedleian Professor of Natural Philosophy and a pre-eminent physician of the Restoration period, he had relatively humble beginnings. He was born in the manor of Great Bedwyn in Wiltshire. His father appears to have been a yeoman farmer and steward of the manor. However, Willis spent most of his life in or around the University of Oxford, when his family moved to North Hinksey, Berkshire, just a few miles outside the University, while he was still young. He was educated in Edward Sylvester's School in town. He entered Christ Church as a servitor (1636), apparently intending to take holy orders. He appears to have had an interest in medical and chemical matters even at this young age. He helped prepare medical recipes for the wife of Canon Thomas Isles of Christ Church ('a knowing woman in physique and surgery') (Aubrey, 1898, pp. 303–304). He was awarded his BA (12 June 1639) and MA (18 June 1642).

While at the University, he established lasting relations with prominent figures in the local community, including Henry Hammond (a canon of Christ Church) and Gilbert Sheldon (the Warden of All Souls) as well as lifelong friendships with his fellow students John Fell (son of the Dean of Christ Church), John Dolben, Richard Allestree, and Ralph Bathurst. The events of civil war struck close to home because the University served as the royalist headquarters during this period (1642–46). Academic activity declined significantly as attentions turned toward political and military matters. Although his friends were all involved in the royalist war effort, Willis did not immediately enlist in the army. He instead retired to his family holdings. However, the war still affected his life. His home lay in a strategic position along both the river and the roadways between Oxford and Abingdon, and numerous battles were fought in the area. Even more importantly, his father and stepmother died (1643) of the epidemic fever that ravaged local military forces. Willis returned to the University about a year later, after suffering frequent raids by parliamentary forces. He enlisted in the royalist army shortly afterwards and appar-

ently served until the University surrendered to parliamentary forces (24 June 1646).

According to Fell, it was during this time that Willis 'turned to the study of Medicine, the Church being destroyed and Divinity together with divines oppressed' (Fell, 1675, sig. b₃v). Apart from Willis being awarded his BM (before the resident parliamentary authorities had consolidated their power), little is known of his activities during the latter half of the 1640s. Correspondence between John Aubrey and John Lydall indicates that Willis apparently had left the University for a year or so around 1648. This was likely to avoid examination by the parliamentary authorities sent to tame the former royalist headquarters. However, Willis was unable to venture far because of his family responsibilities after his parents' deaths. As the eldest son, he was managing his holdings to provide for his eight younger siblings.

Despite his change of career, Willis's religious convictions remained unaltered. He 'followed a religion almost fugitive' as he and his friends struggled to advance the royalist cause and preserve the rites of the abolished Church throughout the 1650s. His medical partner Bathurst helped to secretly ordain Anglican ministers, while Dolben and Allestree acted as couriers between local royalists and the exiled royal courts. Willis was a significant member of this community, hosting religious services conducted by Fell, Allestree, and Dolben according to the 'outlawed' Book of Common Prayer in his rooms opposite Merton College. According to Leoline Jenkins, attendance at these services was as high as 300 people.

Willis's medical career began modestly. Unable to establish a practice for himself within the higher ranks of Interregnum civil society, he practiced medicine as an itinerant physician in the villages and markets around Oxford. He likely found it difficult to compete with other practitioners, because attracting patients depended entirely on his ability to sell himself and his experience. He had little medical training—the University's academic business had all but stopped shortly after he received his MA. A later critic claimed that Willis, while initially such an inexperienced practitioner, 'had been required to beg for remedies from Empirics and foolish women' (Meara, 1665, p. 127). Willis's own demeanor would have exacerbated the situation. Anthony à Wood described him as 'a plain man, a man of no carriage, little discourse, complaisance or society' and Aubrey noted that he 'stammered much' (Wood, 1967, vol. III, p. 1051; Aubrey, 1898, p. 303). Aubrey further claimed that Willis's practice was so meager that he shared a horse with another practitioner as they traveled from market to market.

While working to establish a medical practice, Willis also attempted to foster the patronage relations necessary for his social advancement. His old royalist friends and patrons were of little assistance, but Willis found his skills and experience as a chemist useful. His abilities were known to many of the longtime residents of Oxford. During the late 1640s, he had occasionally acted as chemical assistant to a small group of natural philosophers that gathered in Trinity College. He performed similar duties for the prominent new members of the academic community involved in the natural-philosophical meetings that abounded throughout the decade. He acted as chemical assistant to John Wilkins (Warden, Wadham College), setting up a chemical laboratory in his rooms at Wadham and preparing a variety of chemical recipes. He also assisted William Petty (Tomlins Professor of Anatomy) and participated in the events surrounding the sensational resuscitation of Anne Greene after her supposed execution in 1650. He even introduced Robert Hooke (who worked as his assistant) to Robert Boyle later in the decade.

Diatribae Duae Medico-Philosophicae

Willis's standing within intellectual circles improved greatly during the 1650s. He succeeded in establishing a reputation as a skilled chemist and natural philosopher. In 1656 Samuel Hartlib called him a 'leading and prime man in the Philosophical Club at Oxford' (Hartlib, 1995, 29/5/102A). Toward the close of the decade, Willis evidently wanted to enhance his standing as a physician. His practice had improved enough for him to be able to marry his old friend John Fell's sister Margaret in 1657, but he was still remembered as a struggling physician consulting the urine and dispensing chemical remedies in rural Oxfordshire markets. Petty later recalled 'I could Anno 1656 have returned into England and been at the top of practice in Oliver's Court, when Dr Willis was casting waters at Abington Markett' (Lansdowne, 1928, p. 214). Willis wrote his *Diatribae duae medico-philosophicae* (1659) in an attempt to differentiate himself from other empirical chemical practitioners. He strove to establish that he was a learned physician who aimed to unite theory with empirical practice such that 'reason does not pervert experiences and nature itself and that these do not remove reason from its place' (Willis, 1659, sig. H_4^*). To this end, he introduced a chemical medical philosophy in the first part of the book (*De fermentatione*). He argued that all natural phenomena could be understood and explained according to the actions and fermentation of five different types of chemical particles: spirit, sulfur, salt, earth, and water. He demonstrated in the second part of his book (*De febribus*) how the fermentation of these particles in the blood could explain the causes of fever as well as guide the therapeutic actions of the physician. He reinforced the marriage of philosophical knowledge and practical experience in the final tract (*De urinis*). The urine had long been considered an important diagnostic indicator of the nature of febrile conditions. Willis used his chemical analysis of the urine both to bolster his philosophical and medical beliefs and to justify his therapeutic practices.

Willis's standing within intellectual circles improved greatly following this publication, but this was due more to his devotion to his old friends than to his medical theories. With the Restoration of Charles II in 1660, Willis's friends acquired powerful positions within the University and the body politic. At the instigation of Sheldon, then Warden of All Souls, Bishop of London, and a member of the Privy Council, he was appointed Sedleian Professor of Natural Philosophy and awarded his doctorate in medicine. His medical practice grew significantly during this time. He and the surgeon William Day leased and renovated an old coaching inn, the Angel, for use as a surgery in 1660, and by 1665 Willis was reputed to have the highest salary in Oxford. He was later made a Fellow of the newly established Royal Society (1663) (although he seldom attended their meetings) and an honorary fellow of the College of Physicians (1665).

Anatomy of the Brain and Nerves

In the early 1660s Willis began to perform detailed research into the anatomy of the brain and nerves and the pathology of their disorders. This topic occupied his attention for much of the following decade and was the subject of his next four works. His first book on this topic was *Cerebri anatome* (1664), in which Willis revealed the physical structures responsible for the inner workings of human sensation, motivation, and behavior. Although he directed the investigations, his assistant Richard Lower (1631–91) largely performed the anatomies. Willis showed how the animal economy was driven by the explosive actions of a volatile spirituous substance (called animal spirits) in the nerves. This substance carried information from the sense organs to the brain. It also conveyed the spirits responsible for communicating the dictates of the reason and the passions throughout the body. His account was augmented by lavish anatomical illustrations provided by Christopher Wren. Willis provided a pathology of convulsive neurological diseases three years later in his *Pathologiae cerebri* (1667), which expanded upon his spirituous neurophysiology. He argued that conditions like epilepsy, hysterical passions, and hypochondriacal affections were the result of convulsions caused by the explosion of particles within the muscular parts of the body due to an abundance of highly volatile spirituous particles.

Willis moved to London around the time of the publication of his *Pathologiae cerebri*. This was likely done in order to be able to attend his friend Sheldon after he had suffered from a grave illness. The move greatly enhanced Willis's practice, and he quickly became a highly sought-after physician to the higher ranks of English society. However, his theories faced a number of challenges during the late 1660s. Lower, for example, called the details of his physiology of muscular motion into question, while Nathaniel Highmore (1613–85) criticized his pathology of hysterical passions and hypochondriacal affections. Willis responded to these challenges and defended his convulsive neuropathology in *Affectionum quae dicuntur hystericae & hypochondriacae pathologia spasmodica vindicata* (1670).

Willis's final neurological work was his most ambitious. In *De anima brutorum* (1672), he presented a comprehensive physiology and pathology of the animal soul. This was the 'part' of the body common to man and the beasts, believed to be the physical source of the bodily passions that urged individual creatures to seek out those things (such as food, shelter, and a mate) necessary for the furtherance of animal life. Distempers of the animal soul caused a variety of illnesses that corrupted human thought and behavior, such as melancholy and mania. Willis attributed these illnesses to the excited actions of animal spirits in the nerves. Not surprisingly, cures (whether involving the regulation of the six non-naturals or the prescription of medicines) centered around soothing these excited actions.

Willis's final work was his *Pharmaceutice rationalis* (1674–75), in which he explained the reasons underlying the curative actions of medicines. He described the actions of the stomach and explained how ingested medicaments promoted health by altering the physiological functioning of the animal economy. He also provided detailed accounts of how specific medicines acted upon the individual body parts in the posthumously published second volume.

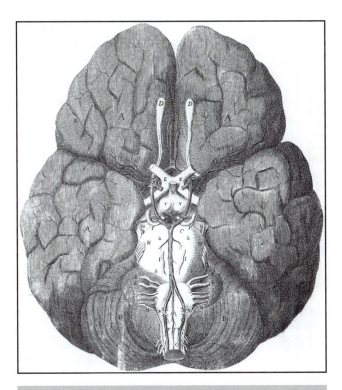

Circle of Willis. Engraving from *Cerebri anatome . . .* London, 1664. Rare Books, Wellcome Library, London.

Willis was interred in Westminster Abbey after an extravagant service costing just under 500 pounds, excluding the cost of the tombstone (as his grandson Browne Willis complained fifty years later) (Wood, 1967, vol. III, pp. 1048–1049 n3). He was survived by his second wife, Elizabeth Calley (1634/5–1709), whom he had married in 1672 (roughly two years after the death of his first wife, Mary), and his children Thomas, Anne, Jane, and Rachel.

Bibliography

Primary: 1676. *Opera omnia* (Geneva); 1684. (Pordage, S., trans.) *Dr Willis's Practice of Physick, Being the Whole Works . . .* (London); 1659. *Diatribae duae medico-philosophicae* (London); 1664. *Cerebri anatome: cui accessit nervorum descriptio et usus* (London); 1667. *Pathologiae cerebri, et nervosi generis specimen* (Oxford); 1670. *Affectionum quae dicuntur hystericae & hypochondriacae pathologia spasmodica vindicata* (London); 1672. *De anima brutorum quae hominis vitalis ac sensitiva est, exercitationes duae* (Oxford); 1674–75. *Pharmaceutice rationalis sive diatriba de medicamentorum operationibus in humano corpore* 2 vols. (Oxford); 1980. (Dewhurst, Kenneth, ed.) *Thomas Willis' Oxford Lectures* (Oxford); 1981. (Dewhurst, Kenneth, ed.) *Willis's Oxford Casebook (1650–52)* (Oxford).

Secondary: Martensen, Robert, 2004. *The Brain Takes Shape: An Early History* (Oxford); Hartlib, Samuel, 1995. 'Ephemerides 1656 Part 4' in *The Hartlib Papers* (1995); Martensen, Robert, 1992. '"Habit of Reason": Anatomy and Anglicanism in Restoration England.' *Bulletin of the History of Medicine* 66: 511–535; Anthony à Wood, 1967. (Bliss, P., ed.) *Athenae oxonienses . . . to Which Are Added the Fasti* (New York) vol. III, pp. 1048–1053; Lansdowne, Henry William Edmund Petty FitzMaurice, ed., 1928. *The Petty-Southwell correspondence, 1676–1687* (London); Aubrey, John, 1898. (Clark, Andrew, ed.) *'Brief Lives.' chiefly of the Contemporaries, set down by John Aubrey, between the Years 1669 & 1696* (Oxford); Jenkins, Leoline, 1854. *The Life of Francis Mansell, D.D. Principal of Jesus College, in Oxford* (London); John Fell, 1675. 'Postscript' in Willis, Thomas, *Pharmaceutice Rationalis* (Oxford) sigs. b₂v–c₂; Meara, Edmund, 1665. *Examen diatribae Thomae Willisy [sic] Doctoris Medici et Professoris Oxoniensis de febribvs* (London); *DSB*; *Munk's Roll*; *Oxford DNB*.

Mike Hawkins

WINKLER, CORNELIS (b. Vianen, the Netherlands, 25 February 1855; d. Hoog-Soeren, the Netherlands, 8 May 1941), *medicine, neuropsychiatry*.

The eldest child of a physician, Winkler went to high school in Amsterdam, studied medicine in Utrecht, where he was influenced by the physiologist and ophthalmologist Franciscus C. Donders (1818–89), and wrote his thesis (*Virus tuberculosum*) in 1879. Following a short employment as a resident in the Hague, Donders invited him to come to Utrecht and become reader of psychiatry. He initially declined, but after a visit to Vienna, where he met Theodor Meynert (1833–92) and Julius Wagner von Jauregg

(1857–1940), he accepted the post. He wished to teach psychiatry and neurology 'in one hand', as Wagner von Jauregg had advised him. During a study tour in southern Germany, Winkler met and was influenced by Ludwig Edinger, Carl Weigert, and Bernhard von Gudden.

As a consequence, Dutch psychiatry became tightly linked to neurology, after the German-Austrian example. At the invitation of the Dutch government, Winkler worked in the Dutch East Indies to investigate the cause of beriberi from 1886 to 1888. After returning, he continued his neuroanatomical research, including cortical ablation experiments on rabbits and dogs. In 1893 he was appointed the first professor of psychiatry and neurology (Utrecht), but because he did not have a clinic at his disposal, he resigned after three years and accepted the new chair of neurology and psychiatry in Amsterdam. In this period he was active in criminal anthropology, a subject on which he published several papers. In 1907 he organized an international congress for neurology, psychiatry, and mental care, where he met many of the great neuroscientists of the time, including Constantin von Monakow (1853–1930), who became his friend. They corresponded, cooperated on several projects, and often met in Amsterdam or in Zurich. In cooperation with anatomist Louis Bolk (1866–1930), Winkler made plans for the foundation of the Central Institute for Brain Research, which was opened in Amsterdam in 1909. Following the death of Karl Heilbronner (1869–1914), who had succeeded in building a modern neuropsychiatric clinic at Utrecht, Winkler returned there, staying until he retired in 1925. He continued to do neuroanatomical work together with E. C. Junius, whom he had married after his first wife, Catharina Wilhelmina Pelgrim, died.

In the early years of his career, Winkler struggled to have psychiatry (in which he included neurology) examined for medical graduation. Neuroanatomy was one of the main subjects of his work. He applied von Gudden's atrophy method to study the course of nerves in the central nervous system. He wrote a five-volume *Handbook of Neurology* (1917–33), which in fact was a book on neuroanatomy. With his pupils he worked on clinical subjects including syringomyelia, aphasia, Parkinson's disease, and the plantar reflex. Several of his own papers dealt with aphasia and functional localization. Winkler and the surgeon Johan Anton Guldenarm (1852–1905) performed brain surgery for tumors, abscesses, and hemorrhages in the 1890s. With respect to the teaching of psychiatry, Winkler kept to the doctrines of Wernicke: 'I taught psychiatry on a biological base.' As an adherent to Meynert's and Wernicke's 'brain psychiatry', Winkler approached psychiatry from a biological point of view, explaining psychiatric disorders as arising from a neuropathological basis. He was opposed to Freud's psychoanalysis. Although he had always been in favor of the combined teaching of psychiatry and neurology, he realized, in the 1920s, that the time had come for both subjects to go their own ways. The first separate chair for neurology in the Netherlands was established in Amsterdam (1923, for Bernard Brouwer, 1881–1949). Winkler may be considered the godfather of Dutch neurology.

Bibliography

Primary: 1918–33. *Opera Omnia* 10 vols. (Haarlem); 1917–33. *Handboek der neurologie. De bouw van het zenuwstelsel* 5 vols. (Haarlem); 1947. (Winkler-Junius, E., ed.) *Herinneringen van Cornelis Winkler 1855–1941* (Arnhem).

Secondary: Koehler, Peter J., 2002. 'C. Winkler 1855–1941' in Fredericks, J. A. M., G. W. Bruyn, and P. Eling, eds., *History of Neurology in the Netherlands* (Amsterdam) pp. 393–401; Koehler, Peter J., and C. Jagella, 2002. 'De correspondentie tussen Winkler en Von Monakow.' *Nederlands Tijdschrift voor Geneeskunde* 145: 2469-2473, 2474-2478; Lhermitte, Jean, and R. Mourgue, 1946–47. 'La vie et oeuvre de Cornélis Winkler.' *L'Encéphale* 1–13.

Peter Koehler

WINSLOW, FORBES BENIGNUS (b. Pentonville, London, England, August 1810; d. Hove, Sussex, 3 March 1874), *psychiatry.*

Winslow was the ninth son of Thomas Winslow, an army officer, and Mary Forbes. His ancestors had settled in the American colonies in the seventeenth century, and Winslow's early education took place in New York as well as in Britain. He studied medicine at University College London and at the Middlesex Hospital, becoming MRCS (1835) and gaining his MD from Aberdeen (1849). He became FRCPEdin (1850) and MRCP (1859). During the 1830s and 1840s he wrote pocket guides for students as well as lecturing and publishing on insanity, notably on suicide and on the value of the criminal insanity plea in legal trials. His business acumen led to the opening of a lucrative private asylum in the late 1840s, the founding of a specialist medico-psychological journal, and his self-promotion (especially through the editing of the journal) as an expert medical witness.

Winslow's skill at self-promotion was matched only by his evangelical stance as to the outright innocence, by virtue of insanity, of those at whose criminal trials he gave key testimonies. This brought him controversy in two famous criminal insanity cases. In the first—the 1843 trial of Daniel McNaghten, who had attempted the assassination of the prime minister, but murdered another man instead—Winslow's zeal in arguing for McNaghten's insanity was marred by the fact that he had never met McNaghten and knew no more about him than had come out in evidence, all the while testifying to McNaghten's state of mind at the time of the act for which he was charged. The trial was a famously controversial one, requiring the Law Lords to question some of what had occurred and to lay down some rules for future use. Some of the Law Lords involved construed Winslow's evidence as too easily making light of the legal, as opposed to the medical, issues at work in the trial, and as being too much the assertion of unproven 'expertise' and thus close to being evidence that should not have been allowed. Later trial judges placed firmer controls on allowing medical evidence regarding insanity, partly because Winslow had in their view overstepped the mark in the McNaghten proceedings.

The Townley trial in 1863, involving a man who cut the throat of his onetime fiancée after she had come to prefer another man, saw Winslow again in the thick of it. His bold assertions as to Townley's insanity were initially unsuccessful, and Townley was sentenced to death. But on appeal some complications led to a respite, and Townley was sent to Bethlem. There, four further medical experts effectively refuted the testimony of Winslow during the trial and deemed Townley to be fully sane and fully culpable, and he was moved again, to Pentonville prison, for execution. Townley committed suicide before the execution took place. This time, Winslow had to defend himself not only against those who thought the full force of the law was being undermined by very inexact medical arguments, but also against other psychiatrists who likewise deemed his criteria for insanity to be too broad and too imprecise.

Winslow wrote endlessly on medico-legal matters, on diseases of the brain, and on drunkenness, and campaigned for separate asylums for inebriates. His controversial and zealous advocacy for this new application of medical expertise was not matched by any political radicalism, as he remained a Conservative all his life.

Bibliography

Primary: 1843. *The Plea of Insanity in Criminal Cases* (London); 1860. *On the Obscure Diseases of the Brain and Mind* (London).

Secondary: Eigen, J. P., 2003. *Unconscious Crime: Mental Absence and Criminal Responsibility in Victorian London* (Baltimore); Eigen, J. P., 1995. *Witnessing Insanity: Madness and Mad-Doctors in the English Court* (New Haven, CT); *Oxford DNB*.

Michael Neve

WINSLØW, JACOB (JACQUES-BÉNIGNE) (b. Odense, Denmark, 17 April 1669; d. Paris, France, 3 April 1760), *medicine, anatomy.*

The eldest of thirteen children of Peder Jacobsen Winsløw, dean of the Lutheran Church in Odense, and Marta Bruun, Winsløw entered university in Copenhagen in 1687 to study for the ministry. While there he developed a keen interest in the natural sciences, chiefly under the influence of the anatomist-physician Caspar Bartholin, the younger (1655–1738). In 1691 he enrolled at the College of Medicine founded by Ole Borch (1626–90) and simultaneously gained practical experience under Johannes de Buchwald (1658–1738), who was reputed to be the best surgeon in Copenhagen. Being somewhat squeamish about the sight of blood, Winsløw concentrated on anatomy and soon became Bartholin's prosector, and later was *anatomicus regius*.

In 1697, after achieving a bachelor of medicine degree, Winsløw received a royal grant that enabled him to study in the Netherlands and then in Paris, where he studied anatomy and surgery under Joseph-Guichard Duverney (1648–1730). In Paris Winsløw became acquainted both with the writings and the person of Jacques-Bénigne Bossuet (1627–1704), who has been called the greatest orator ever to appear in a Christian pulpit, and who was at this time engaged on his own counter-reforming crusade to bring Protestants back to Catholicism. In 1699, under Bossuet's influence, Winsløw converted to Catholicism and took Bénigne as his baptismal name. This terminated his scholarship from the Danish crown, and evidently severed his relations with his Lutheran family. He was now committed to remaining in France.

By 1704, when he was working at the Hôtel Dieu, he had been authorized to practice medicine in Paris, and in that same year became assistant to Duverney in the Jardin du Roi. He began to build a thriving practice, helped by his MD, which was awarded in 1705, his fellowship of the Académie des Sciences in 1708, and his appointments as physician at the Hôpital Général and at Bicêtre in 1709. He was made docteur-régent of the Faculty of Medicine in 1728 and in 1743 became professor of anatomy at the Jardin du Roi. When Winsløw made the dedicatory address upon the opening of a new anatomical theater for the Faculty of Medicine, in 1745, he was widely regarded as the greatest anatomist of his day. He was obliged to resign his professorship in 1758 due to the loss of his hearing.

Winsløw was a prolific author, producing nearly thirty treatises on various aspects of human anatomy between 1711 and 1743, including demonstrations that muscles always work in groups and that monstrous births resulted from faulty development of the embryo, not merely from lesions of a normal fetus. He was also highly influential in renaming the intercostal nerve as the 'grande sympathetique' nerve and in giving rise to the notion of the sympathetic nervous system. The culmination of his work in anatomy was his *Exposition anatomique de la structure du corps humain* (1732), which appeared in many editions both in French and in various translations.

The most influential of his other works was his *Mortis incertae signa* (1740), which was translated into French by Jacques-Jean Bruhier (1742) and subsequently into a number of other languages. In it, Winsløw argued that it was often difficult to be sure that a person really was dead and that there was therefore a real risk that some people would be buried prematurely. He went on to provide a rich compendium of anecdotal evidence. He even claimed that he himself had been presumed dead, and nearly buried, on two occasions, once as a child, and again as a young man. Although Winsløw's book no doubt was only one factor among many, there is no denying that it played a role in the subsequent widespread popular fear of premature burial and in the introduction of measures to prevent it, which flourished right into the next century and beyond.

Bibliography

Primary: 1732. *Exposition anatomique de la structure du corps humain* (Paris); 1740. *Quaestio medico-chirurgica . . . an mortis incertae signa minus incerta a chirurgicis, quam ab aliis experimentis* (Paris).

Secondary: Bondeson, Jan, 2002. *Buried Alive: The Terrifying History of Our Most Primal Fear* (New York); Olry, R., 1996. 'Winsløw's Contributions to Our Understanding of the Cervical Portion of the Sympathetic Nervous System.' *Journal of the History of the Neurosciences* 5: 190–196; Snorrason, Egell, 1969. *L'anatomiste J.-B. Winsløw, 1669–1760* (Copenhagen); *DSB*.

John Henry

WINTROBE, MAXWELL MYER (b. Halifax, Nova Scotia, Canada, 27 October 1901; d. Salt Lake City, Utah, USA, 9 December 1986), *medicine, hematology.*

Wintrobe's family moved from Halifax to Winnipeg, Manitoba, in 1912. Max, an only child, entered the University of Manitoba at age fifteen and medical school at age twenty. He became aware of Johns Hopkins by reading Harvey Cushing's *The Life of William Osler.* Osler became his hero and Wintrobe decided then that he wanted to someday work at Johns Hopkins. He received the MD degree in 1926. Minot and Murphy's monumental report of the successful treatment of pernicious anemia with liver extract was published that same year. Wintrobe obtained a fellowship and began trying to establish an animal model for pernicious anemia. This research project launched him on a lifelong career in hematology.

Wintrobe spent three years at Tulane (1927–30), where he studied nutritional and other anemias, tropical disease, tuberculosis, and various forms of cancer. The chief of medicine, John Musser, suggested that Wintrobe find out about the 'anemia of the South' and whether it really existed. Wintrobe found little information on blood values in normal adults and children. He collected his own data and developed an accurate method for measuring the packed red cell volume (hematocrit). Despite the fact that this method replaced the previously unreliable devices of the 1920s, Wintrobe refused all royalties and applied for no patent. He also developed the red cell indices (MCV, MCH, and MCHC). These direct measurements allowed quantitative classification of anemias and remain in widespread use today.

While in New Orleans, Wintrobe earned a PhD degree. His thesis, 'The Erythrocyte in Man', was accepted in *Medicine.* Alan Chesney, the dean of Johns Hopkins Medical School, was editor of the journal. Wintrobe met Chesney, who offered him a faculty position at Johns Hopkins, thus fulfilling his longstanding desire to go to that institution.

Wintrobe remained at Johns Hopkins from 1930 until 1943. He took over the Division of Clinical Microscopy a generation after Osler, its founder, had left Baltimore. Wintrobe directed second-year and third-year courses in clinical

microscopy, emphasizing the importance of routine examination of blood smears. He trained various persons as lab technicians, including his wife, Becky. At Hopkins Wintrobe expanded his work on normal blood values and the utility of the hematocrit in measuring the erythrocyte sedimentation rate. He was the first to identify a cryoglobulin in blood from a patient with multiple myeloma, demonstrating the temperature-dependent reversible precipitation. Though Wintrobe's attempts to produce pernicious anemia in animals were unsuccessful, his studies advanced many areas of hematology, including the etiology and management of anemias and the diverse manifestations of leukemias and lymphomas. These and other investigative activities led to the publication in 1942 of Wintrobe's landmark monograph, *Clinical Hematology*, which immediately became the most authoritative book in the field. He wrote the entire book himself through six of its editions and acquired an international reputation (the eleventh edition was published in 2004).

In 1943 Wintrobe moved to Salt Lake City to become first chairman of medicine at the University of Utah Medical School, a position he held until 1967. Wintrobe established an excellent department of medicine and a widely respected hematology division at Utah. He received the first extramural research grant from the National Institutes of Health (for research on hereditary muscular dystrophy). This award was renewed annually for thirty-three years. Between 1947 and 1984, 170 graduate students trained in hematology and participated in research activities at Utah. Wintrobe's bibliography contains over 400 publications in professional journals and books. He became a Master of the American College of Physicians in 1973, was elected to the U.S. National Academy of Sciences in 1973, and was awarded the Kober Medal of the Association of American Physicians in 1974.

Wintrobe also served as one of the founding editors of Tinsley Harrison's *Principles of Internal Medicine.* His later literary efforts included two monographs that reflected his longstanding interest in medical history. *Blood, Pure and Eloquent: A Story of Discovery, of People, and of Ideas* appeared in 1980. In this volume Wintrobe and other leading contemporary hematologists who had made major scientific contributions wrote about various topics in blood diseases from a historical perspective. In 1985 Wintrobe published *Hematology, the Blossoming of a Science: A Story of Inspiration and Effort*, which traces the career development of many investigators and teachers in the field through more than 500 biographical sketches.

Wintrobe was fair and decisive, and held strong opinions. He was a kind and understanding mentor. His devotion to Oslerian ideals was lifelong. The Wintrobes had two children, a daughter and a son. Their son was killed in an auto accident.

The explosion of basic science and clinical information about blood disorders that was discovered between 1926 and Wintrobe's death in 1986 was indeed the golden age of hematology. Wintrobe played a major role in defining and conveying this new knowledge. He established hematology as a distinct subspecialty of internal medicine.

Bibliography

Primary: 1930. 'The Erythrocyte in Man.' *Medicine* 9: 195–255; 1942. *Clinical Hematology* (Philadelphia); 1980. *Blood, Pure and Eloquent: A Story of Discovery, of People, and of Ideas* (New York); 1985. *Hematology, the Blossoming of a Science: A Story of Inspiration and Effort* (Philadelphia).

Secondary: Spivak, Jerry L., 2003. 'Annotation: Maxwell Wintrobe, in His Own Words.' *British Journal of Haematology* 121: 224–232; Valentine, William N., 1990. 'Maxwell Myer Wintrobe' in *Biographical Memoirs, National Academy of Sciences* 59: 447–472; Weisse, Allen B., 1984. *Maxwell M. Wintrobe, Conversations in Medicine* (New York) pp. 75–92.

Marvin J. Stone

WISEMAN, RICHARD   (b. London, England, 1620?; d. Bath, England, 1676), *surgery.*

Wiseman was probably the son of Thomas and Elizabeth Wiseman of St Andrew Undershaft in London. In 1637 he was apprenticed to a surgeon in the capital. Thereafter the details of his life are unclear, but he served as a surgeon in the Royalist army in the west of England during the first civil war. After the Royalists were defeated in 1645, he continued serving that cause, accompanying Prince Charles (later Charles II) into exile. In 1650 Wiseman traveled with Charles when the latter allied with the Scots against the English Republic; the surgeon's later publications reveal how he assisted wounded soldiers at the battles of Dunbar (1650) and Worcester (1651). After the latter engagement, Wiseman was captured, and then returned to civilian life. He was granted the freedom of the Barber-Surgeons' Company in 1652, worked at St Thomas's Hospital, London, and entered private practice. However, he apparently continued moving in Royalist circles, for he was briefly imprisoned by Oliver Cromwell's regime in 1654. Thereafter, he seems to have spent some years abroad in Spain, the Caribbean, and the Spanish Netherlands, apparently serving in the Spanish navy. When Charles II was restored to the throne in 1660, Wiseman received his reward. He was made surgeon in ordinary to the King, was promoted to the post of principal surgeon to the King in 1672, and was granted a royal pension. He also prospered within the metropolitan medical world, and was elected to the court of assistants and then as master of the Barber-Surgeons. By the time he died in 1676, he owned property in London, Lincolnshire, and Worcestershire and was worth over £1,600.

His reputation rests primarily on his *Severall Chirurgical Treatises*, published in the year of his death. This ran to seven further editions by 1734 and was sufficiently well-known for the lexicographer Samuel Johnson (1709–84) to commend it. The volume is made up of eight treatises, dis-

cussing tumors, ulcers, diseases of the anus, the King's Evil, wounds, gunshot wounds, fractures, and venereal infections. Many military historians of the English Civil War have drawn upon it, for it vividly describes the wounds suffered by combatants. Its discussion of the King's Evil reveals Wiseman's fervent Royalism, for it emphasizes the Stuarts' ability to cure this condition through the Royal Touch. These 'miraculous' cures were, Wiseman maintained, far more effective than the efforts of any surgeon, and he attacked those of his contemporaries who offered naturalistic explanations of the monarch's apparent ability to cure the disease. The remainder of the book reveals that this partisan spirit co-existed with an empirical approach to medicine. Each treatise describes and defines the condition being discussed, and then provides a large number of descriptions of specific cases. Wiseman acknowledged that he was building on work by previous authors (notably English surgeons such as William Clowes, 1544–1604, and John Woodall, 1570–1643), but emphasized that there remained 'many Gaps' in the practice of surgery and the history of diseases, and that there was much to be learned from adding observations to the fund of knowledge. His numerous case histories were clearly intended to serve this aim. As a result, many commentators have hailed his work as raising the status of surgery.

Bibliography

Primary: 1676. *Severall Chirurgical Treatises . . .* (London); 1977. (intro. Kirkup, J. A.) *Of Wounds, Of Gun-Shot Wounds, of Fractures and Luxations* (Bath) [1676 edn. (London)].

Secondary: Wear, A., 2000. *Knowledge and Practice in English Medicine, 1550–1680* (Cambridge); Donagan, B., 1998. 'The Casualties of War: Treatment of the Dead and Wounded in the English Civil War' in Gentles, Ian, John Morrill, and Blair Worden, eds., *Soldiers, Writers and Statesmen of the English Revolution* (Cambridge) pp. 114–132; *Oxford DNB.*

Mark Jenner

WITHERING, WILLIAM   (b. Wellington, Shropshire, England, 17 March 1741; d. Sparkbrook near Birmingham, England, 6 October 1799), *botany, medicine.*

Withering, son of Edmund Withering, an apothecary, and Sarah Hector, studied classical languages with a local minister and was then apprenticed to a local practitioner. He had relatives on both sides of the family who were medical men, and in 1762 he went to Edinburgh University, where he studied under Alexander Monro *secundus* (1733–1817), John Hope (1725–86), William Cullen (1710–90), Joseph Black (1728–99), John Rutherford (1695–1779), and John Gregory (1729–73). He was an active member of the student organization, the Royal Medical Society, at Edinburgh, and he graduated MD (1766).

Withering began his medical practice in Stafford, but in 1775 he moved to Birmingham. The next few years were busy ones. Within a year Withering was well established as a physician, treating thousands of poor patients for free in addition to maintaining a lucrative private practice that kept him traveling nearly 6,000 miles per year. He married Helena Cookes (1772) and the couple had three children. Helena's interest in botany piqued Withering's interest as well, and in 1776 he published *The Botanical Arrangement of All the Vegetables Naturally Growing in Great Britain*. This was the first such work to be organized according to the Linnean system, and it became the standard English-language account of British plants, going through fourteen editions over the next hundred years. The last edition was published in 1877. Withering's text was thus responsible for the botanical education of the majority of nineteenth-century British scientists. He was recognized in his own lifetime by being elected a Fellow of the Linnean Society (1789).

Withering had a long-standing interest in chemistry, which he developed while a student under Black at Edinburgh. He published articles on the chemical analysis of minerals in both the Edinburgh journal *Medical Commentaries*, and in the *Philosophical Transactions* of the Royal Society. He also carried out chemical analyses of many of the English mineral waters and of the Caldas da Rainha spring while resident in Cintra, Portugal. In his *Experiments and Observations on the Terra Ponderosa* (1784) he published what became the standard chemical procedure for testing for sulfates. As a tribute to his wide-ranging scientific interests, Withering has both a plant—*Witheringia solanacea*—and a mineral—Witherite—named after him.

Withering put his power of careful analysis to good use in his most famous publication, *An Account of the Foxglove and Some of Its Medical Uses* (1795). Foxglove, *Digitalis purpurea*, had a long history as an ingredient in medicine, but it also had an equally long history as a very violent purge. Withering's attention was first called to it by one of his charity patients, who claimed to have been cured of dropsy (ascites) by a kind of herbal tea. On examining the ingredients, Withering suspected that foxglove had been the active medicine, and he began to research its diuretic qualities. He substituted infusions and dried, powdered leaves for the decoctions most commonly used, in order to be able to prescribe precisely measured doses. Though he found he could not cure all cases of dropsy, his results were marked enough that foxglove became a common prescription for a wide range of diseases. His work provided the clinical starting point for later research by nineteenth-century pharmacologists into the precise connection between heart disease and dropsy and into the chemical responsible for foxglove's action on the heart.

Withering was a longstanding member of the Lunar Society of Birmingham. He was elected FRS in 1785 and a foreign corresponding member of the Portuguese Academy of Science in 1795.

Bibliography

Primary: 1776. *The Botanical Arrangement of All the Vegetables Naturally Growing in Great Britain* (Birmingham); 1785. *An Account of the Foxglove, and some of its medical uses; with practical remarks on dropsy, and other diseases* (Birmingham); 1822. (Withering, W.) *The Miscellaneous Tracts of the Late William Withering M.D. F.R.S.* 2 vols. (London).

Secondary: Mann, Ronald D., ed., 1985. *William Withering and the Foxglove* (Lancaster); Withering, William, Jr., 1822. *The Miscellaneous Tracts of the Late William Withering M.D. F.R.S* (London); *DSB*; *Oxford DNB*.

Lisa Rosner

WOODALL, JOHN (b. Castle Street, Warwickshire, England, 1570; d. London, England, 28 August 1643), *surgery, chemical medicine.*

Woodall was the eldest son of Richard Woodall, a small landowner, and of Mary Hall. His early education remains obscure, but he later served as a regimental surgeon on an English military campaign in Normandy (1589–90). Thereafter, he worked as a surgeon for the English merchant community along the Baltic coast and traveled in Europe. In March 1601 he was made free of the Barber-Surgeons' Company in London by apprenticeship. His remaining professional life was spent in the capital—he even remained in residence and treated patients through plague epidemics. He was active in the Barber-Surgeons, holding a succession of posts in the Company, and was elected Master in 1632. He held the position of surgeon to St Bartholomew's Hospital from 1616 until his death and was surgeon to the smaller foundation of the Charterhouse in London between 1614 and 1627.

Woodall's career was not confined to these venerable institutions. He was highly entrepreneurial and keenly interested in the new opportunities presented by the expansion of international trade in the early seventeenth century. He bought shares in the East India Company, the Virginia Company, and the Somers Island Company, and acquired plantation property in Bermuda. His medical activities converged with his investments. In 1613 he was made surgeon-general to the East India Company. This post involved not only serving in the hospital that the Company had established at its dockyard in Blackwall (now Poplar, London), but also overseeing the surgeons appointed on ships going to the East Indies, offering advice about regimen for Company employees abroad, and preparing the chests that Company surgeons would take upon their long voyages. He continued to provide them with medicinal chests until his death. In the 1620s he was also involved in supplying such chests to the Royal Navy. These combined activities made him a wealthy man by the time he died.

It was in this commercial context that Woodall published his most important book—*The Surgions Mate, or a Treatise Discovering Faithfully . . . the Due Contents of the Surgions Chest* (1617). Designed initially as an advice book for East India Company surgeons, subsequent editions sought a broader audience and adopted the alternative subtitle, *Military and Domestic Medicine.* The work included detailed instructions on the treatment of wounds and injuries and on the surgeon's instruments, and also set out advice for shipboard medicine. Woodall emphasized that the surgeon should not be 'fine fingered', neglecting the more distasteful aspects of his work; he thus gave instructions on the treatment of what we would now term rectal prolapse and stressed that the surgeon should provide close stools for those afflicted with the bloody flux or other debilitating diseases. He paid close attention to the range of diseases that afflicted those on long voyages, and gave a long and detailed account of scurvy. Woodall's commentary is particularly notable because he recommended that the crew be provided with 'the juice of Oringes, limes or Lemons' against it.

Woodall was also an avid partisan of new chemical remedies, and published an account of his plague remedy, which was based upon gold. This interest was as much theoretical as empirical. The last section of *The Surgions Mate* is an early and full exposition of chemical medicine and of Paracelsus's tripartite division of the world into salt, sulfur, and mercury. This drew not only on Paracelsus but also on other chemical authors, such as Oswald Croll (*c.* 1560–1609) and Joseph Duchesne (*c.* 1544–1609).

Bibliography

Primary: 1978. (facsimile of 1617 London edn., with introduction by Kirkup, J.) *The Surgions Mate* (Bath).

Secondary: Berlin, M., 2004. 'Experimentation in Shipbuilding in Jacobean London: The English East India Company.' *Journal de la Renaissance* 2: 31–40; Appleby, J. H., 1981. 'New Light on John Woodall, Surgeon and Adventurer.' *Medical History* 25: 251–268; Debus, A. G., 1966. *The English Paracelsians* (New York); *Oxford DNB.*

Mark Jenner

WRIGHT, ALMROTH EDWARD (b. Middleton Tyas, Yorkshire, England, 10 August 1861; d. Farnham Common, Buckinghamshire, England, 30 April 1947), *pathology.*

Wright was one of three sons born to profoundly Protestant parents, Reverend Charles Henry Hamilton Wright and Ebba Johanna Dorothea. Although he upheld their views that women should be subordinate to men and became a vehement opponent of women's rights, Almroth rejected religion outright. He matriculated in modern languages at Trinity College, Dublin (1882) and in medicine (1883), then received a scholarship to study sciences in Germany with prominent scientists. Wright occupied short-term positions in London, Cambridge, and Sydney until 1892, when he was appointed professor of pathology at the RAMC school at Netley, a position he held for ten years.

At Netley, Wright developed a successful typhoid vaccine, but he was beset by critics and skeptics, and in 1902 he angrily resigned to take up a new appointment at St Mary's Hospital, where he remained till his death. About

the same time, he turned from work on prophylactic vaccines to therapeutical vaccines, following a process he called opsonization. Stated simply, Wright and his assistants would remove bacterial matter from patients, grow a culture, kill it, and then vaccinate the patient with the killed vaccine. Wright believed that opsonization stimulated the phagocytes to more effectively destroy bacteria. George Bernard Shaw, a frequent visitor to Wright's laboratory, caricatured the process in *The Doctor's Dilemma* (1906) by having the character representing Wright, Sir Colenso Ridgeon, explain that 'Opsonin is what you butter the disease germs with to make your white corpuscles eat them.' Shaw was not the only skeptic: Wright's theories were deliberately obnoxious to traditional consultants and to university statisticians, both of whom Wright denounced with a disdain that his parents had reserved for Catholics. Indeed, both the statistics and the clinical evidence were dubious, and pathologists began to denounce the laboratory work as well. But in the decade before World War I, Wright's theories were widely popular and St Mary's became a humming center for pathological research on the strength of them. Wright invested the profits from vaccines and from his lucrative private practice into developing one of the largest medical research laboratories in the country at the time, and he trained many outstanding scientists. Unusually for a pathologist, he had designated beds at the hospital, paid for initially from his profits and later by the Medical Research Council. His treatise on laboratory work, *Techniques of the Teat and the Capillary Tube* (1912), became a classic work of reference.

Wright's typhoid vaccine was triumphantly vindicated during World War I, when it probably prevented something like a million cases in the trenches. But his therapeutical vaccines and grandiose plans for reforming British medical science fell increasingly into disrepute after the war, and Wright turned his attention to a treatise on logic, posthumously published, which was intended to expose the stupidity of his enemies once and for all. They, in turn, called him 'Sir Almost Wright' or 'Sir Always Wrong'. His therapeutic vaccines had long since fallen from favor by the time that they were made obsolete by the development of antibiotics, the first of which, penicillin, was discovered in Wright's laboratory by Sir Alexander Fleming (1881–1955).

In 1889 Wright married Jane Georgina Wilson, and they had three children. The marriage was not happy and Wright continued to spend long days in the laboratory to the end of his life. Knighted in 1906, the same year he was elected FRS, Wright was made CB (1915) and KBE (1919).

Bibliography

Primary: 1904. *A Short Treatise on Anti-Typhoid Inoculation* (London); 1912. *Techniques of the Teat and the Capillary Glass Tube* (London) (2nd edn. 1921); 1953. (Romanes, Giles J., ed.) *Alethetropic Logic: A Posthumous Work* (London).

Secondary: Heaman, E. A., 2003. *St Mary's: The History of a London Teaching Hospital* (Montreal and Kingston); Dunnill, Michael, 2000. *The Plato of Praed Street: The Life and Times of Almroth Wright* (London); *DSB; Oxford DNB.*

E. A. Heaman

WU, LIEN-TEH (aka WU LIANDE; NG LEEN-TUCK; TUCK, G. L.) (b. Georgetown, Penang, Malaya [now Malaysia], 10 March 1879; d. Penang, Malaysia, 21 January 1960), *medicine, public health.*

Wu Lien-Teh was the fourth son in the family of eleven of a goldsmith father, Ng Kee-Hock, and mother, Lim Choy-Fan. The family lived in Georgetown, Penang, then a British colony off the northwest coast of the Malay Peninsula (now West/Peninsular Malaysia). He was originally named Ng Leen-Tuck in the Cantonese dialect (Five United Virtues), pronounced Wu Lien-Teh in Mandarin. At school and university an error recorded his name as Gnoh Lean-Teik, and later Gnoh Lean-Tuck. As a civil servant in China, he reverted to Wu Lien-Teh, as he was known in the West.

Wu excelled at Penang Free School, becoming the only recipient of the prestigious Queen's Scholarship for 1896. He went to Emmanuel College, Cambridge, as the first Chinese to read medicine. He won many awards: the Kerslake scholarship (pathology), the Cheadle Gold Medal (medicine), and special prizes in clinical medicine and surgery. In 1899 he gained one of two University scholarships for clinical training at St Mary's Hospital, London. He also served as house physician at the Brompton Hospital for Consumption and Diseases of the Chest, London. An Emmanuel College Research Studentship funded postgraduate work (1902–03) at the Liverpool School of Tropical Medicine under Ronald Ross; at Halle-an-der-Salle, Germany, with Karl Fraenkel; and at Institute Pasteur, Paris, with Elie Mechnikov.

Wu studied the cause of the high rate of tetanus infections among patients given a large dose of gelatin fluid to treat aortic or popliteal aneurysms, concluding that unless the gelatin solution was thoroughly sterilized, there was a high risk of tetanus. He submitted 'The Occurrence of Tetanus Spores in Gelatin' as a Cambridge MD thesis (1905), adding to his BA (1899) and MA, MB, BChir (1903).

A Doctor in British Malaya

Wu decided to take up a Research Studentship from Emmanuel College (1903–04) and work on tropical diseases at the Institute for Medical Research, Kuala Lumpur, having learned from the Colonial Office (London) that although he would easily be accepted into the Colonial Medical Service, he could serve only as an assistant medical officer and not as a medical officer, due to the race barrier. There were no opportunities for non-European medical specialists or research workers.

Toward the end of 1904, Wu returned to his hometown and established a private practice in Chulia Street, buying the dispensary of a British lady doctor. As one of only four non-European practitioners in Georgetown in 1905, his practice flourished, and a prosperous practice allowed Wu to go to Singapore to marry Ruth Huang Shu-Chiung (1883–1937), the second daughter of the pioneer Foochow immigrant to Sarawak, Wong Nai Siong (1849–1924), and sister-in-law of the renowned Straits Chinese leader Dr Lim Boon Keng (1869–1957). Wu and Ruth had three sons. The eldest, Daven Wu Chang-Keng, who also became a doctor, lived to thirty-two. His two other sons, Tommy Wu Chang-Fu and Willy Wu Chang-Ming died at the ages of sixteen years and of six months, respectively. Ruth Huang died in 1937, aged fifty-four. Wu's second marriage to Marie Lee Shu-Chiung resulted in five children: Betty Wu Yu Lin, Ellen Wu Yu Chen, Fred Wu Chang Sheng, John Wu Chang Yun, and Pearl Wu Yu Chu. The girls became teachers, Chang Sheng a barrister, and Chang Yun a doctor.

Youthful and committed, Wu became involved in issues such as promoting female education, removing the queue (pigtail), campaigning against gambling, encouraging physical exercises among boys and girls, and forming literary clubs. Wu, Lim Boon Keng, and Song Ong Siang (1871–1941) edited the *Straits Chinese Magazine* (1897–1907), a quarterly publication hoping to provoke discussion on local concerns such as Straits Chinese identity, the necessity of modern medical practices (e.g., vaccination), the opium controversy, and women's rights.

Inspired by Lim, Wu joined the anti-opium campaign, becoming president and physician-in-chief of the Penang Anti-Opium Association. In March 1906 he organized the inaugural Anti-Opium Conference for the Straits Settlements and the Federated Malay States in Ipoh, Perak. Badly hurt by the increasing successes of the anti-opium campaign, those with opium interests moved against Wu early in 1907. The Senior Medical Officer of Penang, armed with a warrant, embarked on a search for noxious drugs at his dispensary, finding an ounce of tincture of opium in the poison cabinet. Wu claimed this belonged to the previous owner, but he was immediately issued with a summons for illegal possession of a 'deleterious drug' without a government license, based on recent legislation requiring all registered medical practitioners to be licensed 'to buy, keep and use certain specified deleterious drugs' (Wu, 1959, p. 242). The Straits Branch of the British Medical Association refused to defend him, his membership in the Royal Society of Medicine (London) notwithstanding. He engaged the leading British lawyer in Penang, Arthur R. Adams. The court case and subsequent appeal were unsuccessful. Wu was fined $100 (Straits dollars) and ordered to apply for the appropriate license. Adams declined his professional fees.

Despite these difficulties, Wu found himself invited to address the Anti-Opium Conference of 1907 at Queen's Hall, London. He received a standing ovation from the 500-strong audience for a speech outlining the appalling opium menace in the Straits Settlements and proposing sources of revenue other than opium farms that should be considered.

While in Britain, he visited the RAMC, London, and the Military Hospital, Netley, in preparation to take up the offer to become vice-director of the Imperial Army Medical College in Tientsin, made to him by the Grand Councillor Yuan Shih-Kai of the Imperial Chinese government in Beijing.

Plague Fighter

In the autumn of 1908 Wu arrived in Tientsin, where the Imperial Army Medical College had been established to train doctors for the newly created modern Chinese army. In December 1910 the Wai Wu Pu (Ministry of Foreign Affairs) summoned him to Beijing. Councillor Alfred Sze told him of a month-old epidemic disease in Harbin (northern Manchuria) claiming numerous Chinese and Russian lives. To avoid a diplomatic situation, it was imperative that the Imperial Chinese government instigate immediate action against the epidemic. Wu was chosen as the 'expert in bacteriology to proceed to that region to investigate the cause and to suppress it, if possible' (Wu, 1959, pp. 279–280).

On 24 December, Wu and his assistant arrived in Harbin. Over the next four months he established himself as the 'plague fighter', discovering the disease's etiology and successfully suppressing an epidemic 'extending from the far west and north of Manchuria, through the capital [of Beijing] to the provinces of Chihli and Shantung, and finally as far south as Nanking and Shanghai' (Wu, 1959, p. 281).

To ascertain the precise cause of death, it was imperative that a postmortem be performed, but the Chinese opposed dismemberment or interference with a corpse. The opportune death of a Japanese woman, who had been coughing and spitting blood the night before she died, led to a postmortem on 27 December. Wu established that the disease was pneumonic plague, transmitted from person to person. A policy was formulated to suppress the epidemic. All railway, road, and river traffic was strictly controlled and monitored; medical personnel and others in contact with patients, alive or dead, were advised to wear masks to prevent inhalation of bacteria. The death of the French surgeon Mesny, head of the Peiyang Medical College in Tientsin, after only six days of contact with plague patients, spurred public awareness of the need for such precautionary measures.

As the death toll increased in Fuchiatien (a suburb of Harbin), the demand for coffins exceeded supply and orders for direct burial were issued. For more than six weeks, the corpses lay in a mile-long row on the frozen ground. Worse still were corpses in sitting positions, the sick shooed out of their homes to die, who had curled up for warmth. Wu decided on the mass cremation of more than 2,000 corpses in January 1911. Chinese traditions forbidding cremation meant Imperial sanction had to be sought. On 31 January

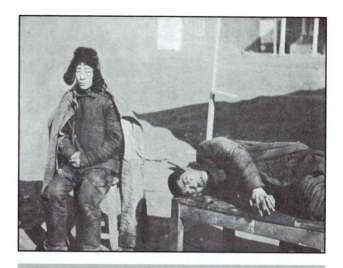

Chinese patients with early and advanced pneumonic plague. Halftone reproduction from *A Treatise on Pneumonic Plague*, Geneva, 1926. Wellcome Library, London.

1911, Imperial China witnessed, perhaps for the first time in five millennia, mass cremation of the dead in Fuchiatien.

The cremations coincided with the start of the Chinese Lunar New Year. People were encouraged to ignite firecrackers inside their homes. The loud bangs were believed to bring good luck and eliminate evil spirits. Sulfur from burning firecrackers also had a salutary effect on the germ-laden dwellings. This date marked the turning point of the anti-plague campaign, with a sustained decrease in deaths thereafter: the last case was recorded on 1 March 1911. By April, the pneumonic plague epidemic was successfully contained after seven months and more than 60,000 deaths.

Wu traced the genesis of the epidemic to the fur trade. The pelt of Mongolian marmots (tarabagans), wild rodents found in Mongolia, Manchuria, and eastern Siberia, could be dyed to imitate sable. Increasing demand encouraged some 10,000 hunters into Manchuria, some from as far away as Shandong (Shantung). Local hunters caught only healthy marmots in the open veldt. Foreign hunters, trying to accumulate as many pelts as possible before winter, turned to digging sick marmots out of their burrows, and also consumed their meat while in the field. Hailar and Manchouli on the Manchurian-Mongolian border and the Manchurian-Siberian divide, respectively, were the main trading centers. There, at local inns, the hunters and others slept huddled together on warm 'kangs', raised heated platforms in rooms with closed windows—ideal conditions for the spread of the pneumonic plague. As the number of cases increased, people panicked and fled along the Chinese Eastern Railway, carrying pneumonic plague with them from Manchouli to as far south as Tsinan, then capital of Shandong Province.

Wu became a popular hero, and detailed the anti-plague campaign in two publications: *Report of the International Plague Conference Held at Mukden, April 1911* (Manila,

1912) and *A Treatise on Pneumonic Plague* (Geneva, 1926). He worked for the Chinese government under the Kuomintang (Nationalist) Party until the mid-1930s, establishing the Harbin-based Manchurian Plague Prevention Service (1912), the Chinese Medical Association (1915), the Central Epidemic Bureau (1919) in Beijing, and the National Quarantine Service (1930), and ultimately worked as the Ministry of Health's chief technical expert (1930). He helped to establish seventeen hospitals, including the Peking (now Beijing) General Hospital, and succeeded somewhat in modernizing China's medical education and services. He also lent his expertise to the League of Nations.

When the Second Sino-Japanese War (1937–45) broke out, Wu decided to return to Malaya and leave his position as surgeon-general to the Republic of China's President, Chiang Kai-shek (1887–1975). He survived the Japanese occupation (1941–45) and for the next two decades ran a private practice at 12 Brewster Road, Ipoh. After the war, he was invited to enter politics as Malaya struggled for independence and also faced a Chinese-led communist insurgency. He declined and continued with his private practice, known as the doctor who dispensed free medical services to the deserving poor. At the age of eighty, he decided to retire and purchased a new house in Penang. Barely a week after moving in, he died.

Visions and Ideals

Wu decried the materialism of private practitioners in Malaya and Singapore. Patients dissatisfied with their treatment changed doctors, and practitioners proceeded with treatment without bothering to consult their predecessor. He felt the ideal of family physicians, with long-standing relationships to their patients, was lacking. He envisaged a less complicated and more economical national health service, like that of Britain. In such a system doctors would have regular and sufficient earnings, reasonable working hours, and sabbaticals for study and travel. He described his utopian model in 'Prospects of Social Medicine in Malaya,' published in the *Medical Journal of Malaya* (1948): 'Medicine will be available to all . . . given by doctors of various nationalities to suit the particular type of people, so that the latter may learn how to keep themselves and their families well, to take the proper kind of food, to submit to regular health examination by specialists in their profession, to have defects . . . repaired before these become serious' (Wu, 1959, p. 577). His profile of an ideal medical doctor was one '. . . keen to do [his] share of lecturing, treating patients, supervising laboratories, performing needed operations, none overworked or over-rich, proud of team work and anticipating the time when [he] may enjoy a holiday, and every five years undertake postgraduate studies in Europe or America with a view to becoming more efficient and useful to the community on [his] return' (Wu, 1959, p. 577).

Bibliography

Primary: 1959. *Plague Fighter: The Autobiography of a Modern Chinese Physician* (Cambridge).

Secondary: Ho, Tak Ming, 2004. 'The Plague Fighter' in Ong, Hean Teik, ed., *To Heal the Sick: The Story of Healthcare and Doctors in Penang, 1786 to 2004* (Penang) pp. 29–33; Ho, Tak Ming, 2000. *Doctors Extraordinaire* (Ipoh); Wu, Yu-Lin, 1995. *Memories of Wu Lien-Teh, Plague Fighter* (Singapore).

Ooi Keat Gin

WU, YOUXING 吳有性 (aka WU, YOUKE 吳有性)
(b. Dongting mountain 又可, Wu county, Jiangsu Province, China, 1582; d. Wu county, Jiangsu Province, China, 1652), *Chinese medicine, epidemiology.*

Wu Youxing is respected among Chinese medical historians as a proto-epidemiologist whose contagionist epidemiology prefigured the germ theory of Koch and others. A Chinese contemporary of Thomas Sydenham (1624–89), Wu similarly wrote on epidemics, fevers, and specific remedies for specific diseases. He also argued for the use of purgatives such as saltpeter and rhubarb, placing him among his contemporaries in the 'Attack and Purge' (*gongxia pai* 攻下派) style of practice attributed to the twelfth-century physician Zhang Congzheng 張從正 (1156–1228). He later became known as the founder of the 'Warm Factor Epidemics' (*wenyi pai* 瘟疫派) medical current and as an influential author in the 'Warm Factor Disorders' (*wenbing xuepai* 溫病學派) current of medicine.

Scant biographical evidence, however, exists about his life. He did not receive a *jinshi* 'elevated scholar' or any other official degree. He published only the *Treatise on Warm Factor Epidemics* (*Wenyi lun* 溫疫論, preface 1642, two volumes, with an appendix *buyi* 補遺, one volume). 'Warm factor' (*wen*) refers to both the perceived cause in Warm or Hot *qi* and the observed fevers of epidemics. The earliest biographical entry in a Wu county history (*Wumen bucheng*, 1803) simply states that he came from Dongting mountain village and wrote the *Treatise on Epidemics* in two volumes with an appendix. Besides the *Treatise on Epidemics*, from his lifetime there is only a stela that lists his name among benefactors commemorating the establishment in 1644 of the Temple of Pure Resolve (*Jing zhi an* 淨志庵). The stela remains in the ruins of the Temple of the Pond of Geese (*E tan miao* 淨志庵) in modern-day East Mountain, a village on the southeast side of Lake Tai about 100 kilometers southwest of Suzhou. An unofficial title as head patriarch (*zuzhang* 族長) follows his name and indicates that he represented the Wu lineage as a patron for the new temple.

From mid-August to mid-September of 1642, Wu Youxing wrote the preface to the *Treatise on Epidemics* in his *Dandan zhai* 淡淡齋 ('insipid studio'). *Dandan* literally means without flavor or tasteless. Wu may have chosen this studio name to suggest his book's central argument: the deadly epidemics of 1641 that swept through Shandong and Hebei in the north to the lower Yangzi provinces in the south had an imperceptible, invisible, yet knowable cause. In classical Chinese medicine, epidemics arose from anomalies in the yearly cycle of six climatic configurations of *qi*: Wind, Cold, Summer Heat, Damp, Dry, and Fire. Wu used the occasion of the 1641–42 epidemics to criticize this configurationist conception of epidemics in favor of a new contagionist perspective. Instead of aberrant configurations of seasonal *qi* (*shiqi* 時氣), he posited formless, invisible, and imperceptible heterogeneous *qi* (*zaqi* 雜氣) as the cause of epidemics. For Wu, heterogeneous *qi*, or deviant *qi* (*liqi* 戾氣), caused the sore throats, fevers, diarrhea, poxes, boils, and rashes of epidemics and ordinary illnesses attributed to seasonal *qi*. Instead of entering through the pores, as did seasonal *qi*, deviant *qi* entered through the mouth and nose. He criticized other physicians for killing their patients with erroneous therapies from the 'Cold Damage' (*shanghan pai* 傷寒派) and 'Warming and Restorative' (*wenbu pai* 溫補派) currents of practice. Wu's conception of pathogenic *qi* challenged the convention of a universal correspondence among cosmic seasonal cycles, the human body, and illness.

In an 1870s report of the medical officers to the Chinese Imperial Maritime Customs service, even the British Surgeon-General, C. A. Gordon, noted Wu's understanding that 'the "poison" of epidemic fevers is taken in at the mouth and nostrils, and is communicable'. Although this new conception of invisible pathogenic *qi* resembled later Western medical concepts of microorganisms and germs, it nevertheless remained embedded in a cosmology in which all phenomena were manifestations of *qi*. Within Chinese medical history, however, Wu's contagionist challenge to traditional configurationist epidemiology represented an indigenous trend of medical skepticism two centuries before Western science compelled Chinese physicians to reevaluate their medical traditions according to imported standards.

Bibliography

Primary: 1642. *Wenyi lun ping zhu* 瘟疫論評注 [*Critical Notes and Annotations on the 'Treatise on Heat Factor Epidemics'*] (comp. Zhejiang zhongyi yanjiusuo, Beijing, 1985); 1803. *Wumen bucheng* 吳門補 (by Qian Siyuan, 1803; ed. by Qian Shiqi, 1820); 1830. *Wumen bucheng* [1970 ed.]: 7/6b. 1884. Gordon, C. A., ed., *An Epitome of the Reports of the Medical Officers to the Chinese Imperial Maritime Customs Service, from 1871–1882* (London) p. 117.

Secondary: Jin Qinglei 金慶雷 and Jin Qingjiang 金慶江, 1993. 'Wu Youxing shengping deng wu kao' 吳有性生平等五考 [Five issues related to the life of Wu Youxing] *Jiangsu zhongyi* 1: 40–41; Yang Jin 楊進, 1988. '*Wenyi lun*' banben ji zhujia 瘟疫論版本及注家 [The Editions and Annotators of the 'Treatise on Heat Factor Epidemics'] *Zhongyihua yishi zazhi* 18(3): 139–141; Dunstan, Helen, 1975. 'The Late Ming Epidemics: A Preliminary Survey.' *Ch'ing-shih wen-t'i* 3(3): 1–59; Shi Changyong 史常永, 1957. 'Shilun chuanranbing xuejia Wu Youke ji qi liqi xueshuo.' 試論傳染病學家吳又可及其戾氣學說 [A Pre-liminary Essay of the Scholar of Contagious Diseases, Wu Youxing, and His Conception of Deviant *qi*] *Yixueshi yu baojian zazhi* 9.3: 180–186; Zhang Qigan 張其淦, ed., 1930. *Mingdai qianyi min shi yong chubian* 明代千遺民詩詠初編 (*Yuyuan congshu*): juan 1: 16a.

Marta E. Hanson

WUCHERER, OTTO EDWARD HENRY (b. Porto, Portugal, 7 July 1820; d. Salvador, Brazil, 7 May 1873), *tropical medicine, public health, helminthology.*

Wucherer was born in Portugal, the son of a German trader and a Dutch mother. Between 1828 and 1830 he lived with his family in the city of Salvador, an important commercial center, the port and capital of Bahia, a province in the northeastern part of what was then the Empire of Brazil (1822–1889). There were many slaves and Afro-descendants. He did his secondary studies in Hamburg (1831–35) and studied medicine at the University of Tübingen (1836–41) with Wilhelm Griesinger, who had a great and permanent influence on Wucherer's career. Wucherer's medical background was influenced by parasitology, by the laboratory medicine then emergent in Germany, and by the social medicine ideas of Rudolf Virchow. He started his professional life working as medical assistant at St Bartholomew's Hospital in London. He then practiced medicine in Lisbon, where his family lived, and went to Brazil in 1843. He worked in small towns in Bahia's inland regions, such as Nazaré and Cachoeira, the latter having a significant concentration of German citizens and an area of cigar manufacturing.

Wucherer settled in Salvador city in 1847, where he attended the German community as a physician and started an important trajectory in medicine and in research. He became the most outstanding and recognized representative of a group of Brazilian and foreign physicians who had settled in Bahia, and which from the 1860s onward, with no formal links to the Schools of Medicine of Bahia and Rio de Janeiro or with the medical establishment of the Empire, was dedicated to studies on the hygiene, anatomo-clinical manifestations, etiology, and parasitology of the tropical diseases that affected the Brazilian population. Wucherer was the most distinguished among the group of physicians who contributed to reformulating the model that had been accepted until then regarding the nosology and etiology of Brazilian diseases, to questioning the rudimentary background of local physicians, and to addressing the lack of European knowledge about public health problems in Brazil. An important characteristic of Wucherer's and his associates' trajectory was that their medical practices attended to the less privileged sectors of the population of Salvador, and not simply to the elites and immigrants' communities.

They developed original works that obtained an international audience, especially their discoveries related to ancylostomiasis, filariasis, and ainhum (a disease that affects black people and is characterized by the strangling of the smaller toe), thus contributing to the debate on the etiology and parasitology of diseases such as beriberi, tuberculosis, leprosy, yellow fever, dracunculiasis, and cholera. The extent and variety of their researches on natural history and medical zoology is exemplified by the publication in 1863 of Wucherer's important essay on local fauna, examining and describing new species of snakes and establishing morphological rules for the identification of poisonous varieties.

From 1865 on Wucherer and his associates began to meet regularly at some of the physicians' residences to discuss the new developments in medicine, and they turned the philanthropic hospital of Santa Casa da Misericórdia into the main locus of clinical, anatomical, pathological, and microscopic investigations. One of the main results of these meetings and the ensuing interchange of ideas was the creation in 1866 of the *Gazeta Médica da Bahia*, one of the most important medical journals of the nineteenth century, in which were published the main works written by members of the group.

Among the fourteen physicians who initially attended the meetings, two stand out for their works and their association with Wucherer. The first is the Scotsman Ligertwood Patterson (1820–82), who graduated in 1841 from the University of Aberdeen, worked with Lister in Edinburgh (1869), and introduced Lister's method into the medical practice in Bahia. He became the physician of the British community in Salvador, and the first meetings of the group took place at his residence. The second is the Portuguese physician José Francisco da Silva Lima (1826–1910), who arrived in Brazil in 1840, received his MD in 1851 from the School of Medicine of Bahia, and produced outstanding research on beriberi and ainhum. The publications and ideas of this group, the Escola Tropicalista Baiana, became more widely known.

Yellow Fever, Cholera, and Medical Theories

Wucherer and his colleagues took an active part in debates about the etiology of diseases, and many times they confronted local and national physicians and authorities. The outburst of yellow fever in Salvador at the end of 1849 generated a confrontation that pitted Patterson, Wucherer, and Silva Lima against the majority of members of the School of Medicine of Bahia and the Council of Public Health. Patterson and Wucherer had observed cases in ships that arrived in Salvador and had clinically diagnosed the first cases in November, indicating that the disease was contagious, although its mode of spread was unknown, and that it was therefore necessary to adopt unpopular quarantine measures. The local medical-sanitarian establishment continued to insist that the disease was of local origin, was not contagious, and would have no serious impact, essentially denying the existence of yellow fever. The debate reached the press, with the accusation made that the foreign physicians were disseminating panic among the population. By the end of 1849, Wucherer was able to make autopsies and anatomic-pathological examinations that convinced him of

scientific evidence for yellow fever. In 1850, together with Patterson, he published in a Salvador newspaper a vehement protest against the authorities' denial that the epidemic was yellow fever and their lack of action about it.

In 1855 a cholera epidemics struck Salvador city. Once again, Wucherer and Patterson were involved both in treating the victims and in the debate about the causes of the disease. Wucherer and his associates assumed the contagionist position, stating that it was the Asian cholera, whereas the health authorities and the majority of the professors at the School of Medicine stated that it was a disease of local and environmental causes. The debate was held in the press, in the School of Medicine, and in the Provincial Governmental Palace. Wucherer and his colleagues were invited, which demonstrates the increasing recognition by the political authorities of their importance.

They criticized the current medical theories, based on the French model, which defended a notion of climatic miasma derived from the combination of precarious living conditions and the tropical humid heat. The so-called 'tropicalists' believed that even if factors concerning environment and hygienic habits were important for the outbreak of a disease, they were not sufficient. More specific factors were needed in order to explain how particular social factors in Brazil, as well as its specific climatic factors, acted to produce diseases.

On the one hand these episodes intensified the animosity between the foreign physicians and the local medical community, whose prestige had been diminished. On the other hand Wucherer and Patterson gained the recognition, sympathy, and confidence of the communities and even of the public authorities, due to their direct involvement in treating the sick and to their courageous participation in the debate about public health. During the 1849 epidemics, Wucherer transformed his residence into an infirmary with over twenty beds, where his own wife died. The epidemics that later struck Bahia and its capital happened in a different medical and scientific context, also transformed by Wucherer and his associates' work and agitation.

Ancylostomiasis, Filariasis, and Helminthology

In several works published in *Gazeta Médica da Bahia* from 1866, Wucherer wrote 'about the disease vulgarly denominated tiredness' and defended, for the first time in Brazil, the parasitic causes of 'intertropical hypoemia', a disease whose climatologic etiology had been thoroughly studied by José Martins de Cruz Jobim, an important doctor and a member of the prestigious Imperial Academy of Medicine in Rio de Janeiro. Drawing on Cruz Jobim's work, Wucherer diagnosed in 1865 an advanced case of hypoemia in a slave who died soon after. In the autopsy, he found, for the first time in Brazil, worms of the species *Anchylostomum duodenale*, which had been identified by Angelo Dubini in 1838. Wucherer's work has the merit of being the first to confirm

Griesinger's findings, which had presented the same ento-zoan as the cause of another anemia, the Egyptian chlorosis.

Wucherer's hypothesis about the role of the *Ancylostomo duodenale* in the production of the 'hypoemia' generated polemics and was rejected by professors of the Schools of Medicine of Bahia and Rio de Janeiro. Some of the members of the Imperial Academy of Medicine questioned the new etiological hypothesis of hypoemia proposed by Wucherer, despite the immediate support that he received from Cruz Jobim, who was then Director of the School of Medicine of Rio de Janeiro.

Another important contribution made by Wucherer was in the study of intertropical hematuria—a disease character-ized by the emission of blood in the urine, which was then called 'lactosis'. In 1866 Wucherer was asked by Griesinger to investigate hematuric patients with the aim of confirming in Brazil the discovery made by Bilharz in 1851 in Egypt. On that occasion, Griesinger himself developed the research on *Distomum hematobium*, renamed *Bilharzia hematobia* by T. Spencer Cobbold. Wucherer's inquiry found nothing in the blood, but he discovered in the urine embryos of an unknown nematode, though none of the eggs described by Bilharz. Having no technical facilities to identify the new worm, he filtered the urine and sent it to Leuckhart. Wucherer isolated in the urine of sick people the larval form of the species later denominated *Wuchereria bancrofti* in honor of him and of the Australian physician Joseph Ban-croft, who discovered the adult filaria. Wucherer's work 'About the Hematuria in Brazil', published in 1869, was his last one in helminthology before his death in 1873.

The investigations made by Wucherer and his followers related to ancylostomiasis and to filariasis were already part of the local traditions expressed by the Schools of Medicine of Bahia and Rio de Janeiro and the Imperial Academy of Medicine. They also reveal the existence of an information network connecting physicians with a growing interest in the role of parasites as disease producers, who were isolated from each other and spread over several continents. In this way, Brazilian physicians and those who had settled in Brazil were able to interact, exchange materials, gain visibility, and engage in dialogue with Griesinger, Leuckhart, Cobbold, Brancfort, and Billarz, among others. The causality of these diseases became the focus of an intense debate and interna-tional interchange between 1866 and 1892. By the end of this period, the field of helminthic parasitology had estab-lished firm methodological and conceptual criteria, and the role of *Ancylostomo duodenalis* and of *Wuchereia bancrofti* in the production of those diseases was fully accepted. In this sense, Otto Wucherer is considered the founder of Brazilian helminthology.

In 1871 Otto Wucherer returned to Germany with his wife and their young son and lived there for one year. Finan-cial difficulties made him return to Salvador and resume clinical medicine to support the family. He died shortly after in May 1873. Wucherer's early death did not stop his col-

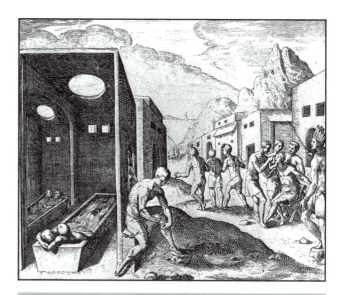

Man extracting a filaria worm from his leg, South America. Etching 1899, Wellcome Library, London.

leagues and followers from carrying on the researches on the biology of parasites, even though they became quite distant from the anatomo-pathological studies associated with the diseases of poverty. By then under the growing influence of germ theory and the development of tropical medicine, they continued to publish the *Gazeta* and to incorporate new members, including professors from the School of Medicine of Bahia such as Raimundo Nina Rodrigues, who is consid-ered to be the founder of legal medicine in Brazil. Wucherer's trajectory and that of the Escola Tropicalista da Bahia is considered as fundamental to the renovation of Bra-zilian medicine in the nineteenth century and to the birth of experimental medicine and as an example of the local knowledge output, in dialogue and accordance with interna-tional scientific development.

Bibliography

Primary: Gazeta Médica da Bahia (1866–1934).

Secondary: Peard, Julyan, 1999. *Race, Place and Medicine, The Idea of the Tropics in Nineteenth-Century Brazilian Medicine* (Durham); Edler, Flávio Coelho, 1999. *A constituição da Medicina Tropical no Brasil Oitocentista: da climatologia à parasitologia médica* (Rio de Janeiro); Coni, Antonio Caldas, 1952. *A Escola Tropicalista Baiana* (Salvador).

Gilberto Hochman and
Flávio Coelho Edler

WUNDERLICH, CARL REINHOLD AUGUST (b. Sulz am Neckar, Germany, 2 August 1815; d. Leipzig, Saxony, Ger-many, 25 September 1877), *medicine.*

Wunderlich was the son of a public health official in Lud-wigsburg whose death in 1824 led the family to move to Stuttgart. There Wunderlich attended school with Wilhelm

Griesinger and Wilhelm Roser, who formed a trio that would go on to study medicine together at Tübingen from 1833 to 1837. He passed his exams in 1838 and occupied an internship at the Katherine Hospital in Stuttgart. Wunderlich received his Habilitation in 1842 and continued his rapid academic promotion in Tübingen, becoming extraordinary professor in 1843 and then in 1846 ordinary professor and director of the Medical Clinic.

Study trips to Paris and Vienna had made it clear to Wunderlich, relatively early on, how Tübingen's medicine was drastically behind the times. Thus, in the reports of these trips that he published in 1841, Wunderlich forcefully argued for the use of physical diagnostic techniques and statistically oriented studies of therapy. He continued this campaign in the editorials of the *Archiv für physiologische Heilkunde* that he founded in 1842 along with his two school friends. This was one of many, albeit ephemeral, journals from the 1840s that argued in favor of a scientific transformation in medicine. However, the program that unified the young generation of physicians broke down in the early 1850s, as the demand for a scientifically based medicine evolved into the formation of new independent disciplines (pathological anatomy, physiological physics, and chemistry). Indeed, Wunderlich found himself in a bitter dispute with Rudolf Virchow over the latter's claim that cellular pathology could serve as the unifying theory for scientific medicine.

In 1850 Wunderlich was appointed professor for specific pathology and therapy and also director of the department of internal medicine at Jakob's Hospital in Leipzig. This busy city hospital was one of the largest in Germany and therefore provided Wunderlich with ideal conditions for continuing his clinical research. Starting in the mid-1850s, Wunderlich introduced the method of measuring patients' temperatures using instruments. Soon he was able to establish its place in the clinical routine. He wanted to fix the 'normal range' of the body temperature, and took thousands of measurements and accumulated millions of items of data. Beyond this, however, he saw this technique as also providing an approach that was comparable to the use of the kymograph in physiology: successive temperature measurements would objectively describe the fever process, thereby allowing the determination of the 'laws of the diseases' and providing the scientific basis for more certain medical practice. Wunderlich had once objected, in his doctoral thesis, to Lucas Schönlein's distinction between abdominal and endemic typhus, but now he arrived at the same result, relying on characteristic fever curves to distinguish between infectious diseases such as cholera, intermittent fever, typhus, etc. In 1868 Wunderlich published his epoch-making *Das Verhalten der Eigenwärme in Krankheiten*, which was translated into many different languages and provided the basis for the modern clinical definition of fever.

Wunderlich's typology of fever curves was rapidly eclipsed by the rise of bacteriology, and the introduction of antibiotics deprived this approach of much of its sense. Nevertheless, his practice of graphically representing the disease process is retained in the customary clinical recording of the patient's temperature curve. The importance of such data, and in particular the relationship between the therapy and the patient's temperature (and pulse, and later blood pressure) has since become deeply entrenched in medical thinking. Even in our modern age of electronic documentation systems, where the temperature curve itself is of no great medical significance, the practice of documentation remains at the base of the communication and organizational structures of today's hospitals.

Bibliography

Primary: 1841. *Wien und Paris. Ein Beitrag zur Geschichte und Beurteilung der gegenwärtigen Heilkunde* (Stuttgart); 1868. *Das Verhalten der Eigenwärme in Krankheiten* (Leipzig) (English edn. 1871).

Secondary: Hess, Volker, 1997. 'Objektivität und Rhetorik. Karl August Wunderlich (1815–1877) und die klinische Thermometrie.' *Medizinhistorisches Journal* 32: 299–319; Schürmann, W. H. T., 1988. *Carl Reinhold Wunderlich und die 'Physiologische Heilkunde'.* MD Thesis, Hannover.

Volker Hess

WUNDT, WILHELM MAXIMILIAN (b. Neckarau, Germany, 16 August 1832; d. Großbothen near Leipzig, Germany, 31 August 1920), *physiology, psychology.*

A physiologist, founder of experimental psychology, and philosopher, Wundt studied natural science, philosophy, and medicine at Tübingen and Heidelberg. In 1855 he graduated MD, and in 1857 he qualified as university lecturer at Heidelberg, where he worked at the physiological institute under Hermann von Helmholtz from 1858 onward. In 1864 he was appointed associate professor at Heidelberg, and in 1871 he was appointed associate professor with a salary. In the winter of 1874 he followed a call to the chair of philosophy at Zurich University, and in 1875 he left for Leipzig University, where he founded the institute for experimental psychology and taught psychology until 1917.

In physiology Wundt was inspired by Hermann von Helmholtz. A productive collaboration developed between the two researchers, leaving Wundt enough time to pursue his own ambitions in sensory-physiological and psychological research despite the demands of teaching. However, in the mid-1860s the teaching duties in physics and physiology at Heidelberg were rather restricting, and Wundt handed in his notice in 1864. Whether conflicts between him and Helmholtz preceded this incident cannot be said. His parliamentary activities in the Zweite Badische Kammer [House of Parliament of Baden] (1866–70) and his commitment to the Heidelberger Arbeiterbildungsverein [Organization for the Education of Workers] would have certainly also reduced his engagement with physiology. In addition, Wundt had begun to turn away from physical physiology and toward physiological and experimental psychology. This new scientific disci-pline emerged toward the end of the nineteenth century. Wundt was one of its early pioneers, who during the course of his scientific career built up and defended experimental psy-chology as a science of experience, establishing the essential basics of 'physiological psychology' as it is quite naturally and successfully practiced nowadays. The name was also the title of his textbook, in two volumes, of 1887.

Starting from a physiological viewpoint, the psychologist can do without philosophical speculation and metaphysical psychology, and turn instead to the experimental methods of natural science. The objects of such psychological investigation are 'contents', which are offered by the consciousness or the imagination in 'inner perception' (sensations, imaginations, acts of will). Fundamental emotional phenomena are acts of will, and drives are the consequences influenced by emotion. Wundt went back to psychophysics, which was a discipline, developed primarily by Gustav Fechner (1801–87), that dealt with the relations between the measurable conditions of the physical environment and its subjective (emotional) experi-ence, and especially with the sensation of colors and brightness. From the observation that, when one is in the dark, differences in brightness can be perceived that are smaller than those dis-tinguishable when one is in the light, it was concluded that a distinct sensory increase (an increase in brightness) has a con-stant relation to the underlying stimulus (the level of light). Fechner further imagined this relation to be continuous and even applicable to the tiniest (infinitesimal) changes, leading to the derivation of the famous Fechner's Law. That law permitted the psychologist to relate differences in the subjective sensation of light, that is, differences in perceived colors, to the light intensity. Fechner's Law is thus not a law in the strict sense of the word, but rather an approach to the experimental evidence. Wundt was fascinated by Fechner's Law and tried to extend it. Instead of seeking a relation between stimulus and reaction, he focused on the relation between stimulus and sensation, an idea that he could never satisfactorily express.

As experimental psychology could record only individual actions, it had to be completed by a descriptive folk psychology, to which Wundt devoted his later years at Leipzig. This disci-pline was geared more or less to 'examine such emotional phe-nomena underlying the general development of human communities and the development of common cultural prod-ucts of general values' (language, religion, myth, customs, and art). Wundt had a strong influence on the historian Karl Lam-precht from Leipzig (1856–1915), whose circle of cultural sci-ence he joined. Whereas Lamprecht tried to examine causalities of social psychology by following psychology, for Wundt psy-chology was the leading discipline of the humanities per se.

Bibliography

Primary: 1858. *Lehre von der Muskelbewegung* (Braunschweig); 1862. *Beiträge zur Theorie der Sinneswahrnehmungen* (Leipzig and Heidelberg); 1863. *Vorlesungen über die Menschen- und Thierseele* 2 vols. (Leipzig) (English edn. 1894); 1865. *Lehrbuch der Physiologie des Menschen* (Erlangen); 1867. *Handbuch der medizinischen Physik* (Erlangen); 1871–76. *Untersuchung zur Mechanik der Nerven und Nervencentren* 2 vols. (Erlangen); 1873–74. *Grundzüge der physiologischen Psychologie* (Leipzig) (English edn. 1904); 1880–83. *Logik* 2 vols. (Stuttgart); 1886. *Ethik* (Stut-tgart) (English edn. 1897); 1889. *System der Philosophie* (Leipzig); 1896. *Grundriß der Psychologie* (Leipzig) (English edn. 1897); 1900. *Völkerpsychologie* (Leipzig); 1912. *Elemente der Völkerpsy-chologie* (Leipzig) (English edn. 1916); 1920. *Erlebtes und Erkanntes* (Stuttgart) [Autobiographical].

Secondary: Wonterra, Maximilian, 2004. *Wilhelm Wundt (1832–1920) und die Anfänge der experimentellen Psychologie* (Leipzig); Lamberti, Georg, 1995. *Wilhelm Maximilian Wundt (1832–1920): Leben, Werk und Persönlichkeit in Bildern und Texten* (Bonn); Chickering, Roger, 1993. *Karl Lamprecht: A German Academic Life (1856–1915)* (Atlantic Highlands, NJ); Oelze, B., 1991. *Wilhelm Wundt: Die Konzeption der Völkerpsychologie* (Münster); Robinson, D. K., 1987. 'Wilhelm Wundt and the Establishment of Experimen-tal Psychology, 1875–1914.' PhD thesis, University of California, (Berkeley); Hiebsch, H., 1977. *Wilhelm Wundt und die Anfänge der experimentellen Psychologie* (Berlin); Boring, E. G., 1950. *A History of Experimental Psychology* (New York) pp. 316–347; Petersen, P., 1925. *Wilhelm Wundt und seine Zeit* (Stuttgart); *DSB*.

Wolfgang U. Eckart

WYNDER, ERNST LUDWIG

WYNDER, ERNST LUDWIG   (b. Herford, Germany, 30 April 1922; d. New York, New York, USA, 14 July 1999), *epidemiology, public health.*

Wynder and his sister Lore, the son and daughter of a phy-sician, Alfred Wynder, and Therese Godfrey Wynder, were born in Herford, Germany. To escape Nazi persecution, the family emigrated to the United States (1938). Ernst became an American citizen (1943) and served in the U.S. Army Intelli-gence Corps from 1943 until 1945. He had obtained a BA from New York University before entering the Army. Subse-quently he obtained a BMed and MD from Washington Uni-versity School of Medicine, graduating in 1950. During and subsequent to his one-year internship at Georgetown Univer-sity Hospital in Washington, D.C., he embarked upon a career of research and advocacy. After internship, his professional affiliations were limited to the Memorial Hospital for Cancer and Allied Diseases, the Sloan-Kettering Institute for Cancer Research in New York City, and the American Health Founda-tion, an independent research center that he founded (1969), located in Valhalla, NY, a few miles north of New York City. The Foundation was dedicated primarily to epidemiological and laboratory research on the etiology and mechanisms of tobacco- and nutrition-related cancers. The Foundation also served as the source and base for Wynder's advocacy of a range of disease prevention policies.

While still a medical student and intern, Wynder carried out a case control study of the association of tobacco smok-ing and lung cancer, the publication of which has long been considered a landmark in the epidemiology of the disease

(Wynder and Graham, 1950). This publication, Wynder's very first, presaged the subsequent course of his career (Doll, 1999). However, in all fairness, it should be noted that a simultaneous publication in the *Journal of the American Medical Association* also reported the association (Levin, Goldstein, and Gerhardt, 1950). These two studies initiated the subsequent plethora of investigations worldwide that culminated in the monumental *Report of the Advisory Committee to the Surgeon General on Smoking and Health* (1964). Wynder's seminal publication and his subsequent continuing research on the relation of tobacco and various cancers made important contributions to that immensely important public health document. Furthermore, he engaged actively in the ensuing debate over the validity of the causal association of tobacco smoking and lung cancer described in the Advisory Committee's *Report* (Wynder, 1961).

At the American Health Foundation, Wynder assembled and led a distinguished group of scientists. Among their most important investigations were the discovery of carcinogenic nitrosamines specific to tobacco and the identification, along with outside collaborators, of benzo(a)pyrine and other carcinogenic polynuclear aromatic hydrocarbons in tobacco tar. Wynder himself expanded his epidemiologic interests to include investigations of nutrition and disease. In continuing case control studies, he repeatedly demonstrated the association between low consumption of saturated fat and low incidence of coronary heart disease, and he advocated dietary modification to achieve the goal of low fat consumption.

After Wynder's death, the Foundation's name was changed to the Institute for Cancer Prevention. Without his strong and inspired leadership, the Institute foundered, and in late 2004 ceased functioning and declared bankruptcy.

Ernst Wynder was an active advocate for public health. He founded and edited the journal *Preventive Medicine*. Under the aegis of the American Health Foundation, he set up the Food and Nutrition Council to educate children in healthy eating habits. He received many awards and recognitions for his multiple contributions. He is also remembered as a kind and generous person.

Bibliography

Primary: 1950. (with Graham, E. A.) 'Tobacco Smoking as a Possible Etiologic Factor in Bronchiogenic Carcinoma. A Study of Six Hundred and Eighty-four Proved Cases.' *Journal of the American Medical Association* 143: 329–336; 1961. 'The Great Debate.'(editorial) *New England Journal of Medicine* 264: 1266.

Secondary: Doll, R., 1999. 'In memoriam: Ernst Wynder (1923–1999).' *American Journal of Public Health* 89: 1798–1799; Levin, M. L., H. Goldstein, and P. R. Gehrhardt, 1950. 'Cancer and Tobacco Smoking; Preliminary Report.' *Journal of the American Medical Association* 143: 336–338.

Warren Winkelstein, Jr.

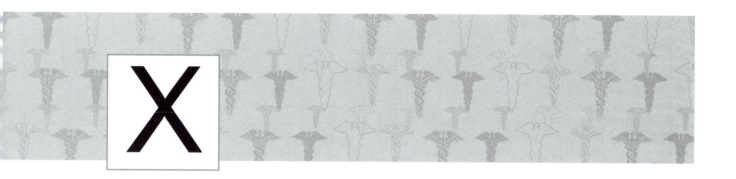

X

XU, SHUWEI 許叔微 **(aka XU, ZHIFU** 許知付**)** (b. Baisha, Zhen prefecture, Jiangsu Province, China, 1079; d. Baisha, China, 1154), *Chinese medicine.*

Xu Shuwei was a Song dynasty (960–1276) physician who came from a poor family. When he was eleven, his father died from a 'seasonal epidemic', followed a few months later by his mother. The inability of physicians to help his ailing parents motivated him to study medicine. His medical career was also facilitated by his repeated failure to pass the civil service examinations until 1132, at the age of fifty-three. Subsequently, he was appointed to a number of teaching positions and acquired the nickname 'Xu the Scholar' 許學士. A prolific writer and compiler, four of his texts have survived to the present.

Xu's perspective on medicine and doctors can be summed up in his own words: 'The physician's Way [Dao] is great. He can nourish life, preserve the body, extend years of life. In sum, he can benefit the world' (preface to *Leizheng puji ben shi fang*). His contributions are multifaceted. He was the first Chinese physician to author a medical text that focuses solely on patients' case histories. He furthered the teaching and dissemination of the cold damage doctrines that had originated in the Han period by compiling a book presenting this knowledge in plain rhyming language. In another book he advanced the integration of cold damage doctrines with the doctrines of classical medicine—Yin, Yang, and the Five Agents. Finally, he compiled a formulary that included innovative formulas drawn from his clinical experience.

Xu's most innovative and intriguing book was *Ninety Discussions on Cold Damage*. In it he assembled ninety case histories based on his patients who had contracted cold damage disorders. Each one included symptoms, diagnosis, differentiating patterns of pathology, and therapy (i.e., medicinal formulas). This is the first compilation in Chinese medicine concentrating on case histories. In subsequent medical literature from the Ming dynasty (1368–1644), this genre became important and common. The organization of the case histories is also significant: all followed a standard pattern. First, Xu provided the important symptoms, next he gave the pulse, and finally, he differentiated the pattern of manifestation, e.g., excessive sweating of the *jueyin* 厥陰 [attenuated Yin tract].

Xu's main interest in medical theory was febrile diseases, or in Chinese terms, cold damage disorders. He greatly revered Zhang Zhongjing's *Treatise on Cold Damage* claiming that 'discussing cold damage disorders without reading Zhongjing's book [the *Treatise*], is like discussing Confucianism without first understanding the six Confucian classics' (preface to *Shanghan bai zheng ge*). Xu claimed that one of the reasons prevailing medical practice harmed rather than helped patients was that physicians either did not have access to the *Treatise* or they did not understand it. In the preface to his *Hundred Mnemonic Verses on Cold*

Damage Manifestations, Xu wrote, 'Hence I took the contents of the *Treatise* and compiled from it one hundred mnemonic poems, each delineating a manifestation type. I did this to make it easier for physicians to study and memorize it [the *Treatise*]' (preface to *Shanghan bai zheng ge*). By creating an easily memorized primer, Xu made an important contribution to the dissemination and popularization of the *Treatise*'s doctrines.

In *Subtleties of Cold Damage Revealed*, Xu discussed seventy-two cold damage manifestation types, detailing the pathogenesis and treatment. He emphasized pulse diagnosis and prescriptions; many of the treatments he offered reflected his clinical experience. Xu claimed that the classical differentiation of pathology according to the Eight Rubrics was the basic category in determining the patterns of disease.

Late in life Xu compiled a formulary, *Original formulary of classified manifestation types for popular relief*, summing up his accumulated clinical knowledge. The formulas in this book were innovative, replacing ancient but commonly used remedies, and they had a significant impact on clinical practice in following generations.

Bibliography

Primary: 1132. *Shanghan bai zheng ge* 傷寒百證歌 [Hundred Mnemonics Verses on Cold Damage Manifestations]; 1132. *Shanghan fa wei lun* 傷寒發微論 [Subtleties of Cold Damage Revealed]; 1132. *Shanghan jiushi lun* 傷寒九十論 [Ninety Discussions on Cold Damage]; 1142. *Leizheng puji ben shi fang* 類證普濟本事方 [Original formulary of classified manifestation types for popular relief].

Secondary: Goldschmidt, Asaf, 1999. 'The Transformations of Chinese Medicine during the Northern Song Dynasty (A.D. 960–1127).' PhD dissertation, University of Pennsylvania (Philadelphia) pp. 105–110.

Asaf Goldschmidt

XUMA, ALFRED BITINI (b. Manzona, Transkei, South Africa, 8 March 1893; d. Soweto, South Africa, 27 January 1962), *general practice.*

The son of well-off Xhosa peasants who had converted to Christianity, Xuma grew up in an environment in which religion and western education were seen as keys to advancement. His success at a missionary primary school in the Transkei spurred him to look abroad for the further education not then available locally to black South Africans. Attracted by the reputation of African American institutions to help their students uplift themselves, he traveled to the United States in 1913 and then paid his own way through high school at the Tuskegee Institute in Alabama by taking on after-hours jobs. This hand-to-mouth existence also characterized the next phases of his education, a BS in agriculture at the University of Minnesota (1917–20), followed by an MD, partly at Marquette University in Milwaukee (1921–23) and partly at Northwestern University in Chicago (1923–26). This he capped with six months' specialized study in obstetrics and gynecology and surgery in Hungary and a brief stint in Scotland to secure the LRCP & S (Edin) and the LRFPS (Glasgow), as his American MD was not recognized in South Africa. To these clinical qualifications he was to add a Diploma in Public Health from the London School of Hygiene and Tropical Medicine in 1938.

Returning to South Africa in 1927 after his fourteen-year odyssey abroad, Xuma brought with him a lifelong commitment to the ideals of self-help and respectability along with a warm appreciation of the fellowship and financial support which Christian benefactors and their organizations had given him.

The general practice which he started in Johannesburg in 1928 was the first such practice run by a local black doctor trained in biomedicine. His patients were primarily poor Africans to whom he offered the benefits of modern medicine in a somewhat didactic manner, but in a language they understood. With a mixture of awe and admiration, they dubbed his house in the African township of Sophiatown 'Empilweni' [place of healing].

What he saw in his daily practice and as part-time medical officer of health in the township of Alexandra strengthened his resolve to speak out in public in favor of full medical training locally for Africans and for better compensation for miners retrenched with silicosis, and against the notion that an attenuated training program would suffice for Africans going to nurse in rural areas. To these positions it was not long before he added a deeper critique of the racially based inequities within South African society and of the need to address related issues such as education, housing, taxation, and wages. His insights led to political involvement, almost inevitable for a man committed to serving 'my Africans' (Gish, 2000, p. 89).

Initially, true to his positive experience of multiracial cooperation in the United States, he associated himself with multiracial, reform-minded organizations in South Africa, but as racial segregation hardened in the mid-1930s, he threw himself into two exclusively black political organizations, the All-Africa Convention and the African National Congress (ANC), of which he became president in 1940.

In this unpaid position Xuma effectively rebuilt the moribund ANC, making it the foremost African political movement in South Africa and thus himself the leading African politician in the country. He formulated 'African Claims in South Africa', a summary of Africans' basic political, social, and economic demands, addressed the United Nations in 1946 to oppose South Africa's wish to annex Namibia, and in 1947 concluded the Doctor's Pact with two fellow doctors-*cum*-politicians (Yusuf Dadoo and Monty Naicker) to facilitate cooperation between the ANC and the leading Indian political movements against the South African government's racially based policies.

Only by burning the candle at both ends was Xuma still able to maintain his practice and his communal medical appointments, which beginning in 1940 also included the headship of a U.S. church–sponsored community clinic south of Johannesburg. The strain on his own health was intense, and by 1945 he was overworked to the point of a nervous breakdown.

By then, however, his unproductive petitioning approach to securing reforms from the government was frustrating many of his younger militant followers in the ANC (such as Nelson Mandela and Walter Sisulu), and in 1949 he was voted out of office. The movement was now headed by another doctor, James Moroka, who opted for more confrontational tactics, and Xuma became marginalized politically. After this he occasionally re-emerged in public—as in the opposition to the forced removal of Africans from Johannesburg's western townships in the mid-

1950s—but essentially he became a respected political has-been. His medical practice returned to the center stage of his life and remained there, even after an apartheid-driven eviction forced him to move to Soweto in 1959, where he had a new Empilweni built.

Xuma married twice, both times to women with strong African American connections. His first wife, Amanda Priscilla Mason (1896–1934) was a Liberian teacher who had been educated in the United States; with her he had two children. His second wife, Madi Hall (1894–1982), was born and bred in the United States.

Bibliography

Secondary: Gish, Steven D., 2000. *Alfred B. Xuma—African, American, South African* (Houndmills and London).

Howard Phillips

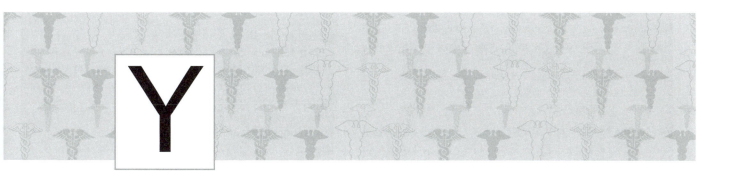

Y

YAJNAVARAHA (fl. Cambodia, tenth century), *traditional Cambodian medicine.*

Yajnavaraha was an influential priest doctor who practiced in tenth-century Angkor, Cambodia. The historical study of ancient Cambodia, both in the pre-Angkor (sixth to ninth centuries) and Angkor (900–1400) periods, has shown that most Brahmin priests at the royal court were extremely influential, combining multiple roles and functions that included King's teacher, performer of sacrifices, doctor, astronomer, astrologer, and political adviser. Most of these priest-doctors were of royal descent, and their title was hereditary.

From his mother's side Yajnavaraha was a Brahmin of royal descent, grandson of King Hashavarman (r. 941–44), who was son of King Yasovarman (r. 889–910) and grandson of King Indravarman (r. 877–89) (Coedes, 1937). In addition to this impressive pedigree, Yajnavaraha learned his arts and his duties from his father Damodara, famous for his command of the *Veda* and *Rg Veda*. Yajnavaraha became the guru of King Jayavarman V (r. 968–1001). His religious and secular contributions to the royal court and assistance to the poor earned him the highest esteem from Jayavarman V, who rewarded him with a parasol of peacock feathers, a gold litter, and other presents. The inscriptions tell us that he was not only well versed in Hindu philosophy such as Yoga (Patanjali), Vaisesika (Kanada), Samkhya (Kapila), and Aksapada, but also in Buddhist doctrines

(Coedes, 1937). He excelled in medicine, music, and astronomy. He had a good command of sacred languages and wrote many dramas for the court artists. He officiated Shivaite rituals at the royal temples. With his young brother Vishnukumara, Yajnavaraha commissioned the erection of a Shivaite temple called Isvarapura (Banteay Srei), located fifteen miles north of Angkor Wat (Coedes, 1937).

He practiced ayurvedic medicine at the royal court and attended the King, members of the royal family, and the families of high-ranking ministers in the traditions of ancient Khmer medicine, which was integrated with knowledge from ayurvedic medicine (Chhem, 2004). Despite his high status, his power, and his duties to the royal family, Yajnavaraha took time to attend 'the poor, the disinherited, the blind, the weak, children, the elders, the sick or other unfortunate people crossing the ocean of suffering [who] flocked in his house everyday' and who sought his medical skills (Coedes 1937). He taught Sanskrit, religious doctrines, and the arts and sciences to his brother Vishnukumara. This pattern of teaching reflects the typical elite Brahmin education, where the teaching is reserved to a few: mainly the King himself, members of the royal house, or members of his own family.

Yajnavaraha was not the only religious scholar at the court of Jayavarman V, but he was certainly the most brilliant and influential. Because of the presence of Yajnavaraha and many other scholars, the reign of this King was one of the most flourishing periods of the intellectual and spiritual life of the Angkor period.

Among the other doctors and scholars was Rajendravaidya, who was known for his mastery of both ayurveda and Dhanurveda (archery) (Sarka, 1968, 39–41). Divakarabhatta, brother-in-law of Jayavarman V, was an expert of Somaveda. Kirtipandita and a Buddhist scholar taught Buddhist doctrines using sacred texts brought from abroad, especially the *Tattvasangrata*, a famous Tibetan manuscript from the eighth century.

Bibliography

Primary: Coedes, George, 1937, 1953, 1954. *Incriptions du Cambodge*, vol. I (Hanoi), vols. V, VI (Paris).

Secondary: Chhem, Rethy, and Michel Antelme, 2004. 'A Khmer Medical Text: "The Treatment of the Four Diseases Manuscript".' *Siksacakr* 6: 33–42; Sarkar, Kumar K., 1968. *Early Indo-Cambodian Contacts: Literary and Linguistic* (Santiniketan and Visva-Bharati).

Rethy Chhem

YAMAGIWA, KATSUSABURŌ (b. Ueda, Shinano domain [now Ueda City, Nagano Prefecture], Japan, 10 April 1863; d. Tokyo, Japan, 2 March 1930), *pathology.*

Yamagiwa Katsusaburō was the third son of Yamamoto Seisaku and his wife Tomo. The father served Ueda *han* as a samurai and was reduced to genteel poverty after the Meiji Revolution. Having received his primary and secondary education in Ueda, in 1879 Katsusaburō was adopted by Yamagiwa Yoshiya in Tokyo. That family had served as physicians to the local daimyo of the Ueda domain and had a private practice in Tokyo at that time. Destined to a career in medicine, Katsusaburō matriculated from the preparatory course of the Medical School of the University of Tokyo in 1880. He married Kaneko, Yoshiya's eldest daughter, in 1884, and he graduated from the Medical School at the head of the class in 1888. In the same year he was appointed as an assistant to the department of pathology. In 1891 Yamagiwa left Japan to study in Germany, following an established course for medical elite at that time. He studied first under Robert Koch (1843–1910) working on tuberculin, then under Rudolf Virchow (1821–1902). It was through the latter's influence that Yamagiwa became interested in the experimental study of cancer. Yamagiwa returned to Japan in 1894, appointed the next year as professor of pathological anatomy at the University of Tokyo. Yamagiwa's early career was thus a paragon of the academic medical elite.

Partly because of his ill health, which prevented Yamagiwa from living the active life of a fashionable practitioner or medical politician, his life was almost entirely devoted to academic research and teaching. His three-volume textbook of general pathology (*Byōrigaku sōron kōgi*) was published in 1895. In 1898 he started researching beriberi, which was then a major concern, particularly in military medicine. It was,

however, his research on cancer conducted during his mature years for which he is now famous. Yamagiwa published a book on cancer of the stomach (*Igan hassei ron*) in 1905. With Yamagiwa one of its leading members, the Japanese Cancer Research Society was founded in 1907 with the help of financial magnate Shibusawa Ei-ichi (1840–1931). In the same year the specialist journal *Gann* [Cancer] was established; it was the third earliest such publication in the world, appearing after similar specialist journals in France (1896) and Germany (1904). Yamagiwa conducted experimental research on cancer in animals, smearing coal tar in the ears of house rabbits for about 100–200 days. The research bore fruit in 1915 in the form of the world's first induced artificial cancer.

Ichikawa Kōichi (1888–1958), a young veterinary surgeon recruited from the Imperial University of Hokkaido, assisted Yamagiwa in these early groundbreaking experiments. He reported the result in a meeting of the Tokyo Medical Society in 1915. The initial reaction of the Japanese medical academia was mixed and was best exemplified in a sarcastic rhyme expressing their suspicion: 'Artificial cancer? Is it a malignant tumor, a false rumor, or a product of an obstinate humor?' But recognition soon followed; in 1918 Yamagiwa was selected an honorary member of the American Cancer Society, and in 1919 he was elected a member of the Imperial Academy of Japan, the highest honor for Japanese scholars. In 1928 the Sophie A. Nordhoff Jung prize was awarded to him. Although he was nominated for a Nobel Prize in medicine, this honor eluded him.

Yamagiwa had suffered from tuberculosis since he was thirty-six years old. During his entire academic career he was virtually an invalid; his life was spent almost entirely in academic teaching and research. He died in 1930 at the age of sixty-seven from acute pneumonia.

Bibliography

Primary: 1916. (with Kōichi, Ichikawa) 'Ueber die künstliche Erzeugnung von Carcinoma.' *Gann* 10 (also published in 1916, *Verh. jap. Path. Ges.* 6: 169–178, 1917, 7: 191–196); 1921. 'Ueber die künstliche Erzeugnung von Terr-Carcinoma und Sarcoma.' *Virchows Archiv* 233; 1937. *Yamagiwa sensei kushū* [Collected Poems of Dr Yamagiwa] (Tokyo).

Secondary: 1970. A special issue of *Shinano Kyōiku* [Shinano Education], No. 1008 (1 November).

Akihito Suzuki

YAMAWAKI, TŌYŌ (b. Kameyama, Tamba domain [now Kyoto Prefecture], Japan, 1705; d. Kyoto, Japan, 24 September 1762), *anatomy, dissection, Ancient Method School* (*Kohōha*).

Yamawaki Tōyō was the son of a physician named Shimizu Tōken, who was originally from Kameyama, just north of Kyoto. He studied medicine in Kyoto with Yamawaki Harunaga, a highly respected physician, and settled in the city with his family. At age nine, Tōyō, who was

Tōken's eldest son, started the study of the Confucian classics; by age thirteen, he could compose prose in classical Chinese. Soon after this, he began studies with Yamawaki Harunaga, who quickly recognized Tōyō's promise. Harunaga was himself the son of a distinguished physician, Yamawaki Harunaka, who had treated the Empress Tōfuku during the previous century and consequently achieved renown. Harunaga, however, lacked a successor, and adopted Tōyō when he reached the age of twenty-two. In this way, Tōyō inherited one of Kyoto's most prestigious medical practices.

The Yamawaki family's medical practice had been based on the theories of Manase Dōsan and his successors, giving it a highly theoretical bent based on the metaphysics of the Chinese Song dynasty (960–1279) Confucian thought. Tōyō, however, had become intrigued by current ideas in Confucianism that emphasized reading the Chinese classics directly, without the interpretations of later thinkers. Soon after the death of his adoptive father, Tōyō started to study under Gotō Konzan (1659–1733), one of the fathers of the Kohōha, or 'Ancient Method School'. Like its contemporaries in Confucian philosophy, this school of medical thought also emphasized the interpretation of classical Chinese texts without the interpretative framework of later medical thinkers. Konzan advocated the close study of the *Shanghanlun* by Zhang Zhongjing (Jp. *Shōkanron* by Chō Chūkei, 196–220), and this work became an important influence on Tōyō's own approach to medicine.

However, it was in Tōyō's own reading of the ancient Chinese classics that he found inspiration for his greatest achievement. His perusal of the *Book of Rites* and the *Book of History*, among other ancient classics, led him to question the veracity of the Chinese traditional anatomy that depicted the human body as being made of up five organs (liver, heart, spleen, lungs, and kidneys) and six viscera (stomach, large intestine, small intestine, gall bladder, bladder, and 'triple burner' or *sanshō*). Instead, he found reference to a nine-organ theory, which included the heart, lungs, liver, gall bladder, bladder, stomach, kidneys, spleen, and intestines; this scheme did not, in other words, differentiate between small and large intestines and dispensed with the abstract triple burner. Moreover, the Kohōha emphasized not only going back to the ancient classics, but also experimentation and verification of theory through empirical means.

Tōyō thus set out to substantiate the nine-organ theory of the body through dissections, but since human dissections were taboo at the time, he dissected river otters instead, based on a then-current assumption that the internal structure of its body was somehow identical to that of the human body. But Tōyō did not accept this assumption without qualification, and he pressed the authorities to allow him to dissect a human body. He succeeded in 1754, when he was allowed to dissect the corpse of a decapitated criminal in Kyoto. While he watched the body opened in front of him, Tōyō had in hand both a traditional anatomy that illustrated the five-organ and six-viscera theory and an illustrated European anatomy text. Based on his observations, he concluded that the dissection clearly demonstrated the validity of the nine-organ theory and wrote the illustrated *Zōhi* [Record of the Organs] to record and explain his observations.

Although Tōyō did not succeed in making the nine-organ theory the accepted anatomical standard, he did start a trend in which physicians conducted a growing numbers of dissections. It was one of these subsequent dissections, conducted by a group led by the physician Sugita Genpaku (1733–1817) that in turn became the stimulus for the first translation of a European medical text into Japanese. In this way Tōyō indirectly contributed to the Japanese adoption of Western medical ideas from the late eighteenth century.

Bibliography

Primary: 1759. *Zōshi* [Record of the Organs] (Kyoto); 1979. (Yoshinori, Ōtsuka, and Yakazu Dōmei, eds.) *Kinsen Kanpō igakusho shūsei* [Collected works of early modern Kanpō medicine] vol. 13. (Tokyo).

Secondary: Okamoto Takashi, 1988. *Kaibō kotohajime: Yamawaki Tōyō no hito to shisō* [The beginnings of anatomy: Yamawaki Tōyō, his life and thought] (Tokyo).

William Johnston

YE, GUI 叶桂 (aka TIANSHI 天士, XIANGYAN 香巖, XIANGYAN 香岩, NANYANG XIANSHENG 南陽先生) (b. Wu county, Suzhou, Jiangsu Province, China, 1667; d. Suzhou, China, 1746), *Chinese medicine.*

Ye Gui is one of the most famous clinicians of eighteenth-century Suzhou, in large part because works attributed to him focused on the vicissitudes of clinical practice and emphasized the individual physician's observations, experience, and flexibility. A collection of his medical case histories (*Linzheng zhinan yi'an* 臨證指南醫案, preface 1766), including an essay on febrile disorders (*Wen re lun* 溫熱論) in a later edition, remain as popular today in Chinese medical practice as they were when first posthumously published. Chinese physicians consider Ye to be one of the main innovators in etiology, diagnosis, and therapy in the Warm Factor Disorder (*wenbing xuepai* 溫病學派) current of medicine developed through the work of Wu Tang 吳瑭 (1758–1836), Wang Shixiong 王士雄 (1808–90), and Zhang Nan 章楠 (fl. 1835) in the nineteenth century. Following the lead of predecessors such as Liu Wansu 劉完素 (1120–1200?), Zhu Zhenheng 朱震亨 (1281–1358), and Wu Youxing 吳有性 (1582–1652), Ye made further distinctions between Cold Damage and Warm Factor disorders. He focused on the hot and damp illnesses prevalent in Suzhou, advocated aromatic stimulants for epidemic fevers instead of conventional Cold Damage treatments, and argued that Warm Factor illnesses do not follow the Six Warps (*liujing* 六經) stages of Cold Damage disorders. They instead transform following the Four Sectors (*sifen* 四分) division of the body from the exterior and more superficial Defensive (*wei* 衛) and (*qi* 氣) sectors to the relatively interior and more serious Constructive (*ying* 營), and Blood (*xue* 血) sectors of the body.

Ye was sufficiently famous as a physician during his life that one of the most prolific poets and literary critics in his region, Shen Deqian 沈德潛 (1673–1769), wrote the eulogy inscribed on his tombstone, which is the earliest and fullest account of Ye's genealogy, medical views, and reputation. The Ye family moved from She county in Anhui Province to Suzhou city in Wu county, possibly with Ye Gui's great-great-grandfather Ye Fengshan 葉封山 or his great-grandfather Ye Longshan 葉龍山 (also a physician), during the early seventeenth century. Planning to pursue a career in government, Ye Gui studied the classics from a tutor and medicine from his father Ye Chaocai 葉朝采 (d. 1679) until his father passed away unexpectedly when Ye was about twelve (thirteen *sui*) years old. To secure a livelihood he turned to medicine, studying first with one of his father's disciples and then allegedly working through another seventeen physicians until he turned eighteen. Following in his grandfather and father's path, Ye became the third generation in a new line of hereditary physicians in Suzhou.

Although a small cottage industry of over forty published texts attributed to Ye Gui developed after his death in 1746, no credible evidence indicates that he published even one medical text during his lifetime. Only two texts published while he lived printed his name on the title page. *Explanations of the Essentials of the 'Treatise on Materia Medica*' (*Bencao jing jie yao* 本草經解要, pr. 1724) lists Ye Gui as the author on the title page and in the two prefaces, but it is more likely that his disciple Wang Yuetian copied the text under Ye's tutelage and used his family's influence to publish it. As a senior disciple of the Suzhou physician Wang Zijie 王子接 (b. 1658) in the early 1730s, Ye collated the *Jiangxueyuan gufang xuan zhu* 絳雪園古方選注 [Crimson Snow Garden Annotations on a Selection of Ancient Formulas] (1732), which Wang Zijie annotated. About twenty years after Ye's death, two of his followers, Hua Nantian 華南田 (1697–1773) and Li Guohua 李國華 (n.d.), compiled the collection of his case records—*Linzheng zhinan yi'an* 臨證指南醫案 (1764) [Medical Case Records as a Guide to Clinical Practice]—that made him famous. Later collections of his medical case histories include the *Zhongfutang yi'an* 種福堂醫案 [Medical Cases of the Hall of Cultivated Fortune] and the *Ye an cunzhen* 葉案存真 [Preserved Genuine Cases of Ye]. These medical case histories have inspired generations of Chinese physicians ever since with their candor, clarity, and range.

Bibliography

Primary: 1724. *Bencao jing jie ya* 本草經解要 [Explanations of Essentials of the 'Treatise on Materia Medica'] (by Yao Qiu 姚球, attrib. Ye Gui 葉桂. *Jigu shanfang* 稽古山方 edition, Beijing); 1732. *Jiangxueyuan gufang xuan zhu* 絳雪園古方選注 [Commentary on Selected Ancient Formulas from the Crimson Snow Garden] (by Wang Zijie 王子接, publisher's preface, 1731, author's preface 1732. *Saoye shanfang* 掃葉山房 edition, Peking Union Medical College). Alternatively titled *Shisan ke gu fang* 十三科古方 [Ancient Formulas for the Thirteen Disciplines]; 1759. '*Ye jun Gui zhuan*' 葉君桂傳 ['Biography of Mr. Ye Gui'], Shen Deqian 沈德潛, in *Guiyu wenchao* 歸愚文鈔 [Selected Writings of Shen Deqian] (repr. Zhou Junfu 周駿富, ed., 1985. *Qingdai zhuanji congkan* 清代傳記叢刊 [Collections of Biographies from the Qing Dynasty] vol. 114: 282–283; vol. 190: 515–517 (Taipei)); 1766. *Linzheng zhinan yian* 臨證指南醫案 [Medical Case Records as a Guide to Clinical Practice] (attrib. Ye Gui 葉桂, eds. Hua Nantian 華南田, Li Guohua 李國華, 1991 (Shanghai)); 1933. *Wuxian zhi* 吳縣誌 [Gazetteer of Wu County] (comp. by Li Genyuan 李根源 (Taipei, 1970) 56 *xia* 11b; 70 *shang* 21b; 75 *shang* 37a.

Secondary: Huang, Yingzhi 黃英志, ed., 1999. *Ye Tianshi yixue quanshu* 葉天士醫學全書. *Ming Qing mingyi quanshu dacheng* series (Beijing); Yang, J. C., 1991. 'Yeh Kuei' in Hummel, Arthur W., ed., *Eminent Chinese of the Ch'ing Period* vol. 2 (Taiwan) pp. 902–903; Zhang, Xiaofang 張孝芳, 1985. 'Ye Gui shixi xiaokao' 葉桂世系小考 ['Short Essay on Ye Gui's Lineage']. *Jiangsu zhongyi zazhi* 11: 3; Lin Gongzheng 林功錚, 1984. 'Yidai mingyi Ye Tianshi' 一代名醫葉天士 ['The Famous Physician of a Generation, Ye Gui'] *YSZZ* 14(2): 82–84.

Marta E. Hanson

YEN, JAMES YANG-CH'U (b. Bazhou, Sichuan Province, China, 26 October 1893; d. New York, New York, USA, 17 January 1990), *public health.*

'Jimmy' Yen was born into a gentry family. He was educated in missionary schools, briefly attended Hong Kong University, and transferred to Yale University in 1916. There he met his future wife, Alice Huie (Xu), whom he married in 1921. On graduation in June 1918, Yen went to France under the auspices of the International Committee of the YMCA to assist with the thousands of coolies in the Chinese Labor Corps recruited by the Allies in World War I. His experiences with these illiterate workers inspired him to develop a simplified system for teaching and writing Chinese. He started with the most basic 1,000 characters and then provided reading materials that used only those.

After the war, Yen returned to Beijing and then went to work in a district of Hebei Province called Dingxian (Ting-hsien). This was to be a 'social laboratory' for what came to be known as the Mass Education Movement (Zhonghua pingmin jiaoyu cijin hui), founded by Yen in 1923. Dingxian had a population of about 400,000, or about one-thousandth of the population of China at that time. Yen and his colleagues first set up a school, then started to teach agriculture and public health. They received assistance in the United States from the Milbank Memorial Fund, the Rockefeller Foundation, and the YMCA. Their public health program also received support from the League of Nations Health Organization.

The public health experiment was set up in 1928 by Yao Xunyuan, who had graduated from the Rockefeller Foundation–funded Peking Union Medical College (PUMC) in 1927. He was succeeded in 1931 by C. C. Chen (Chen Zhiqian) (PUMC 1929), who extended basic health care to the entire population of Dingxian by 1936. Both Yao and Chen had been taught at PUMC by James B. Grant.

At that time, the number of modern trained physicians in China was about one for every 70,000 of population, and almost all of those lived in the cities. At Dingxian, local graduates of the mass education program were elected to be village health workers, and trained to do five things: record births and deaths; vaccinate against smallpox and cholera; give simple treatments from a 'health protection box' (cost: $3), such as antibiotic ointment for trachoma of the eye, disinfectants, and bandages; give health talks with demonstrations and charts prepared by the Health Department of the Mass Education Movement; and maintain a sanitary well in the village. The position of village health worker was unpaid, but the worker gained status and gifts in kind, especially at Chinese New Year. The next level of medical care was the sub-xian Health Station, staffed with a physician and a dresser, in a centrally located village. Here the staff trained and supervised village health workers from up to fifty villages, gave lectures on health, and treated difficult cases passed up to them by the village health workers. The top layer of this system was the Health Center, with a hospital, laboratory, offices, and classrooms in the xian (district) capital. The medical staff there studied rural health problems and conducted supplementary training of medical personnel, epidemic control, school health programs, the training of midwives, and birth control. The total cost for this pilot system of rural health provision was about $36,000, or ten cents per capita in 1936.

During the anti-Japanese war, James Yen evacuated further inland and set up the National College of Rural Reconstruction in November 1940, near Chongqing. C. C. Chen became Commissioner of Public Health for Sichuan Province and adopted the same system to provide primary health care during World War II.

In 1947 James Yen went to the United States to appeal for aid in rebuilding the Chinese rural areas. General George C. Marshall, then U.S. Secretary of State, and President Truman endorsed Yen's plan to assist the Chinese people at the village level, with the result that when Congress passed the China Aid Act in 1948, it provided that up to 10 percent of the $275 million in aid be earmarked for rural reconstruction, and that a Joint Commission on Rural Reconstruction (JCRR) be formed to administer it. The JCRR operated for sixteen months before the Communist takeover. It then moved its operations to Taiwan, where it continued for many years. The Chinese Communist Party's 'barefoot doctor' program of the late 1960s and 1970s was organized along very similar lines, and similar systems of locally funded primary health care delivery were promoted both by the League of Nations in the 1930s and by the United Nations in the 1970s (the People's Republic of China rejoined the UN in 1971).

In 1951 Yen became director of the International Mass Education Movement, with headquarters in the Philippines. In 1960 this organization became the International Institute for Rural Reconstruction. A 1987 United States Presidential End Hunger Award for lifetime achievement cited him for 'developing and disseminating a sustained, integrated program to overcome the root causes of hunger and poverty in the Third World'.

Bibliography

Primary: 1990. (Zhan, Yizhi, ed.) *Yan Yangchu wen ji* [Collected writings of Yan Yangchu (James Yen)] (Chengdu); 1945. (with Buck, Pearl S.) *Tell the People: Talks with James Yen about the Mass Education Movement* (New York); 1967. (with Feliciano, Gregorio M., and the joint staffs of the International Institute of Rural Reconstruction and the Philippine Rural Reconstruction Movement, ed. Price, Harry Bayard) *Rural Reconstruction and Development: A Manual for Field Workers* (New York).

Secondary: Hayford, Charles W., 1990. *To the People: James Yen and Village China* (New York); Lucas, AnElissa, 1982. *Chinese Medical Modernization* (New York).

Bridie Andrews Minehan

YERSIN, ALEXANDRE (b. Lavaux, Vaud Canton, Switzerland, 22 September 1863; d. Nha Trang, Vietnam, 8 February 1943), *medicine, bacteriology.*

Yersin was the youngest of three children raised by his mother in Morges, Switzerland, after the father, a French-speaking Swiss technician, died before Alexandre's birth. Yersin began his medical studies at Lausanne, continued at Marburg, Germany (1884), and went to the Hôtel Dieu in Paris (1885–86). After meeting Emile Roux, Yersin was admitted to the Pasteur Institute in 1887, where he worked on vaccinations against rabies. The next year he defended his medical thesis on tuberculosis, for which he won the bronze medal of the Paris Faculty of Medicine.

The Pasteurians sent Yersin to Berlin in the summer of 1889 to take Robert Koch's course in bacteriology, giving him exposure to the two leading approaches to the new science. Returning to Paris later that year, Yersin worked with Roux on diphtheria and became a naturalized French citizen.

Although he was on the verge of a promising scientific career, the reclusive Yersin in 1890 suddenly fled the Pasteur Institute to travel to Indochina, serving as a ship's doctor to earn his passage. This seemingly reckless decision was to change his life. He began his personal exploration of the interior of Indochina (1891–93), becoming the first French traveler to visit the beautiful plateau and highland country around what became the French town of Dalat.

In 1892, after a meeting with Albert Calmette in Saigon, Yersin joined the French colonial health service. When news of the Hong Kong bubonic plague outbreak of 1894 reached Saigon, French health officials immediately dispatched Yersin to the beleaguered British port.

Yersin arrived three days after a Japanese team headed by Shibasaburō Kitasato, who had studied under Robert Koch in Berlin. The two men have been jointly linked to the discovery of the bacillus which causes bubonic plague. Yersin, however, was the better scientist; much later, his more accurate results eventually resulted in the taxonomic naming of the bacillus *Yersinia pestis* in 1954. Its earlier denomination had been *Pasteurella pestis*.

Yersin's original description of the plague bacillus was concise and correct, whereas Kitasato's contained errors. Only Yersin suggested that rats were a major factor in the transmission of the disease. And only Yersin persisted in plague research, returning to Emile Roux's Paris laboratory in 1895 to develop, along with Amédéé Borrel and Albert Calmette, an anti-plague serum from the blood of horses to boost human immune systems.

Following this stint in Paris, Yersin in 1895 was back in Indochina, where the next year he soon developed a preventive vaccine from a live but attenuated organism. It proved to be of limited value: it only afforded protection for two weeks. Later in 1896 Yersin traveled to plague-infected southern China to try out the Pasteur Institute's anti-plague serum. The next year he appeared in Bombay for the same purpose, but the results in both China and India proved disappointing.

Yersin would rarely return to Europe after 1900. At the request of the Governor General of Indochina, Paul Doumer, Yersin created and directed the new French Medical School in Hanoi between 1902 and 1904. In 1904 he became director of the Pasteur Institute in Nha Trang, which remained his home until his death. Awards came to him from time to time, as in 1927 when he won the Prix Lecomte of the French Academy of Science, and in 1934 when he was named member of the Scientific Council of the Pasteur Institute in Paris and its honorary director. This would require him to make an annual visit to Paris to preside at the institute's general assembly. After his death in 1943, his burial site in Nha Trang became a Vietnamese pilgrimage site.

Bibliography

Primary: 1894. 'La Peste bubonique à Hong Kong.' *Annales de l'Institut Pasteur* 8: 662–667.

Secondary: Mollaret, Henri, and Jacqueline Brossolet, 1985. *Alexandre Yersin, le vainqueur de la peste* (Paris); Howard-Jones, Norman, 1975. 'Kitasato, Yersin and the Plague Bacillus.' *Clio Medica* 10: 23–27; *DSB*.

Myron Echenberg

YI, JEMA 李濟馬 (b. Hamheung, Korea, 1838; d. Hamheung, 1900), *Korean medicine.*

Yi Jema was born in Hamheung, a city in the northern part of Korea. Like all children of the privileged classes, he studied Confucian philosophy, history, and Korean and Chinese literature. He was, however, most interested in medicine, divination according to the tradition of the *Yi jing* 易經 [Classic of Changes], and military strategy. Rather than focusing on external medical treatment, he expressed a profound interest in Heo Jun's 1613 *Dong'uibo'gam* 東醫寶鑑 [Treasured Collections of an Eastern [Korean] Physician] and its emphasis on inner cultivation of the mind and body.

In 1888 Yi Jema took charge of a military office but soon resigned. In 1892 he became a county headman of Jin-Hae, located in the rural south of Korea, where he also practiced medicine. Resigning the post in 1893, he went to Seoul in order to write his own medical book. Completing a first draft of *Dong'ui'susebowon* 東醫壽世保元 [Longevity through the Ages and Preserving the Origin, by an Eastern [Korean] Physician] in 1894, the following year Yi Jema returned to Hamheung, where he remained, making revisions to his work and teaching until he died.

Dong'ui'susebowon established a theory of typologies, which Yi Jema derived from his medical practice. *Sasang* 四象醫學 [four-constitution medicine] is the classification of human beings into four types: *taeyang'in* 太陽人 [those who have an extreme Yang nature], *soyang'in* 少陽人 [those who tend toward a Yang nature], *soeum'in* 少陰人 [those who tend to a Yin nature] and *taeeum'in* 太陰人 [those who have an extreme Yin nature]. According to his observations, for every 10,000 people, more than half are *taeeum'in*; 3,000 are *soyang'in*; 2,000 are *soeum'in*; and only two or three are *taeyang'in*. A person's constitution, determined at birth by the relative qualities and quantities of Yin and Yang in their bodies, would predispose him or her to certain diseases. Even when patients seemed to suffer from the same disease, he argued that the way in which they were treated should depend upon their constitution.

Theorizing his observations about the human body into the four constitutions, Yi Jema reconfigured the traditional correlations of the four organs of lungs, spleen, liver, and kidneys and four sensual organs of ears, eyes, nose, and mouth. In particular, he emphasized the role of negative traits in human temperament, such as self-indulgence, idleness, indulgence in luxury, and greed in long-term illness causation. His solution for sustaining health was a lifelong program for nurturing the mind.

Yi Jema's four-constitution medicine differed from traditional Chinese medicine in three aspects. First, his medicine was body-centered, not symptom-centered. Second, his medicine was based on four immutable constitutional types, not the transformations of the five agents. Third, his medicine was guided by ethical considerations. However, the concept of linking the body surface and human temperament to the inner organs is similar to classical Chinese correspondence medicine, even though the exact correlations are completely different in the two traditions.

The four-volume *Dong'ui'susebowon* was published posthumously in 1901, a year after Yi Jema's death, to widespread acclaim. By reducing a confusion of symptoms to four categories, it became convenient to use in clinical practice. Many Korean nationalists were also delighted to have an indigenous Korean medical system that was apparently independent of Chinese medicine.

Bibliography

Primary: 1901. *Dong'ui'susebowon* 東醫壽世保元 [Longevity through the Ages and Preserving the Origin, by an Eastern [Korean] Physician] (Hamheung).

Secondary: Dongwon, Shin, 2004. *Hoyeolja, Choson'eul Seup'kyok'hada: Momgoa Ui'hak'ui Hankuk'sa* [Cholera Invaded Korea: A Korean History of Body and Medicine] (Seoul); Dujong, Kim, 1966. *Hankuk Ui'hak'sa* [History of Korean Medicine] (Seoul); Sakae, Miki, 1962. *Chosen Igakusi Kyu Sitsubeisi* [History of Korean Medicine and of Disease in Korea] (Osaka).

Dongwon Shin

YLPPÖ, ARVO HENRIK   (b. Akaa, Toijala, Finland, 27 October 1887; d. Helsinki, Finland, 28 January 1992), *pediatrics.*

Ylppö was the oldest of twelve children, the son of Henrik Ylppö, a farmer, and Henriika Maunu. He attended the College Tampereen suomalainen Reaalilyseo from 1898 to 1906 and decided to study medicine. He then attended the Medical faculty of the Imperial Alexander University of Finland in Helsinki from 1906 to 1914. Between 1912 and 1920 Ylppö received his training as a pediatrician at the Kaiserin Auguste Victoria Haus, Charlottenburg in Berlin, the last two years as the chief physician. As a disciple of Leo Langenstein he started his career as a research worker in 1913 with a thesis that clarified the conditions for the development of jaundice in the newborn. Ylppö's conclusion was that the jaundice in the newborn was caused by the immaturity of the liver, which later to a great extent was shown to be true, although the cause was solved about thirty years later when the Rhesus blood group (Rh factor) was found.

Ylppö conducted important research on the diseases of premature infants, a subject which at that time had been little investigated. In an extensive work carried out in Germany in 1919, he ascertained the causes of death in premature infants and demonstrated on the basis of his own autopsies that, among other things, cerebral hemorrhage and inborn anomalies of structure often caused premature death.

Ylppö became particularly famous for his presentations of the classification of premature babies based on weight, which was accepted in 1935 by the American Academy of Pediatrics and which was used all over the world for decades. According to Ylppö, a baby weighing less than 2,500 grams should be classified as a premature. Later a classification based on the weight was abandoned, partly due to other developments in medicine.

When Ylppö returned to Finland, he was already a famous researcher and physician. He was first (1919) appointed a docent and later (1925) a professor in pediatrics at the University of Helsinki, a professorship which he held until 1957, when he retired. Ylppö was very fond of children. In 1925 he married Aino Wegelius (d. 1942) and in 1950 Lea Jokinen; he fathered in all six children.

In 1920 Ylppö also became chief physician of the Children's Castle in Helsinki, a position he held until 1963. At this hospital, founded by the Mannerheim League for Child Welfare, Ylppö started an information bureau for child care in 1922. With this important resource the mortality among suckling babies was lessened. More information bureaus for child care were established all over the country and formed a good base for an established network. Within the framework of the Mannerheim League, Ylppö traveled all over the country, lecturing with wax representations of children's diseases as props.

As head of the Children's Castle he was also a teacher at courses for nursemaids held at the hospital. From the very beginning he appreciated the significance of preventing children's diseases. Therefore he wrote several popular articles and booklets on child care.

As a result of Ylppö's extensive work, the mortality among the suckling babies in Finland has gradually decreased to one of the lowest in the world: under five per 1,000 in 1993.

Ylppö was elected member and honorary member of many scientific societies all over the world and in 1952 he was granted the title of archiater [chief physician]. On his hundredth birthday, still alive, he was honored by a large exhibition and by the issuing of a commemorative stamp.

Bibliography

Primary: Ignatius, J., 2000. 'Lääketieteet' in *Suomen tieteen historia* vol. 3 (Helsinki).

Secondary: 1987. 'Arkkiatri Arvo Ylppö 100 vuotta' in *Suomen Lääkärilehti* 30B.

Hindrik Strandberg

YOSHIMASU, TŌDŌ   (b. Hiroshima, Aki domain [now Hiroshima Prefecture], Japan, 3 March 1702; d. Kyoto, Japan, 9 November 1773), *Ancient Method School, one-poison theory, abdominal diagnosis.*

Yoshimasu Tōdō was born in Aki domain, in what is now Hiroshima Prefecture. He was a descendant of what had previously been a powerful warrior clan, the Hatakeyama, which had been defeated in battle several generations before Tōdō's birth. Following their defeat, his ancestors fled to Kawachi, in the Osaka area, took refuge in the house of a surgeon named Yoshimasu, and thereafter assumed the family name Yoshimasu for themselves and became surgeons who specialized in battlefield wounds. They later moved to Aki and restored the Hatakeyama family name.

Although Tōdō's father was a surgeon, in his youth Tōdō had been infatuated with the martial arts. Before reaching the age of twenty, however, Tōdō realized that there was little practical use for the martial arts in a world without war and that he would have a much better chance of establishing himself by practicing medicine. He then mastered the contemporary craft of surgery but also absorbed a number of the Chinese medical classics, including the *Suwen* and *Nanjing*; he also learned the theories of the Yin and Yang and their influence on the five elements. Tōdō responded to these works with the assertion that if medical theory could not help a physician heal the ill, then its pursuit was of little value.

Kyoto

After finishing a basic education in medicine, Tōdō moved with his parents to Kyoto. There he set out on his own to establish himself as a practicing physician and assumed the family name Yoshimasu. Kyoto was a leading center of medical practice, and without becoming associated with one of the city's more prominent physicians and his school, it was virtually impossible to gain recognition. But Tōdō rejected the most popular medical theories of the time. He found almost everything in the *Suwen* and *Nanjing*, not to mention the works of Goseiha physicians, to be useless in the healing of patients. On the other hand, he did become an enthusiastic proponent of the Chinese classic, the *Shanghanlun* by Zhang Zhongjing (Jp. *Shkanron* by Chō Chūkei, 196–220), as the basis for some of his ideas. Theoretical originality was hardly enough to establish him in the competitive world of Kyoto medicine and Tōdō, almost entirely without patients or students, resorted to making dolls from paper, wood, and plaster in order to make ends meet.

In a stroke of good fortune, however, his doll-making business gave him the break he needed. Tōdō went to the house of a doll wholesaler to deliver some of his wares and found the matron of the house ill. He examined her and the medicine she was taking and said that it would be necessary to remove some of the plaster contained in her medicine. The next day her physician, the renowned Yamawaki Tōyō, heard what Tōdō had recommended and replied that he had been debating whether to include the plaster or take it out of the medicine's formula. Upon hearing Tōdō's recommendation, Tōyō recognized Tōdō's perspicuity as a physician and thereafter recommended him to others in Kyoto. After that, Tōdō became one of the city's leading physicians. He treated numerous patients and taught a large number of students, many of whom went on to become important physicians themselves.

The Ancient Method School

It was in this way that Yoshimasu Tōdō became established as a leading theoretician and practitioner of the Ancient Method School of medicine. He was especially important because of his emphasis on empirical methods. By Tōdō's time, this school had become well established through the work of predecessors, especially Nagoya Gen'i (1628–1696), Gotō Konzan (1659–1733), and Kagawa Shūan (also known as Kagawa Shūtoku, 1683–1755), and his contemporary, Yamawaki Tōyō (1705–1762). Tōdō's impact on Japanese medicine was arguably as great as any of his predecessors in the Ancient Method School.

Tōdō's empiricism had a predecessor in Kagawa Shūan, although it is hard to say whether Shūan's ideas directly influenced Tōdō. By the eighteenth century, Japanese physicians tended to study eclectically the various schools of medicine then current. Few were exclusive in their approaches to either theory or practice. As a consequence, lines of influence are often difficult to draw among physicians at this time. Nevertheless, it is clear that Kagawa Shūan did study for an extended period with Gotō Konzan and that he reinforced several elements of Konzan's approach to medicine—to such an extent that he established a virtually new approach of his own. One was the emphasis on the study of Confucian classics by physicians.

Shūan himself had studied under Itō Jinsai (1627–1705), one of the most renowned scholars of the School of Ancient Learning (Kogakuha). That school's adherents elevated the direct study of the early Chinese classics above the Song dynasty interpretations of those classics. Shūan went radically beyond Tōdō's criticism of established texts, moreover: whereas Tōdō had assailed the use of Song Confucianism and its derivative medical theories, Shūan condemned the standard classics of ancient Chinese medicine, including the *Suwen* and the *Nanjing*, and instead insisted that medical theory be based on the early Chinese classics themselves. Arguably, however, Shūan's most important contribution to Japanese medicine was his empirical approach. In rejecting almost all established theories, he set out to determine the utility of medicinal herbs and dietary treatments through clinical trial and error. He published a three-volume work that explained the uses of 209 different herbs and foods. This work remained an important reference for later physicians, although Shūan's radical approach to medical theory was not nearly as influential. Nevertheless, Yoshimasu Tōdō did share a similar if not total skepticism toward the ancient Chinese medical texts.

Single-Poison Theory and Abdominal Diagnosis

Although Tōdō was considered a member of the Ancient Method School, he had an original approach to medical practice. He completely rejected ideas of Yin, Yang, and the five elements as important to understanding pathology, and instead advocated a single-poison theory. According to this theory, all disease was the result of a single poison. He did not find it necessary to explain the origin of this poison, although he believed that in most cases it was carried in, or was part of, what a person ate or drank. The physician's most important job was to determine the poison's location in the patient's body and apply the proper remedy. Tōdō also rejected the most important diagnostic method of the day, which consisted in examining a patient's pulse for strengths, weaknesses, and other qualities. For him, this was an integral part of the Goseiha methodology, which he saw as pointlessly theoretical. Instead, Tōdō developed a method of abdominal diagnosis in which he visually observed and palpated the abdomen in search of the places where the poison had become stagnant and which in turn suggested the proper therapeutic measures. As he became increasingly important as a teacher, his method of abdominal diagnosis became well known throughout the country.

With his growing popularity, Tōdō wrote numerous medical works that also became influential throughout Japan. One of the most important was his *Yakuchō*, a work on pharmacopoeia. He divided the pharmacopoeia into two groups, one for the maintenance of good health and the promotion of long life, and the other for healing diseases. The former depended on selecting foods, drinks, and medicines that contained no poisons and instead improved a person's strength. The latter, however, required the physician to find the medicine that contained the proper poison that would offset the poison causing disease in the body. Tōdō found the existing works on medicines confused and ill-conceived, and as a consequence set out to examine various medicinals through a process of empirical testing. In this way, his methods strongly resembled those of Kagawa Shūan, although it is not clear whether Tōdō borrowed directly from Shūan.

What is most important is Tōdō's advocacy of experimentation and empirical methods over the previous dependency among many Japanese physicians, even others of the Ancient Method School, on theory and an unquestioning acceptance of Chinese medical texts. However, in that Tōdō's requirement for a medicine to be successful was that it initiate a semi-catatonic state in the patient, it is not clear that he had clear criteria for judging the presence of a poison. When a patient did not slip into such a state, he did not consider the medicine effective. With such powerful medicines, it was inevitable that some of his patients would die while under his care, and in those cases, he simply said that the patient's life had been determined by heaven and that it was not his place to change it.

Yoshimasu Tōdō's Legacy

Tōdō had a number of influential students, many of whom advocated both his empirical approach and his use of abdominal diagnosis. One of his most important students was his son, Yoshimasu Nangai (1750–1813), who expanded his father's approach to assert that qi, blood, and water could all transport poison in the body—but Nangai did not in any way contradict his father's single-poison theory. Tōdō and his approach to medicine also had numerous detractors, including the descendants of Gotō Konzan, who had inherited Konzan's practice and continued to advocate the primacy of the single qi theory of pathology over the single-poison theory of Tōdō. Moreover, during the eighteenth century, the Goseiha continued to have its supporters throughout Japan and by no means was it completely superseded by any advocates of the Ancient Method School. Indeed, even with the rising importance of European medical thought in Japan starting in the late eighteenth century and continuing into the nineteenth, the Goseiha was not quickly eclipsed. Rather there coexisted in Japan during the late eighteenth and most of the nineteenth century a number of distinct and competing approaches to medical theory and practice. None managed to establish the kind of hegemony over medicine that became apparent in modern medicine during the late nineteenth century with the rise of bacteriology, public health, and asepsis.

Despite this plurality of approaches to medical theory and practice, however, it is impossible to deny that Yoshimasu Tōdō and his empirical approach made a profound mark on Japanese medicine, one that helped establish an active receptivity toward empirical methods.

Bibliography

Primary: 1970. Kure Shūzō and Fujikawa Yū, eds., *Tōdō zenshū* [Complete works of Yoshimasu Tōdō] (Kyoto).

Secondary: Fujikawa Yū, 1972. *Nihon igakushi* [Medical history of Japan] (Tokyo).

William Johnston

YOSHIOKA, YAYOI (née **WASHIYAMA**) (b. Hijikata, Shizuoka domain [now Shizuoka Prefecture], Japan, 29 April 1871; d. Tokyo, Japan, 22 May 1959), *women's medical education.*

Yayoi, daughter of Washiyama Yōsai, physician of Kanpō (Japanese-Chinese) medicine, and Mise (née Matsuura), left the rural life for distinction in the metropolis, attended Saisei School, Tokyo (1889–92), and passed the national examinations for a license for medical practice in 1892. She was the twenty-seventh woman doctor under the modern license system. She helped her father's practice back in Shizuoka, moving to Tokyo again in 1895 with an aspiration for further education in the German language in order to study medicine in Germany. In Tokyo, she began a practice of her own. Learning German brought her into an acquaintance with Yoshioka Arata, who had changed his focus from that of a medical student to a German educationalist and schoolmaster. She married Arata in 1895; the union eventually defined her career as an educationalist and administrator, though she continued her practice.

Late nineteenth-century women had sneaked into classes and academies, where they were faced with difficulties because of male chauvinism on the one hand and curious unwelcome attention on the other. The late Meiji era witnessed the tension between the surge in enthusiasm in women's education and its opposition. In 1900 Saisei School, which had been the only institution accepting female medical students, decided to shut the door on women. This exclusion confirmed the need for a medical school for women and led the Yoshiokas to start the Tokyo Women's Medical School in 1900 with four students. She was a useful resource for the school; lecturing in physiology and anatomy, she even offered herself as an object for the students' observation when she gave birth to a boy in 1902.

She was an ambitious school administrator; supported by income from her medical practice, she was always expanding and upgrading the school. Consistently aspiring and thus continually under financial strain, she was audacious in investment opportunities, which eventually turned to her advantage. Her institution was accredited as a medical college in 1912, accepting ninety-five new students and appointed in 1920 as a college whose graduates could be exempt from the national exams for a license. One of her strengths was her use of publicity; she invested in advertising campaigns and grand ceremonies and also in controlling how she was to be represented biographically.

With her abilities in medicine, education, management, and public speaking, she asserted confident and overwhelming leadership, playing significant roles in numerous associations, including women doctors' societies and various wartime associations. She was invited in 1939 by the Nazi Women's Society to visit Germany, where welfare facilities and policies as well as control and discipline impressed her. Her wartime activities resulted in postwar expulsion from public and educational offices between 1947 and 1951. In 1952, when the Yoshiokas' college was renamed Tokyo Women's Medical University, she made a comeback as the president of the university and was honored with an order in 1955 and another posthumously, in addition to two she had received before the war. Though her wish to immortalize herself by mummifying her body was not fulfilled, with her charismatic presence she was arguably the most influential woman in the history of Japanese medicine.

Bibliography

Primary: Kanzaki, Kiyoshi, 1989 [1941]. *Yoshioka Yayoi den* [Biography] (Based on her life, dictated by herself) (Tokyo); Yoshioka, Hiroto, 1969. *Yoshioka Yayoi* (Tokyo); Sakai, Shizu, 2005. *Ai to shisei ni ikiru—Joi Yoshioka Yayoi no tegami* [Selected Letters] (Tokyo); 2000. *Yoshioka Yayoi senshū* [Anthologies] (Tokyo).

Secondary: Enchi, Fumiko, ed., 1978. *Kyōiku bungaku heno reimei* [The Dawn of Education and Literature in Japanese Women's History Series] (Tokyo); Japan Medical Women's Association, 1991. *Nihon joi shi* [History of Women Doctors in Japan] (Tokyo).

Mika Suzuki

YPERMAN, JAN (b. Ypres, Flanders, *c.* 1260–65; d. Ypres, *c.* 1330), *surgery.*

Yperman studied surgery in Paris with Lanfranco of Milan between 1297 and 1303 before returning to his native Ypres, where he was named as a citizen. The town of Ypres then had around 28,000 inhabitants and was one the largest towns in Flanders. He was employed as a salaried surgeon in that city at the hospital founded by Christina Belle in 1276; his wife and daughter (both named Kateline) seem to have been employed in the same hospital. After his return from Paris, his own house may have been outside the city, but beginning in 1313 he occupied a house in Zuutstraat intra muros, near the Belle hospital. He is identified in the records as Magister Jan Yperman. In 1311–12 and 1325 he was employed to accompany the town's militia on military campaigns in Flanders and Brabant. He was appointed a doctor of the sick poor in the city in 1327. The last mention of him in civic records was in 1329.

Apart from the civic records of Ypres, Jan Yperman is known to us through his two surviving written works, a *Surgie* and a work on medicines. The *Surgie* (Latin *Chirurgia*) is a surgical textbook written in Flemish for the sake of his son, who knew no Latin, probably in 1310. The work relies heavily on the Salernitan surgeries of Roger Frugard and the so-called Glosses of the Four Masters, as well as on the later writings of Bruno and his master Lanfranco. After an introduction on the anatomy and physiology of the head (illustrated with a schematic cross-section of the skull), and on the qualities to be looked for in a surgeon, it follows the head-to-toe order of ailments, carefully laid out in seven books. Despite its familiar structure, it is clear that Yperman was no mere compiler, and at a number of points, his own perspective as a practitioner emerges. His techniques in surgery of the skull, in the extraction of arrows, and in techniques of stopping hemorrhaging from blood vessels (he distinguishes arterial and venal bleeding) show that he was not afraid to introduce new ideas based on experience. There are references to cases he treated, such as four men of Ypres suffering from hernia whom he treated successfully with bed rest, diet, and a plaster—rather than cutting with the knife. A number of copies of the *Surgie* survive in Brussels, Cambridge, Ghent, and London. It is evident from other works that his doctrines were followed by other Flemish authorities (for instance Jan Bertrand and Johann Coninck). The *Surgie* was illustrated with a series of images of surgical instruments, for the most part clearly related to those that had entered western surgery through the works of Abulcasis (Al-Zahrāwī).

Yperman was also the author of a *Boec van medicinen,* which is known from a surviving manuscript in the Brussels

Royal Library. This work, like the *Surgie*, builds mostly on Salernitan models, making these older remedies available in the vernacular. It begins with fevers and then considers other disorders, working down to the urinary tract. The *Practica brevis* of Platearius the younger seems to have been the source of much of the humoral medicine in Yperman's work. It is clear that Yperman did not set the kind of boundaries between medicine and surgery that were increasingly to be identified in fourteenth-century France and Italy. Yperman's fame in his own time was considerable, but he was later to be eclipsed by the fifteenth-century popularity of translations of the surgery of Guy de Chauliac in his own country.

Bibliography

Primary: Leersum, E. C. van, 1912. *De 'Cyrurgie' van Meester Jan Yperman* (Leiden); Elaut, L., 1972. *De Medicina van Johan Yperman* (Ghent).

Secondary: Huizenga, E., 2003. *Tussen autoriteit en empirie. De Middelnederlandse chirurgieën in de veertiende en vijftiende eeuw en hun maatschappelijke context* (Hilversum); Keil, Gundolf, 1998. 'Yperman, Jan' in *Lexikon des Mittelalters*, IX, 423–24; Moulin, Daniel, de, 1988. *A History of Surgery: with Emphasis on the Netherlands* (Dordrecht) pp. 60–63.

Peter Jones

YU, YAN 余巖 (aka YU, YUNXIU 余雲岫) (b. Zhejiang, China, 28 October 1879; d. Shanghai, China, 3 January 1954), *medicine, Traditional Chinese Medicine, history of medicine.*

Yu Yan was trained as a modern medical physician. Yet, paradoxically, through his conception and promotion of the 'Chinese medical revolution', he was to exert a long-lasting influence on the twentieth-century history of traditional Chinese medicine.

In 1916, while studying Western medicine at Osaka Medical College, Japan (1908–1911; 1913–1916), Yu published a systematic attack on the ancient Chinese medical classics *Lingshu Shangdui* 靈素商兌 [A Critique of the *Huangdi neijing lingshu* 黃帝內經靈樞 Inner Canon of the Yellow Lord: the Divine Pivot] and *Suwen* 素問 [Basic Questions]. Yu challenged almost every fundamental concept of Chinese medicine from the standpoint of modern Western anatomy and physiology. To his surprise, traditional Chinese doctors did not respond to his attack until much later, when they faced direct threats from the Republican government (1912–49).

After the Republican government created the first Chinese Ministry of Heath in 1929, the National Board of Health unanimously passed Yu's proposal, 'The Abolition of Old-Style Medicine to Remove the Obstacles to Medicine and Public Health'. In the name of the 'Chinese medical revolution', Yu integrated medical policies from various sources: state medicine inspired by Rudolf Virchow (1821–1902), Meiji Japan's (1868–1912) wholesale abolition of traditional medicine, and the nationalist agenda for constructing a modern public health and medical administration infrastructure. Unexpectedly, this resolution mobilized the previously unorganized traditional Chinese doctors into a massive National Medicine movement, leading to a decade-long collective struggle between practitioners of native medicine and of modern biomedicine.

When the National Medicine Institute was established in 1931 and dedicated to the purpose of 'scientizing' Chinese medicine, reform-minded Chinese doctors took Yu's critique as their point of departure. They endorsed his positivist conception of knowledge, such as that Chinese medicine had developed through the accumulation of pre-theory, atomized *jingyan* 經驗 [experience]. Another salient example of Yu's influence was his 'Scientific Research on Nationally-produced Drugs', which presented a reductionist approach that treated Chinese herbs as raw materials outside of their cultural contexts, dismissing both Chinese medical theory and the clinical experience of Chinese doctors. Inspired by the widely acclaimed isolation of ephedrine (for treating asthma) from the Chinese herb *mahuang* 麻黃 (1924), this program became the dominant approach for undertaking scientific research on Chinese medicine. When the Communist government (PRC) in the 1950s decided to promote traditional Chinese medicine, it often labeled the Republican government's nonsupportive medical policy as Yu's policy of 'abolishing Chinese Medicine, preserving Chinese Drugs'.

Paradoxically, Yu played an instrumental role in forming the field of Chinese medical history. In 1925 he published the ground-breaking treatise entitled 'History of the Transformation of the Old-style Chinese Medical Conception of Tuberculosis.' Instead of promoting a new scholarly discipline, Yu regarded medical history as an important enterprise of the Chinese medical revolution. His exemplary article sought to demonstrate that, even though the Chinese had discovered the contagious nature of tuberculosis almost a thousand years before Robert Koch, this important discovery was concealed under philosophical speculation and nonscientific medical theories. In his view, Chinese medical history should strive to simultaneously boost national pride and discredit the still-prevalent notions of Chinese medicine. Being a founding member and a prolific writer of Chinese medical history, Yu helped shape not only the agenda for historical research but also the contemporary understanding of Chinese medicine.

Bibliography

Primary: 1928, 1937. *Yushi Yishu* 余氏醫書 [Mr. Yu's Essays on Medicine] (aka *Yixue Geming Lunwen* 醫學革命論文 [Essays on Medical Revolution]) 3 vols. (Shanghai).

Secondary: Lei, Sean Hsiang-lin, 2002. 'How Did Chinese Medicine Become Experiential? The Political Epistemology of *jingyan*.' *Positions: East Asian Cultures Critique* 10: 333–364; Zhao, Hongjun, 1991. (trans.

Sivin, Nathan) 'Chinese versus Western Medicine: A History of Their Relations in the Twentieth Century.' *Chinese Science* 10: 21–37.

Sean Hsiang-lin Lei

YUN, TIEQIAO 惲鐵憔 (aka SHUJUE 樹珏) (b.
Taizhou, Wujin county, Jiangsu Province, China 1879; d. Shanghai, China, 26 July 1935), *Chinese medicine, pediatrics.*

Yun Tieqiao was born into a scholarly family. After gaining a metropolitan degree in the old education system at the early age of sixteen, he enrolled at the modern Nanyang Public School 南洋公學 in Shanghai (later Jiaotong University 交通大學), graduating in 1906. Fluent in English, Yun Tieqiao taught briefly before joining the Commercial Press in Shanghai (1911) as a translator of English books. Envisaging a literary career for himself, he edited the *Xiaoshuo yuebao* 小說月報 [Short Story Monthly] , publishing Lu Xun's 魯迅 first short story in 1913.

After the tragic death of three of his children from infectious diseases, Yun decided to become a physician in 1916. He studied traditional medicine as an apprentice of Wang Lianshi 汪蓮石, one of Shanghai's foremost teachers at the time. He also engaged in autodidactic studies, reading widely among both Chinese and Western medical texts. In 1920 he opened his own practice in Shanghai. Quickly gaining a reputation as a specialist in pediatrics, Yun was soon invited to teach at various colleges of Chinese medicine. In 1925 he opened his own college, the Tieqiao Chinese Medicine Correspondence School 鐵憔中醫函授學校, teaching over 1,000 students in the following decade. Yun's enduring reputation, however, rests on his ideas about the nature of Chinese medicine. He was a major influence on several generations of physicians in Republican, Maoist, and Dengist China.

Yun's vision of Chinese medicine took shape in the 1920s as he participated in the increasingly hostile polemics between advocates of Chinese medicine and advocates of Western medicine. Advocates of Western medicine argued that, because Chinese medicine was not based on their principles of science, it had forfeited its right to existence in a modern society. These attacks culminated in an unsuccessful attempt to outlaw the education and practice of Chinese medicine in 1929. Yun Tieqiao argued that advocates of Western medicine had a cultural and political bias and that the rejection of Chinese medical doctrines as superstitious mysticism was founded on an unwillingness to engage with Chinese medicine on its own terms. Western anatomy was superior to that propounded in China's ancient medical classics, but the body described and analyzed in these classics was not the anatomical body of Western medicine: it was a body of process and transformation. Traditional Chinese metaphysics—as expressed most cogently in the *Yi jing* 易經 [Book of Changes]—had concerned itself with formulating general principles of transformation. These principles, he argued, were as unchanging as the laws of nature discovered by Western science and therefore as scientific. Yet, in order to remain relevant, they needed to be interpreted for new contexts. The task of the modern physician of Chinese medicine was therefore to translate the principles elucidated in the medical classics into a practice suitable to a modern age.

True to his principles, Yun Tieqiao actively sought to integrate Western physiological, pathological, and pharmacological knowledge into his medical practice. Yet he also warned that the scientization of Chinese medicine advocated by some of his contemporaries was not an effort at serious translation. The translators always risked losing control over the terms according to which their project was to be carried out. Yun Tieqiao thus not only supplied modern Chinese medicine with its ideological foundation; he also foresaw its enduring crisis.

Bibliography

Primary: 1928. *Yaoan yixue congshu* 藥盦醫學從書 [Medical Collection from the Cloister of Medicinals] (Shanghai).

Secondary: Wu Yunbo 吳云波, 1991. 'Yun Tiaqiao de shenghuo yu xueshu sixiang' 惲鐵憔的生活與學術思想 [The life and scholarship of Yun Tieqiao] *Zhonghua yishi zazhi* 中華醫史雜誌 [Chinese Journal of Medical History] 21: 88–93; Zhang Juyong 章巨庸 and Zhang Peishi 章沛時, 1984. 'Xiansheng Yun Tieqiao dui zuguo yixue de wenxian' 先生惲鐵憔對祖國醫學文獻 [Mr. Yun Tieqiao's contribution to our fatherland's medicine] in *Shanghai zhongyi xueyuan* 上海中醫學院, eds., Jindai zhongyi liupai jingyan xuanji 近代中醫流派經驗選集 [Selected Experiences of Chinese Medicine Currents in the Modern Era] (Shanghai) pp. 106–128; Xiao Gong 肖工 and Liu Yanling 劉延伶, 1983. 'Jiechu de zhongyi lilun jia Yun Tieqiao' 杰出的中醫理論佳惲鐵憔 [Yun Tieqiao, outstanding Chinese-medical theorist] *Yixue yu zhexue* 醫學與哲學 [Medicine and Philosophy] 3: 40–43.

Volker Scheid

YUTHOG YONTAN, THE YOUNGER (aka g.YU-THOG YON-TAN MGON-PO GSAR MA) (b. Central Tibet, 1126; d. ?, 1202), *Tibetan medicine.*

Tibetan medical histories discuss two physicians with the name Yuthog Yontan Gonpo (g.Yu-thog yon-tan mgonpo): the earlier, usually dated to the eighth century, is referred to as 'the Elder'; the second, who is dated to the twelfth century, is called 'the Younger'. Each is known as the 'king of physicians'. Traditional accounts consider Yuthog Yontan the Younger to be a reincarnation of the Elder. The Younger is also said to be a descendant of the same family, representing the tradition of passing knowledge through a family lineage, which was (and still is) a very common way to transmit knowledge of Tibetan medical practices.

Many details in the biographical accounts of Yuthog Yontan the Younger allude to biographical details of the Elder. They both evoked tales of highly realized tantric masters. Yuthog Yontan the Elder, to whom the formulat-

ing stages of Tibetan medicine are credited, is most probably a mythical figure whose accounts were constructed at a
later stage in order to give prevalence to the figure of the
Younger.

As legend has it, gods and other supernatural beings
piled the roof (*thog* in Tibetan) of the g.Yu thog family with
turquoise (*g.Yu* in Tibetan). The affluence accumulated in
this way was handed down to the family's descendants.

Yuthog the Elder

Some Tibetan accounts maintain that Yuthog the Elder
was the one who received the teaching of the *Four Tantra*s.
According to these accounts, Yuthog wrote it down and hid
it inside a pillar in the Samye monastery. Yuthog the Elder
is also known for his part in a famous medical debate that
allegedly took place in Tibet in the eighth century. According to the accounts of this debate, the Tibetan King Tri
Song Detsen (Khri srong lde btsan) invited learned doctors
from India, China, Kashmir, Persia, Nepal, Mongolia, Xin-
jiang, and Afghanistan to join a Tibetan doctor in presenting their medical systems in order to establish which
medical system was the supreme one. Yuthog Yontan represented the Tibetan medical system in the debate and won.
While the historical accuracy of this account may be dubious, it illustrates the contacts and likely influences of
Tibetan medicine.

Yuthog the Elder may have been an ordained monk until
the age of eighty, when he is said to have married in order
to propagate the lineage. He is described as an accomplished *siddha*, who could perform psychic feats that exemplified his miraculous powers. He is regarded in the
Tibetan tradition as an emanation of the speech of the
Medicine Buddha. He is said to have visited India three
times in order to compare the Tibetan medical system with
the Indian one. Even though the historicity of his entire
biography is dubious, including his very existence, the biographical details of the person who is considered to be the
father of Tibetan medicine established some of the basic
components of Tibetan physicians and medicine: a fundamental link with religion, a father-son transmission lineage, and a link between medicine and magic. His
biography is an example of the physician saints of Tibet
and of a holy healer, based on the model of the Medicine
Buddha.

Yuthog the Younger

The Tibetan medical accounts pertaining to Yuthog the
Younger state that he began practicing medicine at the age
of eight. His biography, alluding to that of Yuthog the
Elder, recounted that he possessed superhuman powers
and had the ability to perform miracles.

Sources on Yuthog the Younger recount that he traveled
to India six times in order to verify his medical knowledge.

It is said that he studied the *Caraka saṃhitā* and other Sanskrit works in India and wrote twenty treatises on medicine. He is also said to have visited Sri Lanka in order to
study a local version of the *Four Tantras*. As is common in
Tibetan hagiographical works, facts are tightly weaved with
fiction; it is very difficult to establish which is which. But
the Indian link is highly significant: in Tibetan culture in
general, anything Indian is highly revered, and ascribing an
Indian source is often used as an authenticating device.
Other sources also tell us of Yuthog's travels to Persia,
which may not actually have occurred but which reflect his
possible sources of influence.

Yuthog the Younger's most substantial contribution to
Tibetan medicine was his association with the composition
of the *Four Tantras*, Tibetan medicine's most important
text.

The Four Tantras

The origin and history of the *Four Tantras* (*Gyushi,
rGyu-bzhi*) have been the focus of heated debate among
Tibetan scholars for centuries. In one way or another, all
versions link this important text with either Yuthog Yontan
the Elder or the Younger. One of the traditional Tibetan
positions ascribed the text to the Medicine Buddha and
claims it was written down in Sanskrit and then hidden
inside a column of the Samye monastery, to be found when
the time was ripe for its teaching. As such, it is part of what
are known as the 'treasure texts', known in Tibetan as
'terma' (*gter ma*), prevalent in the *Nyingma* (*rnying ma*)
school of Tibetan Buddhism. According to this account, it
was Yuthog the Younger who later 'discovered' the text and
adapted it to the local conditions of Tibet.

Others deny any Sanskrit original and ascribe the text to
a Tibetan author—either the older or the younger Yuthog
Yontan. This view, the most common currently held view
among Tibetan doctors, ascribes the composition of the
text to Yuthog the Younger.

Scholars now agree that the *Four Tantras* are a native
Tibetan text that has incorporated and synthesized elements from the Indian, Chinese, and Greco-Arab medical
systems. This Tibetan synthesis was combined with a Buddhist grounding; indeed, medicine in the Tibetan context is
classified as belonging to the ten 'Buddhist Sciences'. The
Four Tantras are still taught and practiced in Tibetan and
Tibetan influenced regions such as Tibet, Mongolia, Bhu-
tan, and Buryatia (on Lake Baikal, in the former Soviet
Union, among Kalmyk Mongols), and among the exiled
Tibetan community in India.

The basic premise of Tibetan medicine lies in keeping
the three humors (*nyes pa gsum*) in a dynamic balance. The
three humors are wind (*rlung*), bile (*mkhris pa*), and
phlegm (*bad kan*).

The *Four Tantras*, formally titled *Tantra of Secret Instructions on the Eight Branches of the Essence of the Elixir of*

Immortality, are composed of the *Root Tantra*, the *Exegetical Tantra*, the *Instructional Tantra*, and the *Subsequent Tantra*. The *Root Tantra* presents a general outline of the principles of Tibetan medicine, diagnosis and treatments. It discusses the humors and humoral imbalances that give rise to illnesses. Diagnosis is conducted through visual observation, pulse taking, and inquiry. The *Exegetical Tantra* elaborates on the theoretical basis of Tibetan medicine and discusses such topics as embryology, anatomy, channels of the body, pathology, diet and conduct, medication, external therapy, diagnosis, and medical ethics. The third tantra, the *Instructional Tantra,* focuses on the practical application of medical theories, namely the treatment of different types of diseases and humoral imbalances. The fourth tantra, the *Subsequent Tantra*, is a further elaboration on four topics: diagnosis (through pulse examination, urine analysis, and observation of the tongue); the preparation of medicines; inner cleansing procedures; and external therapies such as bloodletting, moxibustion, massage, and minor surgeries.

Yuthog the Younger is also credited with having written an extensive and important commentary on the *Four Tantras* called 'The Eighteen Supplementary Works' (*Cha lag bco brgyad*).

Bibliography

Primary: Lokesh, Chandra, ed., 1968. *Yuthok's Treatise on Tibetan Medicine* (An edition of the *Cha lag bco brgyad* or *The Eighteen Supplementary Works*) (New Delhi); Rechung Rinpoche, 1973. *Tibetan Medicine Illustrated in Original Texts* (London); Dmu dge bsam gtan gyis brtsams, 1985. *g.Yu thog gsar rnying gi rnam thar bzhigs* [The Life Stories of the Older and Younger g.Yu thog] (Leh); *Bdud rtsi snying po yan lag brgyad pa gsang ba man ngag gi rgyud*, 1993. Bod ljongs mi dmangs dpe skrun khang. [rGyud bzhi—The Four Tantras] (Delhi).

Secondary: Karmay, Samten, 1989. 'Vairocana and the rGyud-bzhi.' *Tibetan Medicine* 12: 19–31; Pa sangs, Yon Tan (Pasang Yonten), 1988. *Bod kyi gso ba rig pa'i lo rgyus kyi bang mdzod gyu thog bla ma dran pa'i pho nya* (Leh); Pa sangs, Yon Tan (Pasang Yonten), 1987. 'A History of the Tibetan Medical System.' *Bulletin of the Indian Institute for the History of Medicine* 17: 130–149.

Ronit Yoeli-Tlalim

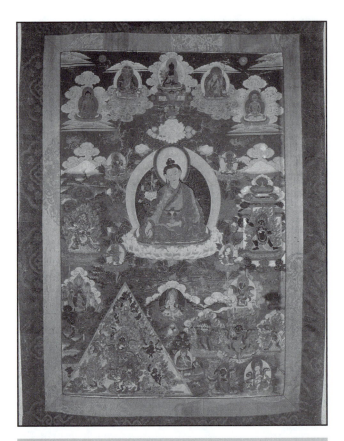

Thangka of Yuthog Yontan Gonpo, who receives the transmission of medical teachings from the Medicine Buddha (sMan-bla, top center). Hayagriva and Vajrapani are to his left and right. Photograph by Mark de Fraeye, Wellcome Photo Library, London.

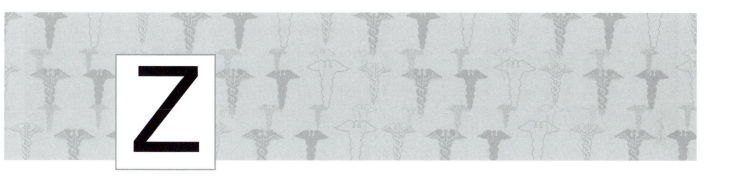

Z

ZACCHIA, PAOLO (b. Rome, Italy, 1584; d. Rome, 1659), *medical jurisprudence.*

Zacchia was the son of Tommaso Zacchia and Giacoma Boncompagna. He began his education with the Fathers of the Scuole Pie, and continued under the Jesuits. In Rome he studied medicine at the Archiginnasio della Sapienza, where he took a degree in medicine. He was also interested in jurisprudence and theology and was a lover of the fine arts and literature. In 1644 Pope Innocent X nominated him as his chief physician and protomedicus of the Papal States, an undertaking he continued under Alexander VII. This position also meant he was the medical expert at the court of the Sacred Roman Rota. He applied himself principally to the study of legal medicine, considerably furthering this branch of studies. He published the first book of his work *Quaestiones medico-legales* in Rome in 1621 and followed this with nine books published between 1625 and 1650.

Quaestiones medico-legales went through several editions and was considered a classic textbook not only in Italy but throughout Europe. It was in effect the first extensive treatise on medical jurisprudence, written not only for physicians but also for jurisconsults (legal experts). The title indicates that the work consisted of questions put by judges to the physician. The work examined all the most important medico-legal problems, starting from those dealing with procreation, marriage, and pregnancy, to those dealing with virginity, rape, impotence, the carrying out of conjugal duties, the duration and period of pregnancy, superfetation (fertilization again after pregnancy, common in some animals including moles), the age and death of the fetus, and the likeness between offspring and their parents. Zacchia stressed the importance of a hydrostatic assay on a dead fetus by floatation, to determine whether it had ever breathed. The book also dealt with injuries to and mutilations of limbs, tortures and punishments, malingering, the professional errors that physicians and pharmacists might make, teratology, miracles, and the precedence between the physician and the jurisconsult.

Zacchia was particularly concerned with mental illnesses, claiming that only a physician was able to judge an individual's mental state. He offered a rather simple and unsophisticated classification of mental deficiency, according to the severity of the defect: the least severe being the obtuse; a rather more severe grade, foolish; the most extreme form, mindless. As for the legal status of the insane, the foolish were excused from the penalties of the law if they committed crimes and they were also debarred from civil actions.

The part that dealt with poisons and poisoning, in effect a systematic treatment of forensic toxicology, was also remarkable. He also looked at sanitary policies, and in particular at environmental hygiene. On the whole, Zacchia proved himself to be a very competent physician and surgeon; he believed that tuberculosis was contagious, claiming that phthisis was a legitimate motive for conjugal separation. The last book was a collection of eighty-five consultations, verdicts, and decisions from the law courts. He also wrote a work on hypochondriasis (1639) in which he identified numerous forms of the condition as well as one on the diet that could be used for Lent (1637). In addition, Zacchia published a poetic translation of the short poem *De ave Phoenice* by Firmiano Lattanzio (1608).

Bibliography

Primary: 1639. *De' mali hipochondriaci* (Rome); 1654. *Quaestiones medico-legales in quibus omnes eae materiae medicae, quae ad legales facultates pertinere videntur, pertractantur et resolvuntur* (Lyon).

Secondary: Pierini, Giovanni, 2001. *Venefici. Dalle 'Quaestiones medico-legalees' di Paolo Zacchia* (Milan); Maeder, Hanspeter, 1981. *Die Frau im 17. Jahrhundert im Spiegel der 'Quaestiones medico-legales' des Paolo Zacchia (1584–1659)*. Inaugural-Dissertation (Bern); Cranefield, Paul F., and Walter Federn, 1970. 'Paulus Zacchias on mental deficiency and on deafness.' *Bulletin of the New York Academy of Medicine* 46: 3–21 [also in Jarcho, Saul, ed., 1976. *Essays and Notes on the History of Medicine* (New York) pp. 118–136].

Giuseppe Ongaro

AL-ZAHRĀWĪ, ABU AL-QĀSIM KHALAF IBN 'ABBĀS (AKA ALBUCASIS) (b. al-Zahrā', near Cordova, Spain, c. 936; d. al-Zahrā', c. 1013), *medicine, surgery.*

Surprisingly little is definitely known of one of the greatest Hispano-Arabic medical practitioners, Zahrāwī.

He was born in al-Zahrā', the royal city near Cordoba, but the additional name al-Ansari, given to him in the manuscripts, shows that his family claimed to have originated in Medina. There is no contemporary evidence for the later stories that make him personal physician to 'Abd ar-Raḥmān III (r. 912–61), his son and successor al-Ḥakam II al-Mustanṣir (r. 961–76), or al-Manṣūr (r. 976–1002). It is supposed that he refrained from mentioning any such appointment out of modesty. All the information about his achievements is collected from his own writings. He operated brilliantly and considered the art of surgery to be one of the decisive skills of a practitioner. He attributed the decline of the art of surgery during his own time to the negligence of the scribes and copyists who produced learned books. He held the ancients in great esteem and drew on their writings, especially those of Paul of Aegina. He also certainly relied upon on his own experience.

Modern scholars ascribe to Zahrāwī the introduction of new practices that continue today, e.g., the use of catgut in abdominal surgery and operations on the pelvis. He introduced to Western medical practice the removal of cataracts, and he laid the foundations for topical cauterization in many surgical operations. He also designed various devices and instruments for surgical treatment and, importantly, drew their images. These included the guillotine and its use, the concealed knife, the trocar for paracentesis (removing fluid that has accumulated in the abdominal cavity), the lithotrite (for crushing stones in the bladder/ urethra), and the vaginal speculum.

His major work, consisting of thirty books (*maqāla*), is the *Kitāb at-taṣrīf li-man 'ajiza 'an al-ta'līf* [The Arrangements. For those who are unable to compile (a manual for themselves)]. Half of the work comprises books on physiology, nosology, and surgical instruments. The book on the instruments and their use has always been of particular interest. It was swiftly translated into Latin by Gerhard of Cremona and was among the first books on medicine to be printed in the fifteenth century. It was subsequently translated into many other European and Oriental languages.

Bibliography

Primary: Spink, M. S., and G. L. Lewis, 1973. *Abulcasis on Surgery and Instruments: A Definitive Edition of the Arabic Text with English Translation and Commentary* (London).

Secondary: Buniyatov, Z. M., 1987. (Foreword to) *Abu-l-Kasim al-Zakhravi. Traktat o khirurgïilinstrumentakh.* Per. s arab. (Moscow); Ullmann, Manfred, 1978. *Islamic Medicine* trans. Watt, Jean (Edinburgh).

Nikolaj Serikoff

ZAKHAR'IN, GRIGORII ANTONOVICH (b. Saratov province, Russia, 8 February 1829; d. Cetine, Serbia, 23 December 1897), *therapeutics.*

Zakhar'in, son of an impoverished landlord and former cavalry officer, Anton Zakhar'in, studied at the Saratov gymnasium and Moscow University from 1847 to 1852. Zakhar'in then worked as a general physician in the faculty clinic for therapeutics, directed by Alexander Ivanovich Over. In 1854 he defended his dissertation on the theme 'De puerperii morbis'. From 1854 to 1859 Zakhar'in was in Europe, where he updated his knowledge in clinical medicine, including pediatrics, gynecology, urology, and otolaryngology. Those with whom he trained included Sergey Petrovich Botkin, Rudolf Virchow, Ludwig Traube, Johann Oppolzer, Ernst-Felix Hoppe-Seyler, and Joseph Skoda in Berlin and Vienna, and Armand Trousseau and Claude Bernard in Paris. His greatest inspiration came from the ideas of Virchow and René Laennec. After returning to Russia in 1860, he lectured on semiotics and general therapeutics at Moscow University. After the death of Over in 1864, Zakhar'in headed the clinics and put into practice the laboratory investigations and the methods of percussion and auscultation for the physical examination of patients. He was a supporter of the differentiation of clinical medicine, reserving in his clinics two wards for children's diseases (1866) and some beds for women's diseases (1875). Zakhar'in read the works of European scientists regularly and was interested in bacteriology in the last years of his life.

In his clinical practice he developed the method of interrogating the patient, gathering details about the patient's life, habits, and heredity. Zakhar'in preferred prolonged interrogations: he could then establish the 'diagnosis morbi' as well as the 'diagnosis aegri' (i.e., the main and attendant diagnoses). Along with Henry Head, he believed that the illnesses of internal organs appear as severe hyperesthesia of certain zones of the dermis or the surface of the body. These became known as Zakhar'in-Head zones.

Zakhar'in worked out methods of differential diagnostics for tuberculosis of the lungs and syphilitic pneumonia and the clinical semiotics for the syphilis of the heart. He also elaborated the classification of tuberculosis of the lungs. He distinguished chlorosis as a special endocrinal disorder caused by nervous disturbance, and he believed that gallstone disease had an infectious nature.

He believed therapeutics must eliminate the cause of disease, but he also used treatment by symptom. He put new cures into practice but only after prolonged examination. In the process of therapeutics he used only one cure, addressing treatment by climate, mineral water, and bloodletting. He recommended his patients maintain strict personal hygiene and diet. Zakhar'in often used calomel as a remedy for diseases of the liver.

Zakhar'in's patients came from the Russian elite and included writers such as Lev (Leo) Tolstoy. Zakhar'in was a physician of Tsar Alexander III, whom he helped in the last days of his life in 1894 in the Crimea. Zakhar'in also sometimes had poor patients, whom he supported materially.

Zakhar'in's creative legacy consists of only forty-four works, six of which were published in France and Germany. His important *Klinicheskie lektsii* [Clinical lectures] (beginning in 1889) were very popular for many years, and he was a talented lecturer. In 1852 Zakhar'in translated into Russian and published eight works of European authors, including those of Virchow and Bernard.

As a scientist Zakhar'in won popularity with his appearance at the Moscow Physical-Medical Society in the 1870s. Zakhar'in preached the building of health resorts within the territory of Russia and he was a supporter of the development of school hygiene.

In the last years of his life Zakhar'in's political views became conservative, and he was often in conflict with Moscow students and liberal professors, including Friedrich Erisman, who reproached him for reactionism, rudeness, and love of money. Morally isolated, Zakhar'in left the university in 1896. Before his death Zakhar'in passed on 500,000 rubles for the building of rural schools in Saratov and Penza provinces and a water system in Serbia.

He founded the Moscow clinical school, from which many important activists of Russian medicine emerged, including therapists Count Nikolai Fedorovich Golubov and Alexei Alexsandroch Ostroumov, pediatrician Nil Fedorovich Filatov, and gynecologist Vladimir Fedorovich Snegirev.

Bibliography

Primary: 1889–94. *Klinicheskie lektsii* [Clinical Lectures] 4 vols. (Moscow) [English trans., 1899 (Boston)]; 1909. *Klinicheskie lektsii i izbrannye stat'i* [Clinical Lectures and Collected Articles] (Moscow).

Secondary: Lushnikov, Aleksandr Georgievich, 1974. *G. A. Zakhar'in (1829–1897)* (Moscow); Gukasian, Aram Grigorievich, 1948. *Grigorii Antonovich Zakhar'in* (Moscow); Golubov, Nikolay Fedorovich, 1927. 'Grigorii Antonovich Zakhar'in.' *Vrachebnoe delo* 3: 161–168.

Dmitry Mikhel

ZAKRZEWSKA, MARIE ELIZABETH   (b. Berlin, Germany, 6 September 1829; d. Boston, Massachusetts, USA, 12 May 1902), *midwifery, medicine, hospital administration.*

Zakrzewska, daughter of Ludwig Martin Zakrzewski, a Prussian civil servant, and Caroline F. W. Urban, a midwife, studied and practiced midwifery at the Royal Charité hospital in Berlin (1850–52) before emigrating to the United States, where she received her MD at Western Reserve College in Cleveland in 1856. She was one of only six women who graduated from this traditionally all-male medical school in the 1850s. She helped Elizabeth (1821–1910) and Emily (1826–1910) Blackwell found and run the New York Infirmary for Indigent Women and Children between 1857 and 1859, and she worked as professor of obstetrics and director of a new clinical department at the New England Female College in Boston from 1859 to 1862. Finally, in 1862, she founded the New England Hospital for Women and Children with the help of many prominent Boston social reformers. There Zakrzewska practiced medicine and trained generations of women physicians until a few years before her death.

Under Zakrzewska's leadership, the New England Hospital grew to be an important symbol of American women's success in challenging the barriers that had been erected to keep them out of the medical profession. Like the New York Infirmary, it was staffed solely by women; it offered medical care to women and children by practitioners of their own sex; and it provided medical students and recent graduates clinical experience at a time when most medical schools and teaching hospitals remained closed to them. Zakrzewska served as resident physician during the first few years of the hospital's existence, as attending physician until 1887, and then as advisory physician until her retirement in 1893, but for all intents and purposes she ran the hospital during this entire period. Committed to orthodox medicine and familiar with the German system of medical education, Zakrzewska had her students charting patient temperatures, pulse rates, and rates of respiration earlier than at most other teaching hospitals. She also implemented hygienic measures that kept the mortality rate from puerperal fever extremely low. As a result, she earned the respect of Boston's medical elite.

Zakrzewska stood out among her female contemporaries (and indeed among many of her male colleagues) for her early praise of German scientific medicine. At a time when most women physicians insisted that they were uniquely positioned to find a balance between sympathy and science, Zakrzewska argued that too much sympathy confused one's ability to make rational decisions, resulting in poor medical care. Her reasons for promoting science, however, went beyond her ideas on proper medical training. A political radical, Zakrzewska viewed science as a weapon in a battle against the antidemocratic forces of religion (especially the Catholic Church) and arbitrary authority.

In her personal life, Zakrzewska flouted middle-class conventions by rejecting the institution of marriage and creating instead a family centered around two individuals: Karl Heinzen, a German radical émigré and political journalist, who (along with his wife and child) shared Zakrzewska's home for twenty years; and Julia A. Sprague, a women's rights reformer, who lived together with Zakrzewska for forty years. For her outspoken views, and for the large number of interns and residents who trained in her hospital, Zakrzewska earned a reputation as one of the most prominent female physicians of the American nineteenth century.

Bibliography

Primary: 1860. (Dall, Caroline Healey, ed.) *A Practical Illustration of "Woman's Right to Labor"* (Boston).

Secondary: Tuchman, Arleen Marcia, 1999. '"Only in a republic can it be proved that science has no sex": Marie E. Zakrzewska (1829–1902) and the Multiple Meanings of Science.' *Journal of Women's History* 11(1): 121–142; Drachman, Virginia G., 1984. *Hospital with a Heart. Women Doctors and the Paradox of Separatism at the New England Hospital 1862–1969* (Ithaca, NY); Vietor, Agnes, ed., 1924. *A Woman's Quest: The Life of Marie E. Zakrzewska M.D.* (New York) (reprinted 1972).

Arleen Marcia Tuchman

ZEISS, HEINRICH (HEINZ) (b. Frankfurt am Main, Germany, 12 July 1888; d. Vladimir, USSR, 31 March 1949), *hygiene, Nazi medicine.*

After attending school Zeiss started his medical studies at Marburg in 1907 and continued at Heidelberg, Freiburg, Berlin, and Munich. At Freiburg he graduated as an MD in 1912. Visiting different universities of the country as Zeiss did was a peregrinatio academica typical for the period before World War I. His first post in 1912 was that of Assistant to Rudolf Otto Neumann at the Institute of Hygiene of Giessen University. He then left for the Friedrichstadt hospital at Dresden. After seven months (1913–14) he volunteered for the Royal Saxon Army, serving as voluntary physician and auxiliary physician of the reserve. He finally received training in tropical medicine at the Hamburg Institute for Tropical Medicine under Martin Mayer (May–July 1914).

With the outbreak of war Zeiss's studies were interrupted. Now twenty-seven years old and a military physician of the reserve, he first went to the Western front in France and then to the Eastern front in Russia. In October 1915 Zeiss was sent to the German military mission in Turkey at the Turkish high command of the military medical service. In spring 1916 he was subordinated to Ernst Rodenwaldt (1878–1965), the consultant hygienist of the 5th Turkish army in Western Asia Minor, and later he occupied the same post under Victor Schilling (1883–1960), the hygienist for the 4th Turkish army in Syria and Western Arabia. In March 1918 Zeiss returned to Dresden, where he continued to serve in the army, until he returned to the Hamburg Institute for Tropical Medicine in March 1919.

The year 1921 was of decisive importance for Zeiss's later life. In September he set out for the Soviet Union as a member of the relief expedition of the German Red Cross, under the direction of Peter Mühlens. Zeiss and Mühlens had met each other during World War I and at the Hamburg Institute for Tropical Diseases. Zeiss was made head of the central authorities for bacteriology of the German Red Cross in Moscow. When the mission ended, and after qualifying as university lecturer for tropical medicine at Hamburg University in 1924, Zeiss entered the Soviet service at the request of N. A. Semashko (1874–1949), high commissioner of the Soviet health system, and functioned as head of the department at the Institute for Chemical and Pharmaceutical Research of the Supreme Economic Council from 1 October 1924 until 30 September 1925. Subsequently, beginning in October 1925, he was in charge of the Microbiological Museum of Living Cultures at the Tarassevitsh Institute for Experimental Therapy and Serum Control under Professor Diatroptov. As head of the museum, Zeiss supervised a considerable collection of living cultures of pathogens. In 1932 he left the Soviet Union.

Even before his departure from the Soviet Union, Zeiss was a member of the DNVP, a party representing national conservative ideas. He sympathized with the Nazi movement under Adolf Hitler during the late 1920s and finally joined the NSDAP in 1931. Internal party politics were not his business, although his ideas on the field of hygiene did closely follow Nazi racial policy, as exemplified in his book *Einführung in die Hygiene und Seuchenlehre* (1936–1943), copublished with Ernst Rodenwaldt. The two scientists are regarded as the fathers of the so-called Geomedizin. In the beginning, this geographical, anthropological, and political view of epidemic and hygienic questions was oriented toward Geopolitics [Haushofer] both in its terminology and its content.

In 1933 Zeiss was appointed associate professor and vice-director of the Berlin Institute of Hygiene. There he was finally called to the chair as full professor in 1937. Beginning in 1934 he was a member of the Scientific Senate for Military Medicine at the Reich Research Council and simultaneously joined the Academy for Military Medicine, linked closely to the military health inspection (Heeressanitätsinspektion). During World War II Zeiss functioned as consultant hygienist in Bulgaria and Greece. Shortly after the war, on 2 November 1945, he was arrested in the Russian part of Berlin. On 10 July 1948 he was accused of espionage against the Soviet Union and was sentenced to twenty-five years of imprisonment. When Zeiss died on 31 March 1949 at Vladimir, USSR, after a chronic infection, he was suffering severely from Parkinson's disease.

Bibliography

Secondary: Weindling, Paul, 1995. 'Heinrich Zeiss' in Eckart, Wolfgang U., and Christoph Gradmann, eds., *Ärztelexikon* (Munich) pp. 389–390; Eckart, Wolfgang U., 2006. 'Creating Confidence: Heinz Zeiss as a Traveller in the Soviet Union, 1921–1932' in Solomon, Susan Gross, ed., *Doing Medicine Together: Germany and Russia between the Wars* (Toronto).

Wolfgang U. Eckart

ZHANG, JIEBIN 張介賓 (aka HUIQING 會卿, JINGYUE 景岳, TONG 通) (b. Shaoxing, Shanyin county, Zhejiang Province, China, 1563; d. Shaoxing, 1640), *Chinese medicine.*

Originally from the southwestern province of Sichuan, Zhang Jiebin's family moved to modern-day Shaoxing in Zhejiang Province, where the Ming government posted his father as a Guard Commander. When he was thirteen *sui* (about twelve), he went to Beijing with his father, who was on official business as an advisor to a high military official. During the late 1570s in Beijing, Zhang began studying medicine with a physician named Jin Ying 金英 (Mengshi 夢石), who advocated restorative formulas for strengthening one's constitutional *qi* (*dabu yuanqi* 大補元氣). Zhang's later emphasis on warming and restorative formulas (*wenbu* 溫補), especially for the kidneys, may well have formed during his early tutelage with Dr Jin.

Following a rather peripatetic life of traveling between Beijing and northeastern China to Korea as well as practicing medicine in Beijing, Zhang moved back to Shaoxing in 1620 (in his late 50s); there he lived his remaining twenty years. In 1624 the Suzhou publisher Tong Yongquan 童湧泉 (c. early seventeenth century) helped Zhang publish his first medical book, an innovative reorganization of chapters in the *Inner Canon of the Yellow Emperor: Basic Questions and Divine Pivot* (c. first century BCE) titled simply the *Leijing* 類經 [Classified Canon]. In the same year, he published two related volumes: the *Leijing fuyi* 類經附翼 [Supplementary Commentary of the Classified Canon] and the *Leijing tuyi* 類經圖翼 [Illustrated Commentary of the Classified Canon]. His commentary on the *Inner Canon* differed from all previous scholarship in that he reorganized the canon along more practical lines and

went beyond commentary and diagrams to refine, change, and develop its myriad concepts. In the earliest biography of Zhang Jiebin, the prolific early-Qing scholar Huang Zongxi 黃宗羲 (1610–95) commented on how popular and erudite the *Classified Canon* was during his time. Zhang wrote two other medical texts, both posthumously published: a comprehensive medical treatise on all diseases titled the *Jingyue quanshu* 景岳全書 [Complete Works of Jingyue] (1700) and a collection of essays on various medical issues titled the *Record of Zhiyi lu* 質疑錄 [(Things) Called into Question] (1688).

Zhang reorganized and created diagrams for the *Inner Canon* in response to a broader medical debate on how limited the *Inner Canon* was for dealing with new contemporary illnesses and regional variations in morbidity. Contemporary scholarship in Han learning that sought to recover the authentic texts of Chinese antiquity from later corruptions inspired some Ming physicians to apply philological methods to separate the authentic Han passages of the *Inner Canon* from later interpolations and revisions. Zhang Jiebin supported the relevance of the *Inner Canon* for present medical practice, yet criticized physicians who oversimplified it and promoted their own biased perspectives. In contrast to his literal-minded contemporaries, who sought a solution to the controversy through recovery of the original passages and structure of the *Inner Canon*, however, Zhang thought that revering the *Inner Canon* was not the same as rigidly adhering to it. He instead reorganized, refined, developed, and diagrammed complex concepts in the *Inner Canon* to facilitate its practical use. He had a ready audience among physicians writing on the *Inner Canon* in south China and literate men purchasing texts on the 'medical canons' (*yijing* 醫經). The emphasis among physicians in the urban centers of Hangzhou and Shaoxing of Zhejiang province during the late Ming was on the classical medical canons of antiquity, especially the *Inner Canon*. Zhejiang province, where Zhang grew up and later returned to practice medicine, was the regional focus of a surge in publications on the *Inner Canon*. Zhang's text was just one of twenty-three new Ming medical texts on the *Inner Canon* that other Zhejiang physicians had published. Well ensconced in the Zhejiang medical community, Zhang Jiebin was a key player in these contemporary debates on the *Inner Canon* and an influential author in the attempt among physicians in his region to recast the *Inner Canon* for the current age.

Bibliography

Primary: 1624. *Leijing* 類經 [Classified Canon], *Leijing fu yi* 類經附翼 [Supplementary Commentary of the Classified Canon], *Leijing tu yi* 類經圖翼 [Illustrated Commentary of the Classified Canon] in Li Zhiyong, ed., 1999. *Zhang Jingyue yixue quan shu* pp. 1–811; 1671. *Nanlei wen'an* 南雷文案 [Literary essays of the Southern Thunder Peak], Huang Zongxi 黃宗羲: 9/5a; 1688. *Zhiyi lu* 質疑錄 [Record of (Things) Called into Question] in

Li Zhiyong, ed., 1999. *Zhang Jingyue yixue quan shu* pp. 1833–1857; 1688. 'Zhang Jingyue zhuan' 張景岳專, in *Zhiyi lu* 質疑錄 [Record of (Things) Called into Question], by Huang Zongxi; 1700. *Jingyue quanshu* 景岳全書 [Complete Works of Jingyue] in Li Zhiyong, ed., 1999. *Zhang Jingyue yixue quan shu* pp. 813–1831; 1728. 'Yishu mingliu liezhuan shisi ming ba' 醫術名流傳十四明八, *juan* 537, in *Gujin tushu jicheng* 古今圖書集成, *yijia lei* 醫家類, ed. Chen Menglei 陳夢雷.

Secondary: Li Zhiyong 李志庸, ed., 1999. *Zhang Jingyue yixue quan shu* 張景岳醫學全書 [Complete Medical Works of Zhang Jingyue], *Ming Qing mingyi quanshu dacheng* 明清名醫全書大成 series (Beijing); Ts'ui, C. H., 1991. 'Chang Chieh-pin' in Hummel, Arthur W., ed., *Eminent Chinese of the Ch'ing Period* vol. 1 (Taiwan) pp. 26–27.

Marta E. Hanson

ZHANG, YUANSU 張元素 (aka JIEGU 潔古) (b. Yishui, Hebei Province, China, 1151; d. ?, 1234), *Chinese medicine, pharmacology.*

Zhang Yuansu was born in turbulent times, as the Jin 金 armies invaded the north of China in 1115 and drove the reigning Song court to the south, where they established their new capital in Hangzhou. Despite having read the Confucian classics at an early age, at twenty-seven he failed the Jinshi 進士 [presented scholar] degree, which would have allowed him entry to the civil service. He did not pursue an official career but focused on studying medicine.

According to medieval and contemporary medical writers, Zhang is credited with important medical innovations during the Song dynasty. He brought the 'empirical' traditions of pharmacotherapy together with the medicine of systematic correspondence and channel theory conceived in the context of acupuncture a millennium before his time. However, his innovations should be understood in the context of a universal effort for the integration of Buddhist and Daoist thinking into the reconfiguration of Confucianism, known as the Neoconfucian movement in the West.

New technologies made possible the printing of 'corrected versions' of canonical texts in large editions. The first two emperors of the Song dynasty actively promoted the compilation of collections of formulas, and official sponsorship of big collections characterized the period. An enhanced level of quality control was met by the introduction of pictures of plants into pharmacological works, thereby fulfilling the standards of a new practical rationalism.

In this spirit Zhang created new formulas on the basis of classical prescriptions, e.g., *Jia jian baitong tang* 加減白通湯 [Scallion Yang-Freeing Variant Decoction] based on the classical *Baitong tang* 白通湯 [Scallion Yang-Freeing Decoction] and *Lizhong tang* 理中湯 [Center-Rectifying Decoction]. His innovative prescriptions followed a system he had devised to categorize herbs according to the Five Agents, describing how each herb had an affinity to, and could exert a strong influence on, a specific acupuncture channel. He also established the concept of the so-called shiyao 使藥 [messenger herb], an ingredient in a complex prescription that could help introduce other herbs into a channel (e.g., *notopterygii rhizoma* for the hand and foot taiyang 手足太陽 channel). He believed that a herb had a very specific affinity to a channel and could also replenish or drain different organs; thus a sour herb such as *paeonia radix alba* had an astringent effect on the lung but also drained the liver in conditions of excess.

The *Yixue qi yuan* 醫學起源 [The source of medicine], Zhang's magnum opus of 1186, summarized his theory of medicine in three chapters: the first contained a theoretical treatise on the Five Agents and the six *qi*; the second was a commentary on the *Huangdi Neijing* 黃帝内經 [Yellow Emperor's Inner Canon]; the third a systematization of materia medica. Forty-three formulas are traditional, and thirty-eight are prescriptions composed by Zhang himself or by his teacher Liu Wansu 劉完素 (1110 or 1120–1200), who is known as the founder of the *hanliang xuepai* 寒涼學派 [cooling school].

Among the eminent physicians of the *Yishui xuepai* 易水學派 [the school of medical thought named after Zhang Yuansu's birthplace] the outstanding student Li Gao 李杲 (1180–1251/2) created an influential Yishui tradition, the *piwei xuepai* 脾胃學派 [Spleen-stomach-school], his *leitmotif* being, 'The inner damage of spleen and stomach is the cause of all [kinds of] diseases.'

Taking into account the political situation in which Zhang formulated his integrated theories of pharmacology, his viewpoint can be interpreted as a stand for political unity faced with the threat of the dissolution of the empire.

Bibliography

Primary: 1186. *Yixue qiyuan* [The source of medicine] Lu Guangming 盧光明 et al., eds., 2000. *Zhonghua yishu jicheng* 中華醫書集成 [Compilation of Chinese medical books] vol. 22.

Secondary: Gu Shengdong 谷勝東, 2003. 'Jin Yuan shiqi shehui yinsu dui fangjixue fazhande yingxiang' 金元時期社會因素對方劑學發展的影響 [The influence of social constituents in the Jin and Yuan period on the development of formula composition]. *Journal of the History of Chinese Medicine* 33: 155–159.

Franz Zehentmayr

ZHU, LIAN 朱璉 (b. Liyang, Jiangsu, China, 1909; d. Nanning, Guangxi, China 18 May 1978), *acupuncture, public health.*

Zhu Lian was a doctor trained in Western medicine who joined the Chinese Communist Party in 1935 and served the Party as deputy leader of the General Health Department of the 129th Division of the Eighth Route Army (八路軍一二九師衛生部). During the time of Yan'an (1935–47), Zhu Lian served as deputy director of the Yan'an China Medical University (延安中国医科大学), head of the General Health Department outpatient section of the

Eighteenth Group Army in Yan'an (延安十八集团军总卫生部), adviser on child welfare to the People's Government of the Shaanxi-Gansu-Ningxia border region, head of the People's Government Ministry of Health in the Shaanxi-Hebei-Shandong-Henan border region, and director of the hospitals in this border region. After Liberation in 1949, Zhu Lian became deputy director of the Maternity and Child Hygiene Section of the Ministry of Health (卫生部妇幼卫生司). She also became deputy director of the Beijing Research Academy of Traditional Chinese Medicine when it was set up in 1955, and head of the Acupuncture Research Center at the same school. She held these positions until 1960, when she was transferred to the Guangxi Autonomous Region to work in public health service.

Zhu Lian is most known for her book *The New Acupuncture* (1951, second edition 1954), a fine hard-bound volume that went through two reprints at a time when publishing was a luxury in a China recovering from over two decades of war. This book set a new precedent in Chinese medical literature as a government-supported volume written by a doctor trained in Western medicine using traditional Chinese healing methods that were rigorously reworked according to the political and scientific precepts of the day.

Responding to a call from Mao Zedong made in the Yan'an base area in 1944 for the 'scientification of Chinese medicine and the popularization of Western medicine (中医科学化, 西医大众化), Zhu Lian set out to raise the level of Chinese medicine by doing away with its feudal, superstitious roots and replacing it with the Soviet scientist Ivan Pavlov's (1849–1936) more politically correct theory of the advanced function of the nerves (高级神经活动). Zhu Lian's medicine was indelibly influenced by war. She discarded the age-long pattern of the flow of the meridians and reorganized the acupuncture points along truncated 'lines (线)' or in 'areas (区)' along the body. The vocabulary and spatial layout used in *The New Acupuncture* reflected the military times during which this medicine was created.

Zhu Lian's new acupuncture was celebrated as the type of medical hybrid that the revolution had called for, but after the establishment of the People's Republic of China in 1949, it soon fell out of favor and a more cautious approach was adopted to interpreting traditional Chinese medical principles.

Bibliography

Primary: 14 March 1949. 'Myself and Acupuncture 我与针灸学.' *People's Daily* 人民日报; 17–18 February 1951. 'The Importance of Acupuncture Therapeutics and its Principles 针灸疗法的重要性及其原理.' *People's Daily* 人民日报; 1951 (2nd ed., 1954). *The New Acupuncture* 新针灸学 (Beijing).

Secondary: Taylor, Kim, 2005. *Chinese Medicine in Early Communist China, 1945–63: A Medicine of Revolution* (London); Li Yun 李云, ed., 1988. *Biographical Dictionary of Chinese Medicine* 中医人民词典 (Beijing); Tang Xuezheng 唐学正, 1951. *A Study of the New Acupuncture* 学习新针灸学 (Beijing).

Kim Taylor

ZHU, ZHENHENG 朱震亨 (aka ZHU, DANXI 朱丹溪)

(b. Wuzhou prefecture, Zhejiang Province, China, 9 January 1282; d. Wuzhou, China, 24 June 1358), *Chinese medicine*.

Zhu Zhenheng was the last and perhaps the greatest of the *Jin Yuan si dajia* 金元四大家 [Four Masters of Medicine in the Jin Yuan], innovators who overturned the orthodoxy of Song state-medicine's prescription art. He is credited with harmonizing the styles of prescription of the other 'masters' into a credible synthesis, while also popularizing a regionally inflected medicine based on North/South differences. In addition, as a native Southerner and a literatus schooled in *Daoxue* 道學, the neo-Confucian philosophy of the Way after Zhu Xi 朱熹, his life served as an influential model for the *ruyi* 儒醫 'scholar physician' ideal. Neo-Confucianism also shaped his reading of the classic *Yellow Emperor's Inner Canon* through the lens of Zhou Dunyi's 周敦頤 cosmology and Zhu Xi's ethics. His medical doctrines and therapeutic strategies were widespread in Jiangnan (Southern) elite practice between the fourteenth and sixteenth centuries, spreading also to Korea and Japan.

Zhu came from a prominent local lineage. After failing the mid-level *juren* 舉人 imperial examinations in his mid thirties, he abandoned classical studies and pursued medicine. Spurred by the ignorance of local physicians, whose practice relied on a few memorized formulas, he traveled to Hangzhou to become the disciple of the reclusive Luo Zhiti 羅知悌 and learned of the Northern 'Jin-Yuan masters'. Back in Wuzhou, he quickly gained fame for combining clinical mastery with respect for textual learning from the medical canon and insistence upon the moral dimensions of bodily self-cultivation—founding doctrines of the 'scholar physician' identity. During his lifetime, his prestige was based less on his success with patients than on his activities for his kin-group and friendships with such leading scholars of the day as Song Lian 宋濂. To these arbiters of local society, Zhu's asceticism and service to the community as a physician were marks of both a gentlemanly self cultivation in humility and the sage pursuit of the Confucian Way in obscurity.

Zhu's therapeutic motto, 'Yang is always in excess; Yin is always deficient,' evoked a Yin Yang body out of balance where, rather than encompassing Yin in a benign hierarchy, Yang power was always a potential source of destructive instability. His was a feminized Southern body—Han, not 'barbarian'—naturally delicate, in which Yin Water (fluids associated with generative centers) needed protection against the Yang internal heat of human desires and emotions as well as against the desiccating force of pathogenic environmental *qi.* In pharmacy, Zhu's signature strategy was to 'nourish Yin and make Fire descend'. Using quotations from the *Yellow Emperor's Inner Canon* to explicate this maxim, Zhu gave ethical significance to two of the classic 'six *qi*' (renamed Princely Fire 君火 and Ministerial Fire 相火) interpreted as primary vitalities governing the heart and consciousness above and kidney and generative energy below. Clinically the maxim taught doctors to prescribe mild and gentle doses designed to preserve the body's fluids. His formulas for phlegm [*tan* 痰] and damp heat [*shishi* 濕熱] were considered well suited to the illnesses of the humid Southeast.

Zhu was not from a hereditary medical family but was self-taught, enhancing his prestige as a 'scholar physician'. He taught what later came to be lineages propagating his school of medical thought. His students included his son and nephew, as well as Dai Shishi 戴士世 and his two sons, Dai Wen 戴溫 and Dai Yuanli 戴原禮. Dai Yuanli (1324–1405), Zhu's favorite, later served the founding Ming emperor as court physician, and his lineage was a leading transmitter of Zhu's teachings to the influential Ming network of Huizhou doctors around Wang Ji 汪機.

Zhu wrote little apart from two medical essays completed in 1347 at the behest of his disciples: *Jufang fahui* 局方發揮 [Exposé of Official Prescriptions], his critique of Song pharmacy; and *Ge zhi yu lun* 格致餘論 [Further Views on Extending Knowledge], the outline of his basic doctrines, including his incorporation of neo-Confucian philosophy into medical cosmology. Over the next 200 years several lineages of his medical followers published compendia based on his pharmacy, while the records of more than 100 of his best-known medical cases found their way into the widely circulated late Ming (1552) anthology of Jiang Guan 江瓘, *Ming yi lei an* 名醫類案 [Classified Case Histories of Famous Doctors]. The major sources for his life are a funerary commemorative essay composed by his friend Song Lian, and a memoir by Dai Liang 戴良, brother and uncle of Zhu's medical disciples.

Bibliography

Primary: 1993–1995. *Collected Medical Works of Zhu Danxi (Danxi yiji* 丹溪醫集) (Compiled by the Literature Research Division of the Zhejiang Provincial Academy of Chinese Medicine 浙江省中醫研究院文獻研究室).

Secondary: Furth, Charlotte, 2006. 'The Physician as Philosopher of the Way: Zhu Zhenheng (1282–1368).' *Harvard Journal of Asian Studies* 66(2); He Shixi 何時希, 1991. *Zhongguo lidai yijia chuanlu* 中國歷代醫家傳錄. 1: 247–258.

Charlotte Furth

ZINNIS, ANASTASIOS (b. Ioannina, Ottoman Empire [now Greece], 1829; d. Athens, Greece, 1899), *pediatrics.*

Zinnis studied pediatrics in Paris between 1856 and 1858 under Eugène Bouchut, Guillot, and Blache. In 1858 he settled in Athens, and the following year he was placed in charge of the newly established State Infant Institution of Athens, which also served as the pediatric clinic of the Athens University Medical School. The State Infant Institution was an early initiative of a philanthropic movement dedicated to protecting the physical and moral well-being of poor abandoned children from the high death rate reducing their numbers. To philanthropic activists, the welfare, care, and education of children who have no record of birth and no formal means of protection constituted an important social mission. Such children were typically regarded with some anxiety as incarnations of future disorder, and many believed it was necessary to transform them into 'apostles' who would stabilize the poor population and 'restore' the lower-class community, thus promoting a more secure public order and social unity.

As chairman of the State Infant Institution, Zinnis systematically recorded the number of infants entering the institution, documenting the phenomenal extent of infant abandonment during the last decades in the nineteenth century. He also closely monitored and studied the mortality rate, causes, and means for combating and reducing the rate of infant abandonment. In 1879 Zinnis became temporary professor at the Athens University Medical School and in 1881 a regular professor.

Zinnis regarded diarrhea as the most lethal illness affecting infants; he supported the notion that teething was the main cause of children's diarrhea, that it was aggravated by high summer temperatures but was due mainly to inadequate breastfeeding, improper diet, and problems of peptic ability during early infancy (i.e., five to six months old). Like other doctors of his time, Zinnis exhorted mothers of well-off families to breastfeed their own children (rather than having the children breastfed by servants), while also joining in a 'true crusade' to abolish superstitions and 'nonsensical everyday practices' of child rearing among of the lower classes.

Zinnis was undoubtedly one of the most prominent researchers of pediatric illnesses in his time and was the founder of pediatrics in Greece. Many of his books (some written in French) received awards from the Paris Medical Academy.

Bibliography

Primary: 1877. *De la mortalité chez les enfants à la mamelle à Athènes* [The infant death rate in Athens] (Athens); 1878. *De la prophylaxie des maladies contagieuses* [On the precaution against contagious children's illnesses] (Athens); 1880. *Étude sur les principales causes léthifères chez les enfants au-dessous de cinq ans, et plus spécialement chez ceux de 0-1 an à Athènes* [Study in relation to the main cause of death of the children in Athens] (Athens); 1881. *Principale cause de l'excessive mortalité chez les enfants-trouvés et moyens d'y remédier* [Main cause of the exceptionally high death rate of the abandoned children and the precaution for prevention] (Athens); 1882. *On the appropriate precautions for prevention of illnesses relating to children's breathing organs* (Athens); 1883. *Du rôle de la dentition dans la pathologie enfantine* [On the effects of tooth growth and its related illness of infants] (Athens); 1885. *Du traitement de la diarrhée chronique chez les enfants* [Treatment of diarrhea in young children] (Athens).

Secondary: Korasidou, Maria, 2002. *When Illness Threatens. Surveillance and Health Control of the Population in Greece of 19th Century* (in Greek) (Athens); Korasidou, Maria, 1995. *The Wretched in Athens and Their Benefactors. Poverty and Philanthropy in the Hellenic Capital City in the 19th Century* (in Greek) (Athens).

Maria Korasidou

IBN ZUHR, ABU MARWĀN 'ABD AL-MALIK (aka AVENZOAR, ABHOMERON ABINÇOAR, ABYMERON AVENZOHAR) (b. Seville, Spain, *c.* 1091; d. Seville, 1162), *medicine.*

Ibn Zuhr is the most renowned member of a prominent family of physicians in al-Andalus (medieval Muslim Spain). He was educated in Islamic law, theology, language, and literature; he began his medical training and practice under his father, Abu l–'Alā' Zuhr (d. 1131). Like him, Abu Marwān b. Zuhr also became the court physician to the Almoravid dynasty. Around 1130 he fell out of favor with the Almoravid ruler, 'Alī b. Yūsuf b. Tashufin. He fled from Seville but was eventually jailed in Marrakesh. When the Almohad dynasty conquered that city in 1147, Ibn Zuhr entered its service and returned to Seville, where he devoted himself to medical practice and teaching, as well as to the composition of books.

Devoted exclusively to medicine, Ibn Zuhr also strictly observed the precepts of the Islamic religion in his practice. His father introduced him early to the study of Galenic and Hippocratic writings, and having sworn the Hippocratic Oath when he still was a young boy, he began to work as his father's assistant and substitute. Ibn Zuhr is traditionally attributed with the first descriptions of mediastinal tumors and abscesses on the pericardium. He is also said to have introduced, or improved, artificial feeding through the gullet or through the rectum, and to have identified the *Sarcoptes scabiei* as the cause of scabies. Likewise, he is known for having recommended tracheotomy, a procedure that when young he performed only once on a goat. Although his discoveries still require a critical assessment, throughout his works Ibn Zuhr shows a particular fondness of pharmacology.

His earliest treatise, the *Kitāb al-Iqtisād fi islāh al-anfūs wa-l-ajsād* [Book of the Golden Mean Regarding the Treatment of Souls and Bodies], is identified with the *Kitāb al-Zinā* [Book on Cosmetics]. Far beyond the usual topics advocated by his predecessors, Ibn Zuhr in this work proposed, in addition to treatments and norms to improve a person's external appearance, surgical operations to remedy congenital or acquired features that affect physical beauty, such as a large nose, extremely thick lips, crooked teeth, tears in the earlobes caused by adornments, and malformations of the thorax. However, it is unlikely that Ibn Zuhr ever performed any of the surgical procedures he described, for he admitted to fainting at the sight of blood. The *Kitāb al-Taysīr fil–mudāwat wa-t-tadbīr* [Book to Facilitate Therapeutics and Regimen], written under the patronage of the Almohad caliph 'Abd al-Mu'min, is his most renowned work. Devoted to pathology and therapy, it was translated into Hebrew and also, in 1281 by John of Capua, into Latin. The Latin version was employed as a textbook in European universities along with works by al-Rāzī and Ibn Sīnā. Ibn Zuhr also wrote a book on dietetics (*Kitāb al-Aghdhiyā*), and several essays on a variety of topics, such as skin diseases (*Risālat fi 'l-baras*), disorders of the kidneys (*Maqala fi 'ilal al-kulā*), the superiority of honey over sugar (*Risala fi tafdīl al-'asal 'alā s-sukkar*), and a short treatise entitled *Kitāb al-Qānūn* [Book of the Norm].

Bibliography

Primary: 1983. (Khuri, Mishil, ed.) *Kitāb al-Taysīr fil–mudāwat wa-t-tadbīr* [Book to Facilitate Therapeutics and Regimen] (Damascus); 1992. *Kitāb al-Aghdhiya* [Book on Foodstuffs] (Arabic edition, with Spanish translation and study by García Sánchez, Expiración) (Madrid); (forthcoming, 2006 *Kitāb al-Iqtisād fi islāh al-anfūs wa-l-ajsād* [Book of the Golden Mean Regarding the Treatment of Souls and Bodies] (Arabic edition, with Spanish translation and study by Kuhne Brabant, Rosa).

Secondary: Kuhne Brabant, Rosa, 1996. '*Zina e islah*. Reflexiones para entender la medicina estética del joven Abu Marwān b. Zuhr.' *Al-Andalus—Magreb* 4: 281–298; Kuhne Brabant, Rosa, 1991. 'Abu Marwān b. Zuhr: un professionel de la médicine en plein XIIème siècle' in *Le Patrimoine Andalous dans la Culture Arabe et Espagnole* (Tunis) pp. 129–141; Kuhne Brabant, Rosa, 1986. 'Aportaciones para esclarecer alguno de los puntos oscuros en la biografía de Avenzoar' in *Actas del XII Congreso de la Unión Europea de Arabistas e Islamólogos (Málaga, 1984)* (Madrid) pp. 433–446.

Cristina Álvarez Millán

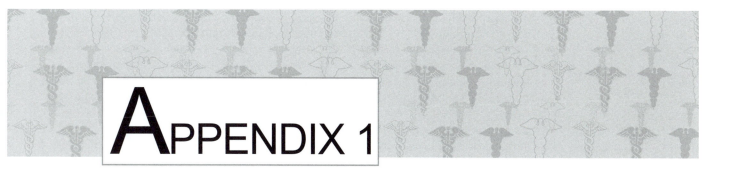

APPENDIX 1

List of Individuals by Country

Afghanistan	Al-Bīrūnī
Algeria	Fanon, Foley, Laveran
Argentina	Aráoz Alfaro, Carrillo, Coni, Favaloro, Grierson, Houssay, Ingenieros, Mazza, Rawson, Sayé i Sempere
Australia	Argyle, W. Armstrong, Balls-Headley, Bancroft, Beaney, Bland, Bryce, Burnet, Burton-Bradley, Cade, Campbell, Cilento, Cleland, Coppleson, Cumpston, D'Arcy, Dunlop, Fairley, Fiaschi, Florey, Gillbee, Gregg, Haire, Halford, Kenny, MacGregor, Mackellar, W. Mackenzie, Macnamara, Manning, Scantlebury Brown, Skirving, Stuart, Thompson, W. Thomson
Austria	Adler, Auenbrugger, Billroth, Breuer, Brücke, Dietl, Frank, A. Freud, S. Freud, Gall, Kaposi, Klein, Krafft-Ebing, Ludwig, Mesmer, Paracelsus, Reich, Rokitansky, Semmelweis, Skoda, Swieten, Wagner-Jauregg, Wenckebach
Belgium	Bordet, Depage, Dodonaeus, Guislain, Helmont, John of Saint-Amand, Palfyn, Pompe van Meerdervoort, Quetelet, Sand, Vesalius, Yperman
Brazil	Barros Barreto, Brazil, Candau, Carrillo, Chagas, Cruz, Fraga, Hackett, Penna, Pinotti, Piso, Ribas, Simond, Soper, Souza, Wucherer
Cambodia	Pen, Yajnavaraha
Canada	Abbott, Banting, Barker, Bethune, Grenfell, Huggins, MacGregor, Macphail, Osler, Penfield, I. Robb, Selye, Wintrobe
Chile	Cruz-Coke Lassabe, Horwitz Barak
China	Bethune, Bian Que, Chen Su Lan, Chunyu Yi, Ding Fubao, Ding Ganren, Fei Boxiong, Ge Hong, Hatem, Hobson, Li Gao, Li Shizhen, Liu Wansu, Lockhart, Manson, Parker, Qian Yi, Sun Simiao, Tao Hongjing, Wang Ji, Wang Weiyi, Wu Lien-Teh, Wu Youxing, Xu Shuwei, Ye Gui, Yen, Yu Yan, Yun Tieqiao, Zhang Jiebin, Zhang Yuansu, Zhu Lian, Zhu Zhenheng

Note

In listing these countries we have tried to make it easy for readers to find coherent groupings, but national boundaries are historically variable. Where the area is clear we have used modern geographical boundaries.

Classical Antiquity	Aëtius, Agnodice, Alcmaeon, Anaximander, Andreas of Carystus, Archagathus, Aretaeus, Aristotle, Asclepiades, Caelius Aurelianus, Celsus, Democedes, Democritus, Diocles, Diogenes, Dioscorides, Empedocles, Erasistratus, Galen, Herophilos, Hippocrates, Machaon, Oribasius, Paul of Aegina, Philistion, Plato, Pliny, Podalirius, Praxagoras, Rufus, Scribonius Largus, Soranus
Colombia	Carrasquilla, Franco, García-Medina, Mutis y Bosio, Perdomo Neira, Vargas Reyes
Costa Rica	Calderón Guardia, Durán Cartín
Croatia	Amatus Lusitanus, Baglivi, Štampar
Cuba	Fernández y Hernández, Finlay y Barres, Gorgas, Guiteras Gener, Pittaluga Fattorini, Reed
Czech Republic	Klebs, Rokitansky, Skoda
Denmark	Bartholin, Fibiger, Finsen, Friderichsen, Gram, Hagedorn, Harpestreng, Hirschsprung, Jerne, Madsen, Panum, Pindborg, Reimann, Salomonsen, Severinus, Stensen, Winsløw
Ecuador	Espejo, Perdomo Neira
England	Abernethy, Addison, Allbutt, Anderson, Arbuthnot, Arderne, G. Armstrong, Baillie, Balint, Balls-Headley, Bancroft, Bateman, Beaney, Beddoes, Beecham, C. Bell, Bennett, Bentley, Bevan, Beveridge, G. Bidloo, Blackley, Blackwell, Bland, Bowlby, Braid, Bright, Bristowe, Brodie, Brown, Brown-Séquard, Browne, Bruce, Brunton, Buchan, Budd, Burkitt, Caius, Carter, Chadwick, Chamberlen, Charnley, Cheselden, G. Cheyne, W. W. Cheyne, Christophers, Clowes, Cochrane, Conolly, Cook, Cooper, Culpeper, Dale, Darwin, Doll, Doniach, Down, C. E. Drew, Duka, Dunglison, Elliotson, Ellis, Fairley, Farr, Fayrer, Fenwick, Ferriar, Ferrier, Fleming, Florey, Floyer, Freeman, A. Freud, S. Freud, Garrod, Gee, Gilbert the Englishman, Gillies, Glisson, Godlee, Gowers, Greenwood, A. Gregory, Grenfell, Gull, Gully, Guthrie, Haire, Halford, Hart, Harvey, Haslam, Hastings, Haygarth, Head, Heberden, Hill, Hobson, Hodgkin, Holloway, G. Holmes, Hope, Horsley, J. Hunter, W. Hunter, Hurst, Hutchinson, Ingen Housz, J. H. Jackson, E. Jenner, W. Jenner, Jex-Blake, John of Gaddesden, A. Jones, R. Jones, Jurin, Kerr, Keynes, King, Klein, Knox, Laing, Lane, Lane-Claypon, Lawrence, Laycock, Leishman, Lettsom, Lewis, Linacre, Lind, Lister, Liston, Lockhart, Lower, Macdonald, J. Mackenzie, M. Mackenzie, Mandeville, Manson, Martin, Maudsley, McGrigor, McKeown, McMichael, Mead, Moynihan, Newman, Newsholme, Nightingale, Osler, J. Paget, R. Paget, Pappworth, Parkes, Parkinson, Percival, Pickering, Pickles, Pott, Prichard, Pringle, Prout, Rajchman, Read, Richard the Englishman, Rivers, Rogers, Ross, Ryle, Sachs, Sanches, Sanderson, Saunders, Scharlieb, Sharp, Sherlock, Shuttleworth, Simon, Smellie, Smirk, T. S. Smith, Snow, Starling, Stephenson, Steptoe, G. Still, Stopes, Sutton, Sydenham, Tait, Thompson, Tredgold, Treves, Trotter, Trowell, Trueta i Raspall, Tuke, D. Turner, J. Turner, Turquet, Underwood, Wakley, M. Warren, Wells, West, Willan, C. Williams, Willis, Winslow, Wiseman, Withering, Woodall, Wright
Egypt	Aḥmad, Bentley, Clot Bey, Griesinger, Ibn al-Haytham, Imhotep, Isaac Israeli, Koch, Mahfouz, Al-Mawṣilī, Meyerhof, Ibn al-Nafīs, E. Warren
Estonia	Baer
Faroe Islands	Finsen, Panum
Fiji	MacGregor
Finland	Mannerheim, Willebrand, Ylppö
France	Alibert, Astruc, Babinski, Baudelocque, Bayle, Bernard, Bernard of Gordon, Bernheim, Bert, Bertillon, Bichat, Boissier de la Croix de Sauvages, Bordeu, Bouchard, Bouchardat, Bourneville, Bovet, Brès, Broca, Brouardel, Broussais, Brown-Séquard, Cabanis, Carrel, Charcot, Chauliac, Civiale, Clot Bey, Corvisart des Marets, Cruveilhier, Davaine, Debré, Déjerine, Delay, Desault, Desgenettes, Despars, Dionis, Du Coudray, Dubois, Duchenne de Boulogne, Dupuytren, Edwards-Pilliet, Esquirol, Fernel, Foley, Fourcroy, Fournier, Gall, Gersdorff, Gilles de Corbeil, Gilles de la Tourette, Girard, Grancher, Guido da Vigevano, Guillain, Haffkine, Hahnemann, Hamburger, Hayem, Henry of Mondeville, Janet, La Mettrie, Lacan, Laennec, Lapeyronie, Larrey, Lasègue, Laveran, Leriche, Littré, A. Louis, P. Louis, Magendie, Magnan, Marie, Marinescu, Mechnikov, Mesmer, Mondor, Moreau de Tours, Morel, Netter, Nicolle, Orfila i Rotger, Paré, Parent-Duchâtelet, Pasteur, Patin, Péan, Percy, Petit, Pinard, Pinel, Pittaluga Fattorini, Portal, Quesnay, Rajchman, Rawson, Rayer, Renaudot, Richerand, Richet, Ricord, Rothschild, Roussy, Roux, Sanches, Sée, Seguin, Simond, Sournia, Spoerry, Tardieu, Tenon, Trousseau, Tzanck, Velpeau, Vicq d'Azyr, Villermé, Vincent, Vulpian, Widal, William of Brescia, Winsløw, Yersin
French Equatorial Africa	Jamot

Gabon	Schweitzer
Germany	Alzheimer, Aschoff, Autenrieth, Baelz, Baer, Bartisch, Basedow, Bauer, Behring, Berger, Bergmann, Billroth, Blaschko, Blumenbach, Bontekoe, Brücke, Brunfels, Büchner, Cohnheim, Conti, Domagk, Ehrlich, Erxleben, Fabricius, Fischer, Frank, Frerichs, Fuchs, Gaaz, Gall, Gersdorff, Goldstein, Graefe, Griesinger, Grotjahn, Hahnemann, Haller, Hata, Hegar, Heister, Henle, Hildegard of Bingen, Hirsch, Hirschfeld, His, Hoffmann, Hufeland, A. Jacobi, Kitasato, Klebs, Klein, Koch, Kraepelin, Krafft-Ebing, Kraus, Kretschmer, La Mettrie, Langenbeck, Laqueur, Leyden, Ludwig, Lust, Mesmer, Meyerhof, Mikulicz-Radecki, Minkowski, Mitscherlich, Moll, Müller, Nissen, Oken, Paracelsus, Pettenkofer, Rabinowitsch-Kempner, Reil, Rösslin, Rolfinck, Rosenbach, Rubner, Rüdin, Sachs, Sauerbruch, Schoenlein, Schwalbe, Schweitzer, Scultetus, Sennert, Siebold, Stahl, Traube, Verschuer, Virchow, C. Vogt, O. Vogt, Wagner, Warburg, Wassermann, Wenckebach, Wier, Wunderlich, Wundt, Ylppö, Zeiss
Ghana	Ampofo, Barnor, De Graft-Johnson, C. Easmon, J. Easmon, Gillman, Noguchi, C. Williams
Goa	Orta
Greece	Belios, Geroulanos, Goudas, Livadas, Papanicolaou, Vouros, Zinnis
Guadalupe	Beauperthuy
Guatemala	Arias de Benavides
Guyana	Beauperthuy
Hawaii	Buck
Hong Kong	Manson
Hungary	Balassa, Balint, Bene, Duka, Korányi, Markusovszky, Semmelweis
India	Abd ul-Hamīd, Aziz, Ballingall, Bentley, Brahmachari, Carter, Choksy, Chopra, Christophers, Dharmendra, Duka, Fayrer, Haffkine, Jhirad, Jivaka, Joshi, M. Ajmal Khān, M. A'zam Khān, Koch, Lad, Leishman, Macdonald, Martin, Morehead, Mukerji, Naidoo, Orta, Pandit, Parkes, Rakhmabai, Ramalingaswami, Ross, Saīd, Scharlieb, Scudder, G. Sen, P. Sen, P. Sharma, T. Sharma, Shukla, Simond, J. Turner, Vaid, Vakil, Varier
Indonesia	Eijkman, Soedarmo, Swellengrebel
Iran	Ibn Māsawayh, Al-Rāzī, Ibn Sīnā
Iraq	Ibn Buṭlān, Ibn al-Haytham, Ibn Māsawayh, Al-Mawṣilī, Ibn al-Tilmīdh
Ireland	Barry, Corrigan, Graves, Sachs, Stokes, Wilde
Islamic/Arabic Medicine	Al-Anṭākī, Ibn al-Bayṭār, Al-Bīrūnī, Ibn Buṭlān, Ibn al-Haytham, Isaac Israeli, Al-Majūsī, Ibn Māsawayh, Al-Mawṣilī, Ibn al-Nafīs, Al-Rāzī, Ibn Rushd, Ibn Sīnā, Ibn al-Tilmīdh, Al-Zahrāwī, Ibn Zuhr
Israel	Ḥaddād, Kark
Italy	Amatus Lusitanus, Aranzio, Aselli, Baglivi, Basaglia, Bassini, Bellini, Benivieni, Berengario da Carpi, Bizzozero, Borelli, Bovet, Bufalini, Cardano, Celli, Cerletti, Cesalpino, Chiarugi, Colombo, Concetti, Constantine the African, Cornaro, Cotugno, Da Monte, De Giovanni, De Sanctis, Del Garbo, Devoto, Dubini, Eustachi, Fabrizi da Acquapendente, Falloppia, Fiaschi, Ficino, Fracastoro, Frank, Frugard, Gariopontus, Gentile da Foligno, Giovannini, Golgi, Grassi, Guido da Vigevano, Hackett, Lancisi, Lanfranc, Lombroso, Malpighi, Mattioli, Mercuriale, Mondino de' Liuzzi, Morgagni, Morselli, Munthe, Mya, Pacini, Perroncito, Peter of Abano, Peter of Spain, Pittaluga Fattorini, Puccinotti, Ramazzini, Rasori, Redi, Rizzoli, Sanarelli, Santorio, Scarpa, Severino, Spallanzani, Taddeo, Tagliacozzi, Tissot, Torrella, Trota, Ugo Benzi, Vallisneri, Valsalva, Vesalius, William of Brescia, William of Saliceto, Zacchia
Jamaica	Barry, Seacole
Japan	Asada, Baelz, Gotō Konzan, Gotō Shinpei, Hanaoka Seishū, Hata, Kitasato, Manase, Miyairi, Mori, Nagayo, Noguchi, Ogata, Ogino Ginko, Pompe van Meerdervoort, L. Richards, Shiga, Siebold, Sugita, Takaki, Yamagiwa, Yamawaki, Yoshimasu Tōdō, Yoshioka Yayoi
Java	Loghem
Kenya	Kasili, Spoerry, Trowell
Korea	Choe Han'gi, Heo, Sejong, Yi Jema
Laos	Suvannavong
Latvia	Bergmann
Lebanon	Ḥaddād, Sournia, Van Dyck, Waldmeier
Liberia	Togba

Lithuania	Rabinowitsch-Kempner
Madagascar	Girard
Malaysia	Danaraj, Gale, C. Williams, Wu Lien-Teh
Mali	Atiman
Malta	Barry, Bruce
Martinique	Fanon
Mauritius	Barry, Brown-Séquard
Medieval Europe	Arderne, Arnald, Bernard of Gordon, Chauliac, Constantine the African, Del Garbo, Despars, Frugard, Gariopontus, Gentile da Foligno, Gilbert the Englishman, Gilles de Corbeil, Guido da Vigevano, Harpestreng, Henry of Mondeville, Hildegard of Bingen, John of Gaddesden, John of Saint-Amand, Lanfranc, Maimonides, Mondino de' Liuzzi, Nicholas of Poland, Peter of Abano, Peter of Spain, Richard the Englishman, Taddeo, Trota, Ugo Benzi, Valesco of Tarenta, William of Brescia, William of Saliceto, Yperman
Mexico	Arias de Benavides, Arroyo Villaverde, Balmis, Bustamante Vasconcelos, Chávez Sánchez, Hernández, Izquierdo Raudón, Liceaga, López Albo, Martínez Báez, Montaña Carranco, Montoya Lafragua, Obrador Alcalde, Rodríguez Lafora
Morocco	Ibn Rushd
Netherlands	Ali Cohen, Beverwijck, G. Bidloo, N. Bidloo, Blankaart, Boerhaave, Bontekoe, Camper, Chamberlen, De Lange, Dodonaeus, Donders, Eijkman, Einthoven, Foreest, Gaubius, Graaf, J. Heurnius, O. Heurnius, Hijmans van den Bergh, Ingen Housz, Jacobs, La Mettrie, Laqueur, Lemnius, Loghem, Mandeville, Piso, Rutgers, Ruysch, Schroeder van der Kolk, Swammerdam, Swellengrebel, Swieten, Sylvius, Tronchin, Wenckebach, Wier, Winkler
New Zealand	Barnett, M. Bell, Buck, Gillies, Gordon, Hercus, King, Liley, G. Robb, Scott, Smirk, A. Thomson
Nigeria	Lambo, MacGregor, Odeku
Norway	Evang, Følling, Hansen, Holst, Refsum, Schiøtz
Pakistan	Khanolkar, Saīd
Panama	Gorgas
Papua New Guinea	Burton-Bradley, Koch, MacGregor
Persia and Persian Empire	Al-Anṭākī, Asaph, Ibn Buṭlān, Al-Majūsī
Peru	Balmis, Carrión, Monge Medrano, Núñez Butrón, Paz Soldán, Unanue
Philippines	Acosta-Sison, Rizal
Poland	Aleksandrowicz, Bieganski, Biernacki, Dietl, Hirschfeld, Hirszfeld, Korczak, Mikulicz-Radecki, Nicholas of Poland, Rajchman, Śniadecki
Portugal	Amatus Lusitanus, Egas Moniz, Orta, Peter of Spain, Sanches, Valesco of Tarenta, Wucherer
Romania	Babeş, Cantacuzino, Ciucă, Marinescu
Russia	Al'tshuller, Baer, Bekhterev, N. Bidloo, Botkin, Briukhonenko, Buial'skii, Burdenko, Dobroslavin, Erisman, Fedorov, Frank, Gaaz, Haffkine, Ilizarov, Inozemtsev, Iudin, Khlopin, Korsakov, P. Louis, Manassein, Mechnikov, Minkowski, Molleson, Negovskii, Ostroumov, Pavlov, Pavlovskii, Pirogov, Pletnev, Pokrovskaia, Rabinowitsch-Kempner, Sanches, Sechenov, Semashko, Semenovskii, Sklifosovskii, Solov'ev, Teziakov, O. Vogt, Zakhar'in, Zeiss
Scotland	Addis, Alison, Arbuthnot, G. Armstrong, Baillie, Ballingall, C. Bell, Bennett, Braid, Brown, Brunton, Buchan, G. Cheyne, W. W. Cheyne, Christison, Cochrane, Cullen, Donald, Ferriar, Ferrier, Fleming, J. Gregory, J. Hunter, W. Hunter, Knox, Laing, Laycock, Lind, Lister, Liston, Livingstone, MacGregor, J. Mackenzie, Manson, McGrigor, McMichael, Monro, Morehead, Orr, Park Ross, Pringle, Simpson, Smellie, Stephenson, Syme, Trotter, Whytt
Serbia	Batut, Djordjević, Kostić, Lazarević, Nešić, Subbotić
Sierra Leone	Boyle, Horton, Johnson, Macdonald
Singapore	Chen Su Lan, Dunlop, Lim Boon Keng
South Africa	Abdurahman, Barnard, Barry, Gale, Gear, Gillman, Gluckman, A. Gregory, Kark, Molema, Moroka, Naidoo, Orenstein, Park Ross, Read, Waterston, Xuma
Spain	Arias de Benavides, Arnald, Arroyo Villaverde, Azúa y Suárez, Balmis, Ibn al-Bayṭār, Bravo de Sobremonte, Calandre Ibáñez, Cardenal Fernández, Casal Julián, Ferrán y Clúa, García Solá, Gimbernat i Arbós, Giovannini, Goyanes Capdevilla, Guilera Molas, Hernández, Jiménez Díaz, Laguna, Lardizábal Dubois, López Albo, Maimonides, Marañón Posadillo, Martínez Vargas, Mercado, Monardes, Mutis y Bosio, Nóvoa Santos, Obrador Alcalde, Orfila i Rotger, Pedro-Pons,

Spain (*cont.*)	Peter of Spain, Piquer Affufat, Pittaluga Fattorini, Puigvert Gorro, Ramón y Cajal, Rodríguez Lafora, Rubio Gali, Ibn Rushd, Sayé i Sempere, Soriano Fischer, Torrella, Trueta i Raspall, Urrutia Guerezta, Valles, Al-Zahrāwī, Ibn Zuhr
Sri Lanka	M. Paul, Wickramarachchi
Sumatra	Loghem, Swellengrebel
Sweden	Acrel, Gullstrand, Holmgren, Huss, Linnaeus, Munthe, Rosén von Rosenstein, Rudbeck, Sandström
Switzerland	Billroth, Bleuler, Bonet, Bovet, Brunfels, Coindet, Conti, De La Rive, Erisman, Fabricius, Forel, Griesinger, Haller, His, Jerne, Jung, Klebs, Kocher, Kubler-Ross, Le Clerc, Ludwig, Meyer, Nissen, Odier, Oken, Paracelsus, Platter, Prevost, Quervain, Reverdin, Rüdin, Tissot, Tronchin, Turquet, Waldmeier
Syria	Ibn al-Bayṭār, Al-Mawṣilī, Ibn al-Nafīs
Taiwan	Gotō Shinpei, Manson
Tanzania	Atiman, Koch, Livingstone
Thailand	Dunlop, Gale, Harinasuta, Jivaka
Tibet	Sangye Gyatso, Yuthog Yontan
Tunisia	Isaac Israeli, Nicolle
Turkey	Al-Anṭākī, Ibn Buṭlān, Nightingale, Nissen, Pirogov, Seacole
Uganda	Bruce, Burkitt, Cook, Gale, Koch, Trowell
Ukraine	Fedorov, Negovskii
United States	Abel, Abt, Addis, Adler, Albright, Baker, Barker, Bartlett, Barton, Battey, Beard, Beaumont, Beck, Beecher, Beers, H. Bigelow, J. Bigelow, Biggs, Billings, Blackwell, Blalock, Bloodgood, Bond, Bowditch, Boyle, Boylston, Brigham, Brown-Séquard, Cabot, Cannon, Carrel, Channing, Chapin, Churchill, Codman, Cole, Coley, Cotton, Councilman, Crile, Cushing, Da Costa, Dameshek, Dandy, Dickinson, Dix, G. Dock, L. Dock, Drake, C. R. Drew, Duhring, Dunglison, Earle, Eddy, Edsall, Emerson, Ewing, Farber, Favaloro, Fishbein, Flexner, Flick, Flint, Frost, Gerhard, Gesell, Gibbon, Goldberger, Goldstein, Gorgas, E. Graham, S. Graham, Grinker, Gross, Guiteras Gener, Hackett, Halsted, Hamilton, Hammond, Hardy, Hatem, Hench, Herrick, O. W. Holmes, Holt, Hooker, Hufnagel, Huggins, J. Jackson, A. Jacobi, M. P. Jacobi, Jarvis, J. Jones, Joslin, Keen, Kellogg, Kelly, Kenny, Kinyoun, Klebs, Kubler-Ross, Lloyd, Long, Lust, C. Mayo, W. Mayo, McBurney, McDowell, Meigs, Menninger, Meyer, Minot, Mitchell, Morgan, S. Morton, W. Morton, C. Mosher, E. Mosher, Mott, Murphy, Newton, Nissen, Noguchi, Nott, Odeku, Orenstein, Osler, B. Palmer, D. Palmer, Papanicolaou, Park, Parker, Parran, J. Paul, Penfield, Pepper, Putnam, Rajchman, Ray, Reed, Reich, A. Richards, D. Richards, L. Richards, I. Robb, Rock, Rush, Sabin, Salk, Sanger, Scribner, Seguin, G. Shattuck, L. Shattuck, Shippen, Sims, N. Smith, T. Smith, Soper, Spock, Squibb, A. Still, Stillé, Sullivan, Taussig, Thayer, S. Thomson, Trall, Trudeau, Van Dyck, Van Hoosen, E. Warren, J. Warren, Waterhouse, Welch, White, D. Williams, Wintrobe, Wynder, Zakrzewska
Uruguay	Morquio, Sanarelli, Sayé i Sempere
Uzbekistan	Al-Bīrūnī, Ibn Sīnā
Venezuela	Balmis, Gabaldón, Razetti
Vietnam	Bert, Lán Ông, Simond, Tuệ Tĩnh, Tùng Tôn Thất, Yersin
Wales	Bevan, Cochrane, R. Jones, Lewis
Zambia	Livingstone

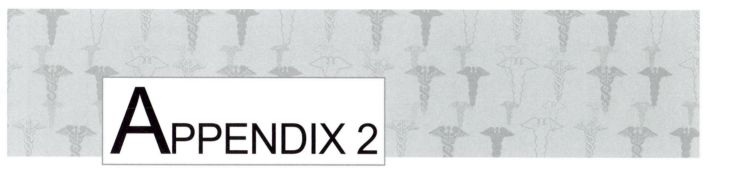

APPENDIX 2

List of Individuals by Fields of Activity

Acupuncture (*see also* Chinese medicine)	Zhu Lian
Addiction medicine	Huss, Kerr, Magnan, Moreau de Tours, Trotter
Administration	*see* Medical administration
Alchemy	Fernel, Paracelsus, Al-Rāzī, Tao Hongjing
Allergy	Blackley, Floyer, Freeman
American Red Cross	*see* Humanitarianism
Analytical psychology	Jung
Anatomy	Abernethy, Alcmaeon, Aranzio, Aretaeus, Aselli, Barker, Bartholin, C. Bell, Bellini, Berengario da Carpi, Beverwijck, Bichat, G. Bidloo, N. Bidloo, Blankaart, Buial'skii, Camper, Cheselden, Colombo, Cooper, Cotugno, Dubini, Dubois, Erasistratus, Eustachi, Fabrizi da Acquapendente, Falloppia, Gimbernat i Arbós, Glisson, Graaf, Guido da Vigevano, Halford, Harvey, Heister, Henle, Herophilos, J. Heurnius, O. Heurnius, His, O. W. Holmes, J. Hunter, W. Hunter, Knox, Lancisi, Lower, Mondino de' Liuzzi, Monro, Morgagni, Müller, Pacini, Palfyn, Platter, Portal, Reil, Rolfinck, Rosén von Rosenstein, Rudbeck, Rufus, Ruysch, Sandström, Scarpa, Scott, Severino, Shippen, Stensen, Sugita, Swammerdam, Valsalva, Vesalius, Vicq d'Azyr, Wilde, Willis, Winsløw, Yamawaki Tōyō
Anesthesia	Beecher, Hanaoka Seishū, Long, W. Morton, Simpson, Snow
Anthropology	Baelz, Baer, Bertillon, Blumenbach, Broca, Buck, Camper, Cleland, De Giovanni, Fischer, Knox, Lombroso, MacGregor, S. Morton, Nott, Prichard, Rivers, Virchow

Notes

The headings used in this appendix are based on those provided by the authors. Some of the categories are modern but include individuals from all periods and cultures. Thus 'pharmacology' groups modern experimentalists with doctors from earlier periods who contributed to knowledge of drugs and their therapeutic uses.

There is no category for 'Medicine'; it would be too large to be meaningful.

'Women in medicine' refers to female pioneers in medicine; later women are treated by specialty not gender.

Demography	Arbuthnot, Bertillon, McKeown
Dentistry (*see also* Odontology)	W. Morton
Dermatology	Addison, Alibert, Azúa y Suárez, Bateman, Blaschko, Duhring, Hutchinson, Kaposi, Rayer, D. Tuner, Tzanck, Willan
Diabetology	Banting, Bouchardat, Doniach, Hagedorn, Joslin
Dietetics (*see also* Nutrition)	Asclepiades, M. Bell, Leyden
Disease classification	Farr
Disease ecology	Burnet
Dissection	*see* Anatomy
Eating disorders	Gull, Lasègue
Eclecticism	Newton
Education (*see also* Medical education)	Korczak, Seguin, Shuttleworth
Egyptian medicine	Imhotep
Electroencephalography	Berger
Embryology	Baer, Empedocles, Fabrizi da Acquapendente, Haller, Harvey, His, Malpighi, Mechnikov, Prevost, Spallanzani, Swammerdam
Endocrinology	Abel, Addison, Albright, Basedow, Brown-Séquard, Coindet, Cruz-Coke Lassabe, Cushing, Doniach, Hagedorn, Horsley, Kocher, Laqueur, Marañón Posadillo, Minkowski, Minot, Starling
Epidemiology	Budd, Burkitt, Carter, Chapin, Cochrane, Doll, Emerson, Finlay y Barres, Frost, Gabaldón, Goldberger, Grassi, Greenwood, Haffkine, Hamilton, Hansen, Heo, Hill, Lán Ông, Lane-Claypon, Loghem, Mazza, McKeown, Panum, Park, J. Paul, Pickles, Puccinotti, Ramazzini, Reed, Sabin, Snow, Solov'ev, Teziakov, Thompson, W. Thomson, Vicq d'Azyr, Wu Youxing, Wynder
Ethics	*see* Philosophy; Medical ethics
Ethnology	*see* Anthropology
Eugenics (*see also* Nazi eugenics)	Mackellar, Pinard
Family medicine	*see* General practice
Family planning	*see* Birth control
Fetal research	Liley
Flying doctor service	Spoerry
Forensic medicine	Brouardel, A. Louis, Orfila i Rotger, Puccinotti, Semenovskii, Tardieu, Zacchia
Forensic psychiatry	Esquirol, Ray, Tardieu, Winslow
Galenism	Patin, Torrella
Gastroenterology	Hurst, Urrutia Guerezta
General practice	Abdurahman, Ampofo, Balint, Breuer, Chen, Gordon, Horton, Jacobs, E. Jenner, Kark, J. Mackenzie, Montoya Lafragua, Naidoo, Parkinson, Pickles, Snow, Xuma
Genetics	De Lange, Garrod
Geography	*see* Medical geography; Natural history
Geology	*see* Natural history
Geriatrics	Floyer, McKeown, M. Warren,
Gynecology	Aëtius, Andreas of Carystus, Balls-Headley, Battey, Caelius Aurelianus, D'Arcy, Dickinson, Donald, Haire, Hegar, Kelly, Mahfouz, Mercado, Ogino Ginko, Papanicolaou, Rock, Scharlieb, Semmelweis, Sims, Soranus, Steptoe, Sun Simiao, Tait, Van Hoosen, Velpeau
Hematology	Aleksandrowicz, Biernacki, Bizzozero, Bryce, Dameshek, Ehrlich, Gowers, Hayem, Herrick, Pittaluga Fattorini, Prevost, Tzanck, Willebrand, Wintrobe
Health administration	*see* Medical administration
Health reform	S. Graham, Kellogg, Lane
Health services research	Cochrane
Helminthology (*see also* Parasitology)	Wucherer
Hepatology	Glisson, Sherlock, Tùng Tôn Thất

Herbalism	Culpeper, Li Gao
High altitude physiology	Monge Medrano
Histology	Bichat, Bizzozero, Calandre Ibáñez, Gillman, Henle, His, Kostić, Ramón y Cajal
Histopathology (*see also* Pathology)	García Solá
History of medicine	Aḥmad, Ali Cohen, Allbutt, Astruc, Billings, Bustamante Vasconcelos, Celsus, Fishbein, Goyanes Capdevilla, Gross, Ḥaddād, Hirsch, Izquierdo Raudón, J. Jones, Le Clerc, Littré, Mead, Meyerhof, Osler, Pliny, Portal, Sournia, Yu Yan
Homeopathy	Blackley, Hahnemann
Hospital architecture	Billings, Tenon
Hospital design	Nightingale
Humanitarianism	Barton, Bethune, Lettsom, Orr, Quervain, Rajchman, Schweitzer
Humoral medicine (modern)	Perdomo Neira
Hydrotherapy	Gully, Trall
Hygiene	Behring, Bouchardat, Brouardel, Celli, Cornaro, Dubini, Erisman, Frank, García-Medina, Grassi, Hippocrates, Hirsch, Holst, Khlopin, Lán Ông, Lancisi, Loghem, Miyairi, Molleson, Parkes, Penna, Pettenkofer, Pokrovskaia, Puccinotti, Rubner, Sanarelli, Sanches, Scharlieb, Teziakov, Zeiss
Hypnotism (*see also* Mesmerism)	Bernheim, Braid, Charcot, Forel
Hysteria	Breuer, Charcot, G. Cheyne, S. Freud
Iatrochemistry (*see also* Chemistry)	Paracelsus, Severinus, Turquet, Woodall
Imaging (*see also* Radiology)	Donald
Immunology	Bordet, Burnet, Ehrlich, Ferrán y Clúa, Freeman, Haffkine, Hirszfeld, Jerne, Jiménez Díaz, Mechnikov, Pasteur, Richet, Roux, Sabin, Sachs, Salk
Individual psychology	Adler
Infant welfare	W. Armstrong, King, Scantlebury Brown
Influenza	Frost
Insulin	*see* Diabetology
International health	Candau, Evang, Horwitz Barak, Lambo, Madsen, Rajchman, Soper, Štampar
Invention	Bland, Carrel, Darwin, Einthoven
Japanese medicine	Asada, Gotō Konzan, Manase, Ogata, Sugita, Yamawaki Tōyō, Yoshimasu Tōdō
Kidney disease	*see* Nephrology
Kinesology	Grierson
Korean medicine	Choe Han'gi, Heo, Sejong, Yi Jema
Laryngology	M. Mackenzie
Legal medicine (*see also* Forensic medicine)	Wakley
Leprology	Beauperthuy, Carter, Dharmendra, Hansen, Hatem, Hutchinson, Khanolkar, Lad, Rogers
Lexicography	Billings, Blankaart, Dunglison, Littré
Literature (*see also* Poetry)	Arbuthnot, Browne, Ferriar, O. W. Holmes, Keynes, Korczak, Macphail, Mitchell, Mondor, Mori, Munthe, Patin, Rizal
Malariology	Belios, Bentley, Celli, Christophers, Fairley, Gabaldón, Golgi, Grassi, Hackett, Harinasuta, Lancisi, Laveran, Livadas, Macdonald, Park Ross, Pinotti, Ross, Soper, Swellengrebel
Maori medicine	Buck
Materialism	Büchner, La Mettrie
Maternal health	Brès, De Graft-Johnson, Gordon, Jhirad, Pinard
Mathematics	Borelli, Plato
Medical administration	Argyle, Dale, Gotō Shinpei, López Albo, Nagayo, Pandit, M. Paul, A. Richards, Suvannavong, Togba, Vulpian, D. Williams, Zakrzewska
Medical botany	Ampofo, Ibn al-Bayṭār, J. Bigelow, Al-Bīrūnī, Blankaart, Boerhaave, Cesalpino, Dioscorides, Dodonaeus, Fuchs, Hernández, Monardes, Orta, Pen, Ruysch
Medical chemistry	*see* Iatrochemistry

Medical education	Anderson, Baelz, Balassa, Batut, Bene, Blackwell, Boerhaave, Brès, Clot Bey, Cook, Coppleson, Corrigan, Cullen, Da Costa, Da Monte, Danaraj, Debré, G. Dock, Drake, Dunglison, Espejo, Flexner, Fourcroy, Fraga, Garrod, Graves, J. Gregory, Halford, Hercus, Hoffmann, O. W. Holmes, W. Hunter, Jex-Blake, John of Saint-Amand, Korányi, Manson, Markusovszky, Meigs, Monro, Montaña Carranco, Morehead, Morgan, Osler, Pappworth, M. Paul, Pedro-Pons, Pepper, Pickering, Pompe van Meerdervoort, Richerand, Rosén von Rosenstein, Rush, Schoenlein, Scott, Scudder, Shippen, Shuttleworth, Siebold, N. Smith, Soriano Fischer, Stillé, Stokes, Stuart, Swieten, Taddeo, Tissot, Traube, Ugo Benzi, Unanue, Vargas Reyes, Vicq d'Azyr, E. Warren, J. Warren, Welch, William of Brescia, D. Williams
Medical entomology	Nott, Ross
Medical ethics	Aristotle, Beecher, J. Gregory, Hooker, Lán Ông, Maimonides, Moll, Pappworth, Percival, Razetti, Rush, Scribonius Largus, Sun Simiao
Medical geography	Drake, Hirsch
Medical journalism	Bourneville, Fishbein, Hart, Macphail, Richerand, Schwalbe, Wakley
Medical jurisprudence	*see* Forensic medicine
Medical philosophy	Bartlett, Bieganski, Büchner, Choe Han'gi, La Mettrie, Mandeville, Patin
Medical publishing	Ding Fubao, Markusovszky
Medical reform	Beddoes, Beveridge, Calderón Guardia, Depage, Fishbein, Flexner, Fourcroy, Hart, Hastings, G. Robb, Wakley
Medical statistics	Bertillon, Greenwood, Hill, P. Louis, Quervain, L. Shattuck
Medical theory	Broussais, Brown, Fernel, Galen, Helmont, Hippocrates, Kraus, Paracelsus, Rasori
Medical transmission	Arnald, Constantine the African
Mental deficiency	Seguin, Tredgold
Mental hygiene	Beers
Mesmerism	Elliotson, Mesmer
Microbiology	Cantacuzino, Cruz, García Solá, Madsen, Noguchi, Pasteur, Ribas
Microscopy	Bennett, Malpighi, Pacini
Midwifery (*see also* Obstetrics)	Agnodice, Du Coudray, Montoya Lafragua, R. Paget, Sharp
Military hygiene	Dobroslavin, Parkes
Military medicine	G. Bidloo, Billings, Burdenko, Coppleson, Desgenettes, Fairley, Foley, Gorgas, Hammond, Larrey, McGrigor, Morgan, Mori, Percy, Pirogov, Pringle, Solov'ev, A. Thomson
Military surgery	Ballingall, Barry, Beaumont, Billings, Burdenko, Djordjević, Fiaschi, Guthrie, J. Hunter, McGrigor, Nešić, Pompe van Meerdervoort, Subbotić
Missionary medicine	Atiman, Cook, Grenfell, Hobson, Livingstone, Lockhart, Parker, Schweitzer, Waldmeier, Waterston
Musicology	Billroth, Al-Rāzī
Natural history	Aristotle, Bancroft, Blumenbach, Casal Julián, Cleland, Darwin, Dodonaeus, Forel, Hernández, Linnaeus, Mutis y Bosio, Oken, Parkinson, Piso, Redi, Vallisneri, Waterhouse
Natural philosophy	Anaximander, Aristotle, Borelli, Cardano, De La Rive, Democedes, Democritus, Diogenes, Empedocles, Fernel, Foreest, Giovannini, Jurin, Ibn al-Nafīs, Oken, Philistion, Pliny, Ibn Rushd, Sylvius
Natural science	Aristotle, Spallanzani, Stensen
Naturopathy	Lust
Naval medicine	Lardizábal Dubois, Lind, Pringle, Trotter, Wagner, Zeiss
Nazi eugenics	Rüdin, Verschuer, Wagner
Nazi medicine	Conti, Rüdin
Nephrology (*see also* Urology)	Addis, Bright, Hamburger, Rayer, A. Richards, Scribner
Neuroanatomy	Gall, Golgi, Ramón y Cajal, C. Vogt, O. Vogt
Neurology	Babinski, Beard, Bourneville, Broca, Brown-Séquard, Cerletti, Charcot, Déjerine, Duchenne de Boulogne, Egas Moniz, Ferrier, Forel, Gilles de la Tourette, Goldstein, Gowers, Griesinger, Grinker, Guillain, Hammond, Head, G. Holmes, Hutchinson, J. H. Jackson, Laycock, Lazarević, Marie, Marinescu, Mitchell, Mitscherlich, Parkinson, Putnam, Ramón y Cajal, Refsum, Rodríguez Lafora, Scarpa, Schroeder van der Kolk, C. Vogt, O. Vogt, Vulpian, Whytt, Willis
Neuropathology	Alzheimer, Bayle, Broca, Charcot, S. Freud, Negovskii
Neurophysiology	Duchenne de Boulogne, Ferrier

Philosophy	Aristotle, Ibn Buṭlān, Cardano, Ficino, Galen, Isaac Israeli, Janet, Peter of Abano, Plato, Al-Rāzī, Ibn Rushd, Ibn Sīnā, Soranus, Taddeo, Valles
Philosophy of medicine	*see* Medical philosophy
Physical diagnosis	Auenbrugger, Cabot, Corvisart des Marets, Elliotson, Flint, Gee, Gerhard, Hope, Laennec, Skoda
Physical therapy	Kenny
Physics	*see* Natural philosophy
Physiology	Abernethy, Alcmaeon, Asclepiades, Autenrieth, Baglivi, Banting, Bartholin, Beaumont, C. Bell, Bellini, Bennett, Bernard, Bert, Bichat, Borelli, Breuer, Briukhonenko, Brown-Séquard, Brücke, Brunton, Cannon, Colombo, Cotugno, Dale, Donders, Dunglison, Eijkman, Einthoven, Erasistratus, Finsen, Golgi, Graaf, Graves, Gullstrand, Halford, Haller, Harvey, Herophilos, O. W. Holmes, Holmgren, Houssay, Izquierdo Raudón, Khlopin, Lane-Claypon, Lawrence, Lower, Ludwig, Magendie, Müller, Panum, Pavlov, Reil, A. Richards, Richerand, Richet, Rubner, Sanderson, Santorio, Sechenov, Selye, Spallanzani, Starling, Stuart, Whytt, Willis, Wundt
Plastic surgery	Gillies, Pirogov, Sauerbruch, Tagliacozzi
Poetry (*see also* Literature)	G. Bidloo, Darwin, Fracastoro, Haller, Redi
Poliomyelitis	Frost, Gear, Kenny, W. MacKenzie, Macnamara, J. Paul, Sabin, Salk
Political activism	*see* Politics
Politics	Bert, Bevan, Bland, Bourneville, Chen, Djordjević, Fourcroy, A. Jacobi, Littré, Molema, Moroka, Rizal, Rush, Spock, Virchow, Wakley, Xuma
Popular medicine	Buchan, G. Cheyne, Cornaro, Culpeper, S. Graham, Hufeland, Kellogg, E. Mosher, Perdomo Neira, Rösslin, Spock, Tissot
Preventive medicine	Hansen, Haygarth, Kark, Pandit, J. Paul, Rosén von Rosenstein
Primary care	*see* General practice
Psychiatric reform	Dix, Esquirol
Psychiatry	Alzheimer, Basaglia, Bayle, Berger, Bleuler, Bourneville, Brigham, Burton-Bradley, Cade, Cerletti, Chiarugi, Conolly, Cotton, De La Rive, De Sanctis, Delay, Down, Earle, Esquirol, Fanon, Forel, Goldstein, Griesinger, Grinker, Guislain, Haslam, Ingenieros, Janet, Jarvis, Jung, King, Korsakov, Kraepelin, Krafft-Ebing, Kretschmer, Kubler-Ross, Lacan, Laing, Lambo, Lasègue, López Albo, Magnan, Mandeville, Manning, Maudsley, Menninger, Meyer, Mitchell, Moreau de Tours, Morel, Morselli, Pinel, Prichard, Puccinotti, Ray, Reil, Rodríguez Lafora, Rüdin, Rush, Schroeder van der Kolk, Seguin, Sullivan, Tredgold, Tuke, Wagner-Jauregg, Waldmeier, Wier, Winkler, Winslow
Psychoanalysis	Adler, Balint, Breuer, Fanon, A. Freud, S. Freud, Jung, Klein, Lacan, Menninger, Mitscherlich, Putnam, Reich, Sullivan
Psychological medicine	Janet
Psychology	Bekhterev, Gall, Lombroso, Pavlov, Sechenov, C. Vogt, O. Vogt, Wundt
Psychophysiology	Cabanis
Psychosomatic medicine	Mitscherlich
Psychotherapy	Bernheim, Goldstein, Moll, Rivers
Public health	Ali Cohen, Alison, Aráoz Alfaro, W. Armstrong, Baker, Balmis, Bancroft, Barnor, Barry, Batut, Belios, Biggs, Billings, Bowditch, Bristowe, Brouardel, Bustamante Vasconcelos, Carrillo, Chadwick, Chagas, Chapin, Chen Su Lan, Choksy, Cilento, Coni, Cruz, Cumpston, Djordjević, Dobroslavin, Durán Cartín, Emerson, Espejo, Evang, Ferriar, Fraga, Gaaz, Gale, García-Medina, Gluckman, Goldberger, Gorgas, Gotō Shinpei, A. Gregory, Guiteras Gener, Hackett, Hatem, Huss, Jarvis, Kinyoun, Laza-rević, Liceaga, Livadas, MacGregor, Mackellar, Madsen, Martínez Báez, Nagayo, Newman, Newsh-olme, Parent-Duchâtelet, Park Ross, Parran, Paz Soldán, Penna, Pinotti, Pokrovskaia, Rajchman, Rawson, Ribas, Sanderson, Semashko, L. Shattuck, Simon, T. S. Smith, Soedarmo, Solov'ev, Souza, Štampar, Swieten, Thompson, Tissot, J. Turner, Unanue, Vicq d'Azyr, Virchow, Welch, Wu Lien-Teh, Wucherer, Wynder, Yen, Zhu Lian
Public health administration	Buck, Chadwick, Newsholme
Rabies	Grancher, Pasteur
Radiology (*see also* Imaging)	Argyle, Boyle, Cannon, Codman, Dandy, Puigvert
Radiotherapy	Guilera Molas

Ranpō medicine	*see* Japanese medicine
Rehabilitation medicine	Caelius Aurelianus, Kenny, W. MacKenzie, Macnamara
Reproductive medicine	Mukerji, Prevost, Rock, Steptoe
Rheumatology	Garrod, Heberden, Hench
Rural medicine	Mazza, Núñez Butrón, Penna
Sanitary science	Nightingale
Sectarian medicine	Eddy, S. Graham, Lloyd, Lust, Newton, B. Palmer, D. Palmer, S. Thomson
Self-experimentation	Carrión
Serological diagnosis	J. Paul, Wassermann, Widal
Serotherapy	Behring, Brazil, Cole, Ehrlich, Roux
Sexology	Beaney, Dickinson, Ellis, Forel, Haire, Hirschfeld, Kostić, Krafft-Ebing, Moll, C. Mosher, Reich, Rutgers, Sanger, Stopes, Trall
Smallpox inoculation	Boylston, Haygarth, Ingen Housz, Jurin, Sutton, Tronchin
Smallpox vaccination	Balmis, J. Jackson, E. Jenner, Waterhouse
Social hygiene	Al'tshuller, Batut, Grotjahn, Semashko, Solov'ev, Štampar
Social medicine	Adler, Celli, Cruz-Coke Lassabe, Frank, Gale, Kark, McKeown, Paz Soldán, Ryle, Sand
Social security	Bevan, Beveridge, Calderón Guardia, Lim Boon Keng
Surf lifesaving	Coppleson
Surgery	Abernethy, Acrel, Amatus Lusitanus, Andreas of Carystus, Aranzio, Archagathus, Arderne, Arias de Benavides, Balassa, Ballingall, Bancroft, Barnett, Bartisch, Bassini, Baudelocque, Bauer, Beaney, Beck, C. Bell, Berengario da Carpi, Bergmann, Bethune, Beverwijck, N. Bidloo, H. Bigelow, Billroth, Bland, Bloodgood, Bond, Boylston, Braid, Broca, Brodie, Buial'skii, Burkitt, Caelius Aurelianus, Camper, Cardenal Fernández, Carrel, Celsus, Chauliac, Cheselden, W. W. Cheyne, Churchill, Civiale, Clowes, Codman, Coley, Colombo, Cooper, Coppleson, Crile, Cushing, Del Garbo, Depage, Desault, Dionis, Djordjević, C. E. Drew, C. R. Drew, Duka, Dunlop, Dupuytren, Durán Cartín, C. Easmon, Fabricius, Fabrizi Da Acquapendente, Fayrer, Fiaschi, Frugard, Geroulanos, Gersdorff, Gilbert the Englishman, Gillbee, Gimbernat i Arbós, Giovannini, Godlee, Graefe, E. Graham, Gross, Guthrie, Halsted, Hanaoka Seishū, Heister, Henry of Mondeville, Hippocrates, Hobson, Horton, J. Hunter, Hutchinson, Ilizarov, Inozemtsev, Iudin, John of Gaddesden, Johnson, Keen, Keynes, Kocher, Lane, Lanfranc, Langenbeck, Lapeyronie, Larrey, Lawrence, Leriche, Lister, Liston, Lockhart, Long, A. Louis, M. Mackenzie, Markusovszky, Martin, C. Mayo, W. Mayo, McBurney, McDowell, Mikulicz-Radecki, Mondor, Morgan, Mott, Moynihan, Murphy, Nicholas of Poland, Nissen, J. Paget, Palfyn, Paracelsus, Paré, Parker, Paul of Aegina, M. Paul, Péan, Percy, Petit, Pirogov, Pott, Quervain, Quesnay, Razetti, Reverdin, Richerand, Rizzoli, G. Robb, Rubio Gali, Sauerbruch, Scarpa, Scudder, Scultetus, Severino, Shippen, Simon, Skirving, Sklifosovskii, N. Smith, Soranus, Subbotić, Syme, Tait, Tenon, Treves, Tùng Tôn Thất, D. Turner, Urrutia Guerezta, Valesco of Tarenta, Vargas Reyes, Velpeau, Vesalius, Wang Ji, E. Warren, J. Warren, Wells, William of Saliceto, D. Williams, Wiseman, Woodall, Yperman, Al-Zahrāwī
Technology	J. Bigelow
Teratology	Abbott, Gregg, Taussig
Terminal care	Saunders
Thai medicine	Jivaka
Thanatology	Kubler-Ross
Theology	Ibn Buṭlān, Gilles de Corbeil, Peter of Spain, Stensen
Therapeutics	Al'tshuller, Botkin, Broussais, Coindet, Dietl, Domagk, Fleming, Galen, P. Louis, Manassein, Ostroumov, Pletnev, Prevost, Sée, Trousseau, Willis, Withering, Zakhar'in
Thermometry	Allbutt, Wunderlich
Thomsonianism	S. Thomson
Tibetan medicine	Sangye Gyatso, Yuthog Yontan
Tissue culture	Carrel
Toxicology	Brunton, Christison, Fayrer, Hamilton, Mitchell, Orfila i Rotger
Traumatology	Ilizarov
Tropical hygiene	Cilento, Fayrer, Macdonald, Martin, Parkes
Tropical medicine	Bentley, Brahmachari, Bruce, Burkitt, Carter, Chagas, Christophers, Cruz, Danaraj, Fairley, Fernández y Hernández, Franco, Gear, Gorgas, Guiteras Gener, Harinasuta, Jamot, Laveran, Leishman, Manson, Morehead, Pandit, Piso, Rogers, C. Williams, Wucherer

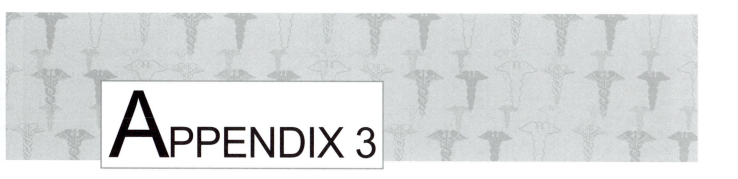

APPENDIX 3

List of Individuals by Birth/Death Dates

Name	Birth/Death Dates	Name	Birth/Death Dates
Machaon	Apocryphal	Asclepiades	fl. 1st century BCE
Podalirius	Apocryphal	Rufus	fl. 1st century BCE
Imhotepc	*c.* 2686–*c.* 2630 BCE	Celsus	fl. 14–37
Anaximander	*c.* 610–545 BCE	Scribonius Largus	fl. 14–54
Democedes	fl. 500 BCE	Pliny the Elder	23/24–79
Bian Que	fl. 6th to 5th century BCE	Dioscorides	fl. 40–80
Jivaka	fl. 6th or 5th century BCE	Aretaeus	fl. 50/100–150/200
Empedocles	*c.* 492–*c.* 432 BCE	Soranus	fl. 100
Alcmaeon	fl. 490–430 BCE	Asaph	fl. 2nd century
Hippocrates	*c.* 460–370 BCE	Galen	129–*c.* 210
Diogenes	fl. 435–400 BCE	Ge Hong	*c.* 283–343/63
Plato	427–348/7 BCE	Oribasius of Pergamon	*c.* 320–390/400
Democritus	fl. 420 BCE	Caelius Aurelianus	fl. late 4th–5th century
Diocles	fl. late 4th century BCE	Tao Hongjing	456–536
Aristotle	384–322 BCE	Aëtius	fl. *c.* 530–560
Philistion	fl. 350 BCE	Sun Simiao	581?–682
Praxagoras	340–320 fl. BCE	Paul of Aegina	fl. 640
Herophilos	*c.* 330–260 BCE	Ibn Māsawayh	*c.* 777–*c.* 857
Erasistratus	*c.* 315–240 BCE	Isaac Israeli	840–932
Andreas of Carystus	fl. after 250–d. 217 BCE	Al-Rāzī	*c.* 865–925/32
Agnodice	fl. 3rd century BCE	Al-Majūsī	900/925–*c.* 994
Archagathus	fl. 219 BCE	Yajnavaraha	fl. 10th century
Chunyu Yi	b. 215 BCE	Al-Zahrāwī	*c.* 936–*c.* 1013

Name	Birth/Death Dates	Name	Birth/Death Dates
Ibn al-Haytham	965–1039/41	Benivieni	1443–1502
Al-Bīrūnī	973–1048/50	Torrella	*c.* 1452–*c.* 1520
Ibn Sīnā	980–1037	Gersdorff	*c.* 1455–*c.* 1529
Wang Weiyi	*c.* 987–*c.* 1067	Linacre	1460?–1524
Al-Mawṣilī	fl. 1010	Berengario da Carpi	*c.* 1460–1530
Ibn Buṭlān	d. 1066	Wang Ji	1463–1539
Constantine the African	d. before 1098/9	Rösslin	*c.* 1465/70–1526
Qian Yi	1032–1113	Fracastoro	1476/8–1553
Gariopontus	fl. *c.* 1035–1050	Dubois	1478–1555
Ibn at-Tilmīdh	*c.* 1074–1165	Cornaro	*c.* 1484–1566
Xu Shuwei	1079–1154	Brunfels	*c.* 1489–1534
Ibn Zuhr	*c.* 1091–1162	Da Monte	1489–1551
Hildegard of Bingen	1098–1179	Paracelsus	1493/4–1541
Frugard	fl. 12th century	Fernel	1497–1558
Trota	fl. 12th century	da Orta	1499?–1568
Liu Wansu	1110/20–1200	Mattioli	1500–1577
Ibn Rushd	1126–1198	Eustachi	*c.* 1500/10–1574
Yuthog Yontan	1126–1202	Fuchs	1501–1566
Maimonides	1138–1204	Cardano	1501–1576
Gilles de Corbeil	*c.* 1140–*c.* 1224	Arias de Benavides	b. 1505
Zhang Yuansu	1151–1234	Lemnius	*c.* 1505–1568
Li Gao	1180–1251	Manase	1507–1594
Harpestreng	d. 1244	Monardes	*c.* 1508–1588
Ibn al-Bayṭār	*c.* 1197–1248	Colombo	*c.* 1510–1559
Gilbert the Englishman	d. *c.* 1250	Caius	1510–1573
Richard the Englishman	fl. 13th century	Paré	*c.* 1510–1590
Peter of Spain	*c.* 1205–1277	Laguna	*c.* 1511–1559
Taddeo	1206/15–1295	Amatus Lusitanus	1511–1568?
William of Saliceto	*c.* 1210–1276/80	Vesalius	1514–1564
Ibn al-Nafīs	*c.* 1213–1288	Wier	1515–1588
John of Saint-Amand	*c.* 1230–1303	Dodonaeus	1517–1585
Lanfranc	d. *c.* 1306	Hernández	*c.* 1517–1587
Nicholas of Poland	*c.* 1235–*c.* 1316	Li Shizhen	1518–1593
Arnald	*c.* 1240–1311	Foreest	1521–1597
Peter of Abano	*c.* 1250–*c.* 1316	Al-Anṭākī	d. 1599
Henry of Mondeville	d. *c.* 1320	Falloppia	1523–1562
William of Brescia	*c.* 1250–1326	Valles	1524–1592
Bernard of Gordon	*c.* 1258–before 1330	Cesalpino	*c.* 1524/5–1603
Yperman	*c.* 1260/65–*c.* 1330	Aranzio	*c.* 1530–1589
Mondino de' Liuzzi	*c.* 1270–1326	Mercuriale	1530–1606
Del Garbo	*c.* 1280–1327	Mercado	1532–1611
Gentile da Foligno	*c.* 1280–1348	Fabrizi da Acquapendente	*c.* 1533–1619
Guido da Vigevano	*c.* 1280–1349	Bartisch	*c.* 1535–1606/7
John of Gaddesden	*c.* 1280–1349	Platter	1536–1614
Zhu Zhenheng	1282–1358	Heo	1539–1615
Chauliac	*c.* 1300–1368	Severinus	1540/42–1602
Arderne	1307/8–*c.* 1380	J. Heurnius	1543–1601
Tuệ Tĩnh	1330–*c.* 1389 or later	Clowes	1543/4–1604
Valesco of Tarenta	d. after 1426	Tagliacozzi	1545–1599
Ugo Benzi	1376–1439	Fabricius	1560–1634
Despars	*c.* 1380–1458	Santorio	1561–1636
Sejong	1397–1450	Zhang Jiebin	1563–1640
Ficino	1433–1499	Woodall	1570–1643

Name	Birth/Death Dates	Name	Birth/Death Dates
Sennert	1572–1637	D. Turner	1667–1734
Turquet	1573–1655	Arbuthnot	1667–1735
O. Heurnius	1577–1652	Ye Gui	1667–1746
Harvey	1578–1657	Baglivi	1668–1707
Helmont	1579–1644	Boerhaave	1668–1738
Severino	1580–1656	Winsløw	1669–1760
Aselli	1581–1625	Mandeville	1670–1733
Wu Youxing	1582–1652	N. Bidloo	1670–1735
Zacchia	1584–1659	G. Cheyne	1671/2–1743
Renaudot	1586–1653	Mead	1673–1754
Beverwijck	1594–1647	Petit	1674–1750
Scultetus	1595–1645	Lapeyronie	1678–1747
Rolfinck	1599–1673	Casal Julián	1680–1759
Glisson	1599–1677	Boylston	1680–1766
Patin	1601–1672	Morgagni	1682–1771
Bravo de Sobremonte	1603–1683	Heister	1683–1758
Browne	1605–1682	Jurin	1684–1750
Borelli	1608–1679	Astruc	1684–1766
Piso	1611–1678	Cheselden	1688–1752
Sylvius	1614–1672	Quesnay	1694–1774
Culpeper	1616–1654	Smellie	1697–1763
Bartholin	1616–1680	Sanches	1699–1783
Wiseman	1620?–1676	Swieten	1700–1772
Bonet	1620–1689	Yoshimasu Tōdō	1702–1773
Willis	1621–1675	Yamawaki Tōyō	1705–1762
Sydenham	1624–1689	Gaubius	1705–1780
Redi	1626–1697	Boissier de la Croix de Sauvages	1706–1767
Malpighi	1628–1694		
Chamberlen	1630/34–after 1720	Rosén von Rosenstein	1706–1773
Rudbeck	1630–1702	Linnaeus	1707–1778
Lower	1631–1691	Pringle	1707–1782
Ramazzini	1633–1714	Haller	1708–1777
Giovannini	1636–1691	La Mettrie	1709–1751
Swammerdam	1637–1680	Tronchin	1709–1781
Stensen	1638–1686	Cullen	1710–1790
Ruysch	1638–1731	Heberden	1710–1801
Sharp	fl. 1641–1671	Piquer Affufat	1711–1772
Graaf	1641–1673	Bond	1713–1784
Bellini	1643–1704	Whytt	1714–1766
Dionis	1643–1718	Pott	1714–1788
Bontekoe	c. 1644–1685	Erxleben	1715–1762
G. Bidloo	1649–1713	Du Coudray	1715?–1794
Floyer	1649–1734	Lind	1715–1794
Blankaart	1650–1704	Acrel	1717–1806
Palfyn	1650–1730	W. Hunter	1718–1783
Le Clerc	1652–1728	G. Armstrong	1719/20–1789
Sangye Gyatso	1653?–1705?	Lán Ông	1720–1791
Lancisi	1654–1720	Bordeu	1722–1776
Gotō Konzan	1659–1733	Camper	1722–1789
Stahl	1659–1734	Auenbrugger	1722–1809
Hoffmann	1660–1742	A. Louis	1723–1792
Vallisneri	1661–1730	J. Gregory	1724–1773
Valsalva	1666–1723	Tenon	1724–1816

Name	Birth/Death Dates	Name	Birth/Death Dates
J. Hunter	1728–1793	N. Smith	1762–1829
Tissot	1728–1797	Hufeland	1762–1836
Buchan	c. 1728–1805	Desgenettes	1762–1837
Spallanzani	1729–1799	Abernethy	1764–1831
Ingen Housz	1730–1799	Haslam	1764–1844
Darwin	1731–1802	Rasori	1766–1837
Mutis y Bosio	1732–1808	Larrey	1766–1842
Monro	1733–1817	Alibert	1768–1837
Sugita	1733–1817	Śniadecki	1768–1838
Mesmer	1734–1815	Cooper	1768–1841
Gimbernat i Arbós	1734–1816	S. Thomson	1769–1843
Brown	1735–1788	De La Rive	1770–1834
Morgan	1735–1789	Bichat	1771–1802
Sutton	1735–1819	McDowell	1771–1830
Shippen	1736–1808	McGrigor	1771–1858
Underwood	1736–1820	Autenrieth	1772–1835
Cotugno	1736–1822	Broussais	1772–1838
Desault	1738–1795	Esquirol	1772–1840
Percival	1740–1804	Coindet	1774–1834
Haygarth	1740–1827	C. Bell	1774–1842
Withering	1741–1799	Bene	1775–1858
Portal	1742–1832	Dupuytren	1777–1835
Lettsom	1744–1815	J. Jackson	1777–1867
Baudelocque	1745–1810	Bateman	1778–1821
Frank	1745–1821	J. Warren	1778–1856
Pinel	1745–1826	Richerand	1779–1840
Rush	1746–1813	Oken	1779–1851
Lardizábal Dubois	1746–1814	Gaaz	1780–1853
Espejo	1747–1795	Laennec	1781–1826
Vicq d'Azyr	1748–1794	Villermé	1782–1863
Odier	1748–1817	G. Shattuck	1783–1854
E. Jenner	1749–1823	Magendie	1783–1855
Scarpa	1752–1832	Brodie	1783–1862
Blumenbach	1752–1840	Lawrence	1783–1867
Balmis	1753–1819	Prout	1785–1850
Percy	1754–1825	Drake	1785–1852
Waterhouse	1754–1846	Beaumont	1785–1853
Fourcroy	1755–1809	Guthrie	1785–1856
Montaña Carranco	1755–1820	Mott	1785–1865
Corvisart des Marets	1755–1821	Ballingall	1786–1855
Parkinson	1755–1824	Prichard	1786–1848
Unanue	1755–1833	Channing	1786–1876
Hahnemann	1755–1843	Orfila i Rotger	1787–1853
Cabanis	1757–1808	P. Louis	1787–1872
Willan	1757–1812	Bufalini	1787–1875
Gall	1758–1828	J. Bigelow	1787–1879
Reil	1759–1813	T. S. Smith	1788–1861
Chiarugi	1759–1820	Bright	1789–1858
Beddoes	1760–1808	Buial'skii	1789–1866
Trotter	1760–1832	Bland	1789–1868
Hanaoka Seishū	1760–1835	Parent-Duchâtelet	1790–1836
Ferriar	1761–1815	Prevost	1790–1850
Baillie	1761–1823	Alison	1790–1859

Name	Birth/Death Dates	Name	Birth/Death Dates
Knox	1791–1862	Moreau de Tours	1804–1884
Elliotson	1791–1868	Parker	1804–1888
Cruveilhier	1791–1874	Seacole	1805–1881
Civiale	1792–1867	Skoda	1805–1881
Meigs	1792–1869	Gross	1805–1884
Baer	1792–1876	Hooker	1806–1867
L. Shattuck	1793–1859	Duchenne de Boulogne	1806–1875
Schoenlein	1793–1864	Bouchardat	1806–1886
Rayer	1793–1867	Beauperthuy	1807–1871
Clot Bey	1793–1868	Ray	1807–1881
Martin	1793–1874	Morehead	1807–1882
Liston	1794–1847	Farr	1807–1883
S. Graham	1794–1851	Huss	1807–1890
Conolly	1794–1866	Gully	1808–1883
Hastings	1794–1866	Vouros	1808–1885
Puccinotti	1794–1872	Bowditch	1808–1892
Addison	1795–1860	Gerhard	1809–1872
Braid	1795–1860	Morel	1809–1873
Wakley	1795–1862	Rizzoli	1809–1880
Barry	1795–1865	Henle	1809–1885
Velpeau	1795–1867	Earle	1809–1892
Graves	1796–1853	O. W. Holmes	1809–1894
Siebold	1796–1866	Ogata	1810–1863
Quetelet	1796–1874	Winslow	1810–1874
Guislain	1797–1860	Pirogov	1810–1881
Schroeder van der Kolk	1797–1862	Langenbeck	1810–1887
Christison	1797–1882	Simpson	1811–1870
Brigham	1798–1849	Budd	1811–1880
Hodgkin	1798–1866	Lockhart	1811–1896
Dunglison	1798–1869	Bennett	1812– 1875
S. Morton	1799–1851	Laycock	1812–1876
Basedow	1799–1854	Trall	1812–1877
Bayle	1799–1858	Seguin	1812–1880
Syme	1799–1870	Davaine	1812–1882
Fei Boxiong	1800–1879	Pacini	1812–1883
Holloway	1800–1883	Flint	1812–1886
Ricord	1800–1889	Snow	1813–1858
Chadwick	1800–1890	Livingstone	1813–1873
Hope	1801–1841	Bernard	1813–1878
Müller	1801–1858	Sims	1813–1883
Trousseau	1801–1867	Stillé	1813–1900
Littré	1801–1881	Dubini	1813–1902
Inozemtsev	1802–1869	M. A'zam Khān	1813–1902
Corrigan	1802–1880	Balassa	1814–1868
Dix	1802–1887	J. Paget	1814–1899
Choe Han'gi	1803–1870	Wilde	1815–1876
Jarvis	1803–1884	Wunderlich	1815–1877
Bartlett	1804–1855	Long	1815–1878
Nott	1804–1873	Markusovszky	1815–1893
Shuttleworth	1804–1877	Asada	1815–1894
Dietl	1804–1878	W. Jenner	1815–1898
Rokitansky	1804–1878	A. Thomson	1816–1860
Stokes	1804–1878	Hobson	1816–1873

Name	Birth/Death Dates	Name	Birth/Death Dates
Vargas Reyes	1816–1873	Lister	1827–1912
Goudas	1816–1882	Korányi	1827–1913
Lasègue	1816–1883	Graefe	1828–1870
Gull	1816–1890	Beaney	1828–1891
Ludwig	1816–1895	Battey	1828–1895
West	1816–1898	Down	1828–1896
Simon	1816–1904	E. Warren	1828–1896
Griesinger	1817–1869	Hammond	1828–1900
Ali Cohen	1817–1889	Sanderson	1828–1905
Brown-Séquard	1817–1894	Hutchinson	1828–1913
Hirsch	1817–1894	A. Still	1828–1917
Semmelweis	1818–1865	Zakhar'in	1829–1897
Traube	1818–1876	Zinnis	1829–1899
Tardieu	1818–1879	Zakrzewska	1829–1902
Newton	1818–1881	Sechenov	1829–1905
Donders	1818–1889	Pompe van Meerdervoort	1829–1908
H. Bigelow	1818–1890	Mitchell	1829–1914
Van Dyck	1818–1895	Péan	1830–1898
Sée	1818–1896	Hirschsprung	1830–1916
Wells	1818–1897	Pen	d. 1919
Pettenkofer	1818–1901	Hegar	1830–1919
W. Morton	1819–1868	A. Jacobi	1830–1919
Parkes	1819–1876	Carter	1831–1897
W. Thomson	1819–1883	Holmgren	1831–1897
Frerichs	1819–1885	His	1831–1904
Brücke	1819–1892	Waldmeier	1831–1915
Squibb	1819–1900	A. Jones	1832–1868
Wucherer	1820–1873	Botkin	1832–1889
Panum	1820–1885	Leyden	1832–1910
Blackley	1820–1900	Fournier	1832–1914
Beecham	1820–1907	Wundt	1832–1920
Nightingale	1820–1910	Perdomo Neira	1833–1874
Bertillon	1821–1883	Bert	1833–1886
Rawson	1821–1890	J. Jones	1833–1896
Virchow	1821–1902	Da Costa	1833–1900
Blackwell	1821–1910	Carrasquilla	1833–1908
Eddy	1821–1910	Finlay y Barres	1833–1915
Barton	1821–1912	Kerr	1834–1899
Pasteur	1822–1895	Klebs	1834–1913
Lad	1824–1874	Horton	1835–1883
Broca	1824–1880	Hart	1835–1898
Gillbee	1824–1885	J. H. Jackson	1835–1911
G. Sen	1824–1896	Magnan	1835–1916
Büchner	1824–1899	Maudsley	1835–1918
Fayrer	1824–1907	Bancroft	1836–1894
Halford	1824–1910	Sklifosovskii	1836–1904
Charcot	1825–1893	Bergmann	1836–1907
Duka	1825–1908	Lombroso	1836–1909
Vulpian	1826–1887	Anderson	1836–1917
Billroth	1826–1894	Allbutt	1836–1925
Bristowe	1827–1895	M. Mackenzie	1837–1892
Tuke	1827–1895	Kaposi	1837–1902
Rubio Gali	1827–1902	Brouardel	1837–1906

Name	Birth/Death Dates	Name	Birth/Death Dates
Bouchard	1837–1915	MacGregor	1846–1919
Keen	1837–1932	E. Mosher	1846–1928
Yi Jema	1838–1900	Fernández y Hernández	1847–1922
Nagayo	1838–1902	Salomonsen	1847–1924
Billings	1838–1913	Perroncito	1847–1936
De Giovanni	1838–1916	Batut	1847–1940
Beard	1839–1883	Trudeau	1848–1915
Cohnheim	1839–1884	Forel	1848–1931
Manning	1839–1903	Baelz	1849–1913
Gee	1839–1911	Déjerine	1849–1917
Liceaga	1839–1920	Osler	1849–1919
Brès	1839–1925	Johnson	1849–1920
Krafft-Ebing	1840–1902	Takaki	1849–1920
Bourneville	1840–1909	Godlee	1849–1925
Jex-Blake	1840–1912	Lloyd	1849–1936
Bernheim	1840–1919	Pavlov	1849–1936
Manassein	1841–1901	Mikulicz-Radecki	1850–1905
Hansen	1841–1912	Rutgers	1850–1924
Kocher	1841–1917	Schiøtz	1850–1927
Balls-Headley	1841–1918	Welch	1850–1934
L. Richards	1841–1930	Richet	1850–1935
Hayem	1841–1933	Lazarević	1851–1891
Dobroslavin	1842–1889	Reed	1851–1902
M. P. Jacobi	1842–1906	Rosenbach	1851–1907
Erisman	1842–1915	Ogino Ginko	1851–1913
Molleson	1842–1920	Scott	1851–1914
Breuer	1842–1925	A. Gregory	c. 1851–1927
Reverdin	1842–1929	Ferrán y Clúa	1851–1929
Pepper	1843–1898	Sandström	1852–1889
Grancher	1843–1907	Pokrovskaia	1852–1921?
Koch	1843–1910	Halsted	1852–1922
Golgi	1843–1926	Durán Cartín	1852–1924
Ferrier	1843–1928	Guiteras Gener	1852–1925
Waterston	1843–1932	Cardenal Fernández	1852–1927
Ostroumov	1844–1908	Morselli	1852–1929
Brunton	1844–1916	Kitasato	1852–1931
Manson	1844–1922	W. W. Cheyne	1852–1932
Bassini	1844–1924	Ramón y Cajal	1852–1934
Mackellar	1844–1926	Kellogg	1852–1943
Djordjević	1844–1930	Treves	1853–1923
Pinard	1844–1934	J. Mackenzie	1853–1925
Tait	1845–1899	Fiaschi	1853–1927
Duhring	1845–1913	Roux	1853–1933
McBurney	1845–1913	Marie	1853–1940
D. Palmer	1845–1913	Gram	1853–1949
Gowers	1845–1915	Korsakov	1854–1900
Mechnikov	1845–1916	Ehrlich	1854–1915
García Solá	1845–1922	Behring	1854–1917
Laveran	1845–1922	Concetti	1854–1920
Scharlieb	1845–1930	Gorgas	1854–1920
Bizzozero	1846–1901	Grassi	1854–1925
Thompson	1846–1915	Babeş	1854–1926
Putnam	1846–1918	Jacobs	1854–1929

Name	Birth/Death Dates	Name	Birth/Death Dates
Rubner	1854–1932	Montoya Lafragua	1859–1938
Councilman	1854–1933	Ellis	1859–1939
Aziz	1855–1911	W. Armstrong	1859–1941
Holt	1855–1924	Janet	1859–1947
Coni	1855–1928	Skirving	1859–1956
Bruce	1855–1931	Finsen	1860–1904
Netter	1855–1936	I. Robb	1860–1910
Winkler	1855–1941	Kinyoun	1860–1919
R. Paget	1855–1948	Einthoven	1860–1927
J. Easmon	1856–1900	Haffkine	1860–1930
Stuart	1856–1920	Holst	1860–1931
Kraepelin	1856–1926	G. Dock	1860–1951
D. Williams	1856–1931	Rizal	1861–1896
Flick	1856–1938	Choksy	1861–1939
S. Freud	1856–1939	W. Mayo	1861–1939
Chapin	1856–1941	Head	1861–1940
Lane	1856–1943	Wright	1861–1947
Carrión	1857–1885	Martínez Vargas	1861–1948
Gilles de la Tourette	1857–1904	Dickinson	1861–1950
Mya	1857–1911	Herrick	1861–1954
Celli	1857–1914	Mori	1862–1922
Horsley	1857–1916	Depage	1862–1925
Murphy	1857–1916	Ribas	1862–1925
Bieganski	1857–1917	Widal	1862–1929
Bekhterev	1857–1927	Gullstrand	1862–1930
Gotō Shinpei	1857–1929	Razetti	1862–1932
Babinski	1857–1932	De Sanctis	1862–1935
Ross	1857–1932	Coley	1862–1936
R. Jones	1857–1933	Moll	1862–1939
Garrod	1857–1936	M. Ajmal Khān	1863–1927
Abel	1857–1938	Mannerheim	1863–1928
Bleuler	1857–1939	Khlopin	1863–1929
Wagner-Jauregg	1857–1940	Schwalbe	1863–1930
Newsholme	1857–1943	Yamagiwa	1863–1930
Fenwick	1857–1947	Cantacuzino	1863–1934
Munthe	1857–1949	Marinescu	1863–1938
Azúa y Suárez	1858–1922	Park	1863–1939
Blaschko	1858–1922	C. Mosher	1863–1940
J. Turner	1858–1922	Yersin	1863–1943
Eijkman	1858–1930	Van Hoosen	1863–1952
Minkowski	1858–1931	Alzheimer	1864–1915
García-Medina	1858–1935	Rivers	1864–1922
Kraus	1858–1936	Thayer	1864–1932
King	1858–1938	Devoto	1864–1936
Edwards-Pilliet	1858–1941	Macphail	1864–1938
Kelly	1858–1943	Sanarelli	1864–1940
Simond	1858–1947	Wenckebach	1864–1940
L. Dock	1858–1956	Crile	1864–1943
Biggs	1859–1923	Rakhmabai	1864–1955
Subbotić	1859–1923	Joshi	1865–1887
Teziakov	1859–1925	Leishman	1865–1926
Grierson	1859–1934	Moynihan	1865–1936
T. Smith	1859–1934	C. Mayo	1865–1939

Name	Birth/Death Dates	Name	Birth/Death Dates
Grenfell	1865–1940	De Lange	1871–1950
Barnett	1865–1946	Foley	1871–1956
Miyairi	1865–1946	Yoshioka Yayoi	1871–1959
Brazil	1865–1950	Cruz	1872–1917
Biernacki	1866–1911	Lust	1872–1945
Wassermann	1866–1925	Rothschild	1872–1947
Ding Ganren	1866–1926	Arroyo Villaverde	1872–1959
Starling	1866–1927	Cole	1872–1966
Nicolle	1866–1936	Hata	1873–1938
Aschoff	1866–1942	Berger	1873–1941
Ewing	1866–1943	Carrel	1873–1944
Meyer	1866–1950	Baker	1873–1945
Atiman	c. 1866–1956	Bentley	1873–1949
Flexner	1866–1959	Nešić	1873–1959
Fibiger	1867–1928	Christophers	1873–1978
Bloodgood	1867–1935	Goldberger	1874–1929
Morquio	1867–1935	Meyerhof	1874–1945
Argyle	1867–1940	Roussy	1874–1948
Barker	1867–1943	Semashko	1874–1949
Abt	1867–1955	Ding Fubao	1874–1952
Geroulanos	1867–1960	Rüdin	1874–1952
Hirschfeld	1868–1935	Egas Moniz	1874–1955
Cabot	1868–1939	Emerson	1874–1957
Penna	1868–1939	Franco	1874–1958
Quervain	1868–1940	Fischer	1874–1967
G. Still	1868–1941	Brahmachari	1875–1946
Rogers	1868–1962	Sauerbruch	1875–1951
Grotjahn	1869–1931	Jung	1875–1961
Cushing	1869–1939	C. Vogt	1875–1962
Abbott	1869–1940	Schweitzer	1875–1965
Codman	1869–1940	Dale	1875–1968
Hijmans van den Bergh	1869–1943	Noguchi	1876–1928
Varier	1869–1944	Solov'ev	1876–1928
Edsall	1869–1945	Urrutia Guerezta	1876–1930
Lim	1869–1957	Cotton	1876–1933
Joslin	1869–1962	Beers	1876–1943
Hamilton	1869–1970	Aḥmad	1876–1946
Adler	1870–1937	Burdenko	1876–1946
Abdurahman	1870–1940	Pittaluga Fattorini	1876–1956
Al'tshuller	1870–1943	Guillain	1876–1961
Newman	1870–1948	Freeman	1876–1962
Willebrand	1870–1949	Goyanes Capdevilla	1876–1964
Cook	1870–1951	G. Holmes	1876–1965
Tredgold	1870–1952	A. Richards	1876–1966
Shiga	1870–1954	Buck	1877–1851
Aráoz Alfaro	1870–1955	Ingenieros	1877–1925
Madsen	1870–1957	W. MacKenzie	1877–1938
O. Vogt	1870–1959	Sachs	1877–1945
Scudder	1870–1960	Sand	1877–1953
Bordet	1870–1961	Cerletti	1877–1963
Rabinowitsch-Kempner	1871–1935	Lane-Claypon	1877–1967
Pletnev	1871–1941	Boyle	1878–1936
Cannon	1871–1945	Korczak	1878–1942

Name	Birth/Death Dates	Name	Birth/Death Dates
Goldstein	1878–1965	Paz Soldán	1885–1972
Loghem	1878–1968	Dandy	1886–1946
Cleland	1878–1971	Mazza	1886–1946
Chagas	1879–1934	Tzanck	1886–1954
Yun Tieqiao	1879–1935	Rodríguez Lafora	1886–1971
Jamot	1879–1937	White	1886–1973
Hurst	1879–1944	Friderichsen	1886–1982
Vincent	1879–1947	Marañón Posadillo	1887–1960
D'Arcy	1879–1950	Acosta-Sison	1887–1970
Yu Yan	1879–1954	Houssay	1887–1971
Leriche	1879–1955	Keynes	1887–1982
Park Ross	1879–1958	Ylppö	1887–1992
Wu Lien-Teh	1879–1960	Wagner	1888–1939
Beveridge	1879–1963	Zeiss	1888–1949
Sanger	1879–1966	Štampar	1888–1958
Orenstein	1879–1972	Kretschmer	1888–1964
Frost	1880–1938	Hagedorn	1888–1971
Laqueur	1880–1947	Hercus	1888–1971
Greenwood	1880–1949	Følling	1888–1973
T. Sharma	c. 1880–1950	Sayé i Sempere	1888–1975
Kenny	1880–1952	Reimann	1888–1979
Cumpston	1880–1954	Girard	1888–1985
Stopes	1880–1958	López Albo	1889–1944
Gesell	1880–1961	Ryle	1889–1950
Fraga	1880–1971	Souza	1889–1951
Orr	1880–1971	Scantlebury Brown	1889–1964
Vaid	1881–1936	Wickramarachchi	1889–1975
Lewis	1881–1945	Fishbein	1889–1976
Addis	1881–1949	Bethune	1890–1939
Fleming	1881–1955	Barros Barreto	1890–1956
B. Palmer	1881–1961	Ḥaddād	1890–1957
Rajchman	1881–1965	Read	1890–1959
Gillies	1882–1960	Briukhonenko	1890–1960
Klein	1882–1960	Calandre Ibáñez	1890–1961
Chopra	1882–1973	Bauer	1890–1978
Mahfouz	1882–1974	Jhirad	1890–1983
Debré	1882–1978	Rock	1890–1984
E. Graham	1883–1957	Banting	1891–1941
Semenovskii	1883–1959	Iudin	1891–1954
Papanicolaou	1883–1962	Gordon	1891–1956
Ciucă	1883–1969	Soriano Fischer	1891–1964
Warburg	1883–1970	Molema	1891–1965
Hirszfeld	1884–1954	Fairley	1891–1966
Hackett	1884–1962	Penfield	1891–1976
Pavlovskii	1884–1965	Moroka	1891–1985
Monge Medrano	1884–1970	Sullivan	1892–1949
Swellengrebel	1885–1970	Haire	1892–1952
Nóvoa Santos	1885–1933	Gregg	1892–1966
Shukla	c. 1885–c. 1945	Parran	1892–1968
Minot	1885–1950	Xuma	1893–1962
Mondor	1885–1962	Coppleson	1893–1965
Pickles	1885–1969	J. Paul	1893–1971
Chen Su Lan	1885–1972	Izquierdo Raudón	1893–1974

Name	Birth/Death Dates	Name	Birth/Death Dates
Soper	1893–1977	Evang	1902–1981
Kostić	1893–1983	Smirk	1902–1991
Cilento	1893–1985	Macdonald	1903–1967
Menninger	1893–1990	Farber	1903–1973
Yen	1893–1990	Gibbon	1903–1973
C. Williams	1893–1992	Gillman	1903–1981
Beck	1894–1971	Spock	1903–1998
Pinotti	1894–1972	C. R. Drew	1904–1950
Livadas	1894–1977	Beecher	1904–1976
Gluckman	1894–1987	Pickering	1904–1980
Martínez Báez	1894–1987	Trowell	1904–1989
Domagk	1895–1964	McMichael	1904–1993
Churchill	1895–1972	Soedarmo	1904–2003
D. Richards	1895–1973	Puigvert Gorro	1905–1990
Khanolkar	1895–1978	Gear	1905–1994
A. Freud	1895–1982	Carrillo	1906–1956
Pandit	1895–1991	P. Sharma	1906–1982
Hench	1896–1965	Hardy	1906–1993
Guilera Molas	1896–1969	Sabin	1906–1993
Verschuer	1896–1969	Naidoo	1906–1998
Balint	1896–1970	Selye	1907–1982
Nissen	1896–1981	Delay	1907–1987
Reich	1897–1957	Bowlby	1907–1990
Bevan	1897–1960	Refsum	1907–1991
M. Warren	1897–1960	Bovet	1907–1992
Bryce	1897–1968	Dunlop	1907–1993
Trueta i Raspall	1897–1977	Mitscherlich	1908–1982
Chávez Sánchez	1897–1979	Aleksandrowicz	1908–1988
Hill	1897–1991	Ampofo	1908–1998
Jiménez Díaz	1898–1967	Abd ul-Hamīd	1908–1999
Florey	1898–1968	Zhu Lian	1909–1978
Pedro-Pons	1898–1971	Cochrane	1909–1988
Bustamante Vasconcelos	1898–1986	Gabaldón	1909–1990
M. Bell	1898–1974	Hamburger	1909–1992
Taussig	1898–1986	Belios	1909–1995
Blalock	1899–1964	Negovskii	1909–2003
Macnamara	1899–1968	Donald	1910–1987
Cruz-Coke Lassabe	1899–1974	Hatem	1910–1988
G. Robb	1899–1974	Pappworth	1910–1994
Burnet	1899–1985	Horwitz Barak	1910–2000
Campbell	1899–1986	Vakil	1911–1974
Conti	1900–1945	Obrador Alcalde	1911–1978
Núñez Butrón	1900–1952	Charnley	1911–1982
Albright	1900–1969	Candau	1911–1983
Dameshek	1900–1969	Burkitt	1911–1993
Calderón Guardia	1900–1970	Jerne	1911–1994
Gale	1900–1976	Kark	1911–1998
M. Paul	1900–1988	Cade	1912–1980
Dharmendra	1900–1991	Tùng Tôn Thất	1912–1982
Grinker	1900–1993	McKeown	1912–1988
Lacan	1901–1981	Doniach	1912–2004
Wintrobe	1901–1986	Doll	1912–2005
Huggins	1901–1997	Steptoe	1913–1988

Name	Birth/Death Dates	Name	Birth/Death Dates
C. Easmon	1913–1994	Ilizarov	1921–1992
Burton-Bradley	1914–1994	Pindborg	1921–1995
Salk	1914–1995	Ramalingaswami	1921–2001
Danaraj	1914–1996	Scribner	1921–2003
P. Sen	1915–1982	Wynder	1922–1999
Togba	1915–2002	Barnard	1922–2001
Stephenson	1916–1967	Favaloro	1923–2000
C. E. Drew	1916–1987	Lambo	1923–2004
Hufnagel	1916–1989	Basaglia	1924–1980
De Graft-Johnson	1917–1985	Fanon	1925–1961
Suvannavong	1917–1985?	Kubler-Ross	1926–2004
Sournia	1917–2000	Odeku	1927–1974
Barnor	1917–2005	Laing	1927–1989
Harinasuta	1918–1999	Fedorov	1927–2000
Spoerry	1918–1999	Liley	1929–1983
Sherlock	1918–2001	Mukerji	1931–1981
Saunders	1918–2005	Kasili	1942–1994
Saīd	1920–1998		

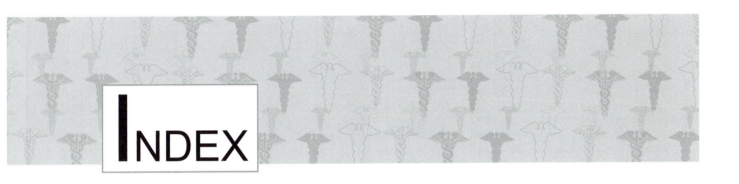

INDEX

Page numbers in **bold** indicate main entries. Entries marked * indicate more complete lists of major fields of activity may be found in Appendix 2.

Index prepared by
Publication Services, Inc.

About the Editors

W. F. BYNUM is Professor Emeritus of the History of Medicine at University College London and was head of the Academic Unit of the Wellcome Unit for the History of Medicine (1973–1996). His publications include the *Dictionary of the History of Science*, *Science and the Practice of Medicine in the 19th Century*, and the *Oxford Dictionary of Scientific Quotations*.

HELEN BYNUM is a freelance historian of science and medicine. She was a Wellcome Trust Lecturer in the History of Medicine at Liverpool (1996–2000). Her publications include *Tropical Medicine in the 20th Century* and *Body and City*.